New Frontiers in Electrocardiography, Cardiac Arrhythmias, and Arrhythmogenic Disorders

New Frontiers in Electrocardiography, Cardiac Arrhythmias, and Arrhythmogenic Disorders

Editors

Paweł T. Matusik
Christian Sohns

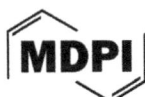

Basel • Beijing • Wuhan • Barcelona • Belgrade • Novi Sad • Cluj • Manchester

Editors
Paweł T. Matusik
Jagiellonian University Medical College
Kraków
Poland

Christian Sohns
Herz- und Diabeteszentrum NRW,
Ruhr-Universität Bochum
Bad Oeynhausen
Germany

Editorial Office
MDPI AG
Grosspeteranlage 5
4052 Basel, Switzerland

This is a reprint of articles from the Special Issue published online in the open access journal *Journal of Clinical Medicine* (ISSN 2077-0383) (available at: https://www.mdpi.com/journal/jcm/special_issues/cardiac_arrhythmias_research).

For citation purposes, cite each article independently as indicated on the article page online and as indicated below:

Lastname, A.A.; Lastname, B.B. Article Title. *Journal Name* **Year**, *Volume Number*, Page Range.

ISBN 978-3-7258-1995-9 (Hbk)
ISBN 978-3-7258-1996-6 (PDF)
doi.org/10.3390/books978-3-7258-1996-6

© 2024 by the authors. Articles in this book are Open Access and distributed under the Creative Commons Attribution (CC BY) license. The book as a whole is distributed by MDPI under the terms and conditions of the Creative Commons Attribution-NonCommercial-NoDerivs (CC BY-NC-ND) license.

Contents

Preface ix

Rafał Król, Michał Karnaś, Michał Ziobro, Jacek Bednarek, Georgios Kollias, Christian Sohns and Paweł T. Matusik
New Frontiers in Electrocardiography, Cardiac Arrhythmias, and Arrhythmogenic Disorders
Reprinted from: *J. Clin. Med.* **2024**, *13*, 2047, doi:10.3390/jcm13072047 1

Piotr Bijak, Vassil B. Traykov, Avi Sabbag, Sergio Conti, Christian Sohns and Paweł T. Matusik
Fever-Induced Brugada Sign: Clue for Clinical Management with Non-Negligible Risk of Sudden Cardiac Death
Reprinted from: *J. Clin. Med.* **2023**, *12*, 3503, doi:10.3390/jcm12103503 6

Magdalena Okólska, Jacek Łach, Paweł T. Matusik, Jacek Pająk, Tomasz Mroczek, Piotr Podolec and Lidia Tomkiewicz-Pająk
Heart Rate Variability and Its Associations with Organ Complications in Adults after Fontan Operation
Reprinted from: *J. Clin. Med.* **2021**, *10*, 4492, doi:10.3390/jcm10194492 9

Krzysztof Ozierański, Agata Tymińska, Marcin Kruk, Beata Koń, Aleksandra Skwarek, Grzegorz Opolski and Marcin Grabowski
Occurrence, Trends, Management and Outcomes of Patients Hospitalized with Clinically Suspected Myocarditis—Ten-Year Perspectives from the MYO-PL Nationwide Database
Reprinted from: *J. Clin. Med.* **2021**, *10*, 4672, doi:10.3390/jcm10204672 20

Chin-Feng Tsai, Yao-Tsung Chuang, Jing-Yang Huang and Kwo-Chang Ueng
Long-Term Prognosis of Febrile Individuals with Right Precordial Coved-Type ST-Segment Elevation Brugada Pattern: A 10-Year Prospective Follow-Up Study
Reprinted from: *J. Clin. Med.* **2021**, *10*, 4997, doi:10.3390/jcm10214997 32

Krzysztof Ozierański, Agata Tymińska, Aleksandra Skwarek, Marcin Kruk, Beata Koń, Jarosław Biliński, et al.
Sex Differences in Incidence, Clinical Characteristics and Outcomes in Children and Young Adults Hospitalized for Clinically Suspected Myocarditis in the Last Ten Years—Data from the MYO-PL Nationwide Database
Reprinted from: *J. Clin. Med.* **2021**, *10*, 5502, doi:10.3390/jcm10235502 47

Sok-Sithikun Bun, Florian Asarisi, Nathan Heme, Fabien Squara, Didier Scarlatti, Philippe Taghji, et al.
Prevalence and Clinical Characteristics of Patients with Pause-Dependent Atrioventricular Block
Reprinted from: *J. Clin. Med.* **2022**, *11*, 449, doi:10.3390/jcm11020449 60

Grzegorz Karkowski, Marcin Kuniewicz, Andrzej Ząbek, Edward Koźluk, Maciej Dębski, Paweł T. Matusik and Jacek Lelakowski
Contact Force-Sensing versus Standard Catheters in Non-Fluoroscopic Radiofrequency Catheter Ablation of Idiopathic Outflow Tract Ventricular Arrhythmias
Reprinted from: *J. Clin. Med.* **2022**, *11*, 593, doi:10.3390/jcm11030593 69

Robert Kowalik, Marek Gierlotka, Krzysztof Ozierański, Przemysław Trzeciak, Anna Fojt, Piotr Feusette, et al.
In-Hospital and One-Year Outcomes of Patients after Early and Late Resuscitated Cardiac Arrest Complicating Acute Myocardial Infarction—Data from a Nationwide Database
Reprinted from: *J. Clin. Med.* **2022**, *11*, 609, doi:10.3390/jcm11030609 80

Miaomiao He, Jie Qiu, Yan Wang, Yang Bai and Guangzhi Chen
Caveolin-3 and Arrhythmias: Insights into the Molecular Mechanisms
Reprinted from: *J. Clin. Med.* **2022**, *11*, 1595, doi:10.3390/jcm11061595 92

Hasina Masha Aziz, Michał P. Zarzecki, Sebastian Garcia-Zamora, Min Seo Kim, Piotr Bijak, Gary Tse, et al.
Pathogenesis and Management of Brugada Syndrome: Recent Advances and Protocol for Umbrella Reviews of Meta-Analyses in Major Arrhythmic Events Risk Stratification
Reprinted from: *J. Clin. Med.* **2022**, *11*, 1912, doi:10.3390/jcm11071912 105

Magdalena Okólska, Grzegorz Karkowski, Marcin Kuniewicz, Jacek Bednarek, Jacek Pająk, Beata Róg, et al.
Prevalence of Arrhythmia in Adults after Fontan Operation
Reprinted from: *J. Clin. Med.* **2022**, *11*, 1968, doi:10.3390/jcm11071968 119

Guan-Yi Li, Fa-Po Chung, Tze-Fan Chao, Yenn-Jiang Lin, Shih-Lin Chang, Li-Wei Lo, et al.
Sinus Node Dysfunction after Successful Atrial Flutter Ablation during Follow-Up: Clinical Characteristics and Predictors
Reprinted from: *J. Clin. Med.* **2022**, *11*, 3212, doi:10.3390/jcm11113212 131

Agata Tymińska, Krzysztof Ozierański, Emil Brociek, Agnieszka Kapłon-Cieślicka, Paweł Balsam, Michał Marchel, et al.
Fifteen-Year Differences in Indications for Cardiac Resynchronization Therapy in International Guidelines—Insights from the Heart Failure Registries of the European Society of Cardiology
Reprinted from: *J. Clin. Med.* **2022**, *11*, 3236, doi:10.3390/jcm11113236 145

Patrycja S. Matusik, Amira Bryll, Agnieszka Pac, Tadeusz J. Popiela and Paweł T. Matusik
Clinical Data, Chest Radiograph and Electrocardiography in the Screening for Left Ventricular Hypertrophy: The CAR_2E_2 Score
Reprinted from: *J. Clin. Med.* **2022**, *11*, 3585, doi:10.3390/jcm11133585 156

Paolo Giovanardi, Cecilia Vernia, Enrico Tincani, Claudio Giberti, Federico Silipo and Andrea Fabbo
Combined Effects of Age and Comorbidities on Electrocardiographic Parameters in a Large Non-Selected Population
Reprinted from: *J. Clin. Med.* **2022**, *11*, 3737, doi:10.3390/jcm11133737 171

Szymon Buś, Konrad Jędrzejewski and Przemysław Guzik
Using Minimum Redundancy Maximum Relevance Algorithm to Select Minimal Sets of Heart Rate Variability Parameters for Atrial Fibrillation Detection
Reprinted from: *J. Clin. Med.* **2022**, *11*, 4004, doi:10.3390/jcm11144004 185

Antonio Oliva, Simone Grassi, Vilma Pinchi, Francesca Cazzato, Mónica Coll, Mireia Alcalde, et al.
Structural Heart Alterations in Brugada Syndrome: Is it Really a Channelopathy? A Systematic Review
Reprinted from: *J. Clin. Med.* **2022**, *11*, 4406, doi:10.3390/jcm11154406 207

Szymon Buś, Konrad Jędrzejewski and Przemysław Guzik
Statistical and Diagnostic Properties of pRRx Parameters in Atrial Fibrillation Detection
Reprinted from: *J. Clin. Med.* **2022**, *11*, 5702, doi:10.3390/jcm11195702 220

Monika Lisicka, Marta Skowrońska, Bartosz Karolak, Jan Wójcik, Piotr Pruszczyk and Piotr Bienias
Heart Rate Variability Impairment Is Associated with Right Ventricular Overload and Early Mortality Risk in Patients with Acute Pulmonary Embolism
Reprinted from: *J. Clin. Med.* **2023**, *12*, 753, doi:10.3390/jcm12030753 237

Sok-Sithikun Bun, Nathan Heme, Florian Asarisi, Fabien Squara, Didier Scarlatti, Pamela Moceri and Emile Ferrari
Prevalence and Clinical Characteristics of Patients with Torsades de Pointes Complicating Acquired Atrioventricular Block
Reprinted from: *J. Clin. Med.* **2023**, *12*, 1067, doi:10.3390/jcm12031067 246

Muneeb Ahmed, Emilie P. Belley-Coté, Yuan Qiu, Peter Belesiotis, Brendan Tao, Alex Wolf, et al.
Rhythm vs. Rate Control in Patients with Postoperative Atrial Fibrillation after Cardiac Surgery: A Systematic Review and Meta-Analysis
Reprinted from: *J. Clin. Med.* **2023**, *12*, 4534, doi:10.3390/jcm12134534 255

Paweł Wałek, Joanna Roskal-Wałek, Patryk Dłubis and Beata Wożakowska-Kapłon
Echocardiographic Evaluation of Atrial Remodelling for the Prognosis of Maintaining Sinus Rhythm after Electrical Cardioversion in Patients with Atrial Fibrillation
Reprinted from: *J. Clin. Med.* **2023**, *12*, 5158, doi:10.3390/jcm12155158 266

Preface

Novel electrocardiographic criteria along with new algorithms to diagnose and treat arrhythmias have been proposed, enabling more personalized patient management, including more rational use of imaging, implantable cardioverter-defibrillators, cardiac resynchronization therapy, and catheter ablation. This progress also concerns the diagnostics, treatment, and classification of arrhythmogenic disorders. Moreover, advancements in imaging and cardiovascular genetics have made better diagnostics and risk stratification possible. However, personalized paths in arrhythmia management are increasingly needed. The Special Issue titled "New Frontiers in Electrocardiography, Cardiac Arrhythmias, and Arrhythmogenic Disorders" in the *Journal of Clinical Medicine* provides updates with recent studies in the field of electrocardiology.

Paweł T. Matusik and Christian Sohns
Editors

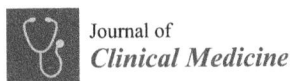

Editorial

New Frontiers in Electrocardiography, Cardiac Arrhythmias, and Arrhythmogenic Disorders

Rafał Król [1], Michał Karnaś [2], Michał Ziobro [2], Jacek Bednarek [1], Georgios Kollias [3], Christian Sohns [4] and Paweł T. Matusik [1,5,*]

1. Department of Electrocardiology, St. John Paul II Hospital, Prądnicka 80, 31-202 Kraków, Poland
2. Faculty of Medicine, Jagiellonian University Medical College, Św. Anny 12, 31-008 Kraków, Poland
3. Ordensklinikum Linz Elisabethinen, Fadingerstraße 1, 4020 Linz, Austria
4. Clinic for Electrophysiology, Herz- und Diabeteszentrum NRW, Georgstr. 11, 32545 Bad Oeynhausen, Germany
5. Department of Electrocardiology, Institute of Cardiology, Faculty of Medicine, Jagiellonian University Medical College, Prądnicka 80, 31-202 Kraków, Poland
* Correspondence: pawel.matusik@wp.eu or pawel.matusik@uj.edu.pl; Tel.: +48-12-614-22-77; Fax: +48-12-614-22-26

Citation: Król, R.; Karnaś, M.; Ziobro, M.; Bednarek, J.; Kollias, G.; Sohns, C.; Matusik, P.T. New Frontiers in Electrocardiography, Cardiac Arrhythmias, and Arrhythmogenic Disorders. *J. Clin. Med.* **2024**, *13*, 2047. https://doi.org/10.3390/jcm13072047

Received: 16 March 2024
Accepted: 25 March 2024
Published: 1 April 2024

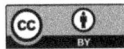

Copyright: © 2024 by the authors. Licensee MDPI, Basel, Switzerland. This article is an open access article distributed under the terms and conditions of the Creative Commons Attribution (CC BY) license (https://creativecommons.org/licenses/by/4.0/).

In recent decades, diagnosing, risk-stratifying, and treating patients with primary electrical diseases, as well as heart rhythm disorders, have improved substantially. Moreover, new clinical classification of rare cardiac arrhythmogenic and conduction disorders and rare arrhythmias has been proposed to facilitate research and simplify differential diagnostics [1]. Significant progress has been made in assessing the genetic background of patients after sudden cardiac arrest [2], and new frontiers have also been reached in the field of stratifying cardiovascular risk and predicting sudden cardiac death. These advances concern the use of novel biomarkers in combination with clinical data [3,4]. Artificial intelligence may also be useful in addressing unmet needs in improving the prediction of sudden cardiac arrest [5]. In current clinical practice, the use of conduction system pacing and subcutaneous implantable cardioverter–defibrillator therapy is increasingly common in patients who require cardiac pacing or sudden cardiac death prevention with the use of implantable cardioverter–defibrillators [6,7]. Importantly, patients at high risk of pacemaker pocket infections or with a lack of upper-extremity venous access may benefit from leadless pacemakers, which may preserve (at least to some extent) atrioventricular synchrony, such as a novel dual-chamber leadless pacemaker system [8,9]. Moreover, there is increasing clinical evidence on the safe extraction of leadless pacemakers with a dwelling time of over 12 months [10].

Important new technologies have been introduced in the field of ablation procedures since cardiac ablations were previously performed with the delivery of direct current shocks to an electrode catheter [11]. Due to the severe complications involved, this was replaced by radiofrequency ablation, which is currently widely used in electrophysiology laboratories. The use of steerable sheaths, contact force sensing (the contact force is positively correlated with the lesion size, steam pops, and thrombus formation), and irrigated tip catheters (larger lesions creation, a lower risk of thrombus and char formation) for ablation has brought about improvements in the field of radiofrequency ablation [12–15]. The catheters may be visualized using fluoroscopy or three-dimensional electroanatomical mapping techniques, limiting or completely omitting the use of X-rays (zero X-ray ablation) and increasing the precision of ablating the arrhythmogenic substrate. Another ablation method is cryoablation, which may be especially valuable in pulmonary vein isolation and in patients with perinodal accessory pathways due to the low risk of persistent iatrogenic atrioventricular block [16]. Moreover, the use of pulse field ablation also holds great promise, which is a novel ablation modality utilizing non-thermal energy and causing irreversible electroporation, leading to cardiac cell death (other cells are less prone to these changes) [17,18]. Among patients who experience recurrent ventricular tachycardias after catheter ablation despite optimal pharmacotherapy or among those who have contraindications to catheter ablation, stereotactic arrhythmia radioablation is a potentially valuable treatment option [19].

In the Special Issue "New Frontiers in Electrocardiography, Cardiac Arrhythmias, and Arrhythmogenic Disorders" of the Journal of Clinical Medicine, readers will find 22 papers (summarized in Table 1) written by authors from around the world (Figure 1). These papers concern a variety of topics in the field of electrocardiology [20–22].

Table 1. Summary of the papers published in the Special Issue "New Frontiers in Electrocardiography, Cardiac Arrhythmias, and Arrhythmogenic Disorders".

Contribution Number	Reference	Type of Publication	Number of Authors/Affiliations	Locations of Authors' Affiliations
1	Bijak, P.; et al. Fever-Induced Brugada Sign: Clue for Clinical Management with Non-Negligible Risk of Sudden Cardiac Death. J. Clin. Med. 2023, 12.	Editorial	6/7	Poland, Bulgaria, Israel, Italy, Germany
2	Bun, S.-S.; et al. Prevalence and Clinical Characteristics of Patients with Torsades de Pointes Complicating Acquired Atrioventricular Block. J. Clin. Med. 2023, 12, 1067.	Article	7/1	France
3	Lisicka, M.; et al. Heart Rate Variability Impairment Is Associated with Right Ventricular Overload and Early Mortality Risk in Patients with Acute Pulmonary Embolism. J. Clin. Med. 2023, 12, 753.	Article	6/2	Poland
4	Buś, S.; et al. Statistical and Diagnostic Properties of pRRx Parameters in Atrial Fibrillation Detection. J. Clin. Med. 2022, 11, 5702.	Article	3/2	Poland
5	Buś, S.; et al. Using Minimum Redundancy Maximum Relevance Algorithm to Select Minimal Sets of Heart Rate Variability Parameters for Atrial Fibrillation Detection. J. Clin. Med. 2022, 11, 4004.	Article	3/2	Poland
6	Giovanardi, P.; et al. Combined Effects of Age and Comorbidities on Electrocardiographic Parameters in a Large Non-Selected Population. J. Clin. Med. 2022, 11, 3737.	Article	6/7	Italy
7	Matusik, P.S.; et al. Clinical Data, Chest Radiograph and Electrocardiography in the Screening for Left Ventricular Hypertrophy: The CAR_2E_2 Score. J. Clin. Med. 2022, 11, 3585.	Article	5/5	Poland
8	Tymińska, A.; et al. Fifteen-Year Differences in Indications for Cardiac Resynchronization Therapy in Inter-national Guidelines—Insights from the Heart Failure Registries of the European Society of Cardiology. J. Clin. Med. 2022, 11, 3236.	Article	11/5	Poland, Spain, Italy, France
9	Li, G.-Y.; et al. Sinus Node Dysfunction after Successful Atrial Flutter Ablation during Follow-Up: Clinical Characteristics and Predictors. J. Clin. Med. 2022, 11, 3212.	Article	16/3	Taiwan
10	Okólska, M.; et al. Prevalence of Arrhythmia in Adults after Fontan Operation. J. Clin. Med. 2022, 11, 1968.	Article	9/7	Poland
11	Kowalik, R.; et al. In-Hospital and One-Year Outcomes of Patients after Early and Late Resuscitated Cardiac Arrest Complicating Acute Myocardial Infarction—Data from a Nationwide Database. J. Clin. Med. 2022, 11, 609.	Article	10/4	Poland
12	Karkowski, G.; et al. Contact Force-Sensing versus Standard Catheters in Non-Fluoroscopic Radiofrequency Catheter Ablation of Idiopathic Outflow Tract Ventricular Arrhythmias. J. Clin. Med. 2022, 11, 593.	Article	7/5	Poland
13	Bun, S.-S.; et al. Prevalence and Clinical Characteristics of Patients with Pause-Dependent Atrioventricular Block. J. Clin. Med. 2022, 11, 449.	Article	9/2	France
14	Ozierański, K.; et al. Sex Differences in Incidence, Clinical Characteristics and Outcomes in Children and Young Adults Hospitalized for Clinically Suspected Myocarditis in the Last Ten Years—Data from the MYO-PL Nationwide Database. J. Clin. Med. 2021, 10, 5502.	Article	8/3	Poland

Table 1. *Cont.*

Contribution Number	Reference	Type of Publication	Number of Authors/Affiliations	Locations of Authors' Affiliations
15	Tsai, C.-F.; et al. Long-Term Prognosis of Febrile Individuals with Right Precordial Coved-Type ST-Segment Elevation Brugada Pattern: A 10-Year Prospective Follow-Up Study. J. Clin. Med. 2021, 10, 4997.	Article	4/3	Taiwan
16	Ozierański, K.; et al. Occurrence, Trends, Management and Outcomes of Patients Hospitalized with Clinically Suspected Myocarditis—Ten-Year Perspectives from the MYO-PL Nationwide Database. J. Clin. Med. 2021, 10, 4672.	Article	7/2	Poland
17	Okólska, M.; et al. Heart Rate Variability and Its Associations with Organ Complications in Adults after Fontan Operation. J. Clin. Med. 2021, 10, 4492.	Article	7/5	Poland
18	Wałek, P.; et al. Echocardiographic Evaluation of Atrial Remodelling for the Prognosis of Maintaining Sinus Rhythm after Electrical Cardioversion in Patients with Atrial Fibrillation. J. Clin. Med. 2023, 12, 5158.	Review	4/3	Poland
19	Aziz, H.M.; et al. Pathogenesis and Management of Brugada Syndrome: Recent Advances and Protocol for Umbrella Reviews of Meta-Analyses in Major Arrhythmic Events Risk Stratification. J. Clin. Med. 2022, 11, 1912.	Review	8/11	Poland, Argentina, Korea, China, the United Kingdom
20	He, M.; et al. Caveolin-3 and Arrhythmias: Insights into the Molecular Mechanisms. J. Clin. Med. 2022, 11, 1595.	Review	5/1	China
21	Ahmed, M.; et al. Rhythm vs. Rate Control in Patients with Postoperative Atrial Fibrillation after Cardiac Surgery: A Systematic Review and Meta-Analysis. J. Clin. Med. 2023, 12, 4534.	Systematic review	15/4	Canada
22	Oliva, A.; et al. Structural Heart Alterations in Brugada Syndrome: Is it Really a Channelopathy? A Systematic Review. J. Clin. Med. 2022, 11, 4406.	Systematic review	21/11	Spain, Italy, The Netherlands

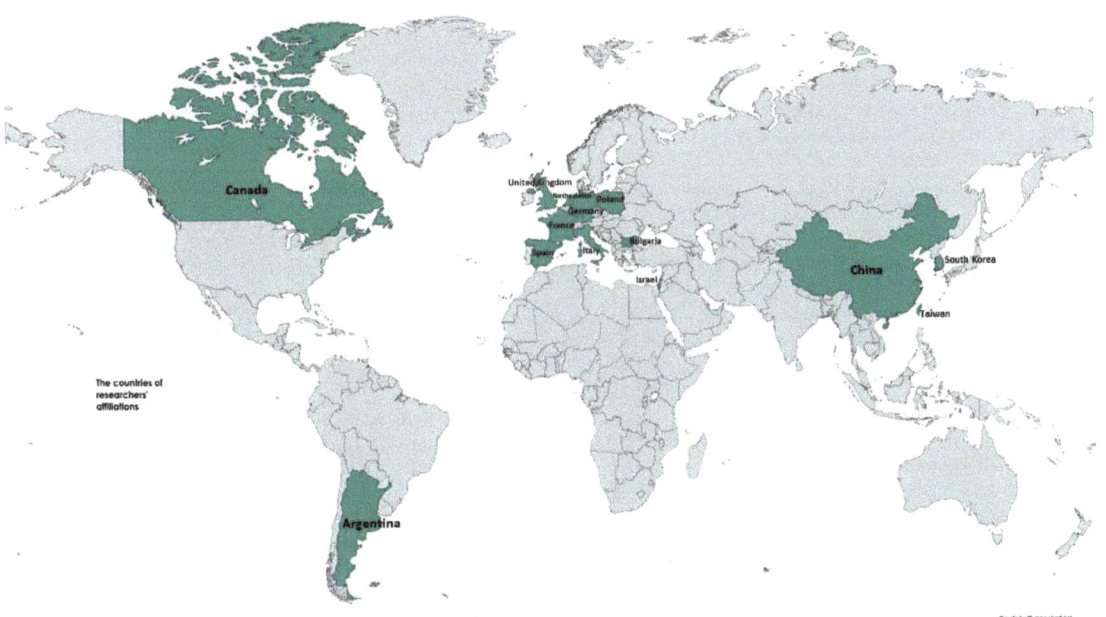

Figure 1. Locations of affiliations of the authors contributing to the Special Issue "New Frontiers in Electrocardiography, Cardiac Arrhythmias, and Arrhythmogenic Disorders".

In the rapidly growing field of electrocardiology, further in-depth analyses of pathogenesis and clinical management, along with important aspects of telehealth, which is promising for the improvement of care [23], are needed. These should include detailed descriptions of case reports and systematic reviews, as seen in other fields of medicine [24,25]. Despite progress, there are gaps in our knowledge of and the clinical care of patients, including those with heart failure, who may benefit from the placement of implantable cardiovascular electronic devices (and their remote monitoring), catheter ablation, or optimized medical therapy [26,27]. Thus, we look forward to reading, reviewing, and/or editing new papers submitted to the Journal of Clinical Medicine, including the new Special Issue "Further Advances in Electrocardiography, Cardiac Arrhythmias, and Arrhythmogenic Disorders".

Author Contributions: Conceptualization, P.T.M.; writing—original draft preparation, R.K., M.K., M.Z., J.B. and P.T.M.; writing—review and editing, G.K., C.S. and P.T.M.; supervision, P.T.M.; funding acquisition, P.T.M. All authors have read and agreed to the published version of the manuscript.

Funding: P.T.M. was supported by the National Science Centre, Poland (grant number 2021/05/X/NZ5/01511); Jagiellonian University Medical College (including grant numbers N41/DBS/000845 and N41/DBS/000517); a Polish Cardiac Society 2018 Scientific Grant in cooperation with Berlin-Chemie/Menarini (sponsor of the grant: Berlin-Chemie/Menarini Poland LLC); and St. John Paul II Hospital.

Acknowledgments: For open access purposes, the authors have applied a CC-BY public copyright license to any Author-Accepted Manuscript (AAM) version arising from this submission. Figure 1 was created using MapChart (mapchart.net).

Conflicts of Interest: R.K. participated in educational activity, which was supported by GE. C.S. received research support and lecture fees from Medtronic, Abbott, Boston Scientific, and Biosense Webster, is a consultant for Medtronic, Boston Scientific, and Biosense Webster, has received grant support from the Else Kröner-Fresenius-Stiftung and Deutsche Herzstiftung. P.T.M. participated in educational activities, which were supported by CIED manufacturers. All remaining authors declare no conflicts of interest. The funders had no role in the design of the study; in the collection, analyses, or interpretation of data; in the writing of the manuscript; or in the decision to publish the results.

References

1. Podolec, P.; Baranchuk, A.; Brugada, J.; Kukla, P.; Lelakowski, J.; Kopec, G.; Rubis, P.; Stepniewski, J.; Podolec, J.; Komar, M.; et al. Clinical classification of rare cardiac arrhythmogenic and conduction disorders, and rare arrhythmias. *Pol. Arch. Intern. Med.* **2019**, *129*, 154–159. [CrossRef] [PubMed]
2. Verheul, L.M.; van der Ree, M.H.; Groeneveld, S.A.; Mulder, B.A.; Christiaans, I.; Kapel, G.F.L.; Alings, M.; Bootsma, M.; Barge-Schaapveld, D.; Balt, J.C.; et al. The genetic basis of apparently idiopathic ventricular fibrillation: A retrospective overview. *Europace* **2023**, *25*, euad336. [CrossRef] [PubMed]
3. Borowiec, K.; Wozniak, O.; Wrobel, A.; Smigielski, W.; Skrzypczynska-Banasik, U.; Kowalik, E.; Lutynska, A.; Hoffman, P.; Biernacka, E.K. A new model for predicting adverse outcomes in arrhythmogenic right ventricular cardiomyopathy. *Pol. Arch. Intern. Med.* **2023**, *133*, 16443. [CrossRef] [PubMed]
4. Matusik, P.T.; Heleniak, Z.; Papuga-Szela, E.; Plens, K.; Lelakowski, J.; Undas, A. Chronic Kidney Disease and Its Impact on a Prothrombotic State in Patients with Atrial Fibrillation. *J. Clin. Med.* **2020**, *9*, 2476. [CrossRef] [PubMed]
5. Holmstrom, L.; Zhang, F.Z.; Ouyang, D.; Dey, D.; Slomka, P.J.; Chugh, S.S. Artificial Intelligence in Ventricular Arrhythmias and Sudden Death. *Arrhythm. Electrophysiol. Rev.* **2023**, *12*, e17. [CrossRef] [PubMed]
6. Mizner, J.; Waldauf, P.; Grieco, D.; Linkova, H.; Ionita, O.; Vijayaraman, P.; Petr, R.; Rakova, R.; Vesela, J.; Stros, P.; et al. A randomized comparison of HBP versus RVP: Effect on left ventricular function and biomarkers of collagen metabolism. *Kardiol. Pol.* **2023**, *81*, 472–481. [CrossRef] [PubMed]
7. Kempa, M.; Budrejko, S.; Tajstra, M.; Syska, P.; Lewandowski, M.; Fabiszak, T.; Michalak, M.; Stanek, A.; Nowak, K.; Mitkowski, P.; et al. Subcutaneous implantable cardioverter-defibrillator therapy in Poland: Results of the Polish S-ICD Registry. *Kardiol. Pol.* **2023**, *81*, 455–462. [CrossRef] [PubMed]
8. Neugebauer, F.; Noti, F.; van Gool, S.; Roten, L.; Baldinger, S.H.; Seiler, J.; Madaffari, A.; Servatius, H.; Ryser, A.; Tanner, H.; et al. Leadless atrioventricular synchronous pacing in an outpatient setting: Early lessons learned on factors affecting atrioventricular synchrony. *Heart Rhythm.* **2022**, *19*, 748–756. [CrossRef]
9. Knops, R.E.; Reddy, V.Y.; Ip, J.E.; Doshi, R.; Exner, D.V.; Defaye, P.; Canby, R.; Bongiorni, M.G.; Shoda, M.; Hindricks, G.; et al. A Dual-Chamber Leadless Pacemaker. *N. Engl. J. Med.* **2023**, *388*, 2360–2370. [CrossRef] [PubMed]

10. Callahan, T.D.T.; Wilkoff, B.L. Extraction of a 5-year-old leadless pacemaker using a competing manufacturer's removal tool. *HeartRhythm Case Rep.* **2023**, *9*, 441–444. [CrossRef]
11. Scheinman, M.M.; Morady, F.; Hess, D.S.; Gonzalez, R. Catheter-induced ablation of the atrioventricular junction to control refractory supraventricular arrhythmias. *JAMA* **1982**, *248*, 851–855. [CrossRef] [PubMed]
12. Gerstenfeld, E.P. Contact force-sensing catheters: Evolution or revolution in catheter ablation technology? *Circ. Arrhythm. Electrophysiol.* **2014**, *7*, 5–6. [CrossRef] [PubMed]
13. Hoffmayer, K.S.; Gerstenfeld, E.P. Contact force-sensing catheters. *Curr. Opin. Cardiol.* **2015**, *30*, 74–80. [CrossRef] [PubMed]
14. Yokoyama, K.; Nakagawa, H.; Shah, D.C.; Lambert, H.; Leo, G.; Aeby, N.; Ikeda, A.; Pitha, J.V.; Sharma, T.; Lazzara, R.; et al. Novel contact force sensor incorporated in irrigated radiofrequency ablation catheter predicts lesion size and incidence of steam pop and thrombus. *Circ. Arrhythm. Electrophysiol.* **2008**, *1*, 354–362. [CrossRef] [PubMed]
15. Mussigbrodt, A.; Grothoff, M.; Dinov, B.; Kosiuk, J.; Richter, S.; Sommer, P.; Breithardt, O.A.; Rolf, S.; Bollmann, A.; Arya, A.; et al. Irrigated tip catheters for radiofrequency ablation in ventricular tachycardia. *Biomed. Res. Int.* **2015**, *2015*, 389294. [CrossRef] [PubMed]
16. Bravo, L.; Atienza, F.; Eidelman, G.; Avila, P.; Pelliza, M.; Castellanos, E.; Loughlin, G.; Datino, T.; Torrecilla, E.G.; Almendral, J.; et al. Safety and efficacy of cryoablation vs. radiofrequency ablation of septal accessory pathways: Systematic review of the literature and meta-analyses. *Europace* **2018**, *20*, 1334–1342. [CrossRef] [PubMed]
17. Verma, A.; Haines, D.E.; Boersma, L.V.; Sood, N.; Natale, A.; Marchlinski, F.E.; Calkins, H.; Sanders, P.; Packer, D.L.; Kuck, K.H.; et al. Pulsed Field Ablation for the Treatment of Atrial Fibrillation: PULSED AF Pivotal Trial. *Circulation* **2023**, *147*, 1422–1432. [CrossRef] [PubMed]
18. Rauber, M.; Manninger, M.; Eberl, A.S.; Scherr, D. Zero-fluoroscopy ablation with multielectrode pulse field ablation system: Case series. *Pacing Clin. Electrophysiol.* **2024**, *47*, 117–120. [CrossRef] [PubMed]
19. Miszczyk, M.; Sajdok, M.; Bednarek, J.; Latusek, T.; Wojakowski, W.; Tomasik, B.; Wita, K.; Jadczyk, T.; Kurzelowski, R.; Drzewiecka, A.; et al. Stereotactic management of arrhythmia-radiosurgery in treatment of ventricular tachycardia (SMART-VT). Results of a prospective safety trial. *Radiother. Oncol.* **2023**, *188*, 109857. [CrossRef] [PubMed]
20. Aziz, H.M.; Zarzecki, M.P.; Garcia-Zamora, S.; Kim, M.S.; Bijak, P.; Tse, G.; Won, H.H.; Matusik, P.T. Pathogenesis and Management of Brugada Syndrome: Recent Advances and Protocol for Umbrella Reviews of Meta-Analyses in Major Arrhythmic Events Risk Stratification. *J. Clin. Med.* **2022**, *11*, 1912. [CrossRef] [PubMed]
21. Ahmed, M.; Belley-Cote, E.P.; Qiu, F.; Belesiotis, P.; Tao, B.; Wolf, A.; Kaur, H.; Ibrahim, A.; Wong, J.A.; Wang, M.K.; et al. Rhythm vs. Rate Control in Patients with Postoperative Atrial Fibrillation after Cardiac Surgery: A Systematic Review and Meta-Analysis. *J. Clin. Med.* **2023**, *12*, 4534. [CrossRef] [PubMed]
22. Bun, S.S.; Heme, N.; Asarisi, F.; Squara, F.; Scarlatti, D.; Moceri, P.; Ferrari, E. Prevalence and Clinical Characteristics of Patients with Torsades de Pointes Complicating Acquired Atrioventricular Block. *J. Clin. Med.* **2023**, *12*, 1067. [CrossRef] [PubMed]
23. Takahashi, E.A.; Schwamm, L.H.; Adeoye, O.M.; Alabi, O.; Jahangir, E.; Misra, S.; Still, C.H.; American Heart Association Council on Cardiovascular Radiology and Intervention; Council on Hypertension, Council on the Kidney in Cardiovascular Disease; Stroke, C. An Overview of Telehealth in the Management of Cardiovascular Disease: A Scientific Statement From the American Heart Association. *Circulation* **2022**, *146*, e558–e568. [CrossRef] [PubMed]
24. Matusik, P.; Mazur, P.; Stepien, E.; Pfitzner, R.; Sadowski, J.; Undas, A. Architecture of intraluminal thrombus removed from abdominal aortic aneurysm. *J. Thromb. Thrombolysis* **2010**, *30*, 7–9. [CrossRef] [PubMed]
25. Rubis, P.; Wisniowska-Smialek, S.; Biernacka-Fijalkowska, P.; Rudnicka-Sosin, L.; Wypasek, E.; Kozanecki, A.; Dziewiecka, E.; Faltyn, P.; Karabinowska, A.; Khachatryan, L.; et al. Left ventricular reverse remodeling is not related to biopsy-detected extracellular matrix fibrosis and serum markers of fibrosis in dilated cardiomyopathy, regardless of the definition used for LVRR. *Heart Vessels* **2017**, *32*, 714–725. [CrossRef] [PubMed]
26. Matusik, P.; Dubiel, M.; Wizner, B.; Fedyk-Lukasik, M.; Zdrojewski, T.; Opolski, G.; Dubiel, J.; Grodzicki, T. Age-related gap in the management of heart failure patients. The National Project of Prevention and Treatment of Cardiovascular Diseases—POLKARD. *Cardiol. J.* **2012**, *19*, 146–152. [CrossRef] [PubMed]
27. Ferrick, A.M.; Raj, S.R.; Deneke, T.; Kojodjojo, P.; Lopez-Cabanillas, N.; Abe, H.; Boveda, S.; Chew, D.S.; Choi, J.I.; Dagres, N.; et al. 2023 HRS/EHRA/APHRS/LAHRS Expert Consensus Statement on Practical Management of the Remote Device Clinic. *Europace* **2023**, *25*, euad123. [CrossRef]

Disclaimer/Publisher's Note: The statements, opinions and data contained in all publications are solely those of the individual author(s) and contributor(s) and not of MDPI and/or the editor(s). MDPI and/or the editor(s) disclaim responsibility for any injury to people or property resulting from any ideas, methods, instructions or products referred to in the content.

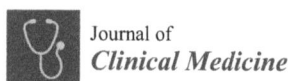

Editorial

Fever-Induced Brugada Sign: Clue for Clinical Management with Non-Negligible Risk of Sudden Cardiac Death

Piotr Bijak [1], Vassil B. Traykov [2], Avi Sabbag [3], Sergio Conti [4], Christian Sohns [5] and Paweł T. Matusik [6,7,*]

[1] Cardiology Outpatient Clinic, The John Paul II Hospital, 31-202 Kraków, Poland
[2] Department of Invasive Electrophysiology and Cardiac Pacing, Acibadem City Clinic Tokuda Hospital, 1407 Sofia, Bulgaria
[3] The Davidai Center for Rhythm Disturbances and Pacing, Chaim Sheba Medical Center, Tel Hashomer 52621, Israel
[4] Department of Cardiology, Electrophysiology Department, ARNAS Ospedali Civico Di Cristina Benfratelli, 90127 Palermo, Italy
[5] Clinic for Electrophysiology, Herz- und Diabeteszentrum NRW, Georgstr. 11, 32545 Bad Oeynhausen, Germany
[6] Department of Electrocardiology, Institute of Cardiology, Faculty of Medicine, Jagiellonian University Medical College, 31-202 Kraków, Poland
[7] Department of Electrocardiology, The John Paul II Hospital, 31-202 Kraków, Poland
* Correspondence: pawel.matusik@wp.eu or pawel.matusik@uj.edu.pl; Tel.: +48-12-614-22-77; Fax: +48-12-614-22-26

Brugada syndrome (BrS) is a primary electrical disease predisposing to ventricular tachyarrhythmias and sudden cardiac death [1]. The optimal diagnostics and risk stratification in patients suspected of having BrS are challenging [2]. A type 1 Brugada electrocardiogram (ECG) pattern is observed in about 2% of patients with fever and is also described in pediatric inflammatory multisystem syndrome related to COVID-19 [3,4]. The current European Society of Cardiology (ESC) guidelines for the management of patients with ventricular arrhythmias and the prevention of sudden cardiac death indicate the necessity to exclude Brugada phenocopies while making a diagnosis of BrS [5]. These guidelines highlight the lower specificity of the type 1 Brugada ECG pattern observed during the sodium channel blocker test or fever [5], but it should be mentioned that these induced Brugada ECG patterns are not considered a BrS phenocopy. In these conditions, genetic testing may be considered, according to a recent expert consensus statement on the state of genetic testing for cardiac diseases [6].

In the Journal of Clinical Medicine Special Issue "New Frontiers in Electrocardiography, Cardiac Arrhythmias, and Arrhythmogenic Disorders", Tsai et al. [7] described a long-term follow-up of a cohort of patients with a fever-induced type 1 Brugada ECG pattern. They included 18 asymptomatic patients without a spontaneous type 1 BrS ECG pattern and no family history of sudden death and 3 symptomatic individuals (two had previous syncopal episodes, while one had aborted sudden cardiac arrest). In the mean follow-up almost 10 years later, none of the asymptomatic patients experienced ventricular arrhythmic events. At the same time, all symptomatic patients experienced cardiac events, including implantable cardioverter-defibrillator therapies (shocks for new arrhythmic events) or sudden death.

Notably, Mizusawa et al. [8] reported the risk of arrhythmic events in patients with fever-induced BrS type 1 ECGs in a relatively large, multicenter, retrospectively collected cohort. In their cohort, the arrhythmic event rate was 3.0%/year in patients with a history of ventricular fibrillation, 1.3%/year in patients with a history of syncope, and 0.9%/year in asymptomatic patients. These results, while possibly derived from a more selected population, emphasize that the risk associated with fever-induced type 1 Brugada ECG is

Citation: Bijak, P.; Traykov, V.B.; Sabbag, A.; Conti, S.; Sohns, C.; Matusik, P.T. Fever-Induced Brugada Sign: Clue for Clinical Management with Non-Negligible Risk of Sudden Cardiac Death. *J. Clin. Med.* **2023**, *12*, 3503. https://doi.org/10.3390/jcm12103503

Received: 24 April 2023
Accepted: 9 May 2023
Published: 16 May 2023

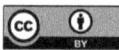

Copyright: © 2023 by the authors. Licensee MDPI, Basel, Switzerland. This article is an open access article distributed under the terms and conditions of the Creative Commons Attribution (CC BY) license (https://creativecommons.org/licenses/by/4.0/).

not negligible (compared to the incidence of sudden cardiac death in the general population of 0.03–0.1%/year [9]).

Moreover, in their paper, Tsai et al. [7] noted that there was an increase in heart rate and a significant shortening of the PR interval during periods of fever. In contrast, QRS duration and QTc intervals were not different during fever, compared to ECGs recorded without this condition in both asymptomatic and symptomatic patients. These data are consistent with the observations of Mizusawa et al. [8]. Interestingly, Mizusawa et al. [8] additionally observed that PR interval, QRS duration, and QTc interval prolonged during the sodium channel blocker challenge, suggesting different mechanisms implicated in their induction.

The association between fever and ECG pattern may be particularly important in light of evidence for inflammation in the right ventricular outflow tract of BrS patients, which may trigger ventricular arrhythmias in predisposed hearts [10].

It should be mentioned that a fever-induced type 1 Brugada ECG pattern may be awarded 3 points in the proposed Modified Shanghai scoring system for the diagnosis of BrS, compared to 3.5 points for a spontaneous type 1 Brugada ECG pattern and 2 points for a sodium channel blocker-induced Brugada type 1 ECG pattern (all at nominal or high leads) [6]. Moreover, the panel of experts for the recent ESC guidelines recommends that an induced type 1 ECG pattern requires other clinical characteristics, including arrhythmic syncope, polymorphic ventricular tachycardia or ventricular fibrillation, and consistent family history to diagnose BrS, contrary to spontaneous type 1 Brugada ECG pattern in patients without other heart diseases [5].

Thus, in line with current ESC guidelines [5], we consider a close follow-up with general recommendations (among others: avoidance of drugs and other substances listed on http://www.brugadadrugs.org (accessed on 24 April 2023) and treatment of fever with antipyretic drugs) of asymptomatic (no arrhythmic syncope/nocturnal agonal respiration) patients with fever-induced type 1 Brugada ECG pattern without documented ventricular arrhythmia and with negative family history (both of BrS and sudden death < 45 years) as the most reasonable approach to clinical management.

Author Contributions: Conceptualization, P.T.M.; writing—original draft preparation, P.B. and P.T.M.; writing—review and editing, V.B.T., A.S., S.C. and C.S.; supervision, P.T.M.; funding acquisition, P.T.M. All authors have read and agreed to the published version of the manuscript.

Funding: P.T.M. is supported by the National Science Centre, Poland (grant number 2021/05/X/NZ5/01511); the Jagiellonian University Medical College; the John Paul II Hospital; and the Ministry of Science and Higher Education stipend for outstanding young scientists.

Acknowledgments: This paper is a result of close clinical and scientific collaboration during a Diploma of Advanced Studies in Cardiac Arrhythmia Management (DAS-CAM). For the purpose of Open Access, the authors have applied a CC-BY public copyright license to any Author Accepted Manuscript (AAM) version arising from this submission.

Conflicts of Interest: The authors declare no conflict of interest. The funders had no role in the design of the study; in the collection, analyses, or interpretation of data; in the writing of the manuscript; or in the decision to publish the results.

References

1. Podolec, P.; Baranchuk, A.; Brugada, J.; Kukla, P.; Lelakowski, J.; Kopec, G.; Rubis, P.; Stepniewski, J.; Podolec, J.; Komar, M.; et al. Clinical classification of rare cardiac arrhythmogenic and conduction disorders, and rare arrhythmias. *Pol. Arch. Intern. Med.* **2019**, *129*, 154–159. [CrossRef] [PubMed]
2. Aziz, H.M.; Zarzecki, M.P.; Garcia-Zamora, S.; Kim, M.S.; Bijak, P.; Tse, G.; Won, H.H.; Matusik, P.T. Pathogenesis and Management of Brugada Syndrome: Recent Advances and Protocol for Umbrella Reviews of Meta-Analyses in Major Arrhythmic Events Risk Stratification. *J. Clin. Med.* **2022**, *11*, 1912. [CrossRef] [PubMed]
3. Adler, A.; Topaz, G.; Heller, K.; Zeltser, D.; Ohayon, T.; Rozovski, U.; Halkin, A.; Rosso, R.; Ben-Shachar, S.; Antzelevitch, C.; et al. Fever-induced Brugada pattern: How common is it and what does it mean? *Heart Rhythm* **2013**, *10*, 1375–1382. [CrossRef] [PubMed]

4. Franke, M.; Ksiazczyk, T.M.; Pietrzak, R.; Werner, B. Incidental diagnosis of Brugada syndrome in two girls hospitalized for pediatric inflammatory multisystem syndrome related to COVID-19 (PIMS-TS). *Kardiol. Pol.* **2022**, *80*, 1045–1046. [CrossRef] [PubMed]
5. Zeppenfeld, K.; Tfelt-Hansen, J.; De Riva, M.; Winkel, B.G.; Behr, E.R.; Blom, N.A.; Charron, P.; Corrado, D.; Dagres, N.; De Chillou, C.; et al. 2022 ESC Guidelines for the management of patients with ventricular arrhythmias and the prevention of sudden cardiac death. *Eur. Heart J.* **2022**, *43*, 3997–4126. [CrossRef] [PubMed]
6. Wilde, A.A.M.; Semsarian, C.; Marquez, M.F.; Shamloo, A.S.; Ackerman, M.J.; Ashley, E.A.; Sternick, E.B.; Barajas-Martinez, H.; Behr, E.R.; Bezzina, C.R.; et al. European Heart Rhythm Association (EHRA)/Heart Rhythm Society (HRS)/Asia Pacific Heart Rhythm Society (APHRS)/Latin American Heart Rhythm Society (LAHRS) Expert Consensus Statement on the state of genetic testing for cardiac diseases. *Europace* **2022**, *24*, 1307–1367. [CrossRef] [PubMed]
7. Tsai, C.F.; Chuang, Y.T.; Huang, J.Y.; Ueng, K.C. Long-Term Prognosis of Febrile Individuals with Right Precordial Coved-Type ST-Segment Elevation Brugada Pattern: A 10-Year Prospective Follow-Up Study. *J. Clin. Med.* **2021**, *10*, 4997. [CrossRef] [PubMed]
8. Mizusawa, Y.; Morita, H.; Adler, A.; Havakuk, O.; Thollet, A.; Maury, P.; Wang, D.W.; Hong, K.; Gandjbakhch, E.; Sacher, F.; et al. Prognostic significance of fever-induced Brugada syndrome. *Heart Rhythm* **2016**, *13*, 1515–1520. [CrossRef] [PubMed]
9. Ha, A.C.T.; Doumouras, B.S.; Wang, C.N.; Tranmer, J.; Lee, D.S. Prediction of Sudden Cardiac Arrest in the General Population: Review of Traditional and Emerging Risk Factors. *Can. J. Cardiol.* **2022**, *38*, 465–478. [CrossRef] [PubMed]
10. Oliva, A.; Grassi, S.; Pinchi, V.; Cazzato, F.; Coll, M.; Alcalde, M.; Vallverdu-Prats, M.; Perez-Serra, A.; Martinez-Barrios, E.; Cesar, S.; et al. Structural Heart Alterations in Brugada Syndrome: Is it Really a Channelopathy? A Systematic Review. *J. Clin. Med.* **2022**, *11*, 4406. [CrossRef] [PubMed]

Disclaimer/Publisher's Note: The statements, opinions and data contained in all publications are solely those of the individual author(s) and contributor(s) and not of MDPI and/or the editor(s). MDPI and/or the editor(s) disclaim responsibility for any injury to people or property resulting from any ideas, methods, instructions or products referred to in the content.

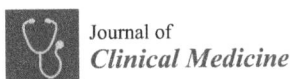

Article

Heart Rate Variability and Its Associations with Organ Complications in Adults after Fontan Operation

Magdalena Okólska [1], Jacek Łach [2], Paweł T. Matusik [3,*], Jacek Pająk [4], Tomasz Mroczek [5], Piotr Podolec [2] and Lidia Tomkiewicz-Pająk [2]

1. Cardiological Outpatient Clinic, Department of Cardiovascular Diseases, John Paul II Hospital, 31-202 Krakow, Poland; m.okolska@interia.pl
2. Department of Cardiac and Vascular Diseases, Institute of Cardiology, Jagiellonian University Medical College, John Paul II Hospital, 31-202 Krakow, Poland; djholter@interia.pl (J.Ł.); ppodolec@interia.pl (P.P.); ltom@wp.pl (L.T.-P.)
3. Department of Electrocardiology, Institute of Cardiology, Faculty of Medicine, Jagiellonian University Medical College, John Paul II Hospital, 31-202 Krakow, Poland
4. Department of Pediatric Heart Surgery and General Pediatric Surgery, Medical University of Warsaw, 02-091 Warsaw, Poland; jacekpajak@poczta.onet.pl
5. Department of Pediatric Cardiac Surgery, Jagiellonian University, 30-663 Krakow, Poland; t_mroczek@hotmail.com
* Correspondence: pawel.matusik@wp.eu; Tel.: +48-12-614-23-81

Citation: Okólska, M.; Łach, J.; Matusik, P.T.; Pająk, J.; Mroczek, T.; Podolec, P.; Tomkiewicz-Pająk, L. Heart Rate Variability and Its Associations with Organ Complications in Adults after Fontan Operation. *J. Clin. Med.* **2021**, *10*, 4492. https://doi.org/10.3390/jcm10194492

Academic Editor: Adrian Covic

Received: 13 August 2021
Accepted: 22 September 2021
Published: 29 September 2021

Publisher's Note: MDPI stays neutral with regard to jurisdictional claims in published maps and institutional affiliations.

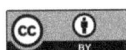

Copyright: © 2021 by the authors. Licensee MDPI, Basel, Switzerland. This article is an open access article distributed under the terms and conditions of the Creative Commons Attribution (CC BY) license (https://creativecommons.org/licenses/by/4.0/).

Abstract: Reduction of heart rate variability (HRV) parameters may be a risk factor and precede the occurrence of arrhythmias or the development of heart failure and complications in people with postinfarct left ventricular dysfunction and after coronary artery bypass grafting. Data on this issue in adults after a Fontan operation (FO) are scarce. This study assessed the association between HRV, exercise capacity, and multiorgan complications in adults after FO. Data were obtained from 30 FO patients (mean age 24 ± 5.4 years) and 30 healthy controls matched for age and sex. HRV was investigated in all patients by clinical examination, laboratory tests, echocardiography, a cardiopulmonary exercise test, and 24-h electrocardiogram. The HRV parameters were reduced in the FO group. Reduced HRV parameters were associated with patients' age at the time of FO, time since surgery, impaired exercise capacity, chronotropic incompetence parameters, and multiorgan complications. Univariate analysis showed that saturated O_2 at rest, percentage difference between adjacent NN intervals of >50 ms duration, and peak heart rate were associated with chronotropic index. Multivariable analysis revealed that all three variables were independent predictors of the chronotropic index. The results of this study suggest novel pathophysiological mechanisms that link HRV, physical performance, and organ damage in patients after FO.

Keywords: heart rate variability; physical performance; Fontan operation; organ complications

1. Introduction

The Fontan operation (FO) is the treatment of choice for patients with single-ventricle congenital heart disease [1]. The aim of this operation is to separate the pulmonary and systemic circulation, and achieve normal or near-normal arterial oxygen saturation. However, over time, cardiac and extra-cardiac complications develop in patients after FO. The literature also provides reports on the development of pathophysiological abnormalities, including abnormal functioning of the autonomic nervous system, altered chemoreceptor activity, and neurohumoral disorders, in this patient population [2–4].

One of the most significant problems in clinical practice during follow-up is identifying patients with a high risk of mortality. Parallel to the use of well-known methods (such as echocardiography), new methods are being developed, but their promising diagnostic or prognostic value is still not fully understood. Assessment of heart rate variability (HRV) is one such method.

A severe decrease in HRV indicates autonomic nervous system (ANS) dysfunction [5]. Decreased HRV may be a risk factor and precede organ complications. Research on patients with postinfarct left ventricular dysfunction indicates a relationship between reduced HRV and the development of heart failure, a higher risk of ventricular arrhythmia, and a worse prognosis [6,7]. HRV reduction is also observed in patients after cardiac surgery [8]. In adults with congenital heart disease, reduced HRV parameters were found among those with tetralogy of Fallot, systemic right ventricle, or cyanotic heart disease and those who underwent aortic coarctation repair or ventricular septal defect closure with right bundle branch block [9–12]. However, only a few studies have analyzed these aspects in patients after FO, and thus the data are limited. Furthermore, literature reports are mostly related to a pediatric population [13–18], while data regarding adult patients are scarce.

Therefore, this study aimed to assess the relationship between HRV parameters, exercise capacity, and multiorgan complications in adults after FO.

2. Materials and Methods

2.1. Study Participants

This was a retrospective study and included 30 adult patients over 18 years of age. All the patients underwent FO as they were diagnosed with functionally single ventricular heart. The patients remained under medical supervision in John Paul II Hospital. The exclusion criteria of the study were as follows: diagnosis of pulmonary artery hypertension requiring vasodilator therapy, asthma, atrial flutter, atrial fibrillation, diabetes, current infection, inflammation, and neoplastic disease, major trauma, pregnancy, use of vitamin K antagonists or beta-blockers, and history of pacemaker placement and alcohol abuse. Healthy, age- and sex-matched volunteers were included in the control group.

All the demographic, anatomic, and clinical data required for the study were obtained from the patients' medical records. Each patient was subjected to a physical examination as well as an assessment of body mass index, ejection fraction of the systemic ventricle, and arterial oxygen saturation. Body mass index was calculated by dividing the weight of the patient (kg) by height (m^2). Oxygen saturation was measured by pulse oximetry while breathing room air.

2.2. Echocardiography

Ejection fraction of the systemic ventricle was assessed using Simpson's method. In addition, valvular competence was evaluated in all the patients by two experienced, independent cardiologists using echocardiography (Vivid 7, GE Medical Systems, Milwaukee, WI, USA), as previously described [19].

2.3. Laboratory Investigations

After overnight fasting for at least 12 h, blood samples were collected from the antecubital vein of patients. The samples were evaluated for the following laboratory parameters that may indicate multi-organ complications: white blood cell count, red blood cell count, hemoglobin concentration, hematocrit, red blood cell distribution width, platelet count, mean platelet volume (MPV), total protein, alanine aminotransferase, aspartate transaminase, gamma-glutamyl transpeptidase (GGTP), alkaline phosphatase, total bilirubin α-fetoprotein, creatinine, cystatin C and N-terminal pro-B-type natriuretic peptide. All of them were assessed by routine laboratory techniques.

2.4. Cardiopulmonary Exercise Test

Exercise tolerance was determined by performing the cardiopulmonary exercise test (CPET) using a modified Bruce protocol (Reynols Medical System, ZAN-600, Hertford, UK). The following parameters were recorded during CPET: blood pressure, rest oxygen saturation (Sat. O_2 rest), 12-lead electrocardiogram, time of exercise, minute ventilation (VE), peak oxygen uptake (VO_2 peak), respiratory exchange ratio (RER), peak ventilatory equivalent of oxygen (VE/VO_2), peak ventilatory equivalent of carbon dioxide (VE/VCO_2), and breathing reserve. VO$_2$ peak was estimated as the highest oxygen uptake at peak exercise (mL/kg/min), and the percentage of the predicted value was calculated. Ventilatory anaerobic threshold was measured using the V-slope method. VE/VO$_2$ was defined as the amount of ventilation needed to uptake a given amount of oxygen, while VE/VCO$_2$ was defined as the amount of ventilation needed to eliminate a given amount of carbon dioxide. RER was calculated by dividing VO$_2$ by VCO$_2$.

2.5. Chronotropic Incompetence

Chronotropic index was determined based on the chronotropic metabolic relationship introduced by Wilkoff et al. [20] and calculated by using the following formula: (peak heart rate − resting heart rate)/(220 − age − resting heart rate). Chronotropic incompetence was defined as a chronotropic index value of <0.8.

Heart rate reserve (HRR) was calculated as the difference between maximal heart rate (HRmax) and peak heart rate. HRmax was determined using the following formula: 220 − age. Accordingly, HRR was calculated as follows: HRR = HRmax − peak heart rate = 220 − age − peak heart rate [21,22].

2.6. Ambulatory 24-h Holter Electrocardiogram

All patients and controls were subjected to standard 24-h electrocardiographic monitoring during daily activity, using a commercially available Holter system. All Holters were reviewed by two experienced observers. All recordings were analyzed using a PC-based Holter system, and those shorter than 21 h were excluded. The predominant rhythm was defined as the one that was present during >50% of the time during the Holter recording.

2.7. Heart Rate Variability

All Holters with available data were reviewed by two experienced analysts to analyze HRV. The beats were classified by automated software as normal, supraventricular extrasystolic, ventricular extrasystolic, those of uncertain origin, or artifacts. The classification was manually reviewed and corrected if necessary. Only normal-to-normal (NN) intervals were included in the HRV analysis.

The following HRV time-domain parameters were measured: standard deviation of all NN intervals (SDNN), standard deviation of the averages of NN intervals in all 5-min segments of the entire recording (SDANN), root mean square of the differences of successive NN intervals (rMSSD), percentage difference between adjacent NN intervals of >50 ms duration (pNN50), and HRV triangular index.

Furthermore, the following HRV frequency parameters were measured: very low frequency (0.017–0.050 Hz); low frequency (0.050–0.150 Hz); and high frequency (0.150–0.350 Hz).

The high frequency component is associated with the activity of the parasympathetic nervous system, and low frequency with both the sympathetic and parasympathetic system. Very low frequency is related to more long-term fluctuations in heart rate [23].

The total power was determined at frequencies ranging from 0.017 to 0.050 Hz. In addition, the low frequency/high frequency ratio was calculated. All spectral indexes were calculated as average data over the complete recording period (up to 24 h). The parameters SDNN, HRV triangular index, total power, and low frequency were assumed to reflect, with some simplification, the overall HRV or activity of both sympathetic and parasympathetic components of the ANS, while the parameters rMSSD, pNN50, and high frequency were directly proportional to the parasympathetic nervous system [23].

2.8. Statistical Analysis

The data distribution was presented as numbers and percentages for categorical variables, means with SDs for normally distributed continuous variables, and medians with lower and upper quartiles (Q1–Q3) for continuous variables with non-normal distribution. The normality of the data distribution was verified using the Kolmogorov–Smirnov test. Quantitative variables of patients who underwent FO and control participants were compared using the two-tailed Student's *t*-test or Mann–Whitney *U* test, whereas qualitative variables were analyzed using the chi-square test. The association between numerical variables was analyzed by calculating the Pearson's correlation or Spearman's rank correlation coefficient. Moreover, the simultaneous influence of Sat. O_2 rest and pNN50 on peak heart rate was assessed using the linear regression model. The results were presented as coefficient (*b*) with 95% confidence interval. The *R*-square value was calculated to describe the goodness-of-fit for the linear regression model. All the analyses were performed using IBM SPSS Statistics for Windows, Version 25.0 (IBM Corp., Armonk, NY, USA). Statistical significance was defined as $p < 0.05$ for the two-tailed test.

3. Results

3.1. Patients' Characteristics

Thirty adult patients who underwent FO were enrolled in the study, including 17 men (57%) with a mean age of 24 ± 5.4 years. These patients did not show any significant difference from the controls with regard to age, sex, and body mass index. The median age of patients at the time of surgery was 3 (Q1–Q3: 2–5) years, the median time after surgery was 19.5 (Q1–Q3: 17–21) years. A total of 19 (64%) patients had fenestration, and 11 (36%) had no fenestration. The mean ejection fraction of the systemic ventricle was 52 ± 9.1%. The baseline characteristics of the study group and the control group are presented in Tables 1 and 2.

Table 1. Baseline characteristics of the study group and controls.

Variables	Fontan Patients (*n* = 30)	Controls (*n* = 30)	*p*-Value
Age, years	24 (5.4)	25.6 (3.8)	0.23
Female sex, *n* (%)	13 (43)	12 (40)	0.95
Height, cm	170 (8.1)	173 (6.9)	0.19
Weight, kg	65.08 (9.7)	69.0 (9.3)	0.85
Body mass index, kg/m^2	22.5 (2.7)	22.7 (2.2)	0.69

Continuous data are presented as mean (SD) and categorical data as number (percentage).

3.2. Laboratory Tests Results

The laboratory parameters determined for the FO group and the control group are presented in Table 3.

Table 2. Baseline characteristics of patients after the Fontan operation.

Variables	Patients (*n* = 30)
Anatomic diagnosis, *n* (%)	
Tricuspid atresia	5 (17)
Pulmonary stenosis/TGA	4 (13)
Right ventricular hypoplasia	11 (36)
Hypoplastic left heart syndrome	5 (17)
Double-outlet right ventricle with left ventricular hypoplasia	3 (10)
Double-inflow left ventricle	1 (4)
Common atrioventricular canal	1 (4)
Systemic ventricle type, *n* (%)	
Left ventricle	24 (80)
Right ventricle	6 (20)

Table 2. Cont.

Variables	Patients (n = 30)
NYHA functional class, n (%)	
I	5 (17)
II	21 (71)
III	4 (12)
IV	0 (0)
Types of Fontan operation, n (%)	
Total cavopulmonary connection, lateral tunnel	29 (96)
Atriopulmonary connection	1 (4)

Abbreviation: NYHA, New York Heart Association; TGA, transposition of great arteries.

Table 3. Laboratory parameters in patients after Fontan procedure and in controls.

Variables	Fontan Group (n = 30)	Controls (n = 30)	p-Value
NT-proBNP, pg/mL	148.0 (96.0–470.0)	24.5 (6.0–35.0)	<0.001
RBC, $10^9/\mu L$	5.5 (0.6)	4.9 (0.5)	<0.001
Hemoglobin, g/dL	18.8 (1.8)	14.7 (1.3)	0.011
Hematocrit, %	47.6 (4.5)	43.0 (3.3)	<0.001
RDW, %	13.2 (12.9–14.4)	12.4 (12.0–12.6)	<0.001
Platelet count, $10^3/\mu L$	164.4 (70.8)	228.2 (38.1)	<0.001
PDW, fL	16.0 (3.2)	12.2 (2.3)	<0.001
MPV, fL	12.0 (1.2)	10.4 (1.0)	<0.001
Cystatin C, mg/L	0.9 (0.2)	0.8 (0.1)	0.009
Creatinine, µmol/L	72.8 (12.9)	77.4 (14.2)	0.19
eGFR, mL/min/1.73 m^2	116.5 (13.6)	112.0 (12.9)	0.26
AST, IU/L	24.0 (20.0–28.0)	19.5 (17.0–22.0)	<0.001
ALT, IU/L	24.0 (19.0–27.0)	20.0 (17.0–23.0)	0.04
GGTP, U/L	61.5 (44.0–117.0)	15.5 (14.0–18.0)	<0.001
Bilirubin, µmol/L	18.3 (10.7–34.0)	12.0 (7.7–17.0)	0.002
α-Fetoprotein, ng/mL	2.5 (1.9–3.6)	2.3 (1.9–3.4)	0.657
ALP, U/L	80.5 (64.0–88.0)	67.0 (55.0–89.0)	0.11
Total protein, g/dL	75.1 (70.2–78.8)	75.0 (73.0–78.6)	0.43
Prothrombin time, s	13.6 (12.6–15.2)	11.9 (11.4–12.0)	<0.001
INR	1.2 (1.2–1.65)	1.0 (0.9–1.1)	<0.001
AST/ALT ratio	1.1 (0.4)	1.0 (0.3)	0.21

Continuous data are presented as mean (SD) or median (Q1–Q3). Abbreviations: ALP, alkaline phosphatase; ALT, alanine aminotransferase; AST, aspartate aminotransferase; AST/ALT ratio, ratio of aspartate transaminase to alanine transaminase; eGFR, estimated glomerular filtration rate; GGTP, γ-glutamyl transpeptidase; INR, international normalized ratio; MPV, mean platelet volume; NT-proBNP, N-terminal pro-B-type natriuretic peptide; PDW, platelet distribution width; RBC, red blood cells; RDW, red cell distribution width.

3.3. CPET Results

The CPET results of patients from the FO group were compared with those from the control group and are presented in Table 4.

Table 4. Cardiopulmonary exercise test results of patients in the Fontan operation group and controls.

Variables	Fontan Group ($n = 30$)	Controls ($n = 30$)	p-Value
Exercise time, min	13.5 (3.4)	16.65 (2.7)	<0.001
Sat. O_2 rest, %	92.0 (89.0–93.0)	97.0 (96.0–98.0)	<0.001
Sat. O_2 exercise, %	87.0 (84.0–89.0)	97.0 (96.0–97.0)	<0.001
Peak VO_2 per kg, mL/kg/min	20.6 (18.2–23.2)	50.9 (46.5–54.1)	<0.001
Peak VO_2, %n	55.0 (48.0–63.0)	97.0 (95.0–98.0)	<0.001
VE	46.0 (35.0–63.0)	123 (97–138)	<0.001
VE/VCO_2, L/L	33.3 (3.9)	26.5 (2.9)	<0.001
RER peak	1.0 (0.08)	1.1 (0.9)	0.01
Chronotropic index	0.55 (0.47–0.62)	0.93 (0.88–0.99)	<0.001
HRR	32.0 (24.0–60.0)	8.0 (1.0–14.0)	<0.001

Continuous data are presented as mean (SD) or median (Q1–Q3). Abbreviations: HRR, heart rate reserve; peak VO_2 per kg, peak oxygen uptake per kilogram; peak VO_2 (%n), percentage of predicted value for peak oxygen uptake; RER peak, peak respiratory exchange ratio; Sat. O_2, oxygen saturation; VE, minute ventilation; VE/VCO_2, peak ventilatory equivalent of CO_2.

3.4. Heart Rate Variability

A significant reduction in HRV was observed in adult patients with Fontan circulation compared with the control subjects (Table 5).

Table 5. Heart rate and HRV in the Fontan patients and control subjects.

Variables	Fontan Patients ($n = 30$)	Controls ($n = 30$)	p-Value
Heart rate, bpm	69.1 (10.4)	80.5 (6.5)	<0.001
Mean NN, ms	922.0 (157.9)	771.57 (59.4)	<0.001
SDNN, ms	121.8 (29.6)	152.74 (23.94)	<0.001
SDANN, ms	111.9 (31.6)	133.63 (25.2)	<0.001
rMSSD, ms	16.5 (10.9–33.5)	32.65 (27.4–43.7)	<0.001
pNN50, ms	6.75 (2.7–13.0)	11.8 (7.2–13.2)	0.018
HRV triangular index, ms	34.5 (11.3)	45.7 (7.8)	<0.001
Very low frequency (ms^2)	301.6 (13.1–491.2)	491.8 (256.2–71.2)	0.030
Low frequency (ms^2)	332.8 (93.4–551.2)	712.3 (538.3–1129.1)	<0.001
High frequency (ms^2)	140.1 (46.1–303.2)	289.0 (156.7–370)	0.019
Total power (ms^2)	861.1 (1.0–1738.0)	1618.7 (957.4–2031)	0.003
Low frequency/high frequency ratio	3.5 (2.5)	4.2 (1.5)	0.190

Continuous data are presented as mean (SD) or median (Q1–Q3). Abbreviations: HRV, heart rate variability; NN, normal-to-normal interval; pNN50, percentage difference between adjacent NN intervals of >50 ms duration; rMSSD, root mean square of the differences of successive NN intervals; SDANN, standard deviation of the averages of NN intervals in all 5-min segments of the entire recording; SDNN, standard deviation of all NN intervals.

The correlations between the HRV parameters and patients' characteristics are presented in Table 6.

Table 6. Correlations between HRV parameters and patient characteristics.

HRV Parameters	Share of the Autonomous Components in the Modulation of HRV Parameters						
	Overall HRV or Sympathetic and Parasympathetic Nervous System Activities				Parasympathetic Nervous System Activity		
	SDNN	HRV Index	Low Frequency	Total Power	rMSSD	pNN50	High Frequency
Group characteristic							
Age at the time of Fontan operation	R = −0.379, *p* = **0.039**	R = −0.250, *p* = 0.183	R = −0.074, *p* = 0.697	R = −0.153, *p* = 0.421	R = 0.270, *p* = 0.149	R = −0.422, *p* = **0.020**	R = −0.047, *p* = 0.805
Age during the study	R = −0.426, *p* = **0.019**	R = −0.217, *p* = 0.25	R = −0.31, *p* = 0.094	R = −0.432, *p* = **0.017**	R = −0.061, *p* = 0.749	R = −0.481, *p* = **0.007**	R = −0.205, *p* = 0.276
Echocardiography							
Ejection fraction of the systemic ventricle	R = 0.584, *p* = **0.001**	R = 0.424, *p* = **0.02**	R = 0.347, *p* = 0.06	R = 0.453, *p* = **0.012**	R = 0.032, *p* = 0.104	R = 0.638, *p* = **0.001**	R = 0.281, *p* = 0.132
Chronotropic parameters							
HRR	R = −0.137, *p* = 0.471	R = −0.411, *p* = **0.023**	R = −0.221, *p* = 0.240	R = −0.264, *p* = 0.159	R = −0.323, *p* = 0.082	R = −0.262, *p* = 0.162	R = −0.193, *p* = 0.307
Chronotropic index	R = 0.220, *p* = 0.243	R = 0.330, *p* = 0.075	R = 0.332, *p* = 0.073	R = 0.333, *p* = 0.072	R = 0.291, *p* = 0.118	R = 0.419, *p* = **0.021**	R = 0.164, *p* = 0.386
CPET parameters							
Exercise time	R = 0.318, *p* = 0.086	R = 0.709, *p* < **0.001**	R = 0.544, *p* = **0.002**	R = 0.45, *p* = **0.013**	R = −0.099, *p* = 0.601	R = 0.440, *p* = **0.015**	R = 0.38, *p* = **0.038**
Peak heart rate	R = 0.262, *p* = 0.163	R = 0.485, *p* = **0.007**	R = 0.384, *p* = **0.036**	R = 0.375, *p* = **0.041**	R = 0.377, *p* = **0.040**	R = 0.394, *p* = **0.031**	R = 0.277, *p* = 0.138
Peak VO$_2$ per kg	R = 0.404, *p* = **0.027**	R = 0.607, *p* < **0.001**	R = 0.394, *p* = **0.031**	R = 0.360, *p* = 0.051	R = 0.142, *p* = 0.453	R = 0.524, *p* = **0.003**	R = 0.290, *p* = 0.119
Peak VO$_2$, %N	R = 0.137, *p* = 0.469	R = 0.541, *p* = **0.002**	R = 0.233, *p* = 0.216	R = 0.185, *p* = 0.328	R = −0.016, *p* = 0.933	R = 0.222, *p* = 0.238	R = 0.077, *p* = 0.687
VE	R = 0.434, *p* = **0.017**	R = 0.369, *p* = **0.045**	R = 0.274, *p* = 0.143	R = 0.249, *p* = 0.184	R = 0.076, *p* = 0.690	R = 0.298, *p* = 0.110	R = 0.377, *p* = **0.04**
VE/VCO$_2$	R = −0.012, *p* = 0.951	R = −0.424, *p* = **0.019**	R = −0.240, *p* = 0.202	R = −0.156, *p* = 0.411	R = 0.119, *p* = 0.530	R = −0.305, *p* = 0.102	R = −0.197, *p* = 0.296
Laboratory tests							
GGTP	R = −0.322, *p* = 0.083	R = −0.245, *p* = 0.192	R = −0.385, *p* = **0.036**	R = −0.346, *p* = 0.061	R = −0.154, *p* = 0.415	R = −0.368, *p* = **0.046**	R = −0.309, *p* = 0.096

Abbreviations: CPET, cardiopulmonary exercise test; GGTP, γ-glutamyl transpeptidase; HRR, heart rate reserve; HRV, heart rate variability; peak VO$_2$ per kg, peak oxygen uptake per kilogram; peak VO$_2$ (%N), percentage of predicted value for peak oxygen uptake; pNN50, percentage difference between adjacent NN intervals of >50 ms duration; rMSSD, root mean square of the differences of successive NN intervals; SDNN, standard deviation of all NN intervals; VE, minute ventilation; VE/VCO$_2$, peak ventilatory equivalent of CO$_2$. Significant results in bold.

3.5. Relationship between HRV, CPET, and Chronotropic Incompetence Parameters

The results of univariate analysis showed that Sat. O$_2$ rest, pNN50, and peak heart rate were associated with chronotropic index (the strongest relationship was observed for peak heart rate (R^2 = 0.54)). The results of multivariable analysis showed that all three variables were significant predictors of chronotropic index, accounting for 70% variability in chronotropic incompetence (Table 7).

Table 7. Association between oxygen saturation at rest, pNN50, peak heart rate, and chronotropic index.

	Univariable Analysis				Multivariable Analysis			
	b	95% CI	p-Value	R^2	b	95% CI	p-Value	R^2
Sat. O_2 rest	0.026	(0.004–0.047)	0.02	0.18	0.021	(0.006–0.035)	0.006	
pNN50	0.016	(0.003–0.029)	0.018	0.19	0.011	(0.003–0.02)	0.013	0.7
Peak heart rate	0.005	(0.003–0.007)	<0.001	0.54	0.004	(0.002–0.006)	<0.001	

Abbreviations: HRR, heart rate reserve; pNN50, percentage difference between adjacent NN intervals of >50 ms duration; Sat. O_2, oxygen saturation; 95% CI, 95% confidence interval; b—coefficient from linear regression; R^2—coefficient of determination.

4. Discussion

This study assessed the association between HRV, exercise capacity, and multi-organ complications in adults after undergoing FO. The findings revealed that patients after FO had significantly reduced HRV, implying a correlation between HRV parameters and age at the time of surgical intervention, the time since operation, reduced exercise capacity, and organ complications.

The activity of the ANS regulates HRV measures. In this study, 70% of patients from the study group showed a significant reduction in HRV parameters. These observations are in accordance with the earlier studies that investigated this issue in pediatric patient groups, but studies on adult groups are scarce [2,14,15,17,24].

In our study, adult patients who underwent FO showed a decrease in HRV parameters. This shows the association between age and reduced HRV. The reduction progressed over time after surgery. Similar observations were presented in the studies by Dahlaqvist et al. [15] and Rydberg et al. [17]. The age of the patient at the time of the surgery plays a crucial role in the pathogenesis of arrhythmias. According to the literature, the best time for surgery in children with single-ventricle heart is up to 4 years of age [25–27]. Decreased HRV parameters were shown in children regardless of the surgical intervention approach utilized (intra-atrial lateral tunnel or extra-cardiac conduit) [15]. The findings of our study may be considered valuable and suggest that special attention should be paid for early qualification of children to FO. This observation is consistent with previous reports, including that of Abbott et al. [28], who proved that an increased preoperative heart rate is associated with an increased perioperative risk of heart damage and mortality.

The CPET results of this study revealed that reduced HRV parameters were associated with chronotropic incompetence and exercise capacity.

Patients who had decreased HRV parameters had lower VO_2 peak and percentage of predicted value of VO_2 peak, and higher VE/VCO_2.

It has been shown that patients with overt heart failure had decreased VO_2 peak and increased VE/VCO_2, which are considered well-established predictors of mortality [29–31]. Furthermore, Kyoto et al. [32] reported a correlation between increased heart rate and decreased VO_2 peak, independent of age, sex, and heart disease. Silvilaired et al. [33] examined patients after tetralogy of Fallot and observed a relationship between the HRV parameters (low frequency and high frequency) and reduced VO_2 peak, which suggested that an impaired ANS response may be responsible for decreased exercise tolerance.

It has also been shown that VE/VCO_2 reflects the relationship between minute ventilation and CO_2 excretion [34]. This study revealed that patients with heart failure exhibited an elevated VE/VCO_2 that was associated with excessive minute ventilation in relation to exercise effort. One of the possible mechanisms explaining this phenomenon is an imbalance between the ANS and excessive sympathetic activity. Previous studies conducted among people with heart failure have shown that an increased ventilation response, expressed as higher VE/VCO_2, independently correlates with all HRV parameters [35].

Impaired chronotropic response is another issue observed in patients who have had FO [30,36]. Patients after FO have higher HRR, achieve shorter exercise time in CPET, and show lower VO_2 peak and higher VE/VCO_2 values. In this study, we attempted to explore whether the knowledge on reduced HRV parameters might be used to predict the occurrence of organ complications. This assumption seems to be justified: our results confirmed that patients with lower pNN50, Sat. O_2 rest, and peak heart rate had chronotropic incompetence and 70% probability of developing heart failure.

In patients after Fontan surgery, liver disorders commonly occur and may cause serious clinical complications [37,38]. In this study, we registered an increased level of GGTP and showed a correlation between GGTP and pNN50. This increased level of GGTP observed in patients after FO could be attributed to liver dysfunction or damage caused by chronic blood stagnation due to increased venous pressure (prevailing in Fontan's circulation). To our knowledge, no studies have so far analyzed the relationship between reduced HRV parameters and liver dysfunction in patients after FO. However, several studies in the literature indicate reduced HRV values in patients with liver fibrosis [39–41]. These studies suggest that ANS dysfunction is associated with poor prognosis in this patient population. Furthermore, Bohogal et al. [41] showed that specific HRV parameters, regardless of the Model for End-Stage Liver Disease score, can predict mortality in patients with cirrhosis. The mechanism of ANS dysfunction in patients with liver fibrosis is still unknown and requires further research. However, the association between HRV and GGTP as observed in our study may be suspected to indirectly indicate the risk of developing liver dysfunction.

Holter ECG monitoring is relatively simple, generally available and non-invasive. It is performed in every patient after FO. HRV parameters have been identified as useful in various clinical scenarios [5,42]. We suppose that decreased HRV parameters may help to identify patients with specific organ complications. Decreased HRV parameters may be a risk of future arrhythmias and may indicate the need for regular follow-up in the case of heart failure development.

This retrospective study has several limitations to be acknowledged. Firstly, the number of patients was small and relatively mixed. Secondly, HRV parameters are highly sensitive to external factors. The norms for the analysis of HRV parameters and prognostically significant reduced values of these parameters in patients with congenital heart disease have not yet been developed. Therefore, further analyses with larger groups of patients are necessary.

5. Conclusions

This study revealed that patients after FO had reduced HRV parameters indicating ANS dysfunction, which was found to be associated with lower exercise tolerance and poor liver function. The data of the study suggest novel pathophysiological mechanisms that link HRV, physical performance, and organ damage in patients after FO.

Author Contributions: Conceptualization, M.O. and L.T.-P.; methodology, M.O., P.T.M. and L.T.-P.; software, M.O. and J.Ł.; validation, M.O., L.T.-P and P.P.; formal analysis, M.O., P.T.M. and J.Ł.; investigation, M.O., L.T.-P. and P.P.; resources, M.O., L.T.-P. and P.P.; data curation, M.O. and J.Ł.; writing—original draft preparation, M.O.; writing—review and editing,: L.T.-P, J.P., P.T.M. and T.M.; visualization, M.O.; supervision, L.T.-P., J.P., T.M. and P.P.; project administration, L.T.-P. and P.P.; funding acquisition, L.T.-P. All authors have read and agreed to the published version of the manuscript.

Funding: This work was supported by a grant of National Science Center (2017/27/B/NZ5/02186), to L.T.-P. The publication of this article was supported by the science found of the John Paul II Hospital, Cracow, Poland (no. FN/21/2021 to M.O).

Institutional Review Board Statement: This study was conducted according to guidelines of Declaration of Helsinki and was approved by the Bioethical Commission at the District Medical Chamber in Cracow (nr. 1072.6120.11.2017).

Informed Consent Statement: All patients gave a written informed consent.

Data Availability Statement: The data presented in this study are available on request from the corresponding author. The data are not publicly available due to planned further publications.

Conflicts of Interest: The authors declare no conflict of interest.

References

1. Baumagartner, H.; De Backer, J.; Babu-Narayan, S.V.; Budts, W.; Chessa, M.; Diller, G.; Lung, B.; Kluin, J.; Lang, I.M.; Meijboom, F.; et al. 2020 ESC Guidelines for the management of adult congenital heart disease. *Eur. Heart J.* **2021**, *42*, 563–645. [CrossRef]
2. Davos, C.H.; Francis, D.P.; Leenarts, M.F.E.; Sing-Chien, Y.; Wei, L.; Davlouros, P.A.; Wensel, R.; Coats, A.J.S.; Piepoli, M.; Sreeram, N.; et al. Global impairment of cardiac autonomic nervous activity late after the Fontan operation. *Circulation* **2003**, *108*, II180–II185. [CrossRef]
3. Kołcz, J.; Tomkiewicz-Pająk, L.; Wójcik, E.; Podolec, P.; Skalski, J. Prognostic significance of neurohumoral factors in early and late postoperative period after Fontan procedure. *Interact. Cardiovasc. Thorac. Surg.* **2011**, *13*, 40–45. [CrossRef] [PubMed]
4. Tomkiewicz-Pająk, L.; Hoffman, P.; Trojnarska, O.; Bednarek, J.; Płazak, W.; Pająk, J.W.; Olszowska, L.; Komar, M.; Podolec, P.S. Long-term follow-up in adult patients after Fontan operation. *Kardiochir. Torakochirurgia Pol.* **2013**, *10*, 357–363.
5. Matusik, P.S.; Matusik, P.T.; Stein, P.K. Heart rate variability in patients with systemic lupus erythematosus: A systematic review and methodological considerations. *Lupus* **2018**, *27*, 1225–1239. [CrossRef] [PubMed]
6. Kleiger, R.E.; Miller, J.P.; Bigger, J.T.; Moss, A.J. Decreased heart rate variability and its association with increased mortality after acute myocardial infarction. *Am. J. Cardiol.* **1987**, *59*, 256. [CrossRef]
7. Nolan, J.; Batin, P.D.; Andrews, R.; Lindsay, S.J.; Brooksby, P.; Mullen, M.; Baig, W.; Flapan, A.D.; Cowley, A.; Prescott, R.J.; et al. Prospective study of heart rate variability and mortality in heart failure. *Circulation* **1998**, *98*, 1510. [CrossRef]
8. Bryniarski, L.; Kawwa, J.; Rajzer, M.; Stolarz, K.; Kawecka-Jaszcz, K. Zmienność rytmu zatokowego serca u pacjentów po zabiegach pomostowania aortalno-wieńcowego-wczesne i późne wyniki rehabilitacji kardiologicznej [Heart rate variability in patients after coronary artery bypass grafting—Early and long term effects of cardiac rehabilitation]. *Przegl. Lek.* **2002**, *59*, 699–702. (In Polish)
9. McLeod, K.A.; Hillis, W.S.; Houston, A.B.; Wilson, N.; Trainer, A.; Neilson, J.; Doig, W.B. Reduced heart rate variability following repair of tetralogy of Fallot. *Heart* **1999**, *81*, 656–660. [CrossRef]
10. Zandstra, T.; Kiès, P.; Maan, A.; Man, S.-C.; Bootsma, M.; Vliegen, H.; Egorova, A.; Mertens, B.; Holman, E.; Schalij, M.; et al. Association between reduced heart rate variability components and supraventricular tachyarrhythmias in patients with a systemic right ventricle. *Auton. Neurosci.* **2020**, *227*, 102696. [CrossRef]
11. Heiberg, J.; Eckerström, F.; Rex, C.E.; Maagaard, M.; Mølgaard, H.; Redington, A.; Gatzoulis, M.; Hjortdal, V.E. Heart rate variability is impaired in adults after closure of ventricular septal defect in childhood: A novel finding associated with right bundle branch block. *Int. J. Cardiol.* **2019**, *274*, 88–92. [CrossRef]
12. Moon, J.R.; Huh, J.; Song, J.; Kang, I.S.; Yang, J.H.; Jun, T.G.; Chang, S.A.; Park, S.W. Depression and heart rate variability in adults with cyanotic congenital heart disease. *Circulation* **2019**, *140*, A13169. [CrossRef]
13. Dahlqvist, J.A.; Wiklund, U.; Karlsson, M.; Hanséus, K.; Strömvall-Larsson, E.; Nygren, A.; Eliasson, H.; Rydberg, A. Sinus node dysfunction in patients with Fontan circulation: Could heart rate variability be predictor for pacemarker implantation? *Pediatr. Cardiol.* **2019**, *40*, 685–693. [CrossRef] [PubMed]
14. Buttera, G.; Bonnet, D.; Iserin, L.; Sidi, D.; Kachaner, J.; Villain, E. Total cavopulmonary and atriopulmonary connection are associated with reduced heart rate variability. *Heart* **1999**, *82*, 704–707. [CrossRef] [PubMed]
15. Dahlaqvist, J.A.; Karlsson, M.; Wiklund, U.; Hörnsten, R.; Strömvall-Larsson, E.; Berggren, H.; Hanséus, K.; Johansson, S.; Rydberg, A. Heart rate variability in children with Fontan circulation: Lateral tunnel and extracardiac conduit. *Pediatr. Cardiol.* **2021**, *33*, 307–315. [CrossRef]
16. Rydberg, A.; Karlsson, M.; Hornsten, R.; Wiklund, U. Can analysis of heart rate variability predict arrhythmia in children with Fontan circulation? *Pediatr. Cardiol.* **2008**, *29*, 50–55. [CrossRef]
17. Rydberg, A.; Rask, P.; Hornstern, R.; Teien, D. Heart rate variability in children with Fontan circulation. *Pediatr. Cardiol.* **2004**, *25*, 365–369. [CrossRef]
18. Bossers, S.S.M.; Duppen, N.; Kapusta, L.; Maan, A.; Duim, A.R.; Bogers Ad, J.J.C.; Hazekamp, M.G.; Iperen, G.; Helbing, W.A.; Blom, N.A. Comprehensive rhythm evaluation in a large contemporary Fontan population. *Eur. J. Cardiothorac. Surg.* **2015**, *48*, 833–840. [CrossRef]
19. Tomkiewicz-Pajak, L.; Podolec, P.; Drabik, L.; Pajak, J.; Kolcz, J.; Plazak, W. Single ventricle function and exercise tolerance in adult patients after Fontan operation. *Acta Cardiol.* **2014**, *69*, 155–160. [CrossRef]
20. Wilkoff, B.L.; Corey, J.; Blackburn, G. A mathematical model of cardiac chronotropic response to exercise. *J. Electrophysiol.* **1989**, *3*, 176–180. [CrossRef]
21. Straburzyńska-Migaj, E. Spiroergometric exercise test. In *Cardiology Handbook of the Polish Cardiac Society*; Ponikowski, P., Hoffmen, P., Witkowski, A., Lipiec, P., Eds.; Via Medica: Gdańsk, Poland, 2019; pp. 87–94. (In Polish)
22. Guazzi, M.; Adams, V.; Conraads, V.; Viviane, C.; Martin, H.; Mezzani, A.; Vanhees, L.; Arena, R.; Fletcher, G.F.; Forman, D.F.; et al. Clinical recommendations for cardiopulmonary exercise testing data assessment in specific patient populations. *Circulation* **2012**, *126*, 2261–2274. [CrossRef]
23. Heart rate variability: Standards of measurement, physiological interpretation, and clinical use. Task Force of the European Society of Cardiology and the North American society of Pacing Electrophysiology. *Circulation* **1996**, *93*, 1043–1065. [CrossRef]

24. Ohuchi, H.; Hasegawa, S.; Yasuda, K.; Yamada, O.; Ono, Y.; Echigo, S. Severely impaired cardiac autonomic nervous activity after the Fontan operation. *Circulation* **2001**, *104*, 1513–1518. Erratum in: *Circulation* **2004**, *109*, 3257.
25. Hofbeck, M.; Koch, A.; Buheitel, G.; Gerling, S.; Rauch, R.; Weyand, M.; Singer, H. Spätpostoperative Herzrhythmusstörungen nach totaler cavopulmonaler Anastomose und ihre Beziehung zum Operationsalter der Patienten [Late postoperative cardiac arrhythmias after total cavopulmonary anastomosis and correlation with age of the patients at operation]. *Z. Kardiol.* **2000**, *89*, 788–794. (In German) [CrossRef]
26. Malec, E.; Zając, A.; Pająk, J. The results of one-stage and two-stage Fontan operation in children with single ventricle. *Kardiol. Pol.* **1998**, *48*, 23–30.
27. Moll, J.A.; Ostrowska, K.; Dobrowolski, J. Diagnostic and therapeutic procedures in single ventricle—Own experience. *Przegląd. Ped.* **2000**, *30*, 140–144.
28. Abbott, T.E.F.; Minto, G.; Lee, A.M.; Pearse, R.M.; Ackland, G.L. POM-HR, POMO-O and OPTIMISE study groups. Elevated preoperative heart rate is associated with cardiopulmonary and autonomic impairment in high-risk surgical patients. *Br. J. Anaesth.* **2017**, *119*, 87–94. [CrossRef]
29. Mantegazza, V.; Apostolo, A.; Hager, A. Cardiopulmonary exercise testing in adult congenital heart disease. *Ann. Am. Thorac. Soc.* **2017**, *14*, S93–S101. [CrossRef]
30. Takken, T.; Blank, A.C.; Hulzebos, E.H.; Van Brussel, M.; Groen, W.G.; Helders, P.J. Cardiopulmonary exercise testing in congenital heart diseases: (Contra)indication and interpretation. *Neth. Heart J.* **2009**, *10*, 385–392. [CrossRef] [PubMed]
31. Myers, J.; Arena, R.; Dewey, F.; Bensimhon, D.; Abella, J.; Hsu, L.; Chase, P.; Guazzi, M.; Peberdy, M.A. A cardiopulmonary exercise testing score for predicting outcomes in patients with heart failure. *Am. Heart J.* **2008**, *156*, 1177–1183. [CrossRef] [PubMed]
32. Kato, Y.; Suzuki, S.; Uejima, T.; Semba, H.; Nagayama, O.; Hayama, E.; Yamashita, T. The relationship between resting heart rate and peak VO2: A comparison of atrial fibrillation and sinus rhythm. *Eur. J. Prev. Cardiol.* **2016**, *23*, 1429–1436. [CrossRef] [PubMed]
33. Silvilairat, S.; Wongsathikun, J.; Sittiwangkul, R.; Pongprot, Y.; Chattipakorn, N. Heart rate variability and exercise capacity of patients with repaired tetralogy of Fallot. *Pediatr. Cardiol.* **2011**, *32*, 1158–1163. [CrossRef] [PubMed]
34. Tomkiewicz-Pajak, L.; Podolec, P.; Kostkiewicz, M.; Tracz, W. Lung function and exercise tolerance in patients with heart failure. *Acta Cardiol.* **2002**, *57*, 80–81. [PubMed]
35. Ponikowski, P.; Chua, T.P.; Piepoli, M.; Banasiak, W.; Anker, S.D.; Szelemej, R.; Molenda, W.; Wrabec, K.; Capucci, A.; Coats, A.J. Ventilatory response to exercise correlates with impaired heart rate variability in patients with chronic congestive heart failure. *Am. J. Cardiol.* **1998**, *82*, 338–344. [CrossRef]
36. Okólska, M.; Skubera, M.; Matusik, P.; Płazak, W.; Pająk, J.; Róg, B.; Podolec, P.; Tomkiewicz-Pająk, L. Chronotropic incompetence causes multiple organ complications in adults after the Fontan procedure. *Kardiol. Pol.* **2021**, *79*, 410–417. [CrossRef]
37. Smaś-Suska, M.; Skubera, M.; Wilkosz, T.; Wryński, T.; Kołcz, J.; Olszowska, M.; Podolec, P.; Tomkiewicz-Pająk, L. Noninvasive assessment of liver status in adult patients after Fontan procedure. *Pol. Arch. Intern. Med.* **2019**, *129*, 181–188. [PubMed]
38. Kaulitz, R.; Haber, P.; Sturm, E.; Schäfer, J.; Hofbeck, M. Serial evaluation of hepatic function profile after Fontan operation. *Herz* **2014**, *39*, 98–104. [CrossRef]
39. Ates, F.; Topal, E.; Kosar, F.; Karincaoglu, M.; Yildirim, B.; Aksoy, Y.; Aladag, M.; Harputluoglu, M.M.; Demirel, U.; Alan, H.; et al. The relationship of heart rate variability with severity and prognosis of cirrhosis. *Dig. Dis. Sci.* **2006**, *51*, 1614–1618. [CrossRef] [PubMed]
40. Mani, A.R.; Montagnese, S.; Jackson, C.D.; Jenkins, C.W.; Head, I.M.; Stephens, R.C.; Moore, K.P.; Morgan, M.Y. Decreased heart rate variability in patients with cirrhosis relates to the presence and degree of hepatic encephalopathy. *Am. J. Physiol. Gastrointest. Liver Physiol.* **2009**, *296*, G330–G338. [CrossRef]
41. Bhogal, A.S.; De Rui, M.; Pavanello, D.; El-Azizi, I.; Rowshan, S.; Amodio, P.; Montagnese, S.; Mani, A.R. Which heart rate variability index is an independent predictor of mortality in cirrhosis? *Dig. Liver Dis.* **2019**, *51*, 695–702. [CrossRef]
42. Marinković, M.; Mujović, N.; Vučićević, V.; Steffel, J.; Potpara, T.S. A square root pattern of changes in heart rate variability during the first year after circumferential pulmonary vein isolation for paroxysmal atrial fibrillation and their relation with long-term arrhythmia recurrence. *Kardiol. Pol.* **2020**, *78*, 209–218. [CrossRef]

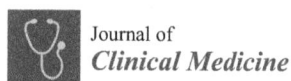

Article

Occurrence, Trends, Management and Outcomes of Patients Hospitalized with Clinically Suspected Myocarditis—Ten-Year Perspectives from the MYO-PL Nationwide Database

Krzysztof Ozierański [1], Agata Tymińska [1,*], Marcin Kruk [2], Beata Koń [2], Aleksandra Skwarek [1], Grzegorz Opolski [1] and Marcin Grabowski [1]

[1] First Department of Cardiology, Medical University of Warsaw, 02-097 Warsaw, Poland; krzysztof.ozieranski@gmail.com (K.O.); S073784@student.wum.edu.pl (A.S.); grzegorz.opolski@gmail.com (G.O.); grabowski.marcin@me.com (M.G.)
[2] National Health Fund, 02-528 Warsaw, Poland; Marcin.Kruk@nfz.gov.pl (M.K.); Beata.Kon@nfz.gov.pl (B.K.)
* Correspondence: agata.tyminska@wum.edu.pl; Tel.: +48-22-5992958; Fax: +48-22-5991957

Abstract: The epidemiology of myocarditis is unknown and based mainly on small single-centre studies. The study aimed to evaluate the current incidence, clinical characteristics, management and outcomes of patients hospitalized due to myocarditis in a general population. The study was registered in ClinicalTrials.gov (NCT04827706). The nationwide MYO-PL (the occurrence, trends, management and outcomes of patients with myocarditis in Poland) database (years 2009–2020) was created to identify hospitalization records with a primary diagnosis of myocarditis according to the International Classification of Diseases and Related Health Problems, 10th Revision (ICD 10), derived from the database of the national healthcare insurer. We identified 19,978 patients who were hospitalized with suspected myocarditis for the first time, of whom 74% were male. The standardized incidence rate of myocarditis ranged from 1.15 to 14 per 100,000 people depending on the age group and was the highest in patients aged 16–20 years. The overall incidence increased with time. The performance of the recommended diagnostic tests (in particular, endomyocardial biopsy) was low. Relative five-year survival ranged from 0.99 to 0.56—worse in younger females and older males. During a five-year follow-up, 6% of patients (3.7% and 6.9% in females and males, respectively) were re-hospitalized for myocarditis. Surprisingly, females more frequently required hospitalization due to heart failure/cardiomyopathy (10.5%) and atrial fibrillation (5%) than compared to males (7.3% and 2.2%, respectively) in the five-year follow up. In the last ten years, the incidence of suspected myocarditis increased, particularly in males. Survival rates for patients with myocarditis were worse than in the general population. Management of myocarditis requires significant improvement.

Keywords: cardiomyopathy; children; endomyocardial biopsy; epidemiology; heart failure; mortality

1. Introduction

Myocarditis is a major cause of heart failure and sudden cardiac death, mainly in children and young adults [1,2]. Myocarditis also constitutes a serious diagnostic and therapeutic problem due to the absence of knowledge gained via systematic investigation. Epidemiological data on the true incidence of myocarditis are lacking, and myocarditis is probably significantly underdiagnosed. The majority of information on the epidemiology, clinical characteristics and outcomes of myocarditis is derived from small single-centre studies [3]. What is more, the published studies offer conflicting results because of the wide variation in diagnostic criteria, hampering accurate estimations of the natural history of myocarditis.

It is important to design multicentre registries for assessing the myocarditis burden on a national or regional level, e.g., the Multicenter Lombardy Registry, which assessed the characteristics, in-hospital management and long-term outcomes of patients with acute myocarditis [4].

Large-scale databases are of particular importance as they may provide relevant information on population trends, demographics and outcomes for a given disease, including the tendencies occurring over a relatively long study period. National data are frequently published with regard to myocardial infarction or heart failure, but there are only single studies on myocarditis. The inpatient database in the United States presented an increasing incidence of hospitalizations due to myocarditis in the years 2007–2014, both in men and women [5]. The Global Burden of Disease 2016 Study (GBD2016) showed a 9% increase in all-age deaths due to myocarditis over a ten year period [6]. GBD2016 also highlighted that observed levels of years of life lost due to cardiomyopathy and myocarditis were much higher than expected, particularly in Eastern and Central Europe [6]. The recently published GBD 2019 showed that disability-adjusted life years and deaths due to cardiomyopathy and myocarditis have significantly increased over the past 30 years [7].

The presented data indicate a pressing need for actual populational data on myocarditis.

Therefore, a nationwide MYO-PL (the occurrence, trends, management and outcomes of patients with myocarditis in Poland) database combining information on all patients with myocarditis was created. In the current study, we aimed to evaluate the incidence, clinical characteristics and outcomes of patients with a hospital-based diagnosis of myocarditis in the last ten years in Poland.

2. Materials and Methods

In this retrospective-prospective study, we used data from the National Health Fund (NHF), which is the only public healthcare insurer in Poland. The NHF reimburses medication and healthcare services provided by healthcare providers (both public and private) with public funds collected from health insurance premiums. In Poland, public health insurance is obligatory for almost all Poles—in December 2019, 88.4% of approximately 38 million Poles had public health insurance and were entitled to obtain healthcare services and medication reimbursed by the NHF. Previously, more data were published based on the NHF database regarding the incidence of acute myocardial infarction [8].

Based on NHF claims data, we derived the healthcare services reported over the years 2009–2020 with a diagnosis of myocarditis—hospitalizations reported with codes I40, I40.0, I40.1, I40.8, I40.9, I41, I41.0, I41.1, I41.2, I41.8, I51.4 and B33.2 according to the International Classification of Diseases and Related Health Problems, 10th Revision (ICD-10). The diagnostic criteria of myocarditis (based on international ICD-10 codes) were clinician-dependent, reflecting routine clinical practice. No other specific inclusion-exclusion criteria were applied, as this is a population database. It should be noted that the criteria for the diagnosis of myocarditis (as well as access to advanced diagnostic procedures, i.e., cardiac magnetic resonance (CMR) and endomyocardial biopsy) have changed over time, making the diagnosis of myocarditis usually a diagnosis of exclusion. Myocarditis should be confirmed by endomyocardial biopsy; however, this is performed only in selected centres worldwide and still not in all patients.

We narrowed the dataset to newly diagnosed myocarditis (first hospitalization), i.e., we included patients for whom no information about the diagnosis of myocarditis was reported in the 400 days preceding hospitalization. For such a group of patients and to establish the baseline characteristics of the patients, data were analyzed 400 days back from the initial diagnosis of myocarditis. Moreover, in-hospital and long-term outcomes were analyzed, including all-cause mortality as well as the occurrence of selected diseases (defined as receiving a service where the selected ICD-10 code was reported) and selected procedures, defined with codes according to International Classification of Diseases, 9th Revision, Clinical Modification (ICD-9-CM) (all ICD codes used in this analysis are presented in a supplementary Table S1). For the follow up, at least a six month period was required. Thus, only patients with a diagnosis of myocarditis between January 2011 and December 2019 were included in the analysis.

To show differences related to the age of patients hospitalized due to myocarditis, the baseline characteristics and long-term outcomes were assessed with regard to age groups.

No ethics approval was required for this study, as it involved the analysis of administrative data. The study complies with the Declaration of Helsinki.

In the study, data from the Central Statistical Office of Poland were also used to refer the obtained results to the population of Poland and to obtain life tables for survival analysis.

Statistical Analysis

The results were presented as means (and standard deviations) or medians (and quartiles) for continuous variables. Ordinal variables were presented as percentages. Associations between study parameters were analyzed using a Pearson chi-square test and a t-test. The observed survival rate was analyzed using the Kaplan–Meier estimates. The relative survival rate (with 95% CIs) was calculated using the Hakulinen method employing single age-specific, year-specific, and sex-specific life tables for the general Polish population. A *p*-value less than 0.05 was considered significant. All tests were two-tailed. Statistical analysis was carried out using R software, version 3.6.1.

3. Results

3.1. Study Population and Clinical Characteristics

During the study period (2011–2019), there were 19,978 patients hospitalized due to myocarditis. The median age of the total cohort was 33 years (32 and 46 years in males and females, respectively). The majority of the patients were male (74%, $n = 14\,870$), regardless of the age group (75.4% and 74.2% in patients aged $\leq$20 and >20 years ($p = 0.14$), respectively).

The incidence of myocarditis was the highest in patients aged 16–20 years (up to 14/100000 in 2016) (Table 1). Two peaks in the overall incidence of myocarditis could be distinguished—in children aged 0–5 years and then in young adults starting from 16–20 years and with a slow decrease from those aged 31–40 years (Figure 1). The overall incidence increased over time, but was driven by a substantial increase in myocarditis incidence in males (Figure 2). The proportion of males was higher in all age groups except patients aged 71–80 and 81+ (Figure 1). In contrast, in females, a slight decrease in the incidence rate was observed over time. Interestingly, the sex distribution of patients with myocarditis was, nevertheless, age-dependent (Figure 1). The proportion of females to males tended to increase with age and was the highest in the oldest age groups.

Most of the clinical characteristics differed between patients aged $\leq$20 and >20 years. Chronic diseases, except for a history of asthma, were more common in the older group. Diagnoses of otolaryngologic and ophthalmic or digestive infectious disease in the prior 6 months were observed more frequently in the younger group. Patients aged $\leq$20 years were more likely to suffer from bradycardia or tachycardia/palpitations, while atrial fibrillation and ventricular tachycardia were more common in those aged >20 years. Most patients were hospitalized in general/cardiology or other hospital wards. On the other hand, approximately 2% of patients required hospitalization in an intensive (cardiac) care unit—more likely for patients $\leq$20 years than for the older group. Reported use of diagnostic procedures, particularly CMR and endomyocardial biopsy, was very low. The main clinical characteristics and management of patients with myocarditis are presented in Table 2.

Table 1. Incidence of patients with myocarditis by the number of 100,000 residents in Poland in a given age group in the years 2011–2019.

Age Group (Years)	Year									p Value [a]
	2011	2012	2013	2014	2015	2016	2017	2018	2019	
0–5	4.27	4.06	4.53	4.14	3.30	2.99	3.24	3.06	2.13	0.000
6–10	1.50	0.99	2.09	1.59	1.09	2.13	1.15	2.42	1.54	0.002
11–15	1.81	1.87	3.37	3.44	3.05	3.45	3.59	3.44	2.88	0.002
16–20	8.79	8.95	11.55	10.60	11.39	14.07	12.51	12.77	12.83	0.000
21–30	7.05	8.72	8.52	10.35	10.41	11.18	10.91	11.09	11.08	0.000
31–40	6.71	7.22	7.35	8.08	8.79	8.39	8.72	8.42	8.99	0.000
41–50	2.94	3.39	4.61	3.89	4.82	4.83	4.82	5.71	5.12	0.000
51–60	3.55	3.41	3.66	3.50	3.00	3.61	3.56	3.91	3.73	0.506
61–70	4.85	3.93	4.51	3.39	3.66	3.91	3.36	3.51	3.29	0.001
71–80	6.85	6.42	6.32	5.10	5.72	4.50	2.87	3.78	3.90	0.000
81+	7.14	7.63	7.66	6.15	6.07	5.11	3.60	3.75	3.61	0.000

[a] A Chi-square test for the independence of the number of patients with myocarditis in a given age group by year.

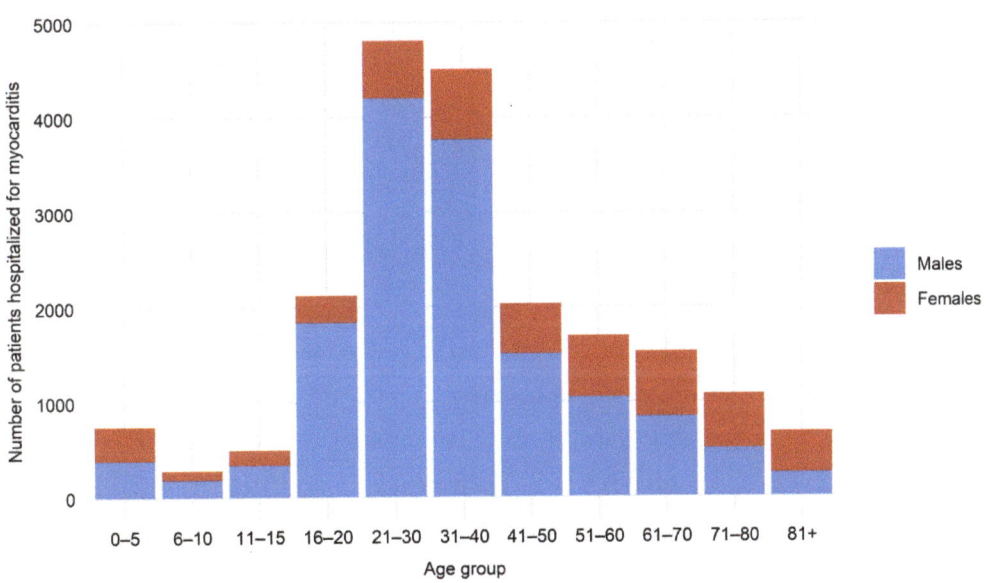

Figure 1. Age and gender distribution of all patients hospitalized for myocarditis in Poland in years 2011–2019. Red—females; blue—males.

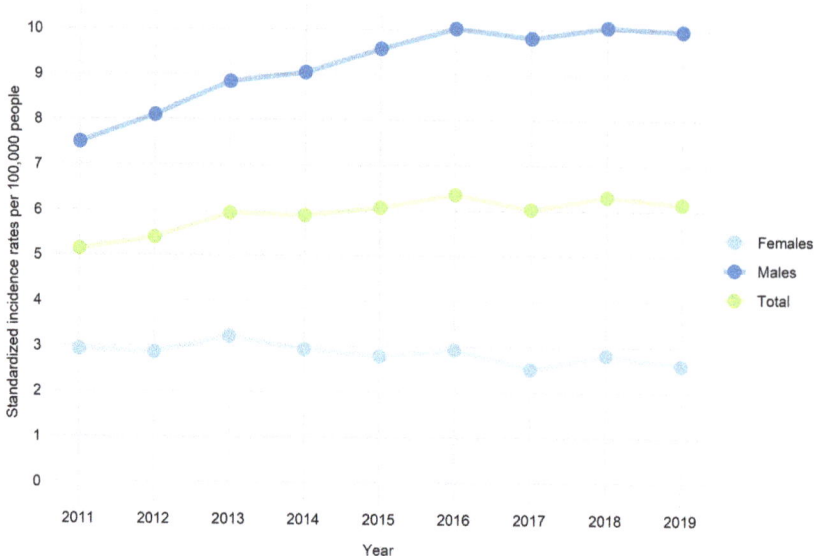

Figure 2. Age-standardized hospitalization rates for myocarditis of males and females by the number of residents in Poland in the years 2011–2019.

Table 2. Clinical characteristics and performed diagnostic procedures in hospitalized patients with myocarditis.

Variable	Total (n = 19,978)	Age ≤20 Years (n = 3659)	Age >20 Years (n = 16,319)	p-Value *
Demographics				
Males, n (%)	14870 (74.4)	2759 (75.4)	12111 (74.2)	0.14
Median Age (IQR) - Total	33 (23–50)	17 (8–19)	37 (29–56)	-
- Females	46 (27–66)	10 (1–16)	54 (36–70)	-
- Males	32 (23–43)	17 (13–19)	35 (28–47)	-
Management				
Hospital ward, n (%) - Cardiology unit	11305 (54.4)	1492 (38.4)	9813 (58.1)	<0.0001
- General ward	5087 (24.5)	1817 (46.8)	3270 (19.4)	<0.0001
- Intensive care unit	263 (1.3)	64 (1.6)	199 (1.2)	0.02
- Intensive cardiac care unit	152 (0.7)	32 (0.8)	120 (0.7)	0.52
- Other	3974 (19.1)	479 (12.3)	3495 (20.7)	<0.0001
Diagnostic procedures, n (%) - C-reactive protein **	8332 (41.7)	1494 (40.8)	6838 (41.9)	0.24
- Brain natriuretic peptides **	2754 (13.8)	475 (13.0)	2279 (14.0)	0.13
- Troponins **	8254 (41.3)	1349 (36.9)	6905 (42.3)	<0.0001

Table 2. Cont.

Variable	Total (n = 19,978)	Age ≤20 Years (n = 3659)	Age >20 Years (n = 16,319)	p-Value *
- Echocardiography ***	16206 (81.1)	3188 (87.1)	13018 (79.8)	<0.0001
- Cardiac Magnetic Resonance ***	3284 (16.4)	563 (15.4)	2721 (16.7)	0.06
- Endomyocardial biopsy ***	142 (0.7)	12 (0.3)	130 (0.8)	0.003
- Endomyocardial biopsy or heart catheterization ***	251 (1.3)	40 (1.1)	211 (1.3)	0.37
- Coronary angiography (invasive or computed tomography) ***	6172 (30.9)	270 (7.4)	5902 (36.2)	<0.0001
Medical history (within up to last 400 days)				
Cardiac Arrhythmias, n (%) - Atrial Fibrillation	788 (3.9)	7 (0.2)	781 (4.8)	<0.0001
- Tachycardia, palpitations	266 (1.3)	63 (1.7)	203 (1.2)	0.03
- Bradycardia	22 (0.1)	12 (0.3)	10 (0.1)	<0.0001
- Atrial extra beat	20 (0.1)	6 (0.2)	14 (0.1)	0.29
- Ventricular extra beat	53 (0.3)	14 (0.4)	39 (0.2)	0.18
- Paroxysmal tachycardia	206 (1.0)	19 (0.5)	187 (1.1)	0.001
- Ventricular tachycardia	48 (0.2)	2 (0.1)	46 (0.3)	0.02
- Ventricular fibrillation	18 (0.1)	2 (0.1)	16 (0.1)	0.63
Chronic coronary syndrome, n (%)	1105 (5.5)	3 (0.1)	1102 (6.8)	<0.0001
Heart failure, n (%)	1173 (5.9)	19 (0.5)	1154 (7.1)	<0.0001
Hypertension, n (%)	3440 (17.2)	53 (1.4)	3387 (20.8)	<0.0001
Diabetes, n (%)	817 (4.1)	17 (0.5)	800 (4.9)	<0.0001
Stroke or transient ischemic attack, n (%)	279 (1.4)	1 (0)	278 (1.7)	<0.0001
Chronic kidney disease, n (%)	210 (1.1)	2 (0.1)	208 (1.3)	<0.0001
Asthma, n (%)	915 (4.6)	227 (6.2)	688 (4.2)	<0.0001
Autoimmune disease, n (%)	267 (1.3)	28 (0.8)	239 (1.5)	0.001
Psychiatric diseases, n (%)	438 (2.2)	44 (1.2)	394 (2.4)	<0.0001
Infectious disease within last 6 months, n (%) Otolaryngologic and eye	6707 (33.6)	1548 (42.3)	5159 (31.6)	<0.0001
Central nervous system	16 (0.1)	4 (0.1)	12 (0.1)	0.71
Respiratory	2867 (14.4)	503 (13.7)	2364 (14.5)	0.26
Digestive	947 (4.7)	200 (5.5)	747 (4.6)	0.02
Urogenital	149 (0.7)	30 (0.8)	119 (0.7)	0.64
Sepsis	73 (0.4)	14 (0.4)	59 (0.4)	0.97
Other	1152 (5.8)	211 (5.8)	941 (5.8)	>0.999

* Comparison between patients aged ≤20 and >20 years old. ** within the index hospitalization. *** within last or proceeding 6 months from diagnosis of myocarditis. IQR—interquartile range; n—number.

3.2. Outcomes

A total of 494 (2.5%) patients died during the index hospitalization (28 (0.8%) and 466 (2.9%) in the groups aged ≤20 and >20 years, respectively). The observed five year survival rate ranged from 0.98 in males aged 0–20 years to 0.26 in males older than 80 years. The relative five-year survival rate, however, ranged from 0.987 to 0.56 in these age-sex groups. Observed and relative survival rates in relation to sex and age are shown in Table 3 (five-year follow up) and Figure 3 (ten-year follow up). Relative survival was associated with age and sex and was higher in younger male age groups than in younger female age groups, while the rate was better in females than in males in older patients. A decline with age and follow-up time in both observed and relative survival rates was observed. Relative survival was substantially less affected by the patient's age than observed survival.

Table 3. Observed and relative survival by sex and age.

Gender	Survival	Age Group				
		0–20	21–40	41–60	61–80	81+
		Observed survival				
Males	1 year	0.990 (0.987–0.994)	0.989 (0.986–0.991)	0.934 (0.924–0.944)	0.802 (0.781–0.823)	0.663 (0.604–0.722)
	3 year	0.985 (0.980–0.990)	0.984 (0.981–0.987)	0.911 (0.899–0.922)	0.697 (0.671–0.722)	0.419 (0.353–0.485)
	5 year	0.980 (0.974–0.986)	0.979 (0.976–0.983)	0.881 (0.867–0.896)	0.589 (0.559–0.619)	0.256 (0.192–0.320)
Females	1 year	0.969 (0.958–0.980)	0.983 (0.976–0.990)	0.930 (0.915–0.944)	0.869 (0.850–0.888)	0.620 (0.575–0.666)
	3 year	0.966 (0.954–0.978)	0.970 (0.960–0.980)	0.913 (0.896–0.929)	0.784 (0.761–0.808)	0.430 (0.382–0.478)
	5 year	0.965 (0.952–0.977)	0.964 (0.952–0.975)	0.900 (0.882–0.918)	0.722 (0.695–0.750)	0.316 (0.268–0.364)
		Relative survival				
Males	1 year	0.994 (0.991–0.997)	0.992 (0.989–0.994)	0.946 (0.937–0.956)	0.845 (0.823–0.866)	0.764 (0.696–0.832)
	3 year	0.990 (0.985–0.994)	0.99 (0.987–0.993)	0.941 (0.929–0.953)	0.800 (0.771–0.829)	0.648 (0.546–0.749)
	5 year	0.987 (0.981–0.992)	0.989 (0.986–0.993)	0.933 (0.918–0.948)	0.750 (0.712–0.787)	0.560 (0.421–0.698)
Females	1 year	0.971 (0.960–0.982)	0.984 (0.977–0.991)	0.941 (0.927–0.955)	0.896 (0.878–0.915)	0.717 (0.665–0.768)
	3 year	0.969 (0.957–0.980)	0.972 (0.963–0.982)	0.931 (0.915–0.947)	0.850 (0.824–0.875)	0.643 (0.572–0.714)
	5 year	0.967 (0.955–0.979)	0.967 (0.956–0.978)	0.928 (0.910–0.946)	0.833 (0.802–0.864)	0.637 (0.542–0.733)

During a five-year follow-up, 6% of the study group (3.7% and 6.9% in females and males, respectively) were readmitted to hospital due to myocarditis. Interestingly, females required hospitalization due to heart failure/cardiomyopathy (10.5%) and atrial fibrillation more frequently (5%) than men (7.3 and 2.2, respectively) in a five-year follow up.

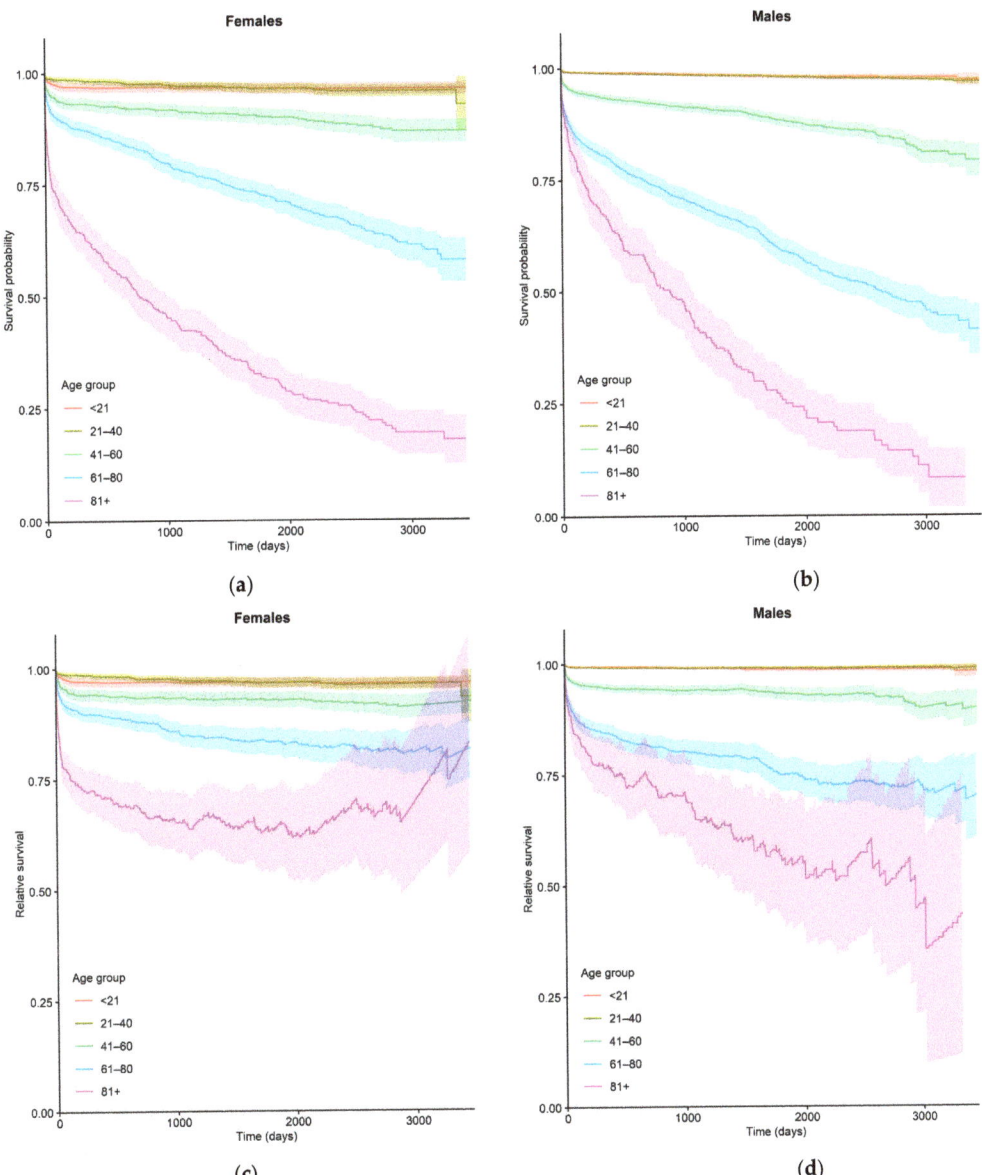

Figure 3. Observed (**a,b**) and relative (**c,d**) ten-year survival rates of patients hospitalized for myocarditis in relation to sex and age.

4. Discussion

Myocarditis is an inflammatory heart disease caused by multiple infectious, non-infectious factors and immune-mediated factors [1]. It presents a challenge in modern cardiology because of the deficit of systematic knowledge of diagnostic and therapeutic modalities. Diagnosis of myocarditis is very demanding and can be reported with multiple ICD-10 codes (I40, I40.0, I40.1, I40.8, I40.9, I41, I41.0, I41.1, I41.2, I41.8, I51.4 and B33.2). The published studies offer conflicting results because of the wide variation in diagnostic criteria (i.e., biopsy proven or not; type of cellular infiltrations; underlying etiology; virus-positive or virus-negative myocarditis; active or chronic inflammation). This was particularly emphasized during the severe acute respiratory syndrome coronavirus 2 pandemic, when many papers with different definitions of myocarditis were published, showing a distorted picture of the true scale of the disease [9,10]. Moreover, in recent years, no large-scale analyses have been conducted, meaning that the current epidemiology of myocarditis is unknown.

This nationwide study includes the unique data of all patients hospitalized with clinician-dependent diagnosis of myocarditis in Poland in the last ten years. It provides new and relevant information with regard to population trends, demographics and the outcomes of patients with myocarditis met in routine clinical practice. This study is particularly important as most of the demographic data for myocarditis derives from small cohort studies hampering accurate estimations of the natural history of myocarditis. During the ten year observation period, myocarditis occurred in patients of all ages with clear predominance in patients aged 16–30 years (Table 1). The overall incidence ranged from 1.15 to 14.07 per 100,000 residents with two peaks—in children aged 0–5 years and then in young adults aged 16–30 years (Figure 1). The age distribution of female patients with myocarditis was notably more stable when compared to male patients. Importantly, we observed an overall increase in myocarditis incidence over time, mainly driven by a substantial increase in myocarditis incidence in male patients (Figure 1).

Previously published data presented similar results that myocarditis was significantly more common in male (approximately 73%) than in female patients [11]. What is more, male patients with myocarditis were noticeably younger than female patients (mean age approximately 34 vs. 49 years, respectively) [11]. Our study showed that the vast majority of patients with myocarditis were male for both children and adults (approximately 74% in both groups aged ≤20 and >20 years). What is more, at the moment of diagnosis, males were several years younger than females (32 vs. 46 years, respectively). Previous studies demonstrated that the incidence of myocarditis was even higher than in our database (1.8–18 per 100,000) [12,13]. There are still no reliable explanations for the increasing incidence of myocarditis. Perhaps it is associated with greater accessibility, mainly to non-invasive tests, such as echocardiography and CMR, or greater awareness of myocarditis. On the other hand, the increased incidence might be related to the greater number of infectious, non-infectious and immune-mediated factors causing myocarditis. To address this question, etiological and pathological analyses should be performed in adequately designed clinical trials.

According to the current criteria of the European Society of Cardiology (ESC), myocarditis should be suspected based on the clinical picture and additional tests (ECG, echocardiography, CMR, troponins) [1]. The diagnosis should be confirmed by endomyocardial biopsy (diagnostic gold standard), but this procedure is infrequently used. Our study showed that the application of ESC criteria for the diagnosis of myocarditis in clinical practice is rare. Non-invasive tests were performed infrequently (troponins—41.3%; echocardiography—81.1%; CMR—16.4%). Ischemic etiology was verified only in 30.9% of patients—significantly more frequently in patients aged >20 years—which was understandable. Endomyocardial biopsy was reported only for a marginal proportion of patients (0.3% vs. 0.8% in patients aged ≤20 and >20 years, respectively). The Nationwide US Inpatient Database (1998–2013) identified 22,299 hospitalization records with a diagnosis of myocarditis and of those, only 798 patients (3.6%) underwent endomyocardial biopsy [12]. What is more, the use of this procedure has been reported as significantly decreasing over time, despite a significant upward trend in the total number of patients with myocarditis [12]. The current ESC recommendations were published in 2013; however, the performance of the recommended diagnostic tests in the observed time period was very low. In particular, the use of endomyocardial biopsy seems to be insufficient. Nowadays, endomyocardial biopsy with current histologic, immunohistochemical and molecular methods provides a diagnosis of certainty in clinically suspected myocarditis and improves differential diagnosis in idiopathic cardiomyopathy or cardiac arrhythmias. It also allows clinicians to establish adequate treatment and monitor the therapy. This indicates that the diagnosis of myocarditis with the use of non-invasive and invasive procedures requires significant improvement.

Myocarditis has been shown in post-mortem studies to be a major cause (up to 42% of cases) of sudden and unexpected death in children and young adults [14,15]. In contrast, a recently published study on autopsies reported that 6% of 14,294 sudden deaths were assigned as being caused by myocarditis [16]. These differences are likely explained by the heterogenicity of the study populations and differences in sudden death, as well as myocarditis definitions and classifications.

Comparison of our database with the Multicenter Lombardy Registry of patients (n = 684) with acute myocarditis, diagnosed either by endomyocardial biopsy or increased troponin plus oedema and late gadolinium enhancement in CMR, shows similar results in the mortality during index hospitalization—2.5 and 3.2%, respectively [4]. Despite the fact that the cited study included patients with fulminant myocarditis (associated with worse prognosis), the difference in hospital mortality is small. This difference may be the result of different inclusion criteria (e.g., exclusion of patients older than 70 years and older than 50 years of age without coronary angiography) and diagnostic procedures, on the basis of which the diagnosis of acute myocarditis was made. Interestingly, a different study on clinically diagnosed acute myocarditis performed on a smaller cohort (n = 322), reported no deaths [17]. This may be due to the relatively high left ventricular ejection fraction (LVEF) in the study cohort. The mean LVEF at presentation was 54 ± 9%. Another prospective study conducted on patients with clinically diagnosed myocarditis (n = 187) investigated mortality in the group of fulminant myocarditis (18.2%) vs. non-fulminant myocarditis patients (0%) [18].

In patients with biopsy-proven myocarditis in long-term observation (the median follow up of 4.7 years), all-cause mortality was 19.2%, while sudden death occurred in 9.9% of cases [19]. Worse outcomes were reported in patients with symptomatic heart failure, reduced LVEF, presence of late contrast enhancement in CMR, malignant ventricular arrhythmias and/or confirmed viral infection in endomyocardial biopsy [20]. In our study, patients with myocarditis had worse survival rates in all age groups than their counterparts in the general population. Our study included a broad spectrum of clinical presentations of myocarditis; therefore, the presented survival rate comprised an average of patients with mild to severe clinical status. The older the age group, the worse the prognosis in comparison to the sex-age-matched general population, although the relative five year survival rate differed in terms of age and sex: In younger age groups, it was better in male patients, while in older age groups female patients had higher survival rates than male patients. It was previously shown that the male sex was associated with a worse course of myocarditis [21]. In the post-mortem study, it was also reported that male patients had a significantly higher risk of sudden death related to myocarditis when compared to female patients [16]. On the other hand, there exists a study showing no sex difference in the rate of major adverse cardiovascular events (MACE) defined as composite of occurrence of congestive heart failure, non-sustained ventricular tachycardia and/or sustained ventricular tachycardia [22]. The vast majority of MACE patients reported in this study had either non-sustained or sustained ventricular tachycardia, and there were no deaths. The exact reason for the mentioned sex differences in the incidence of myocarditis and associated outcomes is unknown.

The survival of patients with myocarditis might be influenced by disease-specific treatment (there is available data about certain effective forms of immunosuppression for biopsy-proven myocarditis) [1,23,24]. Spontaneous or treatment-induced improvement of left ventricular function was observed within a few months of the disease onset in 40–50% to 90% of patients, respectively [3,25]. However, no therapy can yet be approved because of the lack of adequately conducted clinical trials. Data obtained from nationwide databases clearly demonstrate that myocarditis constitutes an emerging challenge for healthcare systems and decisive steps need to be taken to stimulate research in the field.

Limitations

The inclusion of real-life patients allowing for population analyses is an important advantage of this nationwide database; however, it has several limitations that have to be acknowledged. First, in terms of baseline clinical characteristics, the data were limited to 400 days prior to inclusion in the study; therefore, it might be incomplete. Second, errors in ICD-9 and ICD-10 coding and documentation misclassification bias cannot be excluded. Moreover, it is possible that not all diagnoses and procedures may have been reported. There was also an absence of detailed clinical and laboratory data because of the nature of the database. Third, as mentioned above, true myocarditis should be confirmed based on endomyocardial biopsy. However, in the vast majority of cases, it was clinically suspected myocarditis with infrequent use of CMR.

Supplementary Materials: The following are available online at https://www.mdpi.com/article/10.3390/jcm10204672/s1. Table S1: all ICD codes used in this analysis.

Author Contributions: Conceptualization, K.O. and A.T.; methodology, K.O. and A.T.; software, M.K. and B.K.; validation, K.O., A.T., M.K., B.K., A.S., M.G. and G.O.; formal analysis, M.K., B.K., K.O. and A.T.; investigation, K.O. and A.T.; resources, NA; data curation, M.K., B.K. and K.O.; writing—original draft preparation, K.O. and A.T.; writing—review and editing A.S., G.O. and M.G; visualization, M.K. and B.K.; supervision, G.O. and M.G.; project administration, K.O.; funding acquisition, NA. All authors have read and agreed to the published version of the manuscript.

Funding: This research received no external funding.

Institutional Review Board Statement: The study was conducted according to the guidelines of the Declaration of Helsinki. Ethical review and approval were waived for this study, as it involved the analysis of administrative data.

Informed Consent Statement: Patient consent was waived, as it involved the analysis of administrative data.

Data Availability Statement: Data available on request.

Conflicts of Interest: The authors declare no conflict of interest.

References

1. Caforio, A.L.; Pankuweit, S.; Arbustini, E.; Basso, C.; Gimeno-Blanes, J.; Felix, S.B.; Fu, M.; Heliö, T.; Heymans, S.; Jahns, R.; et al. Current state of knowledge on aetiology, diagnosis, management, and therapy of myocarditis: A position statement of the European Society of Cardiology Working Group on Myocardial and Pericardial Diseases. *Eur. Heart J.* **2013**, *34*, 2636–2648, 2648a–2648d. [CrossRef] [PubMed]
2. Tymińska, A.; Ozierański, K.; Caforio, A.L.; Marcolongo, R.; Marchel, M.; Kapłon-Cieślicka, A.; Baritussio, A.; Filipiak, K.J.; Opolski, G.; Grabowski, M. Myocarditis and inflammatory cardiomyopathy in 2021: An update. *Pol. Arch. Intern. Med.* **2021**, *131*, 594–606. [PubMed]
3. Caforio, A.L.; Calabrese, F.; Angelini, A.; Tona, F.; Vinci, A.; Bottaro, S.; Ramondo, A.; Carturan, E.; Iliceto, S.; Thiene, G.; et al. A prospective study of biopsy-proven myocarditis: Prognostic relevance of clinical and aetiopathogenetic features at diagnosis. *Eur. Heart J.* **2007**, *28*, 1326–1333. [CrossRef]
4. Ammirati, E.; Cipriani, M.; Moro, C.; Raineri, C.; Pini, D.; Sormani, P.; Mantovani, R.; Varrenti, M.; Pedrotti, P.; Conca, C.; et al. Clinical Presentation and Outcome in a Contemporary Cohort of Patients with Acute Myocarditis: Multicenter Lombardy Registry. *Circulation* **2018**, *138*, 1088–1099. [CrossRef] [PubMed]
5. Shah, Z.; Mohammed, M.; Vuddanda, V.; Ansari, M.W.; Masoomi, R.; Gupta, K. National Trends, Gender, Management, and Outcomes of Patients Hospitalized for Myocarditis. *Am. J. Cardiol.* **2019**, *124*, 131–136.
6. Collaborators GBDCoD. Global, regional, and national age-sex specific mortality for 264 causes of death, 1980-2016: A systematic analysis for the Global Burden of Disease Study 2016. *Lancet* **2017**, *390*, 1151–1210. [CrossRef]
7. Sacks, D.; Baxter, B.; Campbell, B.; Carpenter, J.S.; Cognard, C.; Dippel, D.; Eesa, M.; Fischer, U.; Hausegger, K.; Hirsch, J.A.; et al. Multisociety Consensus Quality Improvement Revised Consensus Statement for Endovascular Therapy of Acute Ischemic Stroke. *Int. J. Stroke* **2018**, *13*, 612–632. [CrossRef]
8. Wojtyniak, B.; Gierlotka, M.; Opolski, G.; Rabczenko, D.; Ozieranski, K.; Gasior, M.; Chlebus, K.; Wierucki, Ł.; Rutkowski, D.; Dzieła, D.; et al. Observed and relative survival and 5-year outcomes of patients discharged after acute myocardial infarction: The nationwide AMI-PL database. *Kardiol. Pol.* **2020**, *78*, 990–998. [CrossRef]

9. Ozieranski, K.; Tyminska, A.; Jonik, S.; Marcolongo, R.; Baritussio, A.; Grabowski, M.; Filipiak, K.J.; Opolski, G.; Caforio, A. Clinically Suspected Myocarditis in the Course of Severe Acute Respiratory Syndrome Novel Coronavirus-2 Infection: Fact or Fiction? *J. Card. Fail.* **2020**, *27*, 92–96. [CrossRef]
10. Ozieranski, K.; Tyminska, A.; Caforio, A.L.P. Clinically suspected myocarditis in the course of coronavirus infection. *Eur. Heart J.* **2020**, *41*, 2118–2119. [CrossRef]
11. Kyto, V.; Sipila, J.; Rautava, P. The effects of gender and age on occurrence of clinically suspected myocarditis in adulthood. *Heart* **2013**, *99*, 1681–1684. [CrossRef] [PubMed]
12. Elbadawi, A.; Elgendy, I.Y.; Mentias, A.; Ogunbayo, G.O.; Tahir, M.W.; Biniwale, N.; Olorunfemi, O.; Barssoum, K.; Guglin, M. National Trends and Outcomes of Endomyocardial Biopsy for Patients with Myocarditis: From the National Inpatient Sample Database. *J. Card. Fail.* **2018**, *24*, 337–341. [CrossRef]
13. Arola, A.; Pikkarainen, E.; Sipilä, J.O.; Pykäri, J.; Rautava, P.; Kytö, V. Occurrence and Features of Childhood Myocarditis: A Nationwide Study in Finland. *J. Am. Heart Assoc.* **2017**, *6*, e005306. [CrossRef] [PubMed]
14. Gore, I.; Saphir, O. Myocarditis; a classification of 1402 cases. *Am. Heart J.* **1947**, *34*, 827–830. [CrossRef]
15. Basso, C.; Calabrese, F.; Corrado, D.; Thiene, G. Postmortem diagnosis in sudden cardiac death victims: Macroscopic, microscopic and molecular findings. *Cardiovasc. Res.* **2001**, *50*, 290–300. [CrossRef]
16. Lynge, T.H.; Nielsen, T.S.; Gregers Winkel, B.; Tfelt-Hansen, J.; Banner, J. Sudden cardiac death caused by myocarditis in persons aged 1-49 years: A nationwide study of 14 294 deaths in Denmark. *Forensic Sci. Res.* **2019**, *4*, 247–256. [CrossRef] [PubMed]
17. Younis, A.; Matetzky, S.; Mulla, W.; Masalha, E.; Afel, Y.; Chernomordik, F.; Fardman, A.; Goitein, O.; Ben-Zekry, S.; Peled, Y.; et al. Epidemiology Characteristics and Outcome of Patients with Clinically Diagnosed Acute Myocarditis. *Am. J. Med.* **2020**, *133*, 492–499. [CrossRef]
18. Ammirati, E.; Cipriani, M.; Lilliu, M.; Sormani, P.; Varrenti, M.; Raineri, C.; Petrella, D.; Garascia, A.; Pedrotti, P.; Roghi, A.; et al. Survival and Left Ventricular Function Changes in Fulminant Versus Nonfulminant Acute Myocarditis. *Circulation* **2017**, *136*, 529–545. [CrossRef]
19. Grün, S.; Schumm, J.; Greulich, S.; Wagner, A.; Schneider, S.; Bruder, O.; Kispert, E.M.; Hill, S.; Ong, P.; Klingel, K.; et al. Long-term follow-up of biopsy-proven viral myocarditis: Predictors of mortality and incomplete recovery. *J. Am. Coll. Cardiol.* **2012**, *59*, 1604–1615. [CrossRef]
20. Sinagra, G.; Anzini, M.; Pereira, N.L.; Bussani, R.; Finocchiaro, G.; Bartunek, J.; Merlo, M. Myocarditis in Clinical Practice. *Mayo Clin. Proc.* **2016**, *91*, 1256–1266. [CrossRef]
21. McNamara, D.M.; Starling, R.C.; Cooper, L.T.; Boehmer, J.P.; Mather, P.J.; Janosko, K.M.; Gorcsan, J.; Kip, K.E.; Dec, G.W.; IMAC Investigators. Clinical and demographic predictors of outcomes in recent onset dilated cardiomyopathy: Results of the IMAC (Intervention in Myocarditis and Acute Cardiomyopathy)-2 study. *J. Am. Coll. Cardiol.* **2011**, *58*, 1112–1118. [CrossRef] [PubMed]
22. Younis, A.; Mulla, W.; Matetzky, S.; Masalha, E.; Afel, Y.; Fardman, A.; Goitein, O.; Arad, M.; Mazin, I.; Beigel, R. Sex-Based Differences in Characteristics and In-Hospital Outcomes among Patients with Diagnosed Acute Myocarditis. *Am. J. Cardiol.* **2020**, *125*, 1694–1699. [CrossRef]
23. Caforio, A.L.P.; Malipiero, G.; Marcolongo, R.; Iliceto, S. Myocarditis: A Clinical Overview. *Curr. Cardiol. Rep.* **2017**, *19*, 63. [CrossRef]
24. Cheng, C.Y.; Cheng, G.Y.; Shan, Z.G.; Baritussio, A.; Lorenzoni, G.; Tyminska, A.; Ozieranski, K.; Iliceto, S.; Marcolongo, R.; Gregori, D.; et al. Efficacy of immunosuppressive therapy in myocarditis: A 30-year systematic review and meta analysis. *Autoimmun. Rev.* **2021**, *20*, 102710. [CrossRef]
25. Frustaci, A.; Russo, M.A.; Chimenti, C. Randomized study on the efficacy of immunosuppressive therapy in patients with virus-negative inflammatory cardiomyopathy: The TIMIC study. *Eur. Heart J.* **2009**, *30*, 1995–2002. [CrossRef] [PubMed]

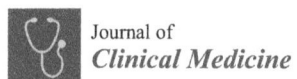

Article

Long-Term Prognosis of Febrile Individuals with Right Precordial Coved-Type ST-Segment Elevation Brugada Pattern: A 10-Year Prospective Follow-Up Study

Chin-Feng Tsai [1,2,*], Yao-Tsung Chuang [1,2], Jing-Yang Huang [3] and Kwo-Chang Ueng [1,2]

1. Division of Cardiology, Department of Internal Medicine, Chung Shan Medical University Hospital, Taichung 40201, Taiwan
2. Institute of Medicine, School of Medicine, Chung Shan Medical University, Taichung 40201, Taiwan; force118chuang@gmail.com (Y.-T.C.); kcueng@gmail.com (K.-C.U.)
3. Department of Medical Research, Chung Shan Medical University Hospital, Taichung 40201, Taiwan; wchinyang@gmail.com
* Correspondence: alberttsai54@hotmail.com; Tel.: +886-4-24739595; Fax: +886-4-24739220

Citation: Tsai, C.-F.; Chuang, Y.-T.; Huang, J.-Y.; Ueng, K.-C. Long-Term Prognosis of Febrile Individuals with Right Precordial Coved-Type ST-Segment Elevation Brugada Pattern: A 10-Year Prospective Follow-Up Study. *J. Clin. Med.* **2021**, *10*, 4997. https://doi.org/10.3390/jcm10214997

Academic Editors: Paweł T. Matusik and Christian Sohns

Received: 19 September 2021
Accepted: 27 October 2021
Published: 27 October 2021

Publisher's Note: MDPI stays neutral with regard to jurisdictional claims in published maps and institutional affiliations.

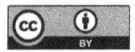

Copyright: © 2021 by the authors. Licensee MDPI, Basel, Switzerland. This article is an open access article distributed under the terms and conditions of the Creative Commons Attribution (CC BY) license (https://creativecommons.org/licenses/by/4.0/).

Abstract: A febrile state may provoke a Brugada electrocardiogram (ECG) pattern and trigger ventricular tachyarrhythmias in susceptible individuals. However, the prognostic value of fever-induced Brugada ECG pattern remains unclear. We analyzed the clinical and extended long-term follow-up data of consecutive febrile patients with a type 1 Brugada ECG presented to the emergency department. A total of 21 individuals (18 males; mean age, 43.7 ± 18.6 years at diagnosis) were divided into symptomatic (resuscitated cardiac arrest in one, syncope in two) and asymptomatic (18, 86%) groups. Sustained polymorphic ventricular tachycardias were inducible in two patients with previous syncope. All 18 asymptomatic patients had no spontaneous type 1 Brugada ECG recorded at second intercostal space and no family history of sudden death. Among asymptomatic individuals, 4 had a total 12 of repeated non-arrhythmogenic febrile episodes all with recurrent type 1 Brugada ECGs, and none had a ventricular arrhythmic event during 116 ± 19 months of follow-up. In the symptomatic group, two had defibrillator shocks for a new arrhythmic event at 31- and 49 months follow-up, respectively, and one without defibrillator therapy died suddenly at 8 months follow-up. A previous history of aborted sudden death or syncope was significantly associated with adverse outcomes in symptomatic compared with asymptomatic individuals (log-rank $p < 0.0001$). In conclusion, clinical presentation or history of syncope is the most important parameter in the risk stratification of febrile patients with type 1 Brugada ECG. Asymptomatic individuals with a negative family history of sudden death and without spontaneous type 1 Brugada ECG, have an exceptionally low future risk of arrhythmic events. Careful follow-up with timely and aggressive control of fever is an appropriate management option.

Keywords: Brugada syndrome; electrocardiogram; fever; genetic disorder; sudden cardiac death; ventricular arrhythmia

1. Introduction

Brugada syndrome is a distinct arrhythmogenic genetic disorder characterized by an ECG pattern of coved-type ST-segment elevation in the right precordial leads (V_1–V_3) at an increased propensity for ventricular fibrillation and the risk of sudden cardiac death [1]. Several non-genetic factors or conditions have been reported to induce Brugada ECG pattern or instead to unmask the concealed form of Brugada syndrome [2–8]. The most frequent finding associated with the Brugada ECG pattern is fever. A febrile state may provoke a Brugada ECG pattern and trigger ventricular tachyarrhythmias in susceptible individuals. However, the prognostic value of Brugada ECG pattern changes observed only during febrile illness remains unclear. Conflicting study results on this association make it uncertain whether fever-induced Brugada ECG pattern bears any relation to the risk of sudden cardiac death. Junttila et al. [4] reported that in most febrile cases with a typical Brugada ECG pattern, sudden cardiac death or malignant arrhythmias developed shortly after the onset of fever regardless of the existence of a predisposing genetic base. In contrast, Adler et al. [8] demonstrated that none of the eight patients presenting with a fever-induced Brugada ECG pattern had arrhythmic events during a 30 ± 13-month follow-up period without antiarrhythmic therapy. Additionally, risk stratification and management of asymptomatic febrile patients with Brugada ECG patterns remain controversial. Some investigators have suggested that patients presenting with a Brugada ECG pattern are at considerably higher risk of sudden cardiac death and that Brugada ECG pattern should be considered a medical emergency [4,7]. However, opponents of this view argue that fever may cause a transient Brugada ECG pattern in susceptible patients who do not have the genetically defined syndrome [2]. Previous studies have demonstrated that asymptomatic individuals, and in particular individuals with only transient ECG abnormalities, are at low risk of sudden cardiac death [9,10]. Therefore, the purpose of this study was to define the clinical relevance and evaluate the risk of ventricular arrhythmias associated with fever-induced Brugada ECG pattern in different clinical situations, and to present extended long-term follow-up data on clinical outcomes in the largest ever reported series of consecutive individuals with fever-induced Brugada ECG pattern.

2. Methods

2.1. Study Population

Consecutive patients admitted to a tertiary university hospital emergency department between May 2009 and May 2014 were screened by weekly review of ECG recordings and all consecutive febrile patients (defined as body temperature >38 °C by tympanic thermometer probe) with a type 1 Brugada ECG pattern characterized by a right bundle branch block and a high take-off >2 mm coved ST-segment elevation, followed by a negative T wave in at least 2 right precordial leads (V_1–V_3) according to the Second Brugada Consensus Conference criteria [3] were included as the analytic sample. Patients with only type 2 or 3 Brugada ECG of lesser degrees or different contours of ST-segment elevation ("saddleback" rather than "coved") were excluded because these findings are not diagnostic and often interpreted inconsistently. All available ECGs of the included patients were independently analyzed by two electrophysiologists (CF Tsai and YT Chuang) and reevaluated after their fevers had subsided. Normalization of Brugada pattern on ECG after resolution of fever confirms the diagnosis of fever-induced Brugada ECG pattern (Figure 1). Patients with a persistent type 1 Brugada ECG after the fever subsided were excluded. In addition, patients with other conditions previously reported to cause similar ECG abnormalities, such as atypical right bundle branch block, acute pericarditis, dissecting aortic aneurysm, electrolyte abnormalities, or mechanical compression of the right ventricular outflow tract, were also excluded [3].

2.2. Study Design and Ethical Considerations

In this prospective cohort study, included patients were categorized into two groups: a symptomatic group that included patients with a history of cardiac arrest or syncope of suspected arrhythmia etiology, and an asymptomatic group that included patients without a personal history of sudden cardiac death or syncope. The human research committee of the study hospital approved the study protocol. All included patients provided signed informed consent to participate in the study.

2.3. Clinical Follow-Up

All patients diagnosed with fever-induced Brugada ECG pattern were prospectively evaluated and followed, at least once, in our institution's arrhythmic clinic after they were discharged directly from the emergency department or from their hospitalization for the index febrile illness.

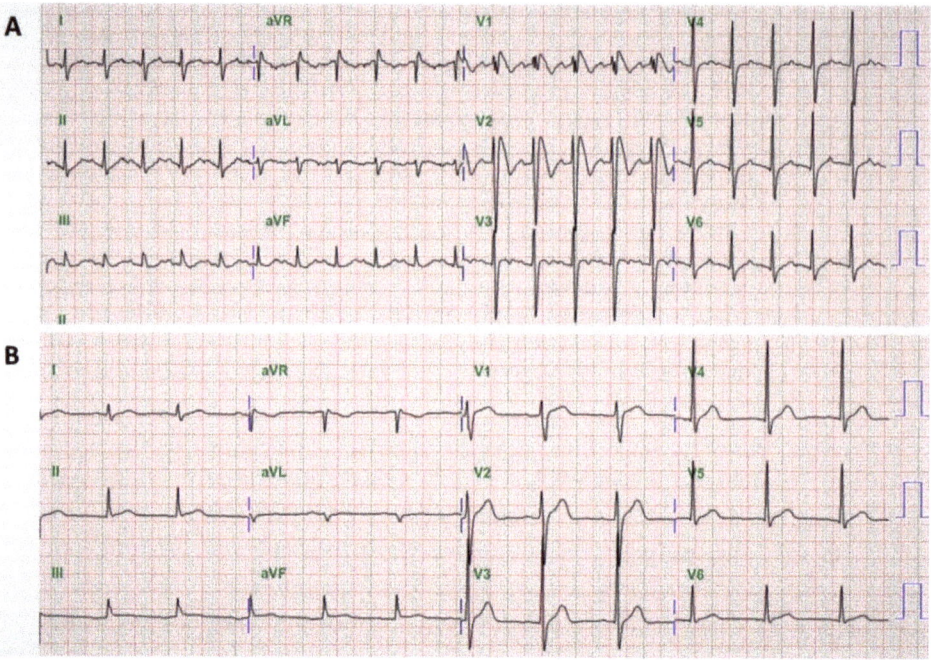

Figure 1. Fever-induced Brugada electrocardiography (ECG) pattern. A 45-year-old man was admitted with diarrhea and abdominal cramps for 2 days. He was febrile (temperature, 40 °C) with tachycardia (pulse, 127 beats/min): (**A**) ECG on admission revealed a right bundle-branch block with coved ST-segment elevation in V_1–V_2 followed by a negative T wave; (**B**) repeated ECG after fever resolved showed normalization of the ST-segment elevation, as well as disappearance of the right bundle-branch block.

Demographic and clinical data of interest were (1) age, (2) gender, (3) presenting symptoms, (4) febrile illness diagnosis, (5) family history of sudden cardiac death, and (6) history of syncope or other arrhythmic symptoms (e.g., severe palpitation, etc.). Routine examinations, including at least echocardiography, excluded any underlying structural heart disease, and laboratory tests excluded acute ischemia and metabolic or electrolyte abnormalities. All patients underwent ECG recordings during the afebrile state at standard lead locations and the high lead position with right precordial leads (V_{1-2}) placed at the second intercostal space to check for the presence of spontaneous type 1 Brugada ECG [3]. All patients were advised to undergo treadmill exercise testing and 24 h Holter monitoring for arrhythmia evaluation. Genetic testing for mutation analysis of the SCN5A gene was also suggested to all included patients. Drug challenge tests and invasive electrophysiological studies were recommended for individuals with positive family or syncopal history, or a spontaneous type 1 Brugada ECG, which may indicate the possible diagnosis of Brugada syndrome. Propafenone or flecainide was used for the class I antiarrhythmic drug challenge [3,11]. The programmed electrical stimulation protocol included a maximum of 3 ventricular extra-stimuli delivered from two ventricular sites (right ventricular apex and outflow tract), with the endpoint being the inducibility of sustained ventricular tachyarrhythmias causing syncope or requiring emergency intervention. An implantable cardioverter-defibrillator (ICD) was strongly recommended for individuals with a history of cardiac arrest and those with inducible ventricular arrhythmias.

Asymptomatic patients with a negative syncope workup or family history of sudden cardiac death were asked to seek a routine cardiac evaluation once annually; if unavailable, all patients were then contacted by phone or letter to determine the status of their arrhythmic symptoms and whether the patient was still alive. All patients were strongly recommended to avoid certain medications responsible for Brugada ECG pattern changes and to receive urgent treatment (e.g., oral paracetamol or a cold compress) for alleviating fever. During the follow-up period, patients were considered to have an arrhythmic event if sudden cardiac death occurred, or when appropriate, ICD shocks or sustained ventricular tachyarrhythmias were documented.

2.4. Statistical Analysis

Paired and unpaired data and survival curve data were analyzed using the SPSS software package (SPSS, Chicago, IL, USA). The time to the first arrhythmic event was depicted with the Kaplan–Meier estimate of the survival function. The difference between the survival curves was tested by the log-rank statistics. Continuous variables are presented as means ± SDs and compared using an unpaired t test or Mann–Whitney U test, depending on data distribution. A value of $p < 0.05$ was considered statistically significant.

3. Results

3.1. Clinical Characteristics of Patient Population

A total of 24 consecutive febrile patients with a type 1 Brugada ECG pattern presented to the emergency department during the study period. Three patients aged 73 ± 4 years were excluded, including one male with gastric cancer with liver metastasis, one male with multiple hepatocellular carcinomas, and one female with pulmonary tuberculosis who experienced in-hospital mortality due to hepatic failure in one and severe sepsis in two, respectively. The study patient population consisted of 21 patients (18 males) with a mean age of 43.7 ± 18.6 years at diagnosis (median, 42 years; range, 21 to 83 years). Mean temperature at the time of the type 1 Brugada ECG recording was 38.9 ± 0.8 °C (range, 38–41 °C) with a mean heart rate of 108 ± 17 beats/min (range, 80–157 beats/min) and a white blood count of $13,080 \pm 4885$ cells/mm^3 (range, 5540–21,440 cells/mm^3) at presentation.

Of the 21 patients with fever-induced Brugada ECG pattern, 19 (90%) presented with symptoms related to fever or an underlying febrile illness, including infectious diseases in 16 patients (3 pneumonia, 3 acute appendicitis, 2 upper respiratory infection, 2 biliary tract infection, 2 urinary tract infection, 1 liver abscess, 1 influenza, 1 infectious diarrhea, 1 infectious colitis), heatstroke in 1 patient, phenytoin-induced Stevens–Johnson disease in 1, and carbon monoxide intoxication in 1 patient (Figure 2). All fever-induced Brugada ECG patterns were incidental findings. Two patients were suspected of having acute coronary syndrome based on an ECG finding of right precordial leads ST-segment elevation; none underwent emergent coronary arteriography because of the absence of any cardiac symptoms and a normal cardiac enzymes level. However, none of the presented ECG cases was identified as type 1 Brugada ECG pattern at the emergency department. Most patients (15 of 19, 79%) were admitted to the medicine or surgery departments to treat their underlying febrile diseases. One patient (male aged 29 years) with the diagnosis of phenytoin-induced Stevens–Johnson disease reported one syncope event leading to a traffic accident and head injury one month prior to admission. He also had a spontaneous type 1 Brugada ECG pattern while afebrile previously. A propafenone drug challenge failed to induce any significant ECG changes. Sustained polymorphic ventricular tachycardia was induced from the right ventricular apex with up to triple extra-stimuli, and an ICD was implanted subsequently under the impression of Brugada syndrome during his index hospitalization. The remaining 18 patients underwent outpatient follow-up in the arrhythmic clinic, and no previous arrhythmias or episodes of syncope or sudden cardiac death were noted in their clinical and familial history. No patients showed up with type 1 Brugada ECG pattern during the afebrile state, and only two patients demonstrated a type 3 Brugada ECG pattern when ECGs were recorded at the high (second) right intercostal space. The results of echocardiography in all and ambulatory Holter monitoring in six patients were unremarkable. All 18 patients refused to undergo an antiarrhythmic drug challenge test or invasive electrophysiologic study, or genetic testing to look for known mutations implicated in Brugada syndrome.

One patient (male aged 79 years) presented with syncope and another patient (male aged 57 years) experienced an episode of ventricular fibrillation and aborted cardiac arrest at presentation to the emergency department. Given their acute cardiac symptoms with new ST-segment elevation, the initial evaluation of these patients was focused on acute pulmonary embolism, aortic dissection, and acute coronary syndrome (Figure 3). Both patients had a normal chest computed tomography study and emergent cardiac catheterization, which revealed normal coronaries and left ventricular systolic function. No family or personal history of syncope or sudden death was found in either patient. In the 79-year-old syncopal patient, the Brugada ECG pattern resolved with defervescence and re-emerged during the propafenone provocation test, and the electrophysiologic testing with standard programmed ventricular stimulation techniques was positive for arrhythmia induction. Although this patient was offered defibrillator implantation, he opted for conservative management. The other patient fulfilled the diagnostic criteria of Brugada syndrome and subsequently received ICD placement during his index hospitalization.

The characteristics of patients between the symptomatic group (with a history of syncope or sudden cardiac death, n = 3) and the asymptomatic group (n = 18) are summarized in Table 1. The age at presentation, body temperature, laboratory data (including WBC, CRP, Na/K) were not significantly different between the symptomatic and asymptomatic groups (p > 0.05).

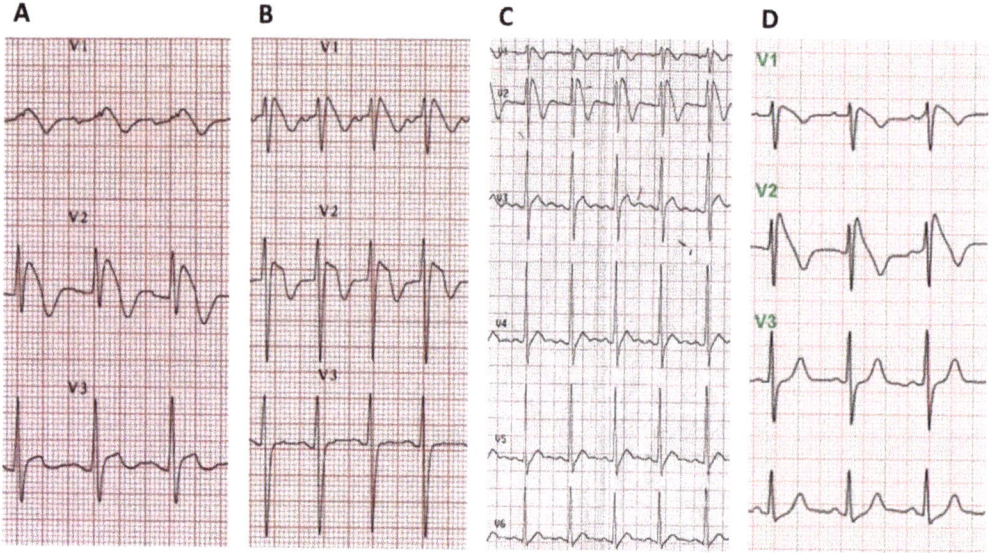

Figure 2. Fever-induced Brugada ECG pattern in different clinical situations. Typical Brugada ECG pattern during the febrile state is evident in different conditions: (**A**) acute tonsilitis in a 25-year-old man (temperature, 39 °C); (**B**) heatstroke in a 24-year-old man (temperature, 41 °C); (**C**) phenytoin-induced Stevens–Johnson disease in a 29-year-old man (temperature, 39.4 °C); (**D**) carbon monoxide intoxication in a 25-year-old female patient (temperature, 38 °C).

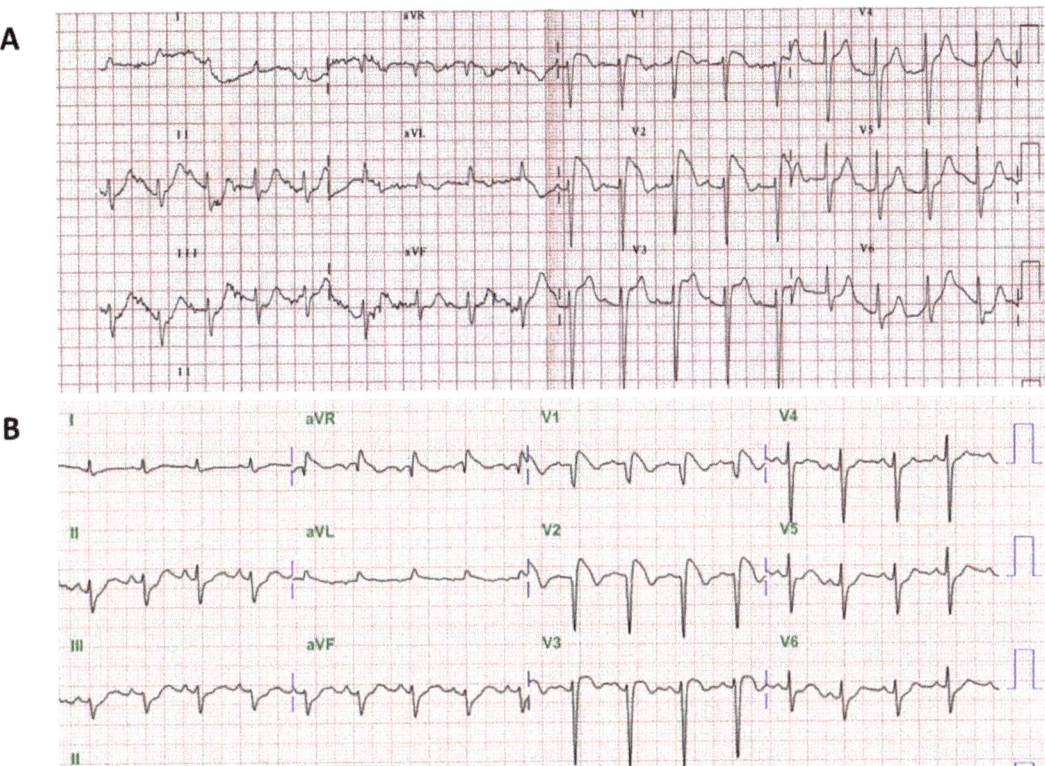

Figure 3. Fever-induced Brugada ECG pattern masquerading as acute coronary syndrome. ECG demonstrated prominent ST-segment elevations in leads V1-3 mimicking anterior wall ST-elevation myocardial infarction in (**A**) a 79-year-old man admitted due to syncope on the roadside and (**B**) a 57-year-old man with out-of-hospital cardiac arrest after resuscitation and recovery of spontaneous circulation.

Table 1. Characteristics of patients between the two groups.

Characteristics	Asymptomatic (n = 18)	Symptomatic (n = 3)	p
Gender	M (15)/F (3)	M (3)	
Age at diagnosis (yr)	42 ± 18	55 ± 25	0.26
Temperature (°C)	38.8 ± 0.8	39.1 ± 0.6	0.54
WBC (cells/mm^3)	12,908 ± 5046	14,113 ± 4503	0.70
C-reactive protein (mg/dL)	8.9 ± 8.4	13.5 ± 6.6	0.38
Sodium (mmol/L)	136 ± 3	137 ± 2	0.80
Potassium (mmol/L)	3.8 ± 0.4	3.7 ± 0.8	0.19
Cardiac symptoms	None	Cardiac arrest (1) syncope (2)	
Programmed ventricular stimulation	NA (0/18)	Polymorphic VT (2/2)	
ICD therapy	None	Two	

Values are presented as mean ± SD. ICD = implantable cardioverter-defibrillator; NA = not available; VT = ventricular tachycardia; WBC = white blood count.

3.2. Effect of Fever on ECG Parameters

ECGs during fever and in the afebrile state were available for analysis in all 21 patients. ECG parameters were measured and compared between the symptomatic group (with a history of syncope or sudden cardiac death, n = 3) and the asymptomatic group (n = 18)

(Table 2). During fever, the heart rate was significantly higher than that at afebrile status in the asymptomatic group (108 ± 20 beats/min vs. 77 ± 7 beats/min; $p < 0.001$) and in the symptomatic group (105 ± 1 beats/min vs. 74 ± 4 beats/min; $p < 0.001$), while the PR interval was significantly shorter than that at afebrile status in the asymptomatic group (159 ± 27 ms vs. 180 ± 21 ms; $p < 0.05$) and in the symptomatic group (149 ± 6 ms vs. 165 ± 13 ms; $p < 0.05$). However, the increase in heart rate and the decrease in PR interval during fever were not significantly different between the symptomatic and asymptomatic groups ($p > 0.05$). QRS duration during fever was not significantly different from that at afebrile status in both the asymptomatic group (102 ± 11 ms vs. 97 ± 8 ms; $p = 0.09$) and the symptomatic group (107 ± 14 ms vs. 90 ± 8 ms; $p = 0.14$). The corrected QT interval during fever was not significantly different from that at afebrile status in both the asymptomatic group (431 ± 42 ms vs. 436 ± 40 ms; $p = 0.74$) and the symptomatic group (453 ± 29 ms vs. 426 ± 24 ms; $p = 0.29$). Changes in QRS duration and corrected QT intervals during fever were not significantly different between the symptomatic and asymptomatic groups ($p > 0.05$).

Table 2. ECG parameters during fever and in the afebrile state between the two groups.

Variable	Asymptomatic ($n = 18$)	Symptomatic ($n = 3$)	p
HR febrile	108 ± 20	105 ± 1	0.77
HR afebrile	77 ± 7	74 ± 4	0.41
Δ HR	31 ± 17	31 ± 3	0.99
PR febrile	159 ± 27	149 ± 6	0.52
PR afebrile	180 ± 21	165 ± 13	0.27
Δ PR	−20 ± 23	−18 ± 9	0.87
QRSd febrile	102 ± 11	107 ± 14	0.54
QRSd afebrile	97 ± 8	90 ± 8	0.21
Δ QRSd	5.8 ± 13	17 ± 14	0.18
QTc febrile	431 ± 42	453 ± 29	0.40
QTc afebrile	436 ± 40	426 ± 24	0.70
Δ QTc	−4.6 ± 44.86	26.3 ± 12.7	0.26

Values are presented as mean ± SD. HR = heart rate (beats/min); PR = PR interval (msec); QRSd = QRS duration or width (msec); QTc = corrected QT interval (msec); Δ = the difference of parameters between febrile and afebrile state.

3.3. Follow-Up Data

Recurrence and Reversibility of Fever-Induced Brugada ECG Pattern

Four patients had a recurrence of type 1 Brugada ECG morphology with repeated febrile episodes (recurrence once in 1, twice in 2, three times in 1). All Brugada ECG pattern anomalies were evident as long as fever was present and vanished once the temperature returned to normal (Figure 4). Neither the etiology nor the height of the fever was able to predict the recurrence and the configuration of the Brugada pattern in these recurrent febrile episodes. The Brugada ECG pattern was not arrhythmogenic in any episode. These patients opted not to pursue any further testing but to return for follow-up of their abnormal ECG findings on an outpatient basis. Given the absence of cardiac symptoms at the recurrent episodes and resolution of the Brugada ECG pattern after the fever subsided, patients were discharged and advised to remember that timely and aggressive control of fever is imperative.

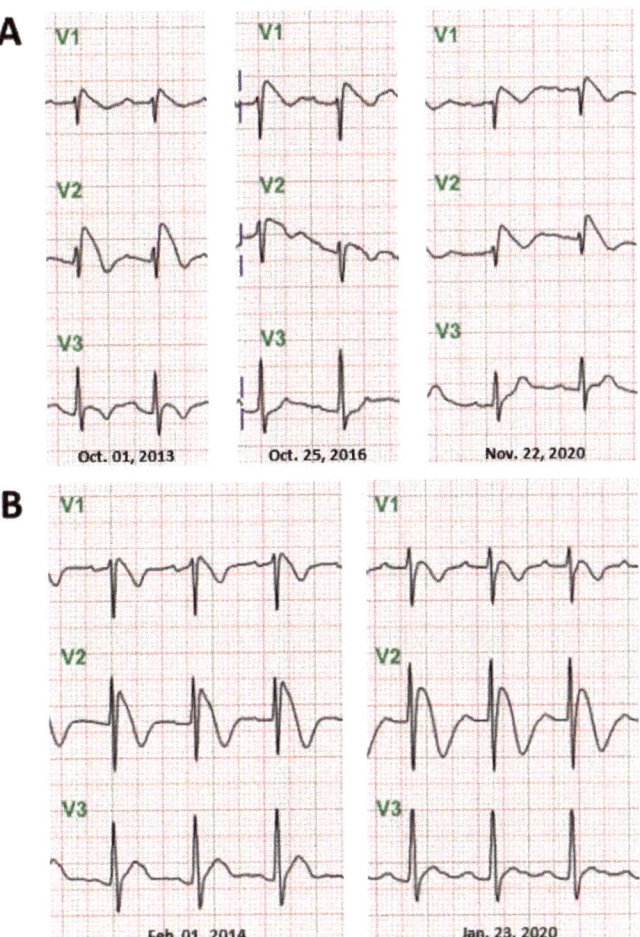

Figure 4. Recurrence of fever-induced Brugada ECG pattern. Admission ECGs displaying recurrences of coved-type ST-segment elevation accompanying repeated febrile episodes in (**A**) an 83-year-old man on 1 October 2013: *Klebsiella pneumoniae* sepsis (temperature, 39.8 °C); on 25 October 2016: upper respiratory tract infection (temperature, 39.2 °C); on 22 November 2020: pneumonia (temperature, 38.5 °C); (**B**) a 21-year-old man on 1 February 2014: infectious diarrhea (temperature, 38.3 °C) and on 23 January 2020: infectious diarrhea (temperature, 38.7 °C).

3.4. Long-Term Outcomes

The mean follow-up period for the entire study population was 116 ± 19 months (range, 84–144 months). During the follow-up period, only one patient with prior cardiac arrest experienced one-time ICD shock for ventricular fibrillation in the afebrile state at a 49-month follow-up. In two patients identified after syncope, one had documented recurrent ventricular tachyarrhythmias requiring ICD interventions (3 events at a 105-month follow-up) and the patient without ICD therapy died unexpectedly at an 8-month follow-up. Among all 18 asymptomatic individuals followed without antiarrhythmic therapy, none had a ventricular arrhythmic event. Differences in outcomes (free of sudden death or ventricular fibrillation events) between the two groups are shown in Figure 5. In the presence of low statistical power because of the limited number of events, having a previous history of aborted sudden cardiac death or syncope was significantly associated with adverse outcomes in symptomatic compared with asymptomatic individuals (log-rank $p < 0.0001$).

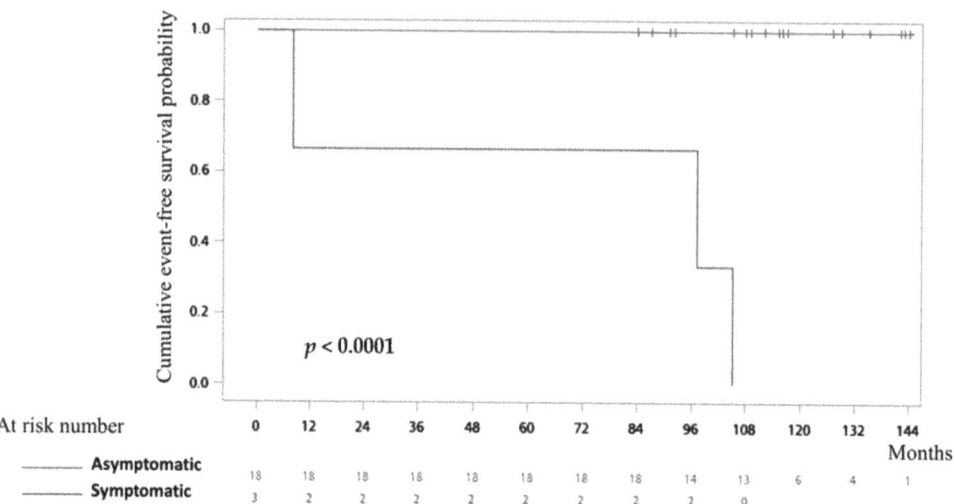

Figure 5. Cumulative survival curves during the follow-up period. Kaplan–Meier analysis of arrhythmic events (sudden cardiac death or documented ventricular fibrillation) during the follow-up depending on clinical presentation with symptomatic (aborted sudden cardiac death or syncope of suspected arrhythmic origin) or asymptomatic individuals when a fever-induced Brugada ECG pattern was identified. The difference between the two groups was statistically significant (log-rank $p < 0.0001$).

4. Discussion

This single-center prospective study demonstrated the outcomes of a cohort of 21 consecutive patients with fever-induced Brugada ECG pattern and, which, to the best of our knowledge, features the longest follow-up to date (median 10-year follow-up; range, 84–144 months). Prospective data were evaluated, reporting the "true" outcomes of fever-induced Brugada ECG pattern in febrile subjects. Results of the present study suggest that the incidental finding of type 1 Brugada ECG in otherwise healthy individuals is seldom recognized by emergency or general physicians. Among subjects with cardiac symptoms, prominent ST elevation at right precordial leads is easily misdiagnosed as an acute coronary syndrome. Our results suggest that clinical presentation or history of aborted cardiac death or syncope is the most important parameter in the risk stratification of febrile patients with type 1 Brugada ECG. In the present study, asymptomatic patients without a family history of sudden death appeared to have a good prognosis. Additionally, the recurrence and reversibility of type 1 Brugada ECG pattern associated with repeated febrile episodes confirm the critical role of fever in uncovering this ECG phenomenon in susceptible individuals. However, the non-arrhythmogenic nature of the ECG phenotype was maintained over time in asymptomatic patients without a history of syncope or sudden cardiac death.

4.1. Recognition of Type 1 Brugada ECG Pattern in Febrile Subjects

Brugada syndrome is a distinct arrhythmogenic disorder widely recognized as an important cause of sudden death in the young and is diagnosed when a patient has a characteristic Brugada type ECG consisting of a coved-type ST elevation in the leads V_{1-3} and documented ventricular tachyarrhythmias or history consistent with ventricular tachyarrhythmias, such as syncope or sudden cardiac death. Therefore, diagnosis of Brugada syndrome is based mainly on the recognition of a putative Brugada pattern on an individual's ECG. The Brugada pattern, on the other hand, can be unmasked by fever and resolve after fever subsides [2–4,7,8]. However, over the past few decades, in the emergency and general internal medicine literature, studies on recognition of fever-induced Brugada ECG patterns have been very limited [12–18]. We confirmed that this peculiar ECG pattern is left unrecognized in patients without cardiovascular symptoms by emergency and internal medicine physicians and surgeons. Instead, the prominent ST elevation in the Brugada ECG pattern may mimic ST-segment elevation myocardial infarction, posting a clinical challenge to emergency and general physicians. This report highlights the importance of recognizing the characteristic Brugada ECG pattern and considering it to be a diagnostic clue for Brugada syndrome. Fever is a common clinical problem and may act as a precipitant for increased susceptibility to potentially fatal ventricular arrhythmias in Brugada syndrome [3,4,7,12]. Therefore, if the Brugada ECG pattern is identified in febrile patients, a detailed patient and family history of syncope or sudden cardiac death is deemed necessary for risk assessment. In the present study, fever-induced Brugada ECG pattern in individuals without clinical or ECG indications of the genetic Brugada abnormality appears to be a relatively benign condition. Among 18 asymptomatic patients, none had a spontaneous type 1 Brugada ECG in the baseline afebrile state and all of them were free of any arrhythmic events at a median follow-up of 116 months. If someone presents with arrhythmic events or syncope during fever, the Brugada syndrome should be considered as a possible diagnosis. Physicians should diagnose syncopal patients with fever cautiously, and repetitive ECG recordings at the higher intercostal spaces may be helpful for enabling a diagnosis [19]. Recording ECGs at higher right intercostal spaces increases the sensitivity of Brugada ECG pattern detection [3,20]. Similar to a prior study [21], only ~10% of subjects in the present study demonstrated a non-diagnostic type 3 Brugada ECG pattern when ECGs were recorded at high right intercostal spaces in the baseline afebrile state.

4.2. Comparison with Previous Studies

The independent clinical significance of the fever-induced Brugada ECG pattern remains unknown. In asymptomatic febrile subjects with a Brugada ECG pattern, the risk of serious arrhythmic events is not well defined. Consistent with the results of an Italian community-based study [22], the risk of future arrhythmic events in asymptomatic febrile individuals without a history of syncope or cardiac arrest is very low, most likely similar to that in the general population. Programmed electrical stimulation seems valuable in patients with a previous syncope. In the present study, two febrile patients with a Brugada ECG pattern and a personal history of syncope were found to have inducible ventricular fibrillation on programmed ventricular stimulation and also experienced a first arrhythmic event at 8- and 31-month follow-up. These results reinforce the notion that clinical presentation is the most important parameter in the risk stratification of febrile patients with a Brugada ECG pattern.

Several studies have demonstrated that fever unmasks or promotes the characteristic Brugada ECG pattern and precipitates ventricular arrhythmias. Junttila et al. [4] reported that in most febrile cases in their series with a typical Brugada ECG pattern, sudden cardiac death or malignant arrhythmias developed shortly after the onset of fever regardless of the existence of a predisposing genetic base. In that study, among the 16 patients with fever-induced type 1 Brugada ECGs, 10 had a history of cardiac arrest or syncope. Additionally, Amin et al. [7] demonstrated that fever precipitated malignant arrhythmias in 18% of patients presenting with cardiac arrest in symptomatic Brugada syndrome. However, in both of these studies, the cardiac arrest occurred mostly at the time of fever presentation, not during the follow-up period. This selection bias may overestimate the long-term arrhythmic risks for febrile patients with an incidental finding of the Brugada ECG pattern. In a large cohort of patients with documented Brugada syndrome, Michowitz et al. [23] showed that ~6% of arrhythmic events were associated with fever and, among these fever-related events, 83% occurred in Caucasian males and 80% presented with aborted cardiac death. A syncopal history and spontaneous type 1 Brugada ECG were noted in 40% and 71%, respectively, of patients with fever-related arrhythmic events. That international multicenter study also confirmed that the involvement of Asians in fever-related arrhythmic events was extremely rare, especially in children. The previous studies described above concluded that patients with Brugada syndrome who develop a fever-induced type 1 ECG are at risk of arrhythmic events. However, in the present study, asymptomatic patients without syncope history or spontaneous type 1 Brugada ECG or family history of sudden cardiac death seldom conform to the diagnosis of Brugada syndrome. The fever-induced Brugada ECG pattern in asymptomatic individuals may be regarded as merely an ECG variant.

A prevalence of 2–4% of fever-induced Brugada ECG patterns in febrile patients referred to the emergency department was reported in two studies, although it was not assessed in this study. Adler et al. [8] reported 8 consecutive patients with fever-induced Brugada ECG patterns who were asymptomatic and remained free of arrhythmic events during 30 months of follow-up. Another study from an endemic area of Brugada syndrome showed that the prevalence of fever-induced Brugada ECG pattern was even higher, up to 5.3%, in febrile male subjects [19]. This estimate, which is dozens of times higher than the known prevalence of Brugada syndrome in the general population, highlights the importance of features distinguishing fever-induced Brugada ECG changes and Brugada syndrome [3]. Mizusawa et al. [24] found that of the 88 asymptomatic patients with fever-induced type 1 Brugada ECG at baseline, 2 patients without evidence of spontaneous type 1 ECG, family cardiac arrest history, or SCN5A mutation experienced sudden cardiac death at the 10- and 75-month follow-up, respectively. Enrollment of non-consecutive cases from an international registry may account for the discrepancies between the study results. The higher event rates in the international registry may be attributable to selection bias stemming from the inclusion of more severely affected patients and families from the 1990s when the syndrome was first described. This study enrolled the largest cohort to date of consecutive febrile patients with Brugada ECG patterns in a single center and reported a very low incidence of arrhythmic events in asymptomatic patients followed for an average of 10 years.

Amin et al. [7] found that, regardless of the cause, fever markedly increased the mean PR/QRS intervals, QTc duration, and ST-segment amplitude in leads V_1 and V_2 for patients with Brugada syndrome. However, inconsistent with a recent study on the relevant ECG markers associated with fever, we found that the PR interval was significantly shorter in the febrile than the afebrile state in both the asymptomatic and symptomatic groups, accompanied by a significant increase in heart rate [24]. Only one asymptomatic patient with diagnosed ruptured acute appendicitis had PR interval prolongation compared with that in the afebrile state (240 ms vs. 190 ms). Febrile illness is a stress-based condition clinically, occurring at an increase in sympathetic activity leading to an increase in heart rate and atrioventricular nodal conduction. Additionally, autonomic influences seem to play an important role in the modulation of the electrophysiology and arrhythmogenesis of Brugada syndrome [25]. ST-segment elevation in the Brugada ECG pattern is mitigated by the administration of beta-adrenergic agonists and is enhanced by parasympathetic agonists such as acetylcholine in experimental and clinical investigations [25,26]. Taken together, these observations show that fever triggers the Brugada ECG phenomenon through the modulatory effect of temperature itself rather than autonomic input.

4.3. Recurrence and Reversibility of Fever-Induced Brugada ECG Pattern

In this study, 4 of 21 patients who presented to the emergency department had recurrent febrile episodes with a total of 12 available ECGs, all of which showed type 1 Brugada ECG pattern regardless of the level and etiology of pyrexia. Furthermore, their classic findings of fever-induced Brugada ECG patterns were reversible with clinical defervescence. These ECG temporal changes demonstrate the direct modulating effect of temperature on the mechanism of the Brugada ECG phenomenon in susceptible individuals. In the setting of Brugada syndrome, mutant sodium channels are shown to be temperature dependent with further impairment occurring at elevated temperature, leading to more evident ECG abnormalities and predisposing to arrhythmias [27]. Patients demonstrating fever-induced Brugada ECG pattern are also likely to be genetically predisposed, although it is not clear whether or to what extent a genetic predisposition may be involved. Insight from cellular electrophysiology suggests that accentuation of the right ventricular action potential notch by a rebalancing of active currents at the end of phase 1 may give rise to the typical Brugada ECG without creating an arrhythmogenic substrate [28,29]. It is possible that a febrile state may modulate the functional expression of ionic currents responsible for the dynamic ECG changes. Fever-induced Brugada ECG pattern may be due to increased susceptibility to fever-induced ECG abnormalities, possibly as a result of an increase in a latent ion channel dysfunction similar to that in drug-induced long QT syndrome. Fever simply unmasks the type 1 Brugada pattern in carriers of this genetically determined arrhythmic disorder. However, further evidence is needed to confirm this postulation. Additionally, recent genetic studies provide new insights on the existence of a pathogenetic link between Brugada syndrome and arrhythmogenic cardiomyopathy. Brugada syndrome may be associated or overlapping with structurally yet not phenotypically expressed cardiomyopathies, such as right ventricular arrhythmogenic cardiomyopathy, hypertrophic cardiomyopathy, and Lamin A/C cardiomyopathy [30,31]. Scheirlynck et al. [32] reported that patients with overlapping phenotypes were associated with a trend toward higher arrhythmic risk. None of the asymptomatic patients in our study underwent cardiac magnetic resonance image or genetic study to address this issue at the follow-up period, and they really showed an exceptionally low future risk of arrhythmic events.

Despite the non-arrhythmogenic nature of all recurrent fever-induced Brugada ECG patterns in asymptomatic patients over a decade-long follow-up period, the lifetime probability of a cardiac event in these patients is not well defined. Careful follow-up is strongly recommended with prompt and aggressive treatment of fever with antipyretics and cold compresses. In addition to being exposed to fever, the Brugada ECG pattern may be unmasked by numerous medications, alcohol and cocaine intoxication, hypokalemia, or other physiologic disruptions [2–5]. The coexistence of multiple trigger factors may possibly cause a more pronounced Brugada ECG phenotype and increase the risk of ventricular arrhythmias. Physicians should be aware of these possible triggers and educate affected patients to avoid them. These cautions were communicated to all of our patients in follow-up at arrhythmic clinics. ICD implantation is the proven effective treatment modality for aborted cardiac arrest survivors and patients with a history of syncope and documented ventricular arrhythmia [3]. However, in asymptomatic individuals with Brugada syndrome, ICD implantation is known to have high complications associated with the procedure and is therefore not recommended, as it has no mortality benefit [33].

4.4. Study Limitations

This study has several limitations, including that febrile groups included in the present study may not necessarily represent the general population because all of them were initially evaluated at an emergency department. ECG is usually not recorded in an otherwise healthy non-cardiac patient presenting to the outpatient clinic with a fever. Additionally, only adults (the youngest man, 21 years old at presentation) were studied because of the independent pediatric emergency room in our hospital. Fever is the most frequent trigger for syncope and sudden death among children with occult Brugada syndrome [34]. However, in a multicenter cohort of Brugada syndrome, Asians with fever-related arrhythmic events were much older than their Caucasian counterparts, and the youngest was 25 years old [23]. Moreover, we only included subjects admitted to the hospital; however, it may be that death during the febrile state in patients not admitted to the hospital had some share of Brugada pattern subjects. This would conflict with the risk of acute cardiac events associated with a febrile Brugada pattern but very unlikely would affect the outcome of those who do not have acute events. One major limitation in evaluating the asymptomatic patient group is that none of these patients chose to undergo the recommended genetic testing, drug challenge testing, or electrophysiological study, which may have further elucidated their condition. The role of programmed ventricular stimulation in risk stratification also has been controversial. In fact, some authors have reported that the inducibility of ventricular tachyarrhythmias by programmed electrical stimulation was not a significant predictor of future arrhythmic events [35,36]. Finally, the results of this study are limited by the low statistical power of the small case series and the limited number of events. Nevertheless, findings of a true consecutive cohort certainly add clinically relevant insights in managing patients with fever-induced Brugada ECG patterns.

5. Conclusions

The present study reported data of a cohort of consecutive patients presenting with fever-induced type 1 Brugada ECG pattern with the longest follow-up reported to date. The lack of cardiac symptoms (syncope, sudden cardiac death) at presentation among asymptomatic patients, with negative personal and family history and without spontaneous type 1 Brugada ECG, suggests an exceptionally low future risk of arrhythmic events. Careful follow-up with a recommendation of timely and aggressive control of the fever is an appropriate option for this patient population.

Author Contributions: Conceptualization, C.-F.T.; methodology, C.-F.T. and Y.-T.C.; validation, C.-F.T., Y.-T.C. and K.-C.U.; formal analysis, J.-Y.H.; investigation, C.-F.T. and Y.-T.C.; resources, C.-F.T.; data curation, C.-F.T., Y.-T.C. and K.-C.U.; writing—original draft preparation, C.-F.T.; writing—review and editing, C.-F.T. and K.-C.U.; supervision, C.-F.T. and K.-C.U.; project administration, C.-F.T.; funding acquisition, C.-F.T. All authors have read and agreed to the published version of the manuscript.

Funding: This work was supported by grants from the National Science Council (NSC) (NSC-101-2314-B-040-017-MY2), Taiwan.

Institutional Review Board Statement: The study was conducted according to the guidelines of the Declaration of Helsinki and approved by the Institutional Review Board of Chung Shan Medical University Hospital (CS 11100).

Informed Consent Statement: Informed consent was obtained from all subjects involved in the study.

Data Availability Statement: The data presented in this study are available on request from the corresponding author.

Conflicts of Interest: The authors declare no conflict of interest.

References

1. Brugada, P.; Brugada, J. Right bundle branch block, persistent ST segment elevation and sudden cardiac death: A distinct clinical and electrocardiographic syndrome: A multicenter report. *J. Am. Coll. Cardiol.* **1992**, *20*, 1391–1396. [CrossRef]
2. Littmann, L.; Monroe, M.H.; Kerns, W.P., 2nd; Svenson, R.H.; Gallagher, J.J. Brugada syndrome and "Brugada sign": Clinical spectrum with a guide for the clinician. *Am. Heart J.* **2003**, *145*, 768–778. [CrossRef]
3. Antzelevitch, C.; Brugada, P.; Borggrefe, M.; Brugada, J.; Brugada, R.; Corrado, D.; Gussak, I.; LeMarec, H.; Nademanee, K.; Perez Riera, A.R.; et al. Brugada syndrome: Report of the second consensus conference: Endorsed by the Heart Rhythm Society and the European Heart Rhythm Association. *Circulation* **2005**, *111*, 659–670. [CrossRef] [PubMed]
4. Junttila, M.J.; Gonzalez, M.; Lizotte, E.; Benito, B. Induced Brugada-type electrocardiogram, a sign for imminent malignant arrhythmia. *Circulation* **2008**, *117*, 1890–1893. [CrossRef] [PubMed]
5. Postema, P.G.; Wolpert, C.; Amin, A.S.; Probst, V.; Borggrefe, M.; Roden, D.M.; Priori, S.G.; Tan, H.L.; Hiraoka, M.; Brugada, J.; et al. Drugs and Brugada syndrome patients: Review of the literature, recommendations, and an up-to-date website (www.brugadadrugs.com). *Heart Rhythm* **2009**, *6*, 1335–1341. [CrossRef]
6. Tsai, C.F.; Wu, D.J.; Lin, M.C.; Ueng, K.C.; Lin, C.S. A Brugada-pattern electrocardiogram and thyrotoxic periodic paralysis. *Ann. Intern. Med.* **2010**, *153*, 848–849. [CrossRef]
7. Amin, A.S.; Meregalli, P.G.; Bardai, A.; Wilde, A.A.M.; Tan, H.L. Fever increases the risk for cardiac arrest in the Brugada syndrome. *Ann. Intern. Med.* **2008**, *149*, 216–218. [CrossRef] [PubMed]
8. Adler, A.; Topaz, G.; Heller, K.; Zeltser, D.; Ohayon, T.; Rozovski, U.; Halkin, A.; Rosso, R.; Ben-Shachar, S.; Antzelevitch, C.; et al. Fever-induced Brugada pattern: How common is it and what does it mean? *Heart Rhythm* **2013**, *10*, 1375–1382. [CrossRef]

9. Priori, S.G.; Napolitano, C.; Gasparini, M.; Pappone, C.; Della Bella, P.; Giordano, U.; Bloise, R.; Giustetto, C.; De Nardis, R.; Grillo, M.; et al. Natural history of Brugada syndrome: Insights for risk stratification and management. *Circulation* **2002**, *105*, 1342–1347. [CrossRef]
10. Delise, P.; Probst, V.; Allocca, G.; Sitta, N.; Sciarra, L.; Brugada, J.; Kamakura, S.; Takagi, M.; Giustetto, C.; Calo, L. Clinical outcome of patients with the Brugada type 1 electrocardiogram without prophylactic implantable cardioverter defibrillator in primary prevention: A cumulative analysis of seven large prospective studies. *Europace* **2018**, *20*, f77–f85. [CrossRef]
11. Shimizu, W.; Antzelevitch, C.; Suyama, K.; Kurita, T.; Taguchi, A.; Aihara, N.; Takaki, H.; Sunagawa, K.; Kamakura, S. Effect of sodium channel blockers on ST segment, QRS duration, and corrected QT interval in patients with Brugada syndrome. *J. Cardiovasc. Electrophysiol.* **2000**, *11*, 1320–1329. [CrossRef] [PubMed]
12. Tan, H.L.; Meregalli, P.G. Lethal ECG changes hidden by therapeutic hypothermia. *Lancet* **2007**, *369*, 78. [CrossRef]
13. Kalra, S.; Iskandar, S.B.; Duggal, S.; Smalligan, R.D. Fever-induced ST-segment elevation with a Brugada syndrome type electrocardiogram. *Ann. Intern. Med.* **2008**, *148*, 82–84. [CrossRef]
14. Alla, V.M.; Suryanarayana, P.G.; Kaushik, M. Temperature twist. *Am. J. Med.* **2010**, *123*, 127–130. [CrossRef] [PubMed]
15. Abbas, H.; Roomi, S.; Ullah, W.; Ahmad, A.; Gajanan, G. Brugada pattern: A comprehensive review on the demographic and clinical spectrum. *BMJ Case Rep.* **2019**, *12*, e229829. [CrossRef] [PubMed]
16. Ortega-Carnicer, J.; Benezet, J.; Ceres, F. Fever-induced ST-segment elevation and T-wave alternans in a patient with Brugada syndrome. *Resuscitation* **2003**, *57*, 315–317. [CrossRef]
17. Dovgalyuka, J.; Holstege, C.; Mattu, A.; Brady, W.J. The electrocardiogram in the patient with syncope. *Am. J. Emerg. Med.* **2007**, *25*, 688–701. [CrossRef] [PubMed]
18. Sharon, M.; Wilson, B.; End, B.; Kraft, C.; Minardi, J. Anterior ST-elevation in a patient with chest pain and fever. *Ann. Emerg. Med.* **2019**, *74*, 782–785. [CrossRef] [PubMed]
19. Rattanawong, P.; Vutthikraivit, W.; Charoensri, A.; Jongraksak, T.; Prombandankul, A.; Kanjanahattakij, N.; Rungaramsin, S.; Wisaratapong, T.; Ngarmukos, T. Fever-induced Brugada syndrome is more common than previously suspected: A cross-sectional study from an endemic area. *Ann. Noninvasive Electrocardiol.* **2016**, *21*, 136–141. [CrossRef]
20. Miyamoto, K.; Yokokawa, M.; Tanaka, K.; Nagai, T.; Okamura, H.; Noda, T.; Satomi, K.; Suyama, K.; Kurita, T.; Aihara, N.; et al. Diagnostic and prognostic value of a type 1 Brugada electrocardiogram at higher (third or second) V1 to V2 recording in men with Brugada syndrome. *Am. J. Cardiol.* **2007**, *99*, 53–57. [CrossRef] [PubMed]
21. Erdogan, O.; Hunuk, B. Frequency of Brugada type ECG pattern in male subjects with fever. *Int. J. Cardiol.* **2013**, *165*, 562–563. [CrossRef] [PubMed]
22. Giustetto, C.; Drago, S.; Demarchi, P.G.; Dalmasso, P.; Bianchi, F.; Masi, A.S.; Carvalho, P.; Occhetta, E.; Rossetti, G.; Riccardi, R.; et al. Risk stratification of the patients with Brugada type electrocardiogram: A community-based prospective study. *Europace* **2009**, *11*, 507–513. [CrossRef] [PubMed]
23. Michowitz, Y.; Milman, A.; Sarquella-Brugada, G.; Andorin, A.; Champagne, J.; Postema, P.G.; Casado-Arroyo, R.; Leshem, E.; Juang, J.J.M.; Giustetto, C.; et al. Fever-related arrhythmic events in the multicenter survey on arrhythmic events in Brugada syndrome. *Heart Rhythm* **2018**, *15*, 1394–1401. [CrossRef]
24. Mizusawa, Y.; Morita, H.; Adler, A.; Havakuk, O.; Thollet, A.; Maury, P.; Wang, D.W.; Hong, K.; Gandjbakhch, E.; Sacher, F.; et al. Prognostic significance of fever-induced Brugada syndrome. *Heart Rhythm.* **2016**, *13*, 1515–1520. [CrossRef]
25. Wichter, T.; Matheja, P.; Eckardt, L.; Kies, P.; Schäfers, K.; Schulze-Bahr, E.; Haverkamp, W.; Borggrefe, M.; Schober, O.; Breithardt, G.; et al. Cardiac autonomic dysfunction in Brugada syndrome. *Circulation* **2002**, *105*, 702–706. [CrossRef]
26. Makimoto, H.; Nakagawa, E.; Takaki, H.; Yamada, Y.; Okamura, H.; Noda, T.; Satomi, K.; Suyama, K.; Aihara, N.; Kurita, T.; et al. Augmented ST-segment elevation during recovery from exercise predicts cardiac events in patients with Brugada syndrome. *J. Am. Coll. Cardiol.* **2010**, *56*, 1576–1584. [CrossRef] [PubMed]
27. Dumaine, R.; Towbin, J.A.; Brugada, P.; Vatta, M.; Nesterenko, D.V.; Nesterenko, V.V.; Brugada, J.; Brugada, R.; Antzelevitch, C. Ionic mechanisms responsible for the electrocardiographic phenotype of the Brugada syndrome are temperature dependent. *Circ. Res.* **1999**, *85*, 803–809. [CrossRef]
28. Wilde, A.A.; Postema, P.G.; Di Diego, J.M.; Viskin, S.; Morita, H.; Fish, J.M.; Antzelevitch, C. The pathophysiological mechanism underlying Brugada syndrome: Depolarization versus repolarization. *J. Mol. Cell. Cardiol.* **2010**, *49*, 543–553. [CrossRef]
29. Antzelevitch, C. The Brugada syndrome: Ionic basis and arrhythmia mechanisms. *J. Cardiovasc. Electrophysiol.* **2001**, *12*, 268–272. [CrossRef]
30. Cerrone, M.; Lin, X.; Zhang, M.; Agullo-Pascual, E.; Pfenniger, A.; Chkourko Gusky, H.; Novelli, V.; Kim, C.; Tirasawadichai, T.; Judge, D.P.; et al. Missense mutations in plakophilin-2 cause sodium current deficit and associate with a Brugada syndrome phenotype. *Circulation* **2014**, *129*, 1092–1103. [CrossRef] [PubMed]
31. Armaroli, A.; Balla, C.; Trabanelli, C.; Selvatici, R.; Brieda, A.; Sette, E.; Bertini, M.; Mele, D.; Biffi, M.; Campo, G.C.; et al. Lamin A/C missense mutation R216C pinpoints overlapping features between Brugada syndrome and laminopathies. *Circ. Genom Precis Med.* **2020**, *13*, e002751. [CrossRef] [PubMed]
32. Scheirlynck, E.; Chivulescu, M.; Lie, Ø.H.; Motoc, A.; Koulalis, J.; de Asmundis, C.; Sieira, J.; Chierchia, G.B.; Brugada, P.; Cosyns, B.; et al. Worse prognosis in Brugada syndrome patients with arrhythmogenic cardiomyopathy features. *JACC Clin. Electrophysiol.* **2020**, *6*, 1353–1363. [CrossRef]

33. Sacher, F.; Probst, V.; Iesaka, Y.; Jacon, P.; Laborderie, J.; Mizon-Gerard, F.; Mabo, P.; Reuter, S.; Lamaison, D.; Takahashi, Y.; et al. Outcome after implantation of a cardioverter-defibrillator in patients with Brugada syndrome: A multicenter study. *Circulation* **2006**, *114*, 2317–2324. [CrossRef]
34. Probst, V.; Denjoy, I.; Meregalli, P.G.; Amirault, J.C.; Sacher, F.; Mansourati, J.; Babuty, D.; Villain, E.; Victor, J.; Schott, J.J.; et al. Clinical aspects and prognosis of Brugada syndrome in children. *Circulation* **2007**, *115*, 2042–2048. [CrossRef]
35. Eckardt, L.; Probst, V.; Smiths, J.P.; Bahr, E.S.; Wolpert, C.; Schimpf, R.; Wichter, T.; Boisseau, P.; Heinecke, A.; Breithardt, G.; et al. Long-term prognosis of individuals with right precordial ST-segment-elevation Brugada syndrome. *Circulation* **2005**, *111*, 257–263. [CrossRef] [PubMed]
36. Priori, S.G.; Gasparini, M.; Napolitano, C.; Della Bella, P.; Ottonelli, A.G.; Sassone, B.; Giordano, U.; Pappone, C.; Mascioli, G.; Rossetti, G.; et al. Risk stratification in Brugada syndrome: Results of the PRELUDE (PRogrammed ELectrical stimUlation preDictive valuE) registry. *J. Am. Coll. Cardiol.* **2012**, *59*, 37–45. [CrossRef] [PubMed]

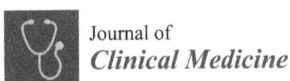

Article

Sex Differences in Incidence, Clinical Characteristics and Outcomes in Children and Young Adults Hospitalized for Clinically Suspected Myocarditis in the Last Ten Years—Data from the MYO-PL Nationwide Database

Krzysztof Ozierański [1], Agata Tymińska [1,*], Aleksandra Skwarek [1], Marcin Kruk [2], Beata Koń [2], Jarosław Biliński [3], Grzegorz Opolski [1] and Marcin Grabowski [1]

1. First Department of Cardiology, Medical University of Warsaw, 02-097 Warsaw, Poland; krzysztof.ozieranski@wum.edu.pl (K.O.); S073784@student.wum.edu.pl (A.S.); grzegorz.opolski@gmail.com (G.O.); grabowski.marcin@me.com (M.G.)
2. National Health Fund, 02-528 Warsaw, Poland; Marcin.Kruk@nfz.gov.pl (M.K.); Beata.Kon@nfz.gov.pl (B.K.)
3. Department of Haematology, Transplantation and Internal Medicine, Medical University of Warsaw, 02-097 Warsaw, Poland; jaroslaw.bilinski@gmail.com
* Correspondence: agata.tyminska@wum.edu.pl; Tel.: +48-22-599-2958; Fax: +48-22-599-1957

Abstract: There is a widespread lack of systematic knowledge about myocarditis in children and young adults in European populations. The MYO-PL nationwide study aimed to evaluate sex differences in the incidence, clinical characteristics, management and outcomes of all young patients with a clinical diagnosis of myocarditis, hospitalized in the last ten years. The study involved data (from the only public healthcare insurer in Poland) of all (n = 3659) patients aged 0–20 years hospitalized for myocarditis in the years 2011–2019. We assessed clinical characteristics, management and five-year outcomes. Males comprised 75.4% of the study population. The standardized incidence rate of myocarditis increased over the last ten years and was, on average, 7.8 and 2.5 (in males and females, respectively). It was the highest (19.5) in males aged 16–20 years. The highest rates of hospital admissions occurred from late autumn to early spring. Most myocarditis-directed diagnostic procedures, including laboratory tests, echocardiography, coronary angiography, cardiac magnetic resonance and endomyocardial biopsy, were performed in a low number of patients, particularly in females. Most patients required rehospitalization for cardiovascular reasons. The results of this large epidemiological study showed an increasing incidence of myocarditis hospitalizations in young patients over last ten years and that it was sex-, age- and season-dependent. Survival in young patients with myocarditis was age- and sex-related and usually it was worse than in the national population. The general management of myocarditis requires significant improvement.

Keywords: cardiomyopathy; endomyocardial biopsy; epidemiology; heart failure; arrhythmias; inflammation

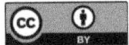

1. Introduction

Myocarditis in children has become an increasingly significant condition over the years. Myocarditis can take various forms, from a mild subclinical course to fulminant acute myocarditis, entailing acute heart failure and being the cause of sudden cardiac death in 4–6% of cases [1–3]. In addition, a number of major complications have been observed, such as dilated cardiomyopathy or clinically significant arrhythmias [4]. The Global Burden of Disease 2016 and 2019 Study (GBD2016 and GBD2019) show a higher-than-expected increase in all-age deaths due to myocarditis over the last decades [5,6]. However, there is still a substantial gap in the current knowledge of the epidemiology, diagnosis, treatment and true course of the disease not only in adults but also in the pediatric/young adult population.

The incidence, management and outcomes of myocarditis in clinical practice in hospitalized patients aged 0–20 years are largely unknown in European populations. There are several nationwide studies investigating myocarditis in pediatric populations; however, there is only one such study performed on a European population [7]. Based on the examples of American or Asian studies, which provided valuable information and conclusions, we believe that big, nationwide databases are of especially high scientific value, as they report real-life, unselected data on the clinical characteristics of patients and on current diagnostic standards.

Several large-scale studies on myocarditis/cardiomyopathy in children have been conducted so far. However, they provide conflicting results due to non-homogenous diagnostic criteria and possible ethnic differences [1–4,7,8]. The available data seem to show an increase in the incidence rate of myocarditis in pediatric patients in the last decade [2]. However, most data were collected prior to 2016 and require updating. What is more, there is little information regarding the sex- and age-related short- and long-term outcomes, without explanation of the possible rationale behind the differences [2,3]. In addition, only one of the abovementioned studies examined the European population, and thus, there is a particular need for studies from this region [7].

Considering the abovementioned lack of knowledge and the rising significance of myocarditis, particularly in the pediatric population, obtaining more population data, particularly from European countries, is highly warranted. In this analysis of a nationwide MYO-PL (the occurrence, trends, management and outcomes of patients with myocarditis in Poland) database containing information about all patients with myocarditis, we aimed to evaluate sex-related differences in the incidence, clinical characteristics, management and long-term outcomes of all real-life, unselected patients aged 0–20 years with a clinical diagnosis of myocarditis hospitalized in Poland in the last ten years.

2. Materials and Methods

The MYO-PL nationwide study gathered data from the National Health Fund (NHF) — the only public healthcare insurer in Poland. The NHF reimburses healthcare services (both public and private) and prescription of medication with public funds. Public health insurance is obligatory for almost all Polish residents. More research results have already been published based on the NHF data regarding the incidence and management of certain diseases [9,10].

Based on the NHF data, we derived hospitalizations due to myocarditis reported in the years 2011–2019 with the following ICD-10 (the International Classification of Diseases and Related Health Problems, 10th Revision) codes: I40, I40.0, I40.1, I40.8, I40.9, I41, I41.0, I41.1, I41.2, I41.8, I51.4 and B33.2 [5]. The diagnostic criteria of myocarditis (based on international ICD-10 codes) were clinician-dependent and reflected routine clinical practice. No other inclusion–exclusion criteria were applied.

The dataset was restricted to the first hospitalization for myocarditis (newly diagnosed patients with a principal (first) diagnosis of myocarditis for whom no information about myocarditis was reported in the 400 days preceding the hospitalization). To establish the baseline clinical characteristics, we analyzed the data for each patient 400 days back dating from the initial diagnosis of myocarditis. In addition, in-hospital and long-term outcomes were analyzed, including all-cause mortality as well as the occurrence of selected diseases (defined as receiving services with specific ICD-10 codes reported) and selected procedures, defined with particular codes following the International Classification of Diseases, 9th Revision, Clinical Modification (ICD-9-CM) (all ICD codes used in this analysis are presented in a Supplementary Table) [6]. The follow-up was assessed for the in-hospital period, 30-days, one-year, three-years, and five-years after discharge. Thus, only patients with a diagnosis of myocarditis between January 2011 and December 2019 were ultimately included in the analysis.

To show age-related differences in patients hospitalized due to myocarditis, baseline characteristics and long-term outcomes were assessed for the following age groups: 0–5,

6–10, 11–15 as well as 16–20 years. Patients aged 0–20 years were included in the study to show age-related differences in children and young adults. The incidence of myocarditis was calculated by the number of residents (per 100,000 people) in Poland in a given age group in the years 2011–2019. Age-standardized hospitalization rates for myocarditis in male and female patients were calculated in relation to the age structure of the Polish population (aged 0–20) from 2011.

No ethics approval was required for this study, as it involved the analysis of administrative data. The study complies with the Declaration of Helsinki.

In the study, data from the Central Statistical Office of Poland was used to relate the obtained results to the Polish population and to build life tables for survival analysis.

Statistical Analysis

The results were presented as means (and standard deviations) or median (and quartiles) for continuous variables. Categorical variables were presented as percentages. The Shapiro–Wilk test was performed to verify the normality of the data distribution. Median values and Mood's median test or mean values and Welsch's *t*-test were used in case of normal and non-normal data distribution, respectively. Associations between the study parameters were analyzed using a Pearson chi-square test and a *t*-test. The observed survival was analyzed using the Kaplan–Meier estimates. The relative survival (with 95% CIs) was calculated using the Hakulinen method employing single age-, year-, and sex-specific life tables for the general Polish population. Logistic regression models were created to report age-adjusted sex differences. A *p*-value less than 0.05 was considered significant. All tests were 2-tailed. Statistical analysis was carried out using R software, version 3.6.1 (Columbus, OH, US)

3. Results

3.1. Incidence of Hospitalizations for Myocarditis and Clinical Characteristics

Medical records of 3659 hospitalized children with a clinical diagnosis of myocarditis were collected between 2011 and 2019. The median age of the total cohort was 17 years (interquartile range 8–19), and was 10 (1–16) years in males and 17 (13–19) years among females ($p < 0.001$). The majority of the patients were male (75.4%, $n = 2759$).

The standardized incidence rate of myocarditis was, on average, 7.8 and 2.5 (in males and females, respectively) and was the highest in males aged 16–20 years. The incidence of myocarditis hospitalizations showed a bimodal distribution, with two peaks: lower in children, aged 0–5 years and higher in young adults, aged 16–20 years (Table 1).

Table 1. The incidence of male and female patients with myocarditis by the number of residents (per 100,000 people) in Poland in a given age group in the years 2011–2019.

Age Group (Years)	Average Incidence	Males Year									*p*-Value [a]	*p*-Value [b]
		2011	2012	2013	2014	2015	2016	2017	2018	2019		
0–5	3.56	4.28	4.43	4.09	4.52	3.46	2.73	2.90	3.40	2.20	0.003	<0.001
6–10	2.09	2.16	1.39	2.61	2.01	1.35	2.83	1.22	3.21	2.04	0.615	0.392
11–15	3.97	2.55	2.43	4.48	4.26	4.00	4.56	4.62	4.82	4.02	0.034	0.005
16–20	19.52	13.90	14.56	19.52	18.16	18.81	23.31	21.98	23.03	22.37	0.001	<0.001

Age Group (Years)	Average Incidence	Females Year									*p*-Value [a]	*p*-Value [b]
		2011	2012	2013	2014	2015	2016	2017	2018	2019		
0–5	3.49	4.26	3.67	5.00	3.73	3.12	3.25	3.60	2.70	2.06	0.009	0.001
6–10	1.11	0.80	0.56	1.54	1.16	0.81	1.39	1.09	1.59	1.02	0.249	0.221
11–15	1.95	1.03	1.28	2.19	2.58	2.05	2.29	2.49	1.98	1.69	0.241	0.148
16–20	3.09	3.46	3.09	3.23	2.70	3.62	4.36	2.57	1.98	2.81	0.324	0.216

[a] Linear regression and [b] P-trend tests for the independence of the number of patients with myocarditis in a given age group by year.

An increase in age-standardized incidence rates of myocarditis hospitalizations over the study period was observed, but it was driven by a substantial increase in the myocarditis incidence rate in males (Figure 1). Conversely, in females, a slight decrease in the incidence rate was seen over time.

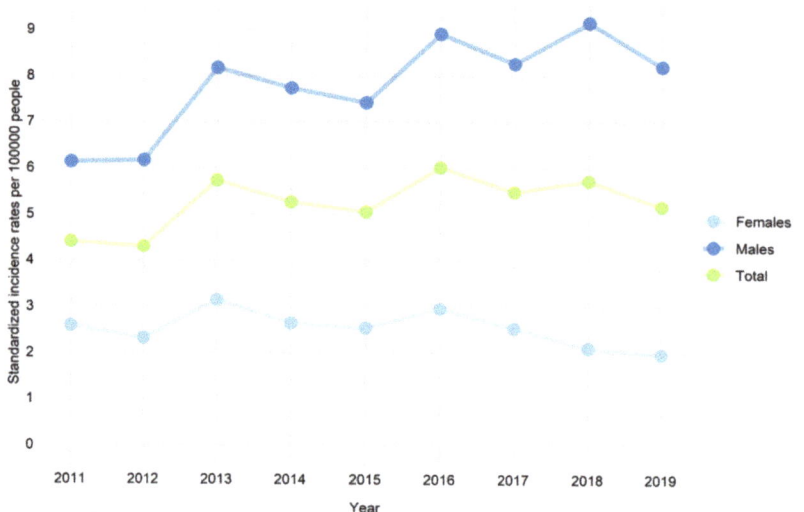

Figure 1. Age-standardized hospitalization rates for myocarditis in male and female patients aged 20 years or younger by the number of residents in Poland (per 100,000 people) in the years 2011–2019.

The incidence rates of myocarditis were higher in males in nearly all age groups and all study years (Table 1). However, the sex difference in the occurrence of myocarditis was clearly age-related. The difference in favour of higher incidence rates of myocarditis in males increased with age and was the highest in patients aged 16–20 years.

We observed a pattern of seasonal changes in the frequency of hospitalizations for myocarditis (Figure 2). The highest rates of hospital admissions occurred from late autumn to early spring (November to April), while the lowest rates were observed in mid-summer (July to August).

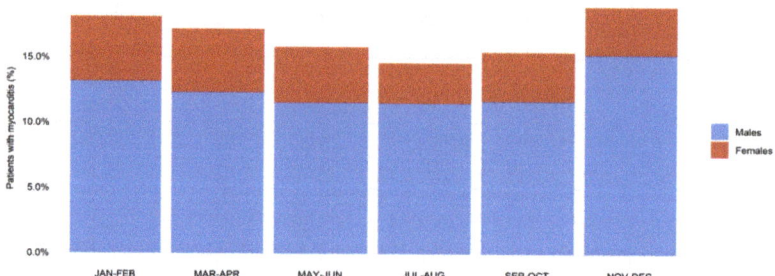

Figure 2. Seasonality of the incidence of male and female patients with myocarditis aged 20 years or younger. Chi-square test for the difference: p-value < 0.001.

Serious cardiac arrhythmias (ventricular tachycardia, ventricular fibrillation and atrial fibrillation) before admission were infrequent both in male and female patients. In females, compared to males, higher rates of tachycardia/palpitations (3.3% vs. 1.2%, respectively) and paroxysmal tachycardia (1.3% and 0.3%, respectively) were observed.

Females were more likely to have had a history of infectious diseases within the last 6 months prior to admission, especially otorhinolaryngologic and/or ophthalmic infections (46.4% vs. 41.0% in males; $p < 0.01$) as well as digestive infections (7.6% vs. 4.8% in males; $p = 0.01$).

3.2. In-Hospital Diagnostic Procedures and Management

Most patients were hospitalized in general wards (internal ward or pediatric department) (49.7%) and in cardiology units (40.7%), but significant sex differences were evident. Males were more frequently admitted to cardiology units (46.4%) in comparison to females (23.3%) who were mostly hospitalized in general wards (59.8% compared to 46.4% in males). Females were more frequently hospitalized in intensive care units (3.8%) than males (1.1%) (Table 2).

Table 2. Clinical characteristics and diagnostic procedures performed in male and female patients aged 20 years or younger hospitalized for myocarditis.

Variable	Total n = 3659	Females n = 900 (24.6%)	Males n = 2759 (75.4%)	OR (95% CI) *	p-Value *
Demographics					
Median Age (IQR)	17 (8–19)	10 (1–16)	17 (13–19)	-	-
Management					
Hospital ward on admission, n (%) - Cardiology unit	1491 (40.7)	210 (23.3)	1281 (46.4)	0.57 (0.47–0.68)	<0.01
General ward (internal ward or pediatric department)	1817 (46.8)	538 (59.8)	1279 (46.4)	1.25 (1.06–1.48)	0.01
Intensive care unit	64 (1.6)	34 (3.8)	30 (1.1)	1.89 (1.12–3.18)	0.02
Intensive cardiac care unit	32 (0.9)	3 (0.3)	29 (1.1)	0.38 (0.11–1.31)	0.13
Other	475 (13.0)	136 (15.1)	339 (12.3)	1.17 (0.93–1.47)	0.18
Diagnostic procedures, n (%) - C-reactive protein **	1494 (40.8)	301 (33.4)	1193 (43.2)	0.79 (0.67–0.93)	<0.01
Troponins **	1349 (36.9)	245 (27.2)	1104 (40.0)	0.73 (0.61–0.87)	<0.01
Brain natriuretic peptides **	475 (13.0)	79 (8.8)	396 (14.4)	0.66 (0.51–0.87)	<0.01
Echocardiography ***	3188 (87.1)	753 (83.7)	2435 (88.3)	0.72 (0.57–0.90)	<0.01
Cardiac Magnetic Resonance ***	563 (15.4)	88 (9.8)	475 (17.2)	0.81 (0.63–1.05)	0.11
Endomyocardial biopsy ***	12 (0.3)	2 (0.2)	10 (0.4)	1.1 (0.23–5.26)	0.91
Endomyocardial biopsy or heart catheterization ***	40 (1.1)	13 (1.4)	27 (1.0)	1.43 (0.70–2.92)	0.32
Coronary angiography (invasive or computed tomography) ***	270 (7.4)	10 (1.1)	260 (9.4)	0.23 (0.12–0.43)	<0.01
Medical history					
Cardiac Arrhythmias, n (%) - Atrial Fibrillation	7 (0.2)	4 (0.4)	3 (0.1)	3.54 (0.71–17.62)	0.12
Tachycardia, palpitations	63 (1.7)	30 (3.3)	33 (1.2)	3.36 (1.97–5.74)	<0.01
Bradycardia	12 (0.3)	4 (0.4)	8 (0.3)	0.81 (0.23–2.79)	0.73
Paroxysmal tachycardia	19 (0.5)	12 (1.3)	7 (0.3)	5.67 (2.10–15.33)	<0.01
Ventricular tachycardia	2 (0.1)	1 (0.1)	1 (0.0)	7.33 (0.44–123.49)	0.17
Ventricular fibrillation	2 (0.1)	0 (0.0)	2 (0.1)	-	0.99
Heart failure, n (%)	19 (0.5)	6 (0.7)	13 (0.5)	1.08 (0.39–3.00)	0.89
Hypertension, n (%)	53 (1.4)	4 (0.4)	49 (1.8)	0.47 (0.17–1.33)	0.16
Diabetes, n (%)	17 (0.5)	4 (0.4)	13 (0.5)	1.70 (0.53–5.43)	0.37
Chronic kidney disease, n (%)	2 (0.1)	1 (0.1)	1 (0.0)	9.36 (0.57–153.2)	0.12
Asthma, n (%)	227 (6.2)	62 (6.9)	165 (6.0)	1.11 (0.81–1.54)	0.51

Table 2. Cont.

Variable	Total n = 3659	Females n = 900 (24.6%)	Males n = 2759 (75.4%)	OR (95% CI) *	p-Value *
Autoimmune disease, n (%)	28 (0.8)	9 (1.0)	19 (0.7)	1.71 (0.73–4.00)	0.21
Psychiatric disease, n (%)	44 (1.2)	9 (1.0)	35 (1.3)	1.39 (0.65–2.99)	0.39
Infectious disease within last 6 months, n (%) - Otolaryngologic and eye	1548 (42.3)	418 (46.4)	1130 (41.0)	1.26 (1.07–1.48)	<0.01
Central nervous system	4 (0.1)	1 (0.1)	3 (0.1)	0.70 (0.07–7.44)	0.77
Respiratory	503 (13.7)	142 (15.8)	361 (13.1)	0.98 (0.78–1.22)	0.85
Digestive	200 (5.5)	68 (7.6)	132 (4.8)	1.58 (1.15–2.19)	0.01
Urogenital	30 (0.8)	11 (1.2)	19 (0.7)	1.12 (0.51–2.47)	0.77
Sepsis	14 (0.4)	4 (0.4)	10 (0.4)	0.81 (0.24–2.72)	0.73
Other	211 (5.8)	68 (7.6)	143 (5.2)	1.33 (0.97–1.83)	0.08
Any	1903 (52.0)	503 (55.9)	1400 (50.7)	1.25 (1.06–1.47)	0.01

* Comparison between sex groups, adjusted for age; ** within the index hospitalization; *** within last or proceeding 6 months from the diagnosis of myocarditis; CI—confidence interval; IQR—interquartile range; n—number; OR—odds ratio.

Most of the myocarditis-directed diagnostic procedures, including laboratory tests, echocardiography, invasive/computed tomography coronary angiography, cardiac magnetic resonance (CMR) or endomyocardial biopsy (EMB), were performed in a low number of patients, especially in females (Table 2). Laboratory studies such as C-reactive protein (43.2% vs. 33.4%; $p < 0.01$), troponins (40% vs. 27.2%; $p < 0.01$) and brain natriuretic peptides (14.4% vs. 8.8%; $p < 0.01$) were more frequently performed in males as compared to females. Males were also more likely to undergo echocardiography (88.3% vs. 83.7%; $p < 0.01$) and/or coronary angiography (9.4% vs. 1.1%; $p < 0.01$) than females. There were no significant sex-related differences in the frequency of CMR and EMB performance, but overall, these procedures were performed in a minority of patients (15.4% and 0.3%, respectively). Consequently, it can be concluded that the etiology of myocarditis remained uncertain in the majority of cases.

The main clinical characteristics and management approaches for patients with myocarditis are presented in Table 2.

3.3. Short- and Long-Term Outcomes

During the five-year observation period, most patients required rehospitalization. The mean number of hospitalizations in a five-year follow-up were 2.8 and 2.0 ($p = 0.001$) for females and males, respectively. Female patients were more frequently hospitalized due to cardiac arrhythmias and cardiomyopathy/heart failure, while male patients were more likely to be rehospitalized for myocarditis (however, there were no statistically significant sex-related differences in the reasons for hospitalization) (Table 3).

There were no differences between male and female patients in the short-term (in-hospital and 30-day) observed mortality regardless of the age group. However, in the long-term follow-up (after five-years), a higher mortality in females compared to males was seen in the group aged 0–5 years (6.4% vs. 1.3% ($p = 0.01$), respectively) (Table 4 and Figure 3). There were no differences in mortality between male and female patients in other age groups. The relative five-year survival rate ranged from 0.96 to 0.99 in males and from 0.95 to 0.99 in females. The relative survival rates in females aged 0–5 and 6–10 years were worse, while in females aged 11–15 and 16–20 years, they were equal/not worse compared with the general population. Relative survival rates in males aged 0–5 years were equal/not worse compared with the general population. In other age groups, the relative survival rates in males were mostly worse than in the general population. Relative survival rates in relation to sex and age are shown in Table 5.

Table 3. Reasons for rehospitalization in the five-year follow-up in patients with myocarditis aged 20 years or younger according to sex.

Reason for Rehospitalization	Females (%)	Males (%)	OR *	95% CI	p-Value
Atrial fibrillation or atrial flutter	0 (0.0)	0 (0.0)	1.00	-	1.00
Ventricular fibrillation, ventricular flutter or cardiac arrest	1 (0.2)	4 (0.3)	0.59	0.06–5.77	0.65
Other cardiac arrhythmias or paroxysmal tachycardia	53 (10.8)	96 (7.2)	1.23	0.84–1.78	0.28
Atrio-ventricular block	4 (0.8)	6 (0.5)	1.79	0.47–6.90	0.40
Autoimmune disease	8 (1.6)	15 (1.1)	1.90	0.76–4.74	0.17
Cardiomyopathy or heart failure	17 (3.5)	31 (2.3)	1.43	0.76–2.71	0.27
Myocarditis	45 (9.1)	158 (11.9)	0.82	0.57–1.18	0.28
Ischemic stroke or transient ischemic attack	0 (0.0)	1 (0.1)	-	-	1.00
Pericarditis	0 (0.0)	1 (0.1)	-	-	1.00
Pulmonary embolism	0 (0.0)	3 (0.2)	-	-	1.00
Embolism or arterial thrombosis	0 (0.0)	1 (0.1)	-	-	1.00
Other reason	284 (57.7)	770 (58.1)	1.03	0.82–1.28	0.82

CI—confidence interval; OR—odds ratio; * females vs. males adjusted for age.

Table 4. Short- and long-term observed mortality of patients aged 20 years or younger hospitalized with myocarditis according to sex and age group.

Follow-Up	Age Group	Mortality (%)		p-Value
		Females	Males	
In-hospital	0–5	2.5%	1.0%	0.21
	6–10	2.1%	1.6%	1.00
	11–15	0.6%	0.9%	1.00
	16–20	0.7%	0.2%	0.40
30 days	0–5	2.5%	1.5%	0.50
	6–10	2.1%	3.2%	0.89
	11–15	1.3%	1.2%	1.00
	16–20	1.1%	0.2%	0.08
1 year	0–5	5.1%	1.9%	0.03
	6–10	4.3%	3.8%	1.00
	11–15	1.9%	1.6%	1.00
	16–20	1.1%	0.3%	0.21
3 years	0–5	5.8%	2.3%	0.04
	6–10	1.5%	3.9%	0.62
	11–15	0.9%	1.7%	0.89
	16–20	1.3%	1.1%	1.00
5 years	0–5	6.4%	1.3%	0.01
	6–10	2.4%	4.7%	0.89
	11–15	1.4%	3.9%	0.55
	16–20	1.9%	1.9%	1.00

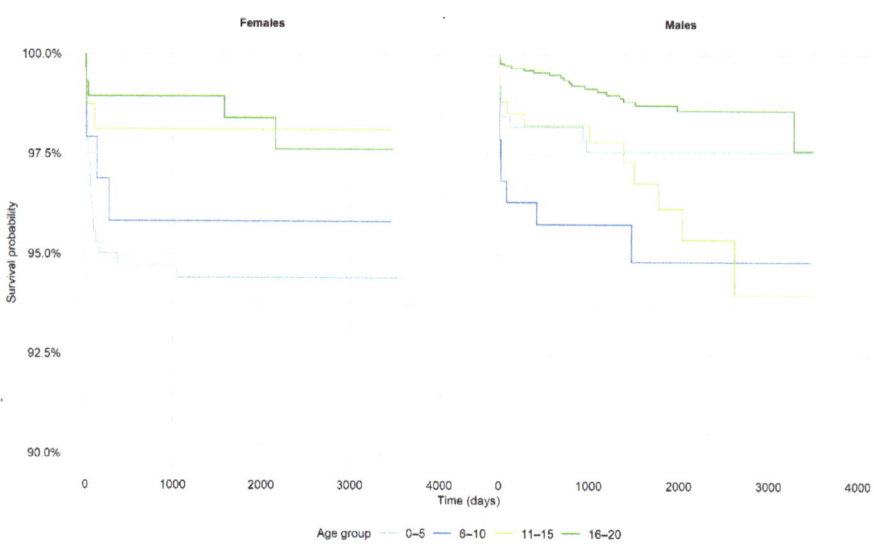

Figure 3. Kaplan–Meier curves for observed mortality in patients hospitalized with myocarditis.

Table 5. Relative survival of patients aged 20 years or younger hospitalized with myocarditis according to sex and age group.

Gender	Outcome	Age Group			
		Relative Survival			
		0–5	6–10	11–15	16–20
Males	30 days	0.99 (0.98–1.00)	0.98 (0.96–0.99)	0.99 (0.98–1.00)	0.998 (0.997–1.00)
	1 year	0.99 (0.98–1.00)	0.97 (0.95–0.996)	0.99 (0.97–0.998)	0.998 (0.995–1.00)
	3 years	0.99 (0.97–1.00)	0.97 (0.94–0.99)	0.98 (0.97–0.997)	0.99 (0.99–0.999)
	5 years	0.99 (0.97–1.00)	0.96 (0.93–0.99)	0.97 (0.94–0.99)	0.99 (0.99–0.998)
Females	30 days	0.98 (0.96–0.99)	0.98 (0.95–1.01)	0.99 (0.97–1.01)	0.99 (0.98–1.00)
	1 year	0.95 (0.93–0.98)	0.96 (0.92–0.998)	0.98 (0.96–1.00)	0.99 (0.98–1.00)
	3 years	0.95 (0.92–0.97)	0.96 (0.92–0.998)	0.98 (0.96–1.00)	0.99 (0.98–1.00)
	5 years	0.95 (0.92–0.97)	0.96 (0.92–0.999)	0.98 (0.96–1.00)	0.99 (0.97–1.00)

4. Discussion

4.1. The Current State of Knowledge and Novelty of the Study

Data on myocarditis in the pediatric population in Europe is highly insufficient. This is especially true for the outcomes of myocarditis and the prognostic factors, which are largely unknown. Most data come from studies on non-European populations, with only one European study based on a nationwide database, performed in Finland few years ago. In Poland, a recent national database provided valuable conclusions about the incidence, presentation and outcomes of myocarditis in the general population [4]. However, these data do not allow for extrapolation for pediatric populations.

This leaves a significant gap in the current general knowledge. MYO-PL is a nationwide study that includes the unique data of all patients aged 0–20 years hospitalized with a clinician-based diagnosis of myocarditis in the last ten years in a large (approx. 38 million people) European country. This study was conducted on what is, to date, the largest European pediatric population. It also presents mostly unknown data regarding sex-related differences and outcomes in short- and long-term follow-up. Moreover, the reduction in the age span of the study groups to 5 years only allows for a better insight into the characteristics of the patients with regard to age groups and displays the age differences more accurately. This database provides up-to-date and comprehensive information concerning the real-life epidemiology, management and long-term course of the disease in daily clinical practice.

What constitutes the novelty of this study is the detailed presentation of the sex-related differences in the incidence, clinical characteristics and outcomes, both short- and long-term. We proved that the overall incidence was higher in males, with the sex-related difference being most accentuated in the group aged 16–20 years.

4.2. Incidence and Patient Characteristics

Previously published research concerning the epidemiology of myocarditis in children in the western population reported the incidence rates spanning a broad spectrum of values. The incidence rates amounted to: 1.95/100,000 person-years in Finland [7], 1.4–2.1/100,000 in Korea [8], 0.8/100,000 in United States (US) [11] and 0.26/100,000 in Japan [4]. The age spans of the investigated groups were 0–15 years, 0–19 years, 0–18 years and 1 month–17 years, respectively. The data were derived from registries [7,8,11] or questionnaires [4] reporting patients hospitalized in the years 2004–2014, 2007–2016, 2007–2016 and 1997–2002, respectively. These studies included patients with a clinical (not EMB-based) diagnosis of myocarditis based on ICD-10 codes (Korean, Finnish and US studies) [7,8] and diagnostic criteria established by the Japanese Circulation Society [4], with no specific exclusion criteria. Importantly, a bimodal age distribution was shown in the studies from Korea and the US by Vasudeva et al. [11], with two peaks occurring, respectively, in infancy and in young adulthood, both in males and females, which is also consistent with the results of our study.

Retrospective data from the registry by Vasudeva et al. suggest a gradual upward tendency of myocarditis hospitalization occurrence with 2898 admissions in 2007 and 3625 in 2014 (27,129 hospitalizations overall during the study period) [12]. A similar increase was observed in a study on patients aged 0–19 years, which demonstrated that the incidence rate increased significantly from 1.4 to 2.1 per 100,000 patients over a nine-year period in the Korean population [8]. Notably, at the study endpoint (2016), the incidence showed a significant sex-related difference (2.5 per 100,000 boys and 1.7 per 100,000 girls, respectively). In our study, we also proved that the increase over time was driven by the male population, mainly at age 16–20, with a slight decrease in the female population. This contrasts with the previous findings by Vasudeva et al. [11], according to which there was a homogenous increase in the incidence in all age and sex groups.

Our study showed progressive male predominance, increasing with age. This is consistent with the previously published studies. In the Korean Study, this difference was demonstrated in groups of patients older than 13 years, whereas in the Finnish Study, as well as in ours, it was detected already in the groups of patients aged 6–11 and 6–10 years, respectively, with a further increase in older patients [7,8]. As the study cohort in the Finnish Study was aged 0–15 years, data limitations need to be considered regarding the young adult population. This problem was addressed in our study by enrolling into the study a group aged 16–20 years, where the sex-related differences turned out to be most pronounced. With regard to the sex-related differences, females were reported to be, on average, younger than males at the disease onset (mean age in females was 10.6 [7] and 6.5 [8], and in males was 12.8 [7] and 9.8 [8]), which was also corroborated in our study (median age was 10 years in females and 17 years in males).

This specific age distribution and predominance of myocarditis occurrence in males is still an unexplained phenomenon that requires further research in order to determine whether it is attributable to a factor that cannot be affected, such as sex-related hormonal balance, or whether it is caused by a possibly modifiable environmental factor.

There are several theories as to what contributes to this distinctive sex-related difference. Some of them suggest a substantial role of sex hormones influencing several components of the immune system. Epidemiological data suggest that estrogen might have a protective character, while testosterone may promote the occurrence of myocarditis. It has been experimentally proven that estrogen and testosterone can modify the reactions of various immune cell populations [13,14]. The influence of genetic factors also needs to be considered. Some authors also attribute these sex-related differences to exercising and physical activity reaching higher intensity among males (particularly relevant in young adulthood) [7].

On the other hand, the infectious factor (mainly viruses) is the most often raised reason for the occurrence of myocarditis [3,15]. In our study, the highest incidence of myocarditis in males was observed from November to April when the impact of infectious etiology of myocarditis might be especially expected. Interestingly, in our study, the frequency of a recent history of an infectious disease was higher in females, while the incidence rate of myocarditis was higher in males, suggesting that possible non-infectious factors may be crucial in the development of a myocardial inflammation. The pathophysiological mechanisms responsible for this specific sex- and age-related distribution remain unknown and require further research.

Furthermore, one may hypothesize that different factors play major roles in US and European populations, as the increase in myocarditis hospitalizations over the years has shown a different pattern. Whereas in the US, a homogenous increase in all age and sex groups was observed, in Europe, the group of young, male adults was especially affected, suggesting the greater role of environmental factors in US, with a more complex etiology (including possibly hormonal and/or immunological changes or influence of physical activity, that are most pronounced during adolescence) in Europe.

The observed higher rate of arrhythmias in females with myocarditis is a so-far uninvestigated phenomenon. Several studies on non-myocarditis patients reported a higher propensity towards arrhythmias (especially supraventricular arrhythmias) in adult females compared to males and linked it with longer rate-corrected QT-intervals in females [16–18]. This has been attributed in many studies to the influence of sex hormones, which does not, however, explain the propensity for arrhythmia in pediatric populations, as hormone differences are less pronounced until puberty [19]. The lower density of ionic currents responsible for early repolarization (mainly K+ channels) in female hearts has been suggested as an underlying cause of the higher observed rate of arrhythmias in females. However, this conclusion is based solely on experiments on rabbit hearts and requires validation in further studies [13,14,20]. It is likely that heart inflammation may aggravate these proarrhythmic mechanisms in females.

4.3. In-Hospital Diagnostic Procedures and Management

We also demonstrated that the application of standard diagnostic procedures required for the confirmation of the diagnosis was generally very low. Interestingly, females were more likely to be admitted to general wards, and not to receive the routine cardiological diagnostic tests (lab tests, echocardiography and coronary angiography) in comparison to males. It should be noted that this tendency of limited testing was more visible in females, even though they more often presented with palpitations and/or tachycardia. In general, the use of golden standard non-invasive (CMR) and invasive (EMB) procedures was marginal. Particularly, the clinical utility of EMB in the diagnosis of myocarditis should be highlighted. EMB provides the confirmation of the diagnosis as well as details on the etiology and type of inflammatory cell infiltration. EMB is associated with a relatively low risk of serious complications (1.9%) as shown in a large retrospective study on a pediatric population [21]. However, the performance of EMB in a center with expertise in this field is strongly recommended [22]. The results of our study confirm that there is a pressing need for the optimization of the diagnostic standards, both in male and female patients, at the level of the healthcare system. Females were more frequently hospitalized in wards other than cardiology wards (i.e., internal ward or pediatric department) and tended to have a worse in-hospital prognosis in most age groups compared to males.

4.4. Outcomes

Short- and long-term outcomes in children and young adults are mostly unknown. The GBD2016 and GBD2019 reports showed a much higher number of life-years lost than expected in the populations of eastern and central Europe [5,6]. In the Finnish study, the overall in-hospital mortality was 1.4%, but the small group of patients precluded statistical analyses of age- and sex-differences [7]. In our study, the in-hospital mortality was lower (<1%) in older (aged over 10 years) than in younger patients (1–2.5%). There were no differences between male and female patients.

In the available literature, there are also no data on long-term outcomes regarding sex-related differences. The Japanese study showed an overall 22.5% mortality (38 out of 169 patients with a one-year follow-up) while the Korean study demonstrated that as many as 30.5% of patients died or had heart transplantation (113 out of 371 patients during the peri-hospital period); however, the latter study included only patients with acute fulminant myocarditis [8]. The strength of our study is in the comprehensive data it provides on five-year outcomes (with data on relative survival based on the total Polish population), rendering it perfect for epidemiological considerations and showing large-scale trends in the outcomes of myocarditis in children and young adults. Compared to the general Polish population, the survival rates in our study tended to be worse in the youngest groups of females (aged 0–5 and 6–10 years) and in the older groups of males. The observed long-term mortality was the highest in patients aged 0–5 years, and was higher in females than in males. There were no differences in other age groups.

The number of rehospitalizations tended to be higher in females, which is a variable that had not been investigated in previous studies. However, there were no significant differences in the reason for hospitalization between male and female patients.

This may be due to the previously described sex differences, encompassing hormonal and immunological differences, which can not only affect the susceptibility to infection and development of the disease, but also the severity and the risk of rehospitalization. Furthermore, the fact that girls are more often hospitalized within general wards may have a negative influence on the quality of care and, consequently, lead to more frequent rehospitalizations.

The importance of this study for public health research is not to be underrated. We demonstrated sex-related differences in the diagnostics and treatment, as well as the outcomes of myocarditis, which provides a unique opportunity for a thoughtful analysis.

With this study, we also provide "hypothesis-generating" material for further research on age- and sex-differences in myocarditis. The main questions remaining to be answered are: 'What makes males more susceptible to myocarditis?' and 'Why is the occurrence of myocarditis age dependent?'. The answers to these questions may also provide more data on true etiological factors (infectious vs. non-infectious and immune-mediated) of myocarditis.

4.5. Diagnosis of Myocarditis in the COVID-19 Era

Results of our study are particularly important and should be discussed in the light of a recent Severe Acute Respiratory Syndrome Coronavirus-2 pandemic. At the moment, the consensus has been reached that it is not a cardiotropic virus and acute myocarditis represented by the viral presence and infiltrates in the myocardium with myocardial injury is rarely observed in the course of Coronavirus Disease 2019 (COVID-19) [15,23]. In individuals with so far uninvestigated predispositions the virus can be a trigger for an immune reaction, leading to immune-mediated myocarditis.

In order to avoid misdiagnosis of myocarditis in patients with COVID-19, we recommend implementing the structured diagnostic algorithm, included in the guidelines created by European Society of Cardiology [24,25]. It should be highlighted that nasal/throat swab tests for COVID-19 in the presence of clinically suspected myocarditis does not allow for establishing the etiology. COVID-19 pandemic did not change the diagnostic path and still EMB/autopsy is a gold standard of confirming the diagnosis.

4.6. Limitations

It is a limitation of the study that the diagnosis of myocarditis was made on the basis of the clinical presentation and auxiliary diagnostic measures, as EMB was very rarely performed, and thus, no histological confirmation was possible. The criteria for the diagnosis of myocarditis (as well as access to advanced diagnostic procedures, i.e., CMR and EMB) have changed over time, making the diagnosis of myocarditis usually a diagnosis of exclusion. Myocarditis should be confirmed by EMB; however, worldwide EMB is performed only in selected centers and still not in the majority of patients. However, the incidence rates of myocarditis presented in our study were in-line with previous similar studies. In contrast to clinical trials, the character of the study is also associated with certain data inaccuracy, dependent on physicians reporting the diseases and procedures using ICD codes. Due to the fact that data were extracted from the national health care payer, we were not able to neither verify each diagnosis nor provide exact results of diagnostic tests, which is a limitation inherent to this type of data collection. Nevertheless, while analyzing myocarditis, one needs to base the observations on real-life data of unselected patients, as standards from clinical trials rarely correspond to routine clinical practice.

5. Conclusions

The results of this large epidemiological study showed an increasing incidence of myocarditis in children and young adults over the last ten years, and that it was sex-, age- and season-dependent. It also made it clear that the management of myocarditis requires significant improvement at the national level. The overall survival in young patients with myocarditis was age- as well as sex-related, and was usually worse than in the general population. The observed mortality was the worst in the youngest females.

Supplementary Materials: The following are available online at https://www.mdpi.com/article/10.3390/jcm10235502/s1, Table S1: International Classification of Diseases and Related Health Problems, 10th Revision (ICD-10); ICD 9th Revision, Clinical Modification (ICD-9-CM); NHF billing codes.

Author Contributions: Conceptualization, K.O. and A.T.; methodology, K.O. and A.T.; software, M.K. and B.K.; validation, K.O., A.T., M.K., B.K., A.S., J.B., M.G. and G.O.; formal analysis, M.K., B.K., K.O. and A.T.; investigation, K.O. and A.T.; resources, NA; data curation, M.K., B.K. and K.O.; writing—original draft preparation, K.O., A.T., A.S and J.B.; writing—review and editing G.O. and M.G; visualization, M.K. and B.K.; supervision, G.O. and M.G.; project administration, K.O.; funding acquisition, NA. All authors have read and agreed to the published version of the manuscript.

Funding: This research received no external funding.

Institutional Review Board Statement: The study was conducted according to the guidelines of the Declaration of Helsinki. Ethical review and approval were waived for this study, as it involved the analysis of administrative data.

Informed Consent Statement: Patient consent was waived as this study involved the analysis of administrative data.

Data Availability Statement: Data are available on request.

Conflicts of Interest: The authors declare no conflict of interest.

References

1. Lynge, T.H.; Nielsen, T.S.; Winkel, B.G.; Tfelt-Hansen, J.; Banner, J. Sudden cardiac death caused by myocarditis in persons aged 1–49 years: A nationwide study of 14,294 deaths in Denmark. *Forensic Sci. Res.* **2019**, *4*, 247–256. [CrossRef]
2. Vos, A.; van der Wal, A.C.; Teeuw, A.H.; Bras, J.; Vink, A.; Nikkels, P.G.J. Cardiovascular causes of sudden unexpected death in children and adolescents (0–17 years): A nationwide autopsy study in the Netherlands. *Neth. Heart J.* **2018**, *26*, 500–505. [CrossRef] [PubMed]
3. Tymińska, A.; Ozierański, K.; Caforio, A.L.P.; Marcolongo, R.; Marchel, M.; Kapłon-Cieślicka, A.; Baritussio, A.; Filipiak, K.J.; Opolski, G.; Grabowski, M. Myocarditis and inflammatory cardiomyopathy in 2021: An update. *Pol. Arch. Intern. Med.* **2021**, *131*, 594–606. [CrossRef] [PubMed]

4. Saji, T.; Matsuura, H.; Hasegawa, K.; Nishikawa, T.; Yamamoto, E.; Ohki, H.; Yasukochi, S.; Arakaki, Y.; Joo, K.; Nakazawa, M. Comparison of the Clinical Presentation, Treatment, and Outcome of Fulminant and Acute Myocarditis in Children. *Circ. J.* **2012**, *76*, 1222–1228. [CrossRef] [PubMed]
5. Moraga, P. Global, regional, and national age-sex specific mortality for 264 causes of death, 1980–2016: A systematic analysis for the Global Burden of Disease Study 2016. *Lancet* **2017**, *390*, 1151–1210.
6. Roth, G.A.; Mensah, G.A.; Johnson, C.O.; Addolorato, G.; Ammirati, E.; Baddour, L.M.; Barengo, N.C.; Beaton, A.Z.; Benjamin, E.J.; Benziger, C.P.; et al. Global Burden of Cardiovascular Diseases and Risk Factors, 1990–2019: Update from the GBD 2019 Study. *J. Am. Coll. Cardiol.* **2020**, *76*, 2982–3021. [CrossRef]
7. Arola, A.; Pikkarainen, E.; Sipilä, J.; Pykäri, J.; Rautava, P.; Kytö, V. Occurrence and Features of Childhood Myocarditis: A Nationwide Study in Finland. *J. Am. Heart Assoc.* **2017**, *6*, e005306. [CrossRef] [PubMed]
8. Kim, J.; Cho, M.-J. Acute Myocarditis in Children: A 10-year Nationwide Study (2007–2016) based on the Health Insurance Review and Assessment Service Database in Korea. *Korean Circ. J.* **2020**, *50*, 1013–1022. [CrossRef]
9. Wojtyniak, B.; Gierlotka, M.; Opolski, G.; Rabczenko, D.; Ozierański, K.; Gąsior, M.; Chlebus, K.; Wierucki, L.; Rutkowski, D.; Dziełak, D.; et al. Observed and relative survival and 5-year outcomes of patients discharged after acute myocardial infarction: The nationwide AMI-PL database. *Kardiol. Pol.* **2020**, *78*, 990–998. [CrossRef]
10. Ozierański, K.; Tymińska, A.; Kruk, J.; Koń, B.; Skwarek, A.; Opolski, G.; Grabowski, M. Occurrence, Trends, Management and Outcomes of Patients Hospitalized with Clinically Suspected Myocarditis—Ten-Year Perspectives from the MYO-PL Nationwide Database. *J. Clin. Med.* **2021**, *10*, 4672. [CrossRef] [PubMed]
11. Vasudeva, R.; Bhatt, P.; Lilje, C.; Desai, P.; Amponsah, J.; Umscheid, J.; Parmar, N.; Bhatt, N.; Adupa, R.; Pagad, S.; et al. Trends in Acute Myocarditis Related Pediatric Hospitalizations in the United States, 2007–2016. *Am. J. Cardiol.* **2021**, *149*, 95–102. [CrossRef]
12. Shah, Z.; Mohammed, M.; Vuddanda, V.; Ansari, M.W.; Masoomi, R.; Gupta, K. National Trends, Gender, Management, and Outcomes of Patients Hospitalized for Myocarditis. *Am. J. Cardiol.* **2019**, *124*, 131–136. [CrossRef]
13. Liu, X.K.; Katchman, A.; Drici, M.D.; Ebert, S.N.; Ducic, I.; Morad, M.; Woosley, R.L. Gender difference in the cycle length-dependent QT and potassium currents in rabbits. *J. Pharmacol. Exp. Ther.* **1998**, *285*, 672–679. [PubMed]
14. Liu, X.-K.; Wang, W.; Ebert, S.N.; Franz, M.R.; Katchman, A.; Woosley, R.L. Female Gender is a Risk Factor for Torsades de Pointes in an In Vitro Animal Model. *J. Cardiovasc. Pharmacol.* **1999**, *34*, 287–294. [CrossRef] [PubMed]
15. Ozieranski, K.; Tyminska, A.; Jonik, S.; Marcolongo, R.; Baritussio, A.; Grabowski, M.; Filipiak, K.J.; Opolski, G.; Caforio, A.L. Clinically Suspected Myocarditis in the Course of Severe Acute Respiratory Syndrome Novel Coronavirus-2 Infection: Fact or Fiction? *J. Card. Fail.* **2021**, *27*, 92–96. [CrossRef] [PubMed]
16. Rodriguez, L.M.; de Chillou, C.; Schläpfer, J.; Metzger, J.; Baiyan, X.; van den Dool, A.; Smeets, J.L.; Wellens, H.J. Age at onset and gender of patients with different types of supraventricular tachycardias. *Am. J. Cardiol.* **1992**, *70*, 1213–1215. [CrossRef]
17. Yarnoz, M.J.; Curtis, A.B. More reasons why men and women are not the same (gender differences in electrophysiology and arrhythmias). *Am. J. Cardiol.* **2008**, *101*, 1291–1296. [CrossRef] [PubMed]
18. Wolbrette, D.; Naccarelli, G.; Curtis, A.; Lehmann, M.; Kadish, A. Gender differences in arrhythmias. *Clin. Cardiol.* **2002**, *25*, 49–56. [CrossRef] [PubMed]
19. Pham, T.V.; Rosen, M.R. Sex, hormones, and repolarization. *Cardiovasc. Res.* **2002**, *53*, 740–751. [CrossRef]
20. Pham, T.V.; Sosunov, E.A.; Gainullin, R.Z.; Danilo, P., Jr.; Rosen, M.R. Impact of sex and gonadal steroids on prolongation of ventricular repolarization and arrhythmias induced by I(K)-blocking drugs. *Circulation* **2001**, *103*, 2207–2212. [CrossRef]
21. Pophal, S.G.; Sigfusson, G.; Booth, K.L.; Bacanu, S.-A.; Webber, S.A.; Ettedgui, J.A.; Neches, W.H.; Park, S.C. Complications of endomyocardial biopsy in children. *J. Am. Coll. Cardiol.* **1999**, *34*, 2105–2110. [CrossRef]
22. Cooper, L.; Baughman, K.L.; Feldman, A.M.; Frustaci, A.; Jessup, M.; Kuhl, U.; Levine, G.N.; Narula, J.; Starling, R.C.; Towbin, J.; et al. The role of endomyocardial biopsy in the management of cardiovascular disease: A Scientific Statement from the American Heart Association, the American College of Cardiology, and the European Society of Cardiology Endorsed by the Heart Failure Society of America and the Heart Failure Association of the European Society of Cardiology. *Eur. Heart J.* **2007**, *28*, 3076–3093. [CrossRef] [PubMed]
23. Task Force for the management of COVID-19 of the European Society of Cardiology (2021). ESC Guidance for the Diagnosis and Management of Cardiovascular Disease during the COVID-19 Pandemic: Part 2-Care Pathways, Treatment, and Follow-Up. *Eur. Heart J.* **2021**, *16*, ehab697. [CrossRef]
24. Caforio, A.L.; Pankuweit, S.; Arbustini, E.; Basso, C.; Gimeno-Blanes, J.; Felix, S.B.; Fu, M.; Heliö, T.; Heymans, S.; Jahns, R.; et al. Current state of knowledge on aetiology, diagnosis, management, and therapy of myocarditis: A position statement of the European Society of Cardiology Working Group on Myocardial and Pericardial Diseases. *Eur. Heart J.* **2013**, *34*, 2636–2648. [CrossRef]
25. McDonagh, T.A.; Metra, M.; Adamo, M.; Gardner, R.S.; Baumbach, A.; Böhm, M.; Burri, H.; Butler, J.; Čelutkienė, J.; Chioncel, O.; et al. Corrigendum to: 2021 ESC Guidelines for the diagnosis and treatment of acute and chronic heart failure: Developed by the Task Force for the diagnosis and treatment of acute and chronic heart failure of the European Society of Cardiology (ESC) With the special contribution of the Heart Failure Association (HFA) of the ESC. *Eur. Heart J.* **2021**, ehab670. [CrossRef]

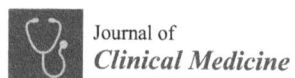

Article

Prevalence and Clinical Characteristics of Patients with Pause-Dependent Atrioventricular Block

Sok-Sithikun Bun [1,*], Florian Asarisi [1], Nathan Heme [1], Fabien Squara [1], Didier Scarlatti [1], Philippe Taghji [2], Jean-Claude Deharo [2], Pamela Moceri [1] and Emile Ferrari [1]

[1] Cardiology Department, Pasteur University Hospital, Côte-d'Azur University, 06000 Nice, France; asarisi.f@chu-nice.fr (F.A.); heme.n@chu-nice.fr (N.H.); squara.f@chu-nice.fr (F.S.); scarlatti.d@chu-nice.fr (D.S.); moceri.p@chu-nice.fr (P.M.); ferrari.e@chu-nice.fr (E.F.)
[2] Cardiology Department, Timone University Hospital, 13385 Marseille, France; philippetaghji@hotmail.com (P.T.); jean-claude.deharo@ap-hm.fr (J.-C.D.)
* Correspondence: sithi.bun@gmail.com; Tel.: +33-492-033-377

Abstract: Background: In patients with complete atrioventricular block (AVB), the prevalence and clinical characteristics of patients with pause-dependent AVB (PD-AVB) is not known. Our objective was to assess the prevalence of PD-AVB in a population of patients with complete (or high-grade) AVB. Methods: Twelve-lead electrocardiogram (ECG) and/or telemonitoring from patients admitted (from September 2020 to November 2021) for complete (or high-degree) AVB were prospectively collected at the University Hospital of Nice. The ECG tracings were analyzed by an electrophysiologist to determine the underlying mechanism of PD-AVB. Results: 100 patients were admitted for complete (or high-grade) AVB (men 55%; 82 ± 12 years). Arterial hypertension was present in 68% of the patients. Baseline QRS width was 117 ± 32 ms, and mean left ventricular ejection fraction was 56 ± 7%. Fourteen patients (14%) with PD-AVB were identified, and presented similar clinical characteristics in comparison with patients without PD-AVB, except for syncope (which was present in 86% versus 51% in the non-PD-AVB patients, $p = 0.01$). PD-AVB sequence was induced by: Premature atrial contraction (8/14), premature ventricular contraction (5/14), His extrasystole (1/14), conduction block in a branch (1/14), and atrial tachycardia termination (1/14). All patients with PD-AVB received a dual-chamber pacemaker during hospitalization. Conclusion: The prevalence of PD-AVB was 14%, and may be underestimated. PD-AVB episodes were more likely associated with syncope in comparison with patients without PD-AVB.

Keywords: pause-dependent atrioventricular block; high-grade atrioventricular block; prevalence; syncope; pacemaker

1. Introduction

Pause-dependent atrioventricular block (PD-AVB) can be defined as a paroxysmal and complete AVB whose mechanism is "bradycardia-dependent". An early description of bradycardia-dependent AVB was made in 1971 by Coumel et al. [1], and a few years later, the mechanism of PD-AVB was reported by Rosenbaum et al. [2]. Although some recent publications use the term phase 4 AVB, a controversy still exists about the exact mechanism of PD-AVB. [3] Actually, a recent report suggested the possible functional nature of PD-AVB related to concealed retrograde conduction in non-diseased His–Purkinje structures [4]. Nevertheless, despite the existence of variable triggers, "pause-dependency" remains the common hallmark. PD-AVB occurrence is related to the inactivation of sodium channels due to spontaneous depolarization within diseased His–Purkinje fibers, during a post-compensatory pause, followed by inability to conduct electrical impulses due to a very low resting membrane potential (phase 4 of action potential). This mechanism may be distinguished from other types of complete AVB. In 2009, Lee et al. proposed a classification of complete AVB in four types: Acquired AVB, vagally-mediated AVB,

Citation: Bun, S.-S.; Asarisi, F.; Heme, N.; Squara, F.; Scarlatti, D.; Taghji, P.; Deharo, J.-C.; Moceri, P.; Ferrari, E. Prevalence and Clinical Characteristics of Patients with Pause-Dependent Atrioventricular Block. J. Clin. Med. 2022, 11, 449. https://doi.org/10.3390/jcm11020449

Academic Editors: Paweł T. Matusik and Christian Sohns

Received: 12 December 2021
Accepted: 14 January 2022
Published: 16 January 2022

Publisher's Note: MDPI stays neutral with regard to jurisdictional claims in published maps and institutional affiliations.

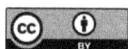

Copyright: © 2022 by the authors. Licensee MDPI, Basel, Switzerland. This article is an open access article distributed under the terms and conditions of the Creative Commons Attribution (CC BY) license (https://creativecommons.org/licenses/by/4.0/).

congenital heart block, and paroxysmal AVB, the later referring to PD-AVB [5]. Recently, the different triggers of PD-AVB have been well described: Premature atrial contraction (PAC), premature ventricular contraction (PVC), supra-ventricular tachycardia termination, sinus rhythm slowdown [6].

PD-AVB is considered a rare entity, but the prevalence of 4AVB is not known. The purpose of this study was to assess the incidence and the clinical characteristics of patients with PD-AVB in a population of patients admitted into a cardiac care unit for complete (or high-grade) AVB.

2. Materials and Methods

All patients admitted at the cardiac care unit of the University Hospital of Nice from September 2020 to November 2021 for complete (or high-grade) AVB were included in this single-center prospective observational study, and their electrocardiograms (ECGs) were systematically collected. Complete AVB but also high-grade (including 2 to 1) AVB were confirmed on 12-lead surface and/or telemetry monitoring by one experienced electrophysiologist (S.-S.B.). Patients with vagally-mediated AVB (Figure 1) defined by gradual slowing of the sinus rate (PP interval lengthening) and AV conduction (prolonging PR) usually seen before complete AVB occurrence, were excluded from this analysis.

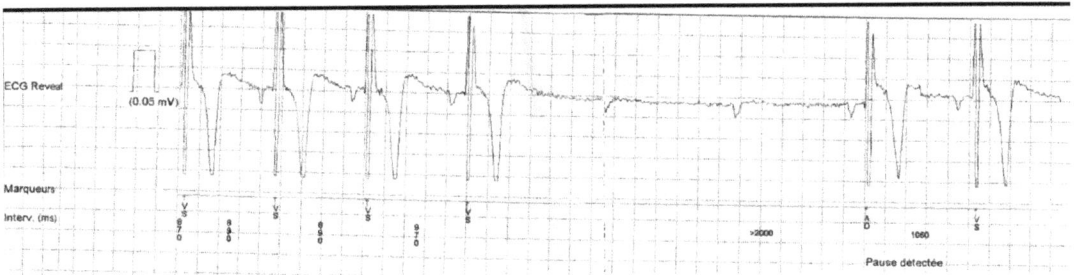

Figure 1. Example of patient presenting with vagally-mediated complete AVB recorded with an implantable loop recorder. One can notice the gradual PP lengthening before the occurrence of complete AVB, but also during the absence of the QRS complexes. A PR interval prolongation is also visible before AVB occurred, with the PR interval after resolution of the block slightly longer than PR before the block. This type of AVB mechanism was excluded from the study. AVB: atrioventricular block.

AVB were classified as permanent if complete (or high-grade) AVB was present all along the period of the hospitalization stay during cardiac monitoring, or intermittent if complete (or high-grade) AVB was observed in alternation with 1:1 conduction (eventually facilitated by isoproterenol infusion). To avoid any confusion with previous studies, the term "paroxysmal" will not be used in our study and will be discussed later.

The clinical and electrocardiographic characteristics of the patients were analyzed; episodes of PD-AVB were classified according to their initiation mechanism. All patients gave their written informed consent for the pacemaker implantation (if needed). The study was approved by the institutional review board.

Statistical Analysis

The statistical analysis was made with Excel (San Diego, CA, USA). Categorical variables are described as numbers and percentages. Continuous variables are described as mean ± SD for variables with normal distributions or as median with range for variables not normally distributed.

3. Results

During the inclusion period, 100 patients were admitted for complete (or high-grade) AVB (men 55%; 82 ± 12 years). Arterial hypertension was present in 68% of the patients.

Baseline QRS width was 117 ± 32 ms, and mean left ventricular ejection fraction was 56 ± 7%. Fourteen patients (14%) with PD-AVB were identified, and presented similar clinical characteristics in comparison with patients without PD-AVB except for syncope (present in 86% versus 51% in the non-4AVB patients) (Table 1). PD-AVB sequence was induced by: Premature atrial contraction (8/14), as shown in Figure 2; premature ventricular contraction (5/14), as seen in Figure 3; His extrasystole (1/14); conduction block in a branch (1/14); and atrial tachycardia termination (1/14), as shown in Figure 4. The mean duration of asystoly during the PD-AVB episode was 5.1 ± 3 s (1.6–10 s). The mean number of consecutive non-conducted p waves during the PD-AVB episode was 8 ± 4 (range 3–15). Patients with PD-AVB represented one third of the total number ($n = 43$) of patients with intermittent complete AVB. Baseline conduction disturbances in patients with intermittent complete AVB are presented in Table 1. All of the patients with PD-AVB received a dual-chamber pacemaker during hospitalization. After a mean follow-up of 6 ± 7 months, the mean percentage of ventricular pacing was 89.2 ± 30% in this population (complete AVB present except for two, one with initial baseline normal QRS, and the other with bifascicular block); versus 73.4 ± 39% in the non-PD-AVB group ($p = 0.31$).

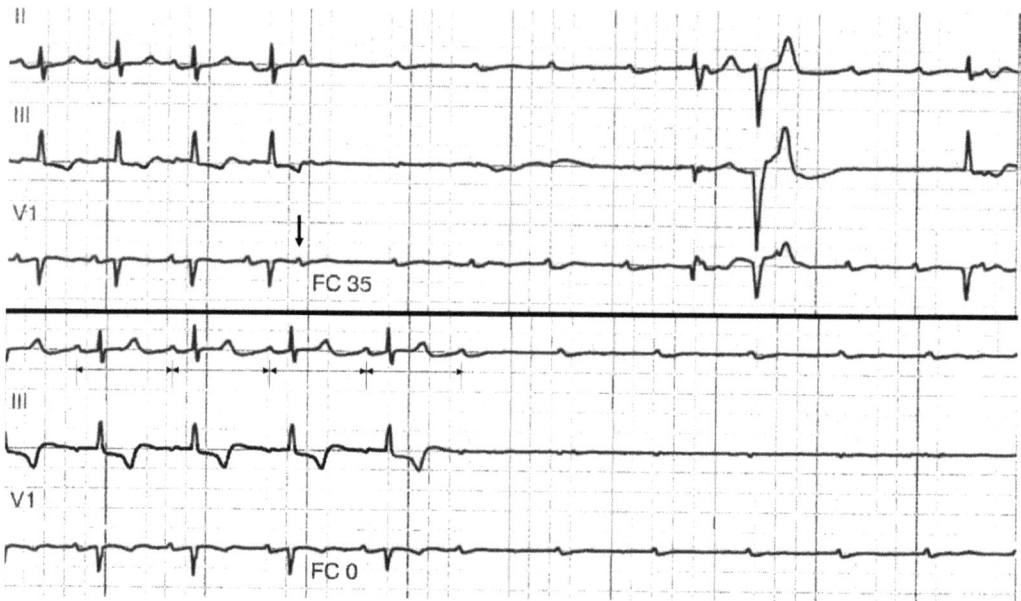

Figure 2. Example of patient presenting with PD-AVB initiated by a premature atrial contraction, recorded on a telemetry strip (upper panel). Another episode could be recorded in the same patient (patient 5 from Table 2), but without any macroscopic variation of the PP intervals preceding the complete AVB (lower panel).

Table 1. Characteristics of patients with pause-dependent atrioventricular block.

	PD-AVB [1] (n = 14)	Non-PD-AVB (n = 86)	p
Age	84 ± 6 (71–96)	82 ± 12 (57–102)	0.22
Men, n (%)	9 (64)	46 (53)	0.45
Syncope	12 (86)	44 (51)	0.01
Arterial hypertension, n (%)	10 (71)	58 (67)	0.77
LVEF (%) [2]	55 ± 10	56 ± 7	0.57
Mean QRS duration (ms)	132 ± 27	117 ± 32	0.15

Table 1. Cont.

	PD-AVB [1] (n = 14)	Non-PD-AVB (n = 86)	p
PR interval (ms)	230 ± 36	199 ± 43	0.10
RBBB [3]/LBBB [4]/Normal QRS, n (%)	RBBB = 3 (22) RBBB/LAFB [5] = 3 (22) RBBB/LPFB [6] = 2 (14) LBBB = 2 (14) Normal = 4 (28)	RBBB = 2 (7) RBBB/LAFB = 4 (14) RBBB/LPFB = 5 (17) LBBB = 5 (17) Normal = 12 (41) Isolated LAFB = 1 (4)	0.16 0.34 0.80 0.80 0.42
Baseline corrected QT interval (ms)	453 ± 44	470 ± 53	0.64
Tpeak-Tend (ms)	114 ± 48	117 ± 45	0.69

[1] PD-AVB: pause-dependent atrioventricular block. [2] LVEF: left ventricular ejection fraction. [3] RBBB: right bundle branch block. [4] LBBB: left bundle branch block. [5] LAFB: left anterior fascicular block. [6] LPFB: left posterior fascicular block.

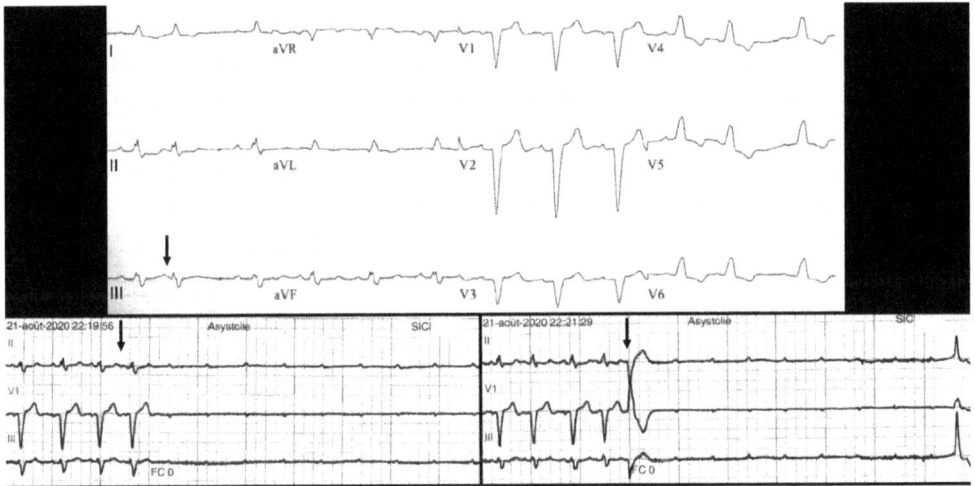

Figure 3. Example of two mechanisms of pause-dependent atrioventricular block seen within the same patient (patient 10 in Table 2). Baseline twelve-lead ECG shows sinus rhythm with complete left bundle branch block and a conducted premature atrial contraction (PAC). Another timely-appropriate PAC then induced PD-AVB (left lower image). Another PD-AVB episode was recorded after a premature ventricular contraction (lower right image).

Table 2. Summary of published cases of pause-dependent atrioventricular block.

Author	Sex	Age (y)	Baseline QRS Width (ms)	Symptom	Mechanism	Outcome
Lee S, 2009 [5]	NA n = 30	69	123 ± 32	Syncope (75%)	PAC [1] (30%) PVC [2] (23%) His extrasystole (10%) Other (37%)	Pacemaker
Atreya AR, 2015 [7]	Male	NA [3]	96	Syncope	PAC	Pacemaker
Georger F, 2015 [8]	Male	74	NA	Syncope	AT termination	Pacemaker
Shesana M, 2017 [9]	Male	45	130	Syncope	PAC	Pacemaker
Bansal R, 2017 [10]	Female	79	Narrow	Near-syncope	PVC	Pacemaker

Table 2. Cont.

Author	Sex	Age (y)	Baseline QRS Width (ms)	Symptom	Mechanism	Outcome
Prasada S, 2019 [11]	Male	81	130	None	PVC	Pacemaker
Uhm JS, 2018 [6]	Male	72	Narrow	Syncope	Vagally-mediated	Pacemaker
	Male	73	NA	Asymptomatic	PVC	Pacemaker refused
	Male	69	Narrow	Syncope	PVC	No pacemaker
	Male	68	NA	Dizziness	PAC	Pacemaker
	Male	71	Narrow	Syncope	AT termination	Pacemaker
Du W, 2020 [3]	Male	76	130	Dizziness	PVC	Pacemaker
Our series, 2022	Female	96	134	Asymptomatic	Block in branch	Pacemaker
	Male	88	156	Syncope	PAC	Pacemaker
	Female	87	112	Syncope	PAC	Pacemaker
	Female	91	124	Heart failure	PVC	Pacemaker
	Female	91	74	Syncope	PVC	Pacemaker
	Female	79	122	Syncope	PAC	Pacemaker
	Male	84	156	Syncope	PAC	Pacemaker
	Male	90	170	Syncope	PAC	Pacemaker
	Male	83	160	Syncope	PVC	Pacemaker
	Male	86	144	Syncope	PAC/PVC	Pacemaker
	Male	76	140	Syncope	AFl [4] termination/PVC	Pacemaker
	Male	72	115	Syncope	PVC/SR acceleration [5]	Pacemaker
	Male	81	96	Syncope	His extrasystole	Pacemaker
	Male	71	152	Syncope	PAC	Pacemaker

[1] PAC: premature atrial contraction. [2] PVC: premature ventricular contraction. [3] NA: non-available. [4] AFl: atrial flutter. [5] SR: sinus rhythm.

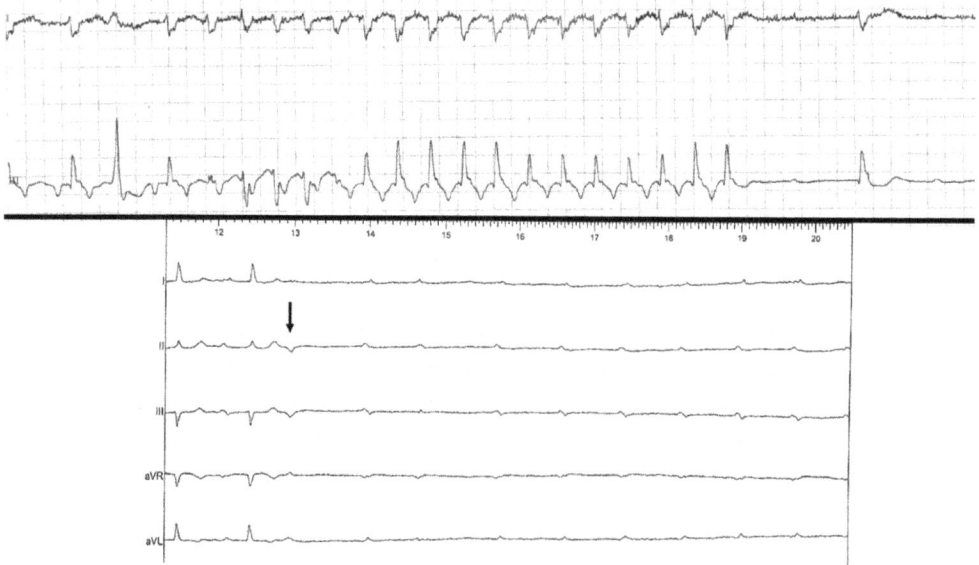

Figure 4. Example of two other mechanisms of pause-dependent atrioventricular blocks. The telemetry strips show a counterclockwise isthmus-dependent flutter termination followed by PD-AVB (upper panel). In the same patient (11 from Table 2), another episode could be recorded, induced by a premature ventricular contraction. Surface ECG showed a PD-AVB episode induced by a His extrasystole (arrow) as shown by the retrograde P wave visible (lower panel). A blocked premature atrial contraction may not be ruled out (patient 13 in Table 2).

4. Discussion

Our study is the first to report the prevalence of PD-AVB in a population of patients admitted into a cardiac care unit for complete (or high-grade) AVB. While 4AVB was considered a rare phenomenon, our study demonstrates a prevalence of 14%, reaching one third if considering only patients with intermittent complete (or high-grade) AVB. Our cohort of patients is representative of the prevalence of complete (or high-grade) AVB in a University center with medium-to high-volume activity. Isolated descriptions or case reports/case series have been published concerning PD-AVB, without further information about its prevalence [7]. In our study population, no specific clinical or electrocardiographic characteristics could be related to the occurrence of PD-AVB, in comparison with other patients with complete AVB. Syncope was significantly more frequently present in patients with PD-AVB, in comparison with patients without PD-AVB (86 versus 51%, $p = 0.01$). To the best of our knowledge, our series is the second largest described with PD-AVB to date. Of note, a recent case reported the possibility for conduction block to occur within a bundle branch, and not within the AV node itself [12]. All previously published cases are summarized in Table 2 [8].

Interestingly, our study is the first to report double distinct mechanisms recorded within the same patient. Four patients presented with two distinct mechanisms of PD-AVB: One patient had PVC-induced PD-AVB and a second episode without significant increase in the PP intervals before AVB (from 690 to 710 ms), and without PR prolongation (Figure 2); another patient presented PD-AVB sequences induced by PAC, and later by PVC (Figure 3); the third patient presented an episode triggered by atrial flutter termination and PVC-induced PD-AVB; the last patient presented PVC-induced PD-AVB and another recorded episode with sinus rhythm acceleration (tachycardia-dependent AVB) (Figure 5). Uhm et al. reported a dual mechanism in a patient presenting PD-AVB episodes induced by a PAC, and SVT termination, but the later episode included the intervention of a temporary pacemaker (not spontaneous) [6].

Lee et al. reported the largest bicentric series to date of paroxysmal AVB. Nevertheless, both tachycardia-dependent AVB [5] and idiopathic paroxysmal AVB were not clearly individualized in this initial description. Actually, a few years later, Brignole et al. described a rare entity, and reported a series of 18 patients with idiopathic paroxysmal AVB, whose mechanism is related to adenosine hypersensitivity [13,14].

To summarize, our suggestion for paroxysmal AVB classification may be as follows:

(1) "Extrinsic" vagally-mediated AVB characterized by significant PR prolongation or Wenckebach before initiation of AVB, gradual slowing of the sinus rate (PP interval), resumption of AV conduction with sinus acceleration, PP interval prolongation during ventricular asystole. Often, a shortening of the PR interval compared to the last PR interval with AV conduction before an AV block can be observed (upon withdrawal of the vagal effect). A clinical history suggestive of heightened vagal tone is present.

(2) "Idiopathic" paroxysmal AVB involving a younger population (mean age 55 ± 19 years) without cardiac and ECG abnormalities, without progression to persistent forms of AVB, and with efficacy of cardiac pacing. AVB occurs with abrupt onset and delayed emergence of an adequate escape rhythm without PP cycle lenghthening or PR interval prolongation. A low baseline adenosine plasma level was found in this specific population. This entity should remain a diagnosis of exclusion.

(3) "Intrinsic" AVB (suggesting AV conduction disease), which may be divided into four categories: Congenital heart block; tachycardia-dependent AVB; PD-AVB; and finally other acquired AVB when the preceding features/conditions are lacking (non-PD-AVB group in our study) as shown in Figure 6. Progressive cardiac conduction disease may be integrated into this last category, and refers to primary genetic degenerative diseases of genetic origin (several mutations have been described, such as in SCN5A of the cardiac sodium channel) [9]. Combined AVB initiation circumstances may be encountered in this "intrinsic" AVB group.

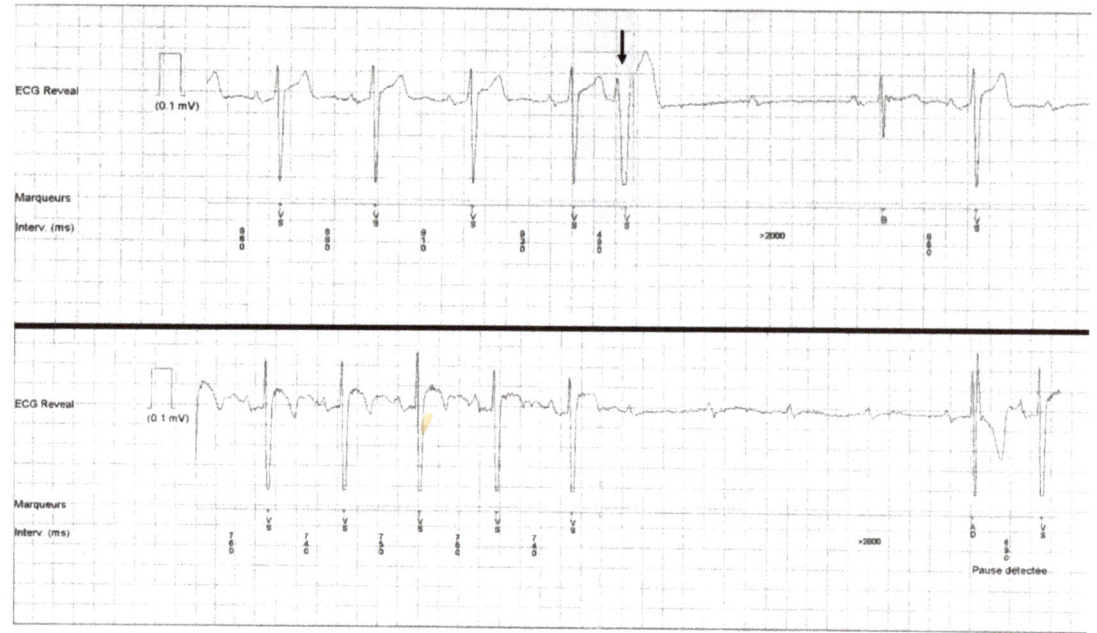

Figure 5. Example of pause-dependent atrioventricular block induced by a premature ventricular contraction (arrow), and recorded with an implantable loop recorder. In the same patient, another episode was preceded by sinus rhythm acceleration (from 760 to 740 ms) corresponding to tachycardia-dependent atrioventricular block.

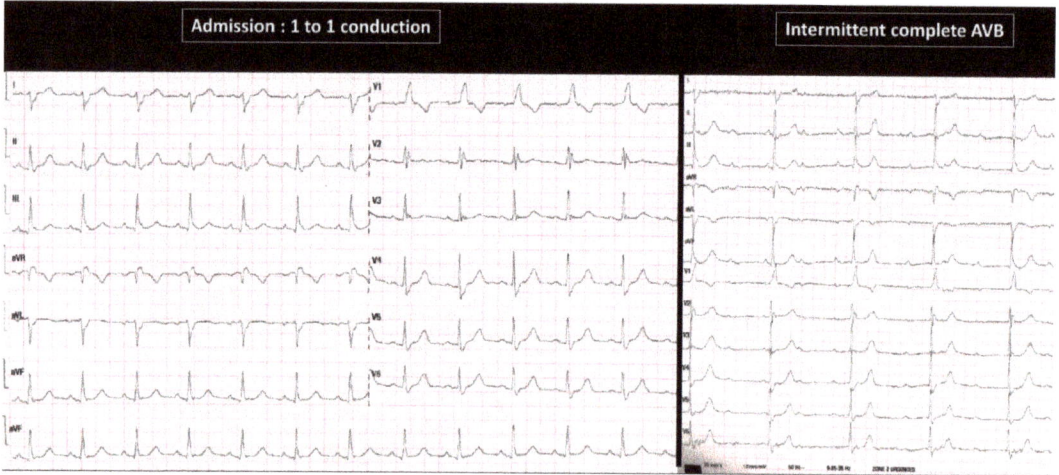

Figure 6. Twelve-lead ECG from an 82 year-old female patient admitted at the emergency department for syncope with cerebral traumatism. The initial ECG shows sinus rhythm with 1 to 1 atrioventricular conduction and complete right bundle branch block associated with left fascicular posterior block. During ECG monitoring at the cardiac care unit, the patient developed an intermittent complete "intrinsic" AVB episode. No trigger of PD-AVB was found in this patient, who was included in the non-PD-AVB group.

The main differences that may be seen between our population and Lee's report are that their population was significantly younger than ours (69 versus 84 ± 6 years-old) with thinner QRS duration (123 ± 32 versus 132 ± 27 ms in our series). The authors also reported that PAC was the main trigger of PD-AVB in 30% of the cases, PVC in 23%, His extrasystole in 10%, and other variable mechanisms in 37%. Our results are in line with the literature, because PAC were also found to be the most prominent trigger (two thirds).

Of note, in our series, two patients out of 14 with PD-AVB underwent a transcatheter aortic valve intervention (TAVI) in their past medical history. According to the latest European guidelines, early permanent cardiac pacing may be recommended in the case of transient high-grade AVB during TAVI in patients with pre-existing RBBB [15,16]. Actually, transitory AVB may usually be encountered during rapid ventricular pacing before valve expansion. In this case, permanent pacemaker implantation could then be discussed if baseline RBBB was present before the intervention. For patients with newly-developed LBBB, an ambulatory ECG monitoring or electrophysiological study may be considered.

Limitations

This is a monocentric study with a limited number of patients. True prevalence of PD-AVB could have been underestimated. No electrophysiological study was performed in this elderly population with an indication of permanent cardiac pacing (syncope present in 80% of the cases). Electrophysiological study is usually not recommended in the setting of symptomatic complete AVB [16].

Of note, all our patients with PD-AVB received a dual-chamber pacemaker (with exclusive right ventricular septal lead position). PD-AVB (once identified) usually occurs in diseased His–Purkinje systems. Further studies are needed to confirm the usefulness/superiority of conduction system pacing in these patients, as recently reported by Du et al. [4].

5. Conclusions

The prevalence of 4AVB was 14%, and may be underestimated. PD-AVB episodes were more likely associated with syncope in comparison with patients without PD-AVB. These patients may elicit multiple triggers of PD-AVB.

Author Contributions: Conceptualization, S.-S.B.; methodology, S.-S.B. and P.T.; validation, S.-S.B.; formal analysis, S.-S.B.; investigation, F.A. and N.H.; writing—original draft preparation, S.-S.B.; writing—review and editing, P.T.; visualization, J.-C.D., F.S. and D.S.; supervision, P.M. and E.F. All authors have read and agreed to the published version of the manuscript.

Funding: This research received no external funding.

Institutional Review Board Statement: The study was conducted according to the guidelines of the Declaration of Helsinki, and approved by the Institutional Review Board of Nice University Hospital (protocol code SB-CHU22).

Informed Consent Statement: Informed consent was obtained from all subjects involved in the study. Written informed consent has been obtained from the patient(s) to publish this paper.

Conflicts of Interest: The authors declare no conflict of interest.

References

1. Coumel, P.; Fabiato, A.; Waynberger, M.; Motte, G.; Slama, R.; Bouvrain, Y. Bradycardia-dependent atrio-ventricular block. Report of two cases of A-V block elicited by premature beats. *J. Electrocardiol.* **1971**, *4*, 168–177. [CrossRef]
2. Rosenbaum, M.B.; Elizari, M.V.; Levi, R.J.; Nau, G.J. Paroxysmal atrioventricular block related to hypopolarization and spontaneous diastolic depolarization. *Chest* **1973**, *63*, 678–688. [CrossRef] [PubMed]
3. El-Sherif, N.; Jalife, J. Paroxysmal atrioventricular block: Are phase 3 and phase 4 block mechanisms or misnomers? *Heart Rhythm* **2009**, *6*, 1514–1521. [CrossRef] [PubMed]
4. Du, W.; Xu, J.; Li, S.F.; Yu, B. The functional atrioventricular block caused by a premature ventricular beat from His-Purkinje system: Electrophysiological insights in permanent peri-left bundle branch area pacing. *Heart Rhythm Case Rep.* **2020**, *6*, 601–604. [CrossRef] [PubMed]
5. Lee, S.; Wellens, H.J.; Josephson, M.E. Paroxysmal atrioventricular block. *Heart Rhythm* **2009**, *6*, 1229–1234. [CrossRef] [PubMed]

6. Uhm, J.S.; Joung, B.; Pak, H.N.; Lee, M.H. Various triggers of phase 4 block. *Heart Rhythm Case Rep.* **2018**, *4*, 197–199. [CrossRef] [PubMed]
7. Atreya, A.R.; Cook, J.R.; Fox, M.T. Pause-dependent paroxysmal phase-4 atrioventricular block. *BMJ Case Rep.* **2015**, *16*, bcr2015211801. [CrossRef] [PubMed]
8. Georger, F.; De Roy, L.; Sorea, C.; Albenque, J.P.; Boveda, S.; Belhassen, B. Unusual mechanism of complete atrioventricular block following atrial flutter ablation. *Heart Rhythm Case Rep.* **2015**, *1*, 369–372. [CrossRef] [PubMed]
9. Shenasa, M.; Josephson, M.E.; Wit, A.L. Paroxysmal atrioventricular block: Electrophysiological mechanism of phase 4 conduction block in the His-Purkinje system: A comparison with phase 3 block. *Pacing Clin. Electrophysiol.* **2017**, *40*, 1234–1241. [CrossRef] [PubMed]
10. Bansal, R.; Mahajan, A.; Rathi, C.; Mehta, A.; Lokhandwala, Y. What is the mechanism of paroxysmal atrioventricular block in a patient with recurrent syncope? *J. Arrhythmia* **2019**, *35*, 870–872. [CrossRef] [PubMed]
11. Prasada, S.; Nishtala, A.; Goldschlager, N. Prolonged Ventricular Asystole. *Circulation* **2019**, *139*, 2798–2801. [CrossRef] [PubMed]
12. Maxwell, N.; Dryer, M.M.; Baranchuk, A.; Vinocur, J.M. Phase 4 block of the right bundle branch suggesting His-Purkinje system involvement in Lyme carditis. *Heart Rhythm Case Rep.* **2020**, *7*, 112–116. [CrossRef] [PubMed]
13. Brignole, M.; Deharo, J.C.; De Roy, L.; Menozzi, C.; Blommaert, D.; Dabiri, L.; Ruf, J.; Guieu, R. Syncope due to idiopathic paroxysmal atrioventricular block: Long-term follow-up of a distinct form of atrioventricular block. *J. Am. Coll. Cardiol.* **2011**, *58*, 167–173. [CrossRef] [PubMed]
14. Deharo, J.C.; Brignole, M.; Guieu, R. Adenosine hypersensitivity and atrioventricular block. *Herzschrittmacherther Elektrophysiol.* **2018**, *29*, 166–170. [CrossRef] [PubMed]
15. Mangieri, A.; Laricchia, A.; Montalto, C.; Palena, M.L.; Fisicaro, A.; Cereda, A.; Sticchi, A.; Latib, A.; Giannini, F.; Khokhar, A.A.; et al. Patient selection, procedural planning and interventional guidance for transcatheter aortic valve intervention. *Minerva Cardiol. Angiol.* **2021**, *69*, 671–683. [CrossRef] [PubMed]
16. Glikson, M.; Nielsen, J.C.; Kronborg, M.B.; Michowitz, Y.; Auricchio, A.; Barbash, I.M.; Barrabés, J.A.; Boriani, G.; Braunschweig, F.; Brignole, M.; et al. 2021 ESC Guidelines on cardiac pacing and cardiac resynchronization therapy. *Eur. Heart J.* **2021**, *42*, 3427–3520. [CrossRef] [PubMed]

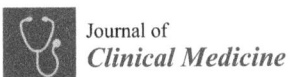

Article

Contact Force-Sensing versus Standard Catheters in Non-Fluoroscopic Radiofrequency Catheter Ablation of Idiopathic Outflow Tract Ventricular Arrhythmias

Grzegorz Karkowski [1], Marcin Kuniewicz [1,2], Andrzej Ząbek [1], Edward Koźluk [3], Maciej Dębski [4], Paweł T. Matusik [1,5,*] and Jacek Lelakowski [1,5]

1. Department of Electrocardiology, The John Paul II Hospital, 31-202 Kraków, Poland; gkarkowski@interia.pl (G.K.); kuniewiczm@gmail.com (M.K.); andrzej_j_z@poczta.onet.pl (A.Z.); jacek.lelakowski@uj.edu.pl (J.L.)
2. Department of Anatomy, Jagiellonian University Medical College, 31-008 Kraków, Poland
3. Department of Cardiology, Medical University of Warsaw, 02-097 Warsaw, Poland; ekozluk@vp.pl
4. Department of Cardiology, Norfolk and Norwich University Hospital, University of East Anglia, Norwich NR4 7TJ, UK; maciekdebski@gmail.com
5. Department of Electrocardiology, Institute of Cardiology, Jagiellonian University Medical College, 31-008 Kraków, Poland
* Correspondence: pawel.matusik@uj.edu.pl; Tel.: +48-12-614-2277

Abstract: Background: Adequate contact between the catheter tip and tissue is important for optimal lesion formation and, in some procedures, it has been associated with improved effectiveness and safety. We evaluated the potential benefits of contact force-sensing (CFS) catheters during non-fluoroscopic radiofrequency catheter ablation (NF-RFCA) of idiopathic ventricular arrhythmias (VAs) originating from outflow tracts (OTs). Methods: A group of 102 patients who underwent NF-RFCA (CARTO, Biosense Webster Inc., Irvine, CA, USA) of VAs from OTs between 2014 to 2018 was retrospectively analyzed. Results: We included 52 (50.9%) patients in whom NF-RFCA was performed using CFS catheters and 50 (49.1%) who were ablated using standard catheters. Arrhythmias were localized in the right and left OT in 70 (68.6%) and 32 (31.4%) patients, respectively. The RFCA acute success rate was 96.1% ($n = 98$) and long-term success during a minimum 12-month follow-up (mean 51.3 ± 21.6 months) was 85.3% ($n = 87$), with no difference between CFS and standard catheters. There was no difference in complications rate between CFS ($n = 1$) and standard catheter ($n = 2$) ablations. Conclusions: There is no additional advantage of CFS catheters use over standard catheters during NF-RFCA of OT-VAs in terms of procedural effectiveness and safety.

Keywords: contact force; non-fluoroscopic ablation; outflow tracts; premature ventricular contractions; ventricular arrhythmias

Citation: Karkowski, G.; Kuniewicz, M.; Ząbek, A.; Koźluk, E.; Dębski, M.; Matusik, P.T.; Lelakowski, J. Contact Force-Sensing versus Standard Catheters in Non-Fluoroscopic Radiofrequency Catheter Ablation of Idiopathic Outflow Tract Ventricular Arrhythmias. *J. Clin. Med.* 2022, 11, 593. https://doi.org/10.3390/jcm11030593

Academic Editors: Christian Sohns and Bernhard Rauch

Received: 15 December 2021
Accepted: 21 January 2022
Published: 25 January 2022

Publisher's Note: MDPI stays neutral with regard to jurisdictional claims in published maps and institutional affiliations.

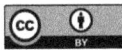

Copyright: © 2022 by the authors. Licensee MDPI, Basel, Switzerland. This article is an open access article distributed under the terms and conditions of the Creative Commons Attribution (CC BY) license (https://creativecommons.org/licenses/by/4.0/).

1. Introduction

The non-fluoroscopic (NF) radiofrequency catheter ablation (RFCA) of idiopathic ventricular arrhythmias (VAs) from outflow tracts (OTs) has a good effectiveness and safety profile, but arrhythmia recurrence is not uncommon and may be observed in 4–12.5% of the patients [1–5]. Activation mapping of ventricular OTs arrhythmias reveals focal origin in most cases. Besides precise mapping, procedural success depends on good ablation lesion formation. Multiple factors influence the optimal creation of lesions, some of which are operator-dependent and include the type of energy source (e.g., cryoablation, radiofrequency current), power setting, application duration, catheter tip orientation or catheter type and size. Importantly, adequate contact between the catheter tip and tissue plays an essential role in lesion formation [3,6,7]. Inadequate contact force (CF) will decrease lesion size and reduce ablation effectiveness [8]. On the other hand, excessive CF might lead to mechanical injury or tissue overheating, causing steam pop, which is a life-threatening complication [9,10]. Traditionally, evaluation of optimal CF has been based on operator-dependent parameters such as tactile feedback, visual assessment of catheter motion and physical parameters such as impedance drop, tip temperature value or electrogram amplitude change during application. Unfortunately, those parameters have a poor correlation with real CF during application and have a limited role in clinical practice [6,8]. Introduction and validation of contact force-sensing catheters (CFS) capable of real-time catheter tip–tissue contact force measurement have helped optimize lesion formation and increase procedural safety [11,12]. The benefits of CFS catheters have been previously proven in atrial fibrillation (AF) RFCA [11–13]. Due to outflow tract anatomy and ventricular tissue thickness, especially in septal location, such as left ventricular (LV) summit, optimal CF is theoretically very desirable, especially in the NF procedure. However, published data are contradictory and recent studies revealed no advantage of CFS guidance in fluoroscopic RFCA compared to standard open irrigated catheters of OT-VAs [14,15]. Due to the increasing role of NF-RFCA, we aimed to evaluate the potential benefits of open irrigated CFS catheters in RFCA of idiopathic VAs from OTs without fluoroscopy guidance.

2. Materials and Methods

2.1. Patients

We retrospectively analyzed a group of 102 patients who between 2014 and 2018 underwent NF-RFCA of premature ventricular contractions (PVC) from OTs. Procedures were performed or supervised by operators experienced in NF and fluoroscopic RFCA. NF-RFCA was defined as ablation performed without use of fluoroscopy (zero-fluoroscopy). The choice of catheter type was left to the decision of the operator. Patients listed for RFCA had idiopathic, symptomatic VAs with high daily PVC burden (generally minimum 10% PVC per day) from the right or left ventricular OT (RVOT or LVOT), including arrhythmias originating from aortic cusps. Antiarrhythmic medications were suspended 48 h before the ablation. None of the patients was on amiodarone or sotalol before ablation. The CFS catheters were used for mapping and ablation in 52 patients, while standard catheters were without CFS in the remaining 50 patients. All patients provided written consent to undergo the procedure. The local ethics committee waived the need for their opinion to perform the study due to the retrospective character of the project (L.dz.OIL/KBL/82/2021). The study protocol conformed to the ethical guidelines of the 1975 Declaration of Helsinki.

2.2. Mapping and Ablation Protocol

All ablations were guided by CARTO electroanatomic mapping system (Biosense Webster Inc., Diamond Bar, CA, USA). In standard catheter group, 3.5 mm open irrigated tip catheters (Biosense Webster Navistar Thermocool) were used, while in the remaining patients 3.5 mm open irrigated-tip catheters with CFS (Thermocool SmartTouch®, Biosense Webster, Irvine, CA, USA) were used. The setting of RF application parameters: energy in RVOT 30–40 Wats (W), in LVOT 20–30 W, the flow of irrigation: of 15–30 mL/min, time of application (60 s), temperature limits (max 45 °C) were the same in both groups. RF applications were performed at the CF target in the CFS group, i.e., between 10–30 g. To determine the PVC origin, activation mapping was used to look for the earliest endocardial potential advancing QRS during PVC. Additionally, in the earliest activation spot, pace-mapping was applied to confirm PVC localization with PVC compatibility of at least 95% of the complexes analyzed by electrophysiological recording system (LABSYSTEM™ PRO, Boston Scientific, Marlborough, MA, USA) with as low as possible pacing output (1–2 mV/0.5 ms over pacing capture loss, max. pacing output 12 mV/0.5 ms), Figure 1.

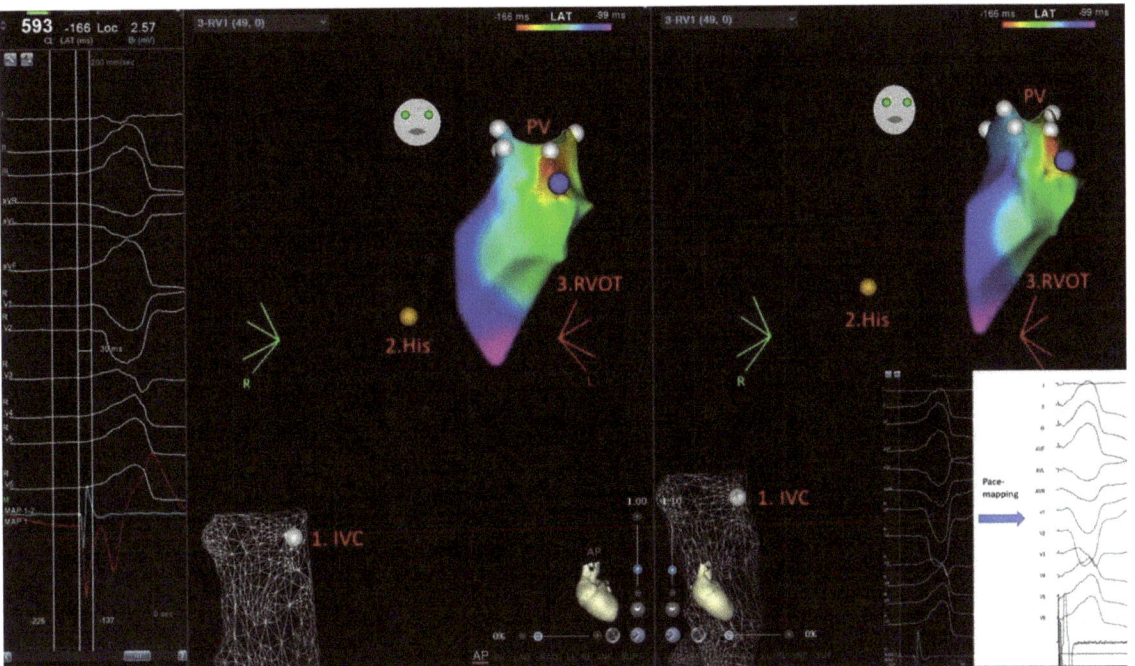

Figure 1. A. Activation map of premature ventricular contraction (PVC) from right ventricular outflow tract-RVOT (CARTO Biosense Webster Inc., Irvine, CA, USA) performed without fluoroscopy. First stage of the procedure is FAM of IVC and CF sensor calibration (if used). Second stage is His potential (yellow dot) localization and performance of respiratory gating. The third stage is performance of point-by-point activation mapping supported with pace-mapping. In showed case, earliest endocardial potential advancing PVC-QRS-30 ms (with automatic reference annotation)–spot of RF application, blue dot-a spot of optimal pace-mapping with compatibility with PVC > 95%. White dots–PV marked. AP and RAO projections. Abbreviations: CF, contact force; FAM, fast anatomical mapping; IVC, inferior vena cava; PVC, premature ventricular contraction; PV, pulmonary valve.

The technique of NF-RFCA was described previously [5]. CFS catheters were calibrated to set the baseline value before mapping and ablation in inferior vena cava (1–2 cm below right atrium) or in descending aorta (1–2 cm below aortic arch), depending on venous or arterial approach.

During the RFCA of RVOT-VAs, a single or double (for coronary sinus diagnostic electrode) femoral vein puncture was performed. In left-sided arrhythmias, single femoral artery access was obtained. In some cases, both right and left access was used. The procedure was performed under local anesthesia or conscious sedation, if necessary.

The acute (short-term) efficacy of RFCA was defined as no recurrent PVCs after 15 min from the last RF application. The patients were challenged with isoproterenol only in those cases where PVCs required pharmacological induction before ablation. A minimum 12-month follow-up period was required. Long-term efficacy was defined as a significant arrhythmia reduction (over 80% reduction of arrhythmia burden) after at least three months in repeated 24-h ECG monitoring (every 6–12 months). Antiarrhythmic medication was not continued after ablation, except beta-blockers or calcium blockers if used for another indication, i.e., hypertension. Antiarrhythmics were introduced in the case of symptomatic arrhythmia recurrence. All necessary medical follow-up data (12 lead ECG, 24-h Holter ECG, repeat ablation information) were obtained from outpatient medical records.

2.3. Twenty-Four-Hour Holter Monitoring and Echocardiography

Twenty-four-hour Holter ECG monitoring was performed before ablation, three months after RF ablation, and at least once a year after this period. ECG recordings were performed according to the Polish Cardiac Society Guidelines [16].

Transthoracic echocardiography (TTE) was performed in all patients. Exams were done with Vivid S6 (GE Healthcare, Chicago, IL, USA) device, according to the European Association for Cardiovascular Imaging (EACVI) and Polish guidelines at the time of patient enrollment [17].

2.4. Statistical Analysis

Continuous variables are presented as means and standard deviations (SD) or medians and interquartile ranges, as appropriate, and were compared using the Student's t-test or the Mann–Whitney U test. Categorical variables are expressed as absolute numbers and frequencies and were compared with the chi-square test, including Yates' correction for continuity or Fisher's exact test. The graphic presentation of the long-term premature ventricular contraction ablation success is shown using Kaplan–Meier curves, which were compared using the log-rank test. All statistical tests were 2-tailed, and a $p < 0.05$ was considered statistically significant. Data were analyzed using IBM SPSS Statistics Version 25.0 software (IBM Corp, Armonk, NY, USA).

3. Results

3.1. Baseline Patients' Characteristic

The study included 102 patients, 52 (50.9%) had CFS guided RFCA and 50 (49.1%) RFCA using standard catheters. In 2014, only standard catheters were used for RFCA, but from 2016, CFS catheters started to be used more often than standard ones. The distribution of used catheter types during the years is presented in Figure 2.

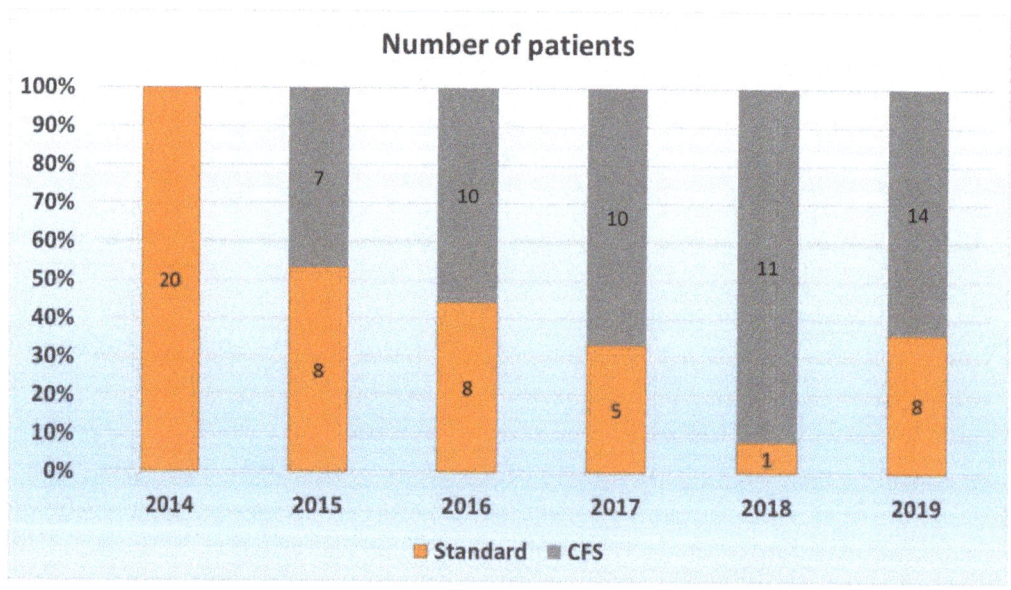

Figure 2. Distribution of ablation catheters type over time. Abbreviations: CFS—contact force-sensing.

The mean age of the patients was 43.4 years (SD 14.8); 63 (61.8%) were female. PVCs were originating from RVOT and LVOT in 70 (68.6%) and 32 (31.4%) patients, respectively. In 17 cases (16.7%), the procedure was performed as a re-do ablation (5 cases (10.0%) in standard group and 12 cases (23.1%) in CFS group, $p = 0.132$). The patients' age, comorbidities such as hypertension, coronary artery disease, and diabetes mellitus, and history of AF and medical therapy at baseline and during follow-up were similar in CFS and standard catheter groups. Detailed patients' baseline characteristics are presented in Table 1.

Table 1. Patient characteristics.

Variable	Total (n = 102)	Standard Catheter Ablation (n = 50)	CFS Catheter Ablation (n = 52)	p-Value
Age (years)	42.0 (32.7–55.0)	42.0 (32.7–53.5)	42.0 (32.2–55.7)	p = 0.987
Female, n (%)	63 (61.8)	29 (58.0)	34 (65.4)	p = 0.443
RVOT PVCs origin, n (%)	70 (68.6)	35 (70)	35 (67.3)	p = 0.770
LVOT PVCs origin, n (%)	32 (31.4)	15 (30)	17 (32.7)	
Hypertension, n (%)	27 (26.5)	13 (26.0)	14 (26.9)	p = 0.916
History of CAD, n (%)	12 (11.8)	6 (12.0)	6 (11.5)	p = 0.942
Diabetes mellitus, n (%)	5 (4.9)	4 (8.0)	1 (1.9)	p = 0.200
Presence of CIED, n (%)	2 (2.0)	2 (4.0)	0 (0.0)	p = 0.238
History of AF, n (%)	2 (2.0)	0 (0.0)	2 (3.8)	p = 0.495
Invasive correction of atrial septal defect *, n (%)	2 (2.0)	1 (2.0)	1 (1.9)	p > 0.99
Beta blocker, n (%)	26 (25.5)	12 (24.0)	14 (26.9)	p = 0.735
Calcium-channel blocker **, n (%)	3 (2.9)	2 (4.0)	1 (1.9)	p = 0.614
Propafenone, n (%)	11 (10.8)	7 (14.0)	4 (7.7)	p = 0.305
Number of antiarrhythmic drugs after ablation	0.0 (0.0–1.0)	0.0 (0.0–1.0)	0.0 (0.0–1.0)	p = 0.605

Data are presented as median (Q1–Q3) or number (percentage). Abbreviations: AF—atrial fibrillation; BMI—body mass index, CAD—coronary artery disease; CIED—cardiac implantable electronic device; CFS—contact force-sensing. * Interatrial septal occluder or surgical correction, ** Verapamil or diltiazem.

3.2. Procedural Characteristic and Ablation Effectiveness

The median procedural time was 85 min (Q1–Q3 65.0–100.7 min) and was significantly longer in the CFS group (90.0 min, Q1–Q3 70.0–120.0 min) compared with the standard catheter group (80.0 min, Q1–Q3 65.0–90.0 min) ($p = 0.029$). Notably, neither the site of the procedure (RVOT/LVOT) nor procedural time varied significantly between groups (Table 2).

Table 2. Procedural parameters and complications.

Parameter	Total (n = 102)	Standard Catheter Ablation (n = 50)	CFS Catheter Ablation (n = 52)	p-Value
Duration of procedure (min)	85.0 (65.0–100.7)	80.0 (65.0–90.0)	90.0 (70.0–120.0)	p = 0.029
Duration of procedure in only RVOT ablation site (min)	80.0 (60.0–106.2)	70.0 (65.0–85.0)	85.0 (60.0–120.0)	p = 0.074
Duration of procedure in only LVOT ablation site (min)	90.0 (76.2–100.0)	90.0 (75.0–96.0)	96.0 (76.0–125.0)	p = 0.261
Re-ablation at baseline, n (%)	17 (16.7)	5 (10)	12 (23.1)	p = 0.132
Use of isoproterenol, n (%)	21 (20.6)	11 (22.0)	10 (19.2)	p = 0.730
Overall acute success, n (%)	98 (96.1)	48 (96.0)	50 (96.2)	p > 0.99
RVOT acute success, n (%)	68 (97.1)	34 (97.1)	34 (97.1)	p > 0.99
LVOT acute success, n (%)	30 (93.7)	14 (93.3%)	16 (94.1)	p > 0.99
Overall long-term success, n (%)	87 (85.3)	41 (82.0)	46 (88.5)	p = 0.357
RVOT long-term success, n (%)	61 (87.1)	29 (82.9)	32 (91.4)	p = 0.477
LVOT long-term success, n (%)	26 (81.2)	12 (80.0)	14 (82.3)	p > 0.99
Complications, n (%)	3 (2.9)	2 (4.0)	1 (1.9)	p = 0.614
Duration of follow-up (months)	52.5 (34.5–69.5)	69.5 (46.2–77.5)	40.0 (24.0–56.7)	p < 0.001

Data are presented as median (Q1–Q3) or number (percentage). Abbreviations: CFS—contact force-sensing; LVOT—left ventricular outflow tract; RVOT—right ventricular outflow tract.

The overall acute success was 96.1% ($n = 98$), and it did not differ between CFS (96.2%) and standard (96.0%) RFCA ($p > 0.99$) in the whole group and in patients with RVOT or LVOT arrhythmia origin considered separately (Table 2 and Figure 3).

In the follow-up of 51.3 months (SD 21.6 months), long-term success was achieved in 85.3% ($n = 87$) of patients, and there was no difference between patients ablated using CFS (88.5%) and standard (82.0%) catheters ($p = 0.357$). The long-term success of RFCA was similar in CFS and the standard catheter group and did not depend on LVOT or RVOT PVCs origin (Figure 4).

In addition, there was no significant difference in long-term success between standard and CFS catheters (Figure 5).

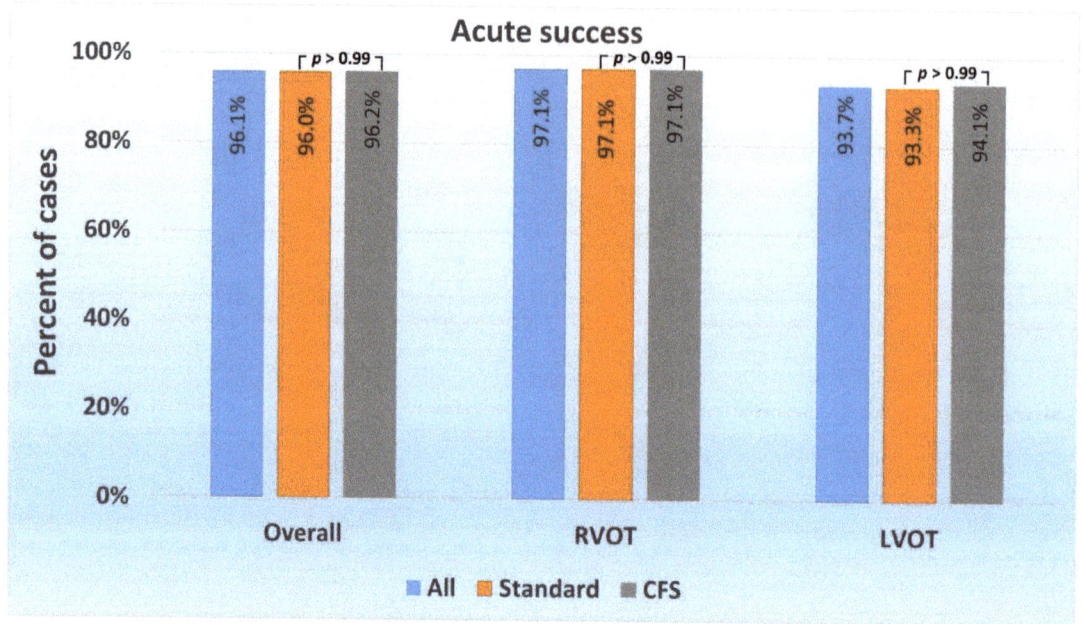

Figure 3. Premature ventricular contraction ablation acute success according to catheter type and arrhythmia localization. Abbreviations: CFS—contact force-sensing; LVOT—left ventricular outflow tract; RVOT—right ventricular outflow tract.

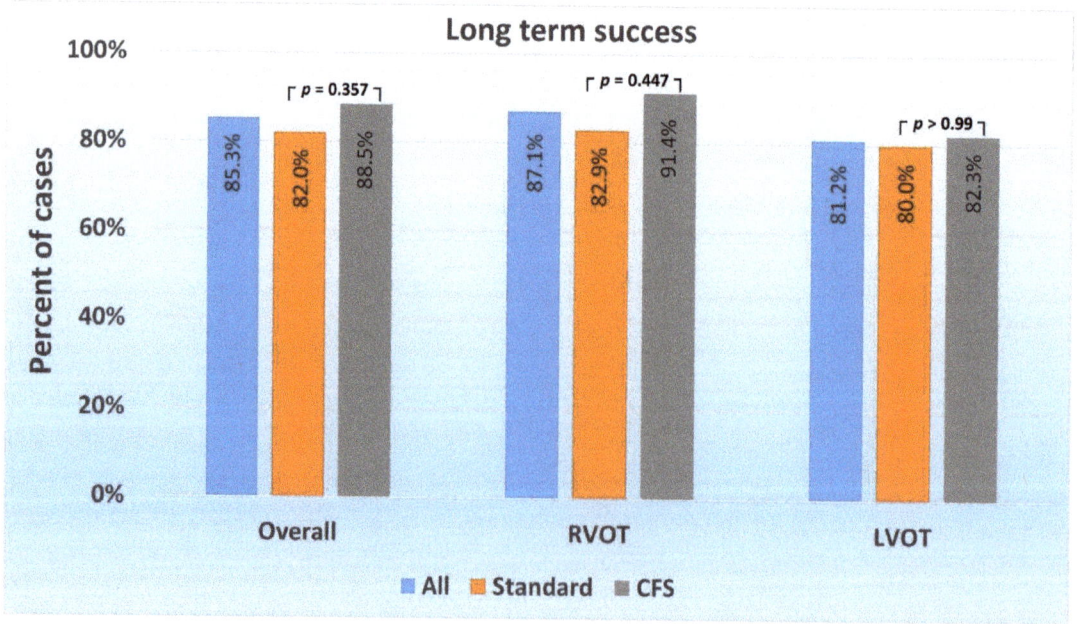

Figure 4. Premature ventricular contraction ablation long-term success according to catheter type and arrhythmia localization. Abbreviations: CFS—contact force-sensing; LVOT—left ventricular outflow tract; RVOT—right ventricular outflow tract.

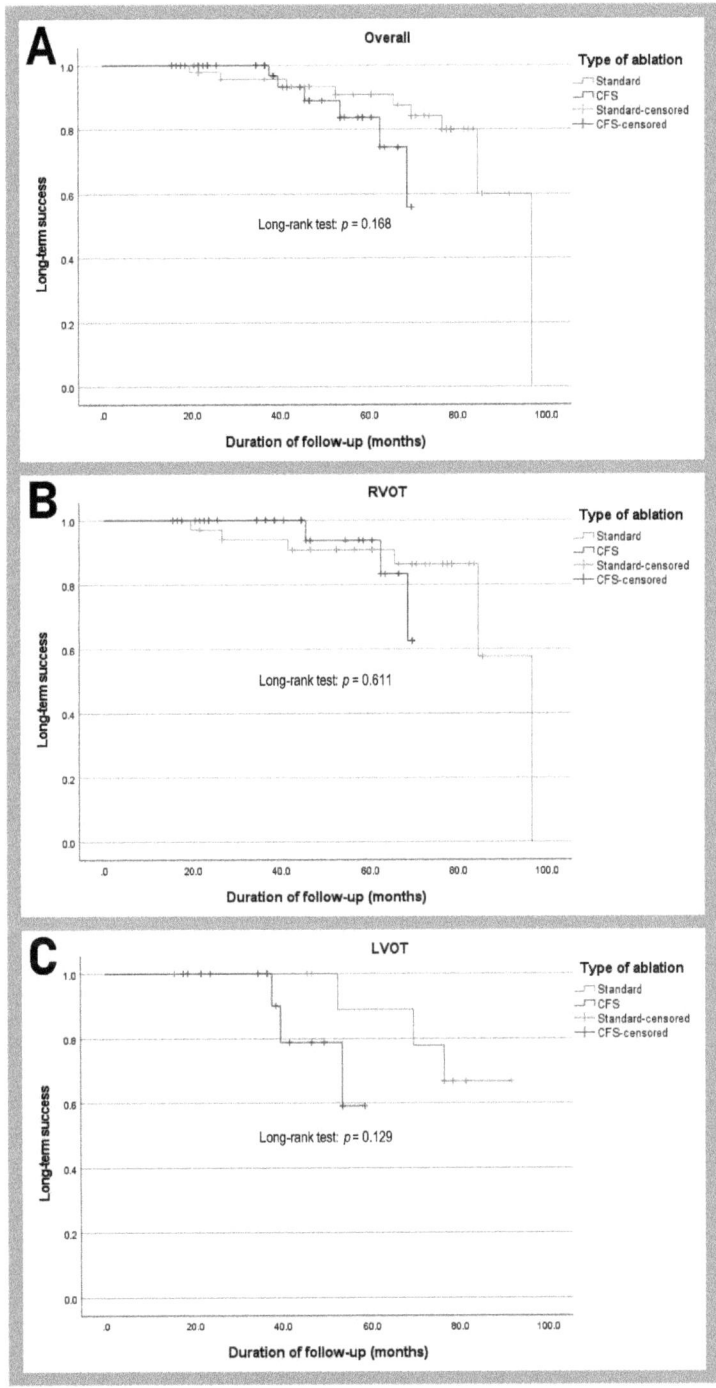

Figure 5. Kaplan–Meier curves of the long-term ablation success of the premature ventricular contractions according to catheter type and arrhythmia localization. (**A**) overall, (**B**) RVOT group, (**C**) LVOT group. Abbreviations: CFS—contact force-sensing; LVOT—left ventricular outflow tract; RVOT—right ventricular outflow tract.

However, the median follow-up was significantly shorter in the CFS group than in the standard catheter group (40.0 months vs. 69.5 months, $p < 0.001$). Detailed results are presented in Table 2.

3.3. Complications

There was no difference in complication rate between CFS and standard catheter ablations ($p > 0.99$). However, there were three (2.9%) major perioperative complications: one pseudoaneurysm after femoral artery access in standard catheters group (treated by thrombin injection) and two patients developed pericarditis in CFS catheters group. In one case after ablation in the aortic root and in the second case after ablation in the tricuspid valve region. In one case, pericarditis required pharmacotherapy. In the second case, despite medication use (ibuprofen and colchicine), the patient required pericardiocentesis two weeks later due to the symptomatic pericardial effusion (sub-acute perforation could not be excluded).

4. Discussion

To the best of our knowledge, this is the first study evaluating the role of CFS catheters in RFCA OT-VAs without fluoroscopy. Recent publications have demonstrated the safety and efficacy of NF-RFCA in OT arrhythmias, but the role of CFS catheters in this setting is unknown [1,4,5]. The results of our study show no advantages of CFS over standard catheters in NF-RFCA of OT-VAs, in keeping with previous publications concerning the same arrhythmia type but performed with fluoroscopy guidance [14,15,18]. Reichlin et al. [14] and Abraham et al. [15] compared the effectiveness and safety of CFS vs. standard catheters and showed similar outcomes in LVOT and RVOT arrhythmia ablation. In other studies, the use of CFS catheters only shortened a procedural, fluoroscopy and ablation time [18]. Conversely, we observed a longer procedural time in the CFS guidance group which might be explained by often time-consuming attempts to achieve intended CF (>10 g) with relatively stiffer CFS catheters compared to standard ones and also time needed for CFS catheters calibration, which should be done after CFS catheter introduction and every time when the operator makes a decision to map and/or ablate another ventricle during NF-RFCA of OT-VAs. Nevertheless, the lack of apparent benefit of CFS catheters in OT-VAs seems surprising if we consider the well-studied advantages of CFS catheters in RFCA of AF. TOCCATA [19] was the first study that showed the value of optimal CF on pulmonary vein isolation effectiveness. All patients treated with an average CF of <10 g experienced AF recurrences, unlike patients with CF > 20 g who were free of AF in 12-month follow-up. Furthermore, TOCCASTAR, a prospective randomized multicenter trial, confirmed the usefulness of CFS catheters and the correlation between optimal CF and pulmonary vein isolation effectiveness. Notably, the improved procedural outcomes were evident when >90% of applications were in the optimal range with a minimum of 10 g. For VA ablation there is lack of such strong data indicating a clear CF cut off needed for procedural outcome improvement. In a recent retrospective study by Abraham et al. [15] (CFS catheters $n = 75$ vs. standard catheters $n = 75$), the median CF was 12.0 (9.5–18.5) g and did not differ significantly between acute success and failure. Larger studies regarding optimal CF in VAs ablation would be valuable. Besides CF value, used CFS catheters provide information on catheter tip direction and angle in relation to cardiac tissue (pointing vector). Standard catheters, used in the current study, show only the information on tip direction relative to the operator coded by color of the catheter, which is less intuitive and clear.

Acute and long-term pulmonary vein isolation efficiency depends mainly on durable, transmural and continuous (dense) ablation lines in the left atrium, while a fundamental goal is an optimal lesion formation for RF ablation. Distinctly for idiopathic OT-VAs, lesion transmurality is not usually necessary for ablation success. Moreover, it is nearly impossible to achieve it even with a high CF. Additionally, a curvier catheter route to RVOT or LVOT and, connected with it, more difficult mapping process compared to transseptal (straight) left atrium access might favor stiffer CFS catheters in AF ablations. Based on the present findings and recently published data, we speculate that the most critical step in idiopathic OT-VAs is a very detailed mapping process. It appears that CFS guidance impacts neither this process nor RF application efficiency to a significant degree. However, in a case of questionable PVC origin (RVOT or LVOT), information of appropriate CF during unsuccessful RF application might be useful, pointing towards the necessity for further mapping in other localizations (another OT) or use of an epicardial approach due to deep (from the endocardium) PVC origin. The epicardial region is mainly reached via the venous system using a coronary sinus. Deep arrhythmia foci rarely require ablation from the left and right OTs or with simultaneous bipolar ablation. In contrast, during substrate mapping in patients with structural heart disease, point acquisition requires sufficient CF to create an adequate voltage map without false low-voltage zones [20]. The minimum value of optimal CF during the systolic/diastolic phase (to obtain contact) has been estimated at 9 g and 8 g for RV and LV, respectively [20].

The CFS technology should also provide safety during RFCA. In NF-RFCA the operator relies only on catheter visualization in 3 D mapping systems and information of real-time CF might be potentially very important. Excessive CF during mapping and ablation might produce cardiac or vessel injury leading to massive bleeding or tamponade. Those major complications are rare but potentially life-threatening. Real-time CF measurement gives the operators (especially those inexperienced) confidence throughout the process of catheter insertion, mapping and RF application, mainly when RFCA is performed without fluoroscopy guidance, but we showed that it did not impact on procedural safety. Standard catheters are less stiff and more steerable with the right level the CF information. In an ex vivo swine model study, Shah et al. [21] defined lower minimum perforating forces in the right and left ventricle, at 159 g and 227 g, respectively. Those values were lower in previously ablated tissue, and, additionally, time to perforation was shorter when catheters were introduced by a steerable long sheath [21]. Otherwise, in VAs ablations, increasing CF and power during RF application might cause steam pops and lead to cardiac perforation, embolic stroke and ventricular septal defect, which have been reported to be more likely than mechanical perforation [22,23].

According to Akca et al.'s meta-analysis concerning different types of ablations, the impact of CFS catheters on procedural safety was demonstrated only in AF [24]. Additionally, in the TOCCATA study, cardiac perforation was linked to excessive CF based on blinded CFS measurements [19]. On the contrary, in previously published data and our study results, there is no evidence of the significant implication of the CFS catheter on safety during ventricular RFCA, independent of the presence of structural heart disease, arrhythmia localization, or fluoroscopy use [14,15,18,24–26]. Novel techniques are introduced in cardiac electrophysiology [27]. The use of non-fluoroscopic imaging during catheter ablation is more frequently used than before [28,29]. It may be speculated that CFS catheters might be of special value in this setting in patients with congenital heart disease, while in the case of ventricular arrhythmias originating from left ventricle, there may be limited additional benefit in patients with left ventricular hypertrophy.

Limitations of the Study

The primary study limitation is a relatively small patient group (especially those with LVOT PVCs origin). There was a trend towards higher success rate using CFS catheters during RVOT-VA ablations, which was not statistically significant probably due to a relatively small group of investigated patients. The study had retrospective design and there was no randomization of ablations using CFS catheters and standard catheters. Furthermore, an important limitation of this study was that the decision of using CFS or standard catheters was based on the choice of each operator. The proportion of CFS catheters has generally increased during recent years and is not equal to standard catheters in particular years. Additionally, there is no information on CF during applications but only the targeted value of optimal contact and the number of RF applications in both groups (power and time settings were the same).

5. Conclusions

The results of our study show no additional advantages of CFS catheters during NF-RFCA of OT-VAs compared to standard catheters regarding procedural effectiveness and safety.

Author Contributions: Conceptualization, G.K., M.K.; methodology, G.K, M.K., E.K. and A.Z.; formal analysis, G.K., A.Z. and P.T.M.; investigation, G.K., M.K., E.K.; resources, G.K., M.K., A.Z., E.K.; data curation; G.K., M.K.; writing—original draft preparation, G.K., M.K., A.Z., E.K.; writing—review and editing, G.K., M.K., A.Z., E.K., M.D., P.T.M. and J.L.; visualization, G.K., M.K., A.Z.; supervision, A.Z., P.T.M. and J.L.; project administration, G.K.; funding acquisition, G.K., P.T.M., J.L. All authors have read and agreed to the published version of the manuscript.

Funding: This article was supported by the science fund of the John Paul II Hospital, Cracow, Poland (no. FN/25/2021 to P.M.).

Institutional Review Board Statement: The institutional ethics committee approved the study protocol. The study protocol conformed to the ethical guidelines of the 1975 Declaration of Helsinki.

Informed Consent Statement: Not applicable.

Data Availability Statement: The authors confirm that the data supporting the findings of this study are available within the article.

Conflicts of Interest: G.K. and M.K. have received travel expenses coverage and EP training course fee from Biosense Webster (Johnson & Johnson), E.K. has received proctor fee and conference grants form Biosense Webster (Johnson & Johnson). The other authors declare no conflict of interest.

References

1. Zhu, T.Y.; Liu, S.R.; Chen, Y.Y.; Xie, L.Z.; He, L.W.; Meng, S.R.; Peng, J. Zero-fluoroscopy catheter ablation for idiopathic premature ventricular contractions from the aortic sinus cusp. *Nan Fang Yi Ke Da Xue Xue Bao* **2016**, *36*, 1105–1109. [PubMed]
2. Koźluk, E.; Gawrysiak, M.; Piątkowska, A.; Lodziński, P.; Kiliszek, M.; Małkowska, S.; Zaczek, R.; Piątkowski, R.; Opolski, G.; Kozłowski, D. Radiofrequency ablation without the use of fluoroscopy—In what kind of patients is it feasible? *Arch. Med. Sci.* **2013**, *9*, 821–825. [CrossRef] [PubMed]
3. Kozluk, E.; Rodkiewicz, D.; Piątkowska, A.; Opolski, G. Safety and efficacy of cryoablation without the use of fluoroscopy. *Cardiol. J.* **2018**, *25*, 327–332. [CrossRef] [PubMed]
4. Styczkiewicz, K.; Ludwik, B.; Śledź, J.; Lipczyńska, M.; Zaborska, B.; Kryński, T.; Deutsch, K.; Morka, A.; Kukla, P.; Styczkiewicz, M.; et al. Long-term Follow-Up and Comparison of Techniques in Radiofrequency Ablation of Ventricular Arrhythmias Originating from the Aortic Cusps (AVATAR Registry). *Pol. Arch. Intern Med.* **2019**, *29*, 399–407. [CrossRef]
5. Karkowski, G.; Kuniewicz, M.; Koźluk, E.; Chyży, T.; Ząbek, A.; Dusza, M.; Lelakowski, J. Non-fluoroscopic radiofrequency catheter ablation of right and left sided ventricular arrhythmias. *Postepy Kardiol. Interwencyjnej* **2020**, *16*, 321–329. [CrossRef]
6. Zheng, X.; Walcott, G.P.; Hall, J.A.; Rollins, D.L.; Smith, W.M.; Kay, G.N.; Ideker, R.E. Electrode impedance: An indicator of electrode-tissue contact and lesion dimensions during linear ablation. *J. Interv. Card. Electrophysiol.* **2000**, *4*, 645–654. [CrossRef]
7. Wittkampf, F.H.M.; Nakagawa, H. RF catheter ablation: Lessons and lesions. *Pacing Clin. Electrophysiol.* **2006**, *29*, 1285–1297. [CrossRef]
8. Kumar, S.; Morton, J.B.; Lee, G.; Halloran, K.; Kistler, P.M.; Kalman, J.M. High incidence of low catheter-tissue contact force at the cavotricuspid isthmus during catheter ablation of atrial flutter: Implications for achieving isthmus block. *J. Cardiovasc. Electrophysiol.* **2015**, *26*, 826–831. [CrossRef]
9. Yokoyama, K.; Nakagawa, H.; Shah, D.C.; Lambert, H.; Leo, G.; Aeby, N.; Ikeda, A.; Pitha, J.V.; Sharma, T.; Lazzara, R.; et al. Novel Contact Force Sensor Incorporated in Irrigated Radiofrequency Ablation Catheter Predicts Lesion Size and Incidence of Steam Pop and Thrombus. *Circ. Arrhythm. Electrophysiol.* **2008**, *1*, 354–362. [CrossRef]
10. Seiler, J.; Roberts-Thomson, K.C.; Raymond, J.M.; Vest, J.; Delacretaz, E.; Stevenson, W.G. Steam pops during irrigated radiofrequency ablation: Feasibility of impedance monitoring for prevention. *Heart Rhythm* **2008**, *5*, 1411–1416. [CrossRef]
11. Sarkozy, A.; Shah, D.; Saenen, J.; Sieira, J.; Phlips, T.; Boris, W.; Namdar, M.; Vrints, C. Contact force in atrial fibrillation: Role of atrial rhythm and ventricular contractions: Co-Force Atrial Fibrillation Study. *Circ. Arrhythm. Electrophysiol.* **2015**, *8*, 1342–1350. [CrossRef] [PubMed]
12. Lin, H.; Chen, Y.H.; Hou, J.W.; Lu, Z.Y.; Xiang, Y.; Li, Y.G. Role of contact force-guided radiofrequency catheter ablation for treatment of atrial fibrillation: A systematic review and meta-analysis. *J. Cardiovasc. Electrophysiol.* **2017**, *28*, 994–1005. [CrossRef] [PubMed]
13. Reddy, V.Y.; Dukkipati, S.R.; Neuzil, P.; Natale, A.; Albenque, J.P.; Kautzner, J.; Shah, D.; Michaud, G.; Wharton, M.; Harari, D.; et al. Randomized, Controlled Trial of the Safety and Effectiveness of a Contact Force-Sensing Irrigated Catheter for Ablation of Paroxysmal Atrial Fibrillation: Results of the TactiCath Contact Force Ablation Catheter Study for Atrial Fibrillation (TOCCASTAR) Study. *Circulation* **2015**, *132*, 907–915. [CrossRef]

14. Zhou, J.; Qu, F.; Sang, X.; Wang, X.; Nan, R. Impact of contact force sensing technology on outcome of catheter ablation of idiopathic premature ventricular contractions originating from the outflow tracts. *Europace* **2021**, *23*, 603–609. [CrossRef]
15. Ábrahám, P.; Ambrus, M.; Herczeg, S.; Szegedi, N.; Nagy, K.V.; Salló, Z.; Osztheimer, I.; Széplaki, G.; Tahin, T.; Merkely, B.; et al. Similar outcomes with manual contact force ablation catheters and traditional catheters in the treatment of outflow tract premature ventricular complexes. *Europace* **2021**, *23*, 596–602. [CrossRef] [PubMed]
16. Baranowski, R.; Bieganowska, K.; Cygankiewicz, I.; Guzik, P.; Kurpesa, M.; Lelonek, M.; Maciejewska, M.; Miszczak-Knecht, M.; Piotrowicz, E.; Szydło, K.; et al. Wytyczne dotyczące wykonywania długotrwałych rejestracji EKG. Stanowisko grupy ekspertów Sekcji Elektrokardiologii Nieinwazyjnej i Telemedycyny Polskiego Towarzystwa Kardiologicznego. *Kardiol. Pol.* **2013**, *71* (Suppl. IX), 225–241. (In Polish) [CrossRef]
17. Steeds, R.P.; Garbi, M.; Cardim, N.; Kasprzak, J.D.; Sade, E.; Nihoyannopoulos, P.; Popescu, B.A.; Stefanidis, A.; Cosyns, B.; Monaghan, M.; et al. 2014–2016 EACVI Scientific Documents Committee; 2014–2016 EACVI Scientific Documents Committee. EACVI appropriateness criteria for the use of transthoracic echocardiography in adults: A report of literature and current practice review. *Eur. Heart J. Cardiovasc. Imaging* **2017**, *18*, 1191–1204. [CrossRef]
18. Zhao, Z.; Liu, X.; Gao, L.; Xi, Y.; Chen, Q.; Chang, D.; Xiao, X.; Cheng, J.; Yang, Y.; Xia, Y.; et al. Benefit of contact force–guided catheter ablation for treating premature ventricular contractions. *Tex. Heart Inst. J.* **2020**, *47*, 3–9. [CrossRef]
19. Reddy, V.Y.; Shah, D.; Kautzner, J.; Schmidt, B.; Saoudi, N.; Herrera, C.; Jaïs, P.; Hindricks, G.; Peichl, P.; Yulzari, A.; et al. The relationship between contact force and clinical outcome during radiofrequency catheter ablation of atrial fibrillation in the Toccata study. *Heart Rhythm* **2012**, *9*, 1789–1795. [CrossRef]
20. Mizuno, H.; Vergara, P.; Maccabelli, G.; Trevisi, N.; Eng, S.C.; Brombin, C.; Mazzone, P.; Della Bella, P. Contact force monitoring for cardiac mapping in patients with ventricular tachycardia. *J. Cardiovasc. Electrophysiol.* **2013**, *24*, 519–524. [CrossRef]
21. Shah, D.; Lambert, H.; Langenkamp, A.; Vanenkov, Y.; Leo, G.; Gentil-Baron, P.; Walpoth, B. Catheter tip force required for mechanical perforation of porcine cardiac chambers. *Europace* **2011**, *13*, 277–283. [CrossRef] [PubMed]
22. Ikeda, A.; Nakagawa, H.; Lambert, H.; Shah, D.C.; Fonck, E.; Yulzari, A.; Sharma, T.; Pitha, J.V.; Lazzara, R.; Jackman, W.M. Relationship between catheter contact force and radiofrequency lesion size and incidence of steam pop in the beating canine heart: Electrogram amplitude, impedance, and electrode temperature are poor predictors of electrode-tissue contact force and lesion size. *Circ. Arrhythm. Electrophysiol.* **2014**, *7*, 1174–1180. [PubMed]
23. Schönbauer, R.; Sommer, P.; Misfeld, M.; Dinov, B.; Fiedler, L.; Huo, Y.; Gaspar, T.; Breithardt, O.A.; Hindricks, G.; Arya, A. Relevant ventricular septal defect caused by steam pop during ablation of premature ventricular contraction. *Circulation* **2013**, *127*, e843. [CrossRef] [PubMed]
24. Akca, F.; Janse, P.; Theuns, D.A.; Szili-Torok, T. A prospective study on safety of catheter ablation procedures: Contact force guided ablation could reduce the risk of cardiac perforation. *Int. J. Cardiol.* **2015**, *179*, 441–448. [CrossRef] [PubMed]
25. Capulzini, L.; Vergara, P.; Mugnai, G.; Salghetti, F.; Abugattas, J.P.; El Bouchaibi, S.; Iacopino, S.; Sieira, J.; Enriquez Coutiño, H.; Ströker, E.; et al. Acute and one year outcome of premature ventricular contraction ablation guided by contact force and automated pacemapping software. *J. Arrhythm.* **2019**, *35*, 542–549. [CrossRef] [PubMed]
26. Hendriks, A.A.; Akca, F.; Dabiri Abkenari, L.; Khan, M.; Bhagwandien, R.; Yap, S.C.; Wijchers, S.; Szili-Torok, T. Safety and Clinical Outcome of Catheter Ablation of Ventricular Arrhythmias Using Contact Force Sensing. *J. Cardiovasc. Electrophysiol.* **2015**, *26*, 1224–1229. [CrossRef]
27. Guckel, D.; Niemann, S.; Ditzhaus, M.; Molatta, S.; Bergau, L.; Fink, T.; Sciacca, V.; El Hamriti, M.; Imnadze, G.; Steinhauer, P.; et al. Long-Term Efficacy and Impact on Mortality of Remote Magnetic Navigation Guided Catheter Ablation of Ventricular Arrhythmias. *J. Clin. Med.* **2021**, *10*, 4695. [CrossRef]
28. Deutsch, K.; Ciurzyński, M.; Śledź, J.; Zienciuk-Krajka, A.; Mazij, M.; Ludwik, B.; Stec, P.; Wileczek, A.; Pruszczyk, P.; Stec, S. Association between the geographic region and the risk of familial atrioventricular nodal reentrant tachycardia in the Polish population. *Pol. Arch. Intern Med.* **2021**, *131*. [CrossRef]
29. Fadhle, A.; Hu, M.; Wang, Y. The safety and efficacy of zero-fluoroscopy ablation versus conventional ablation in patients with supraventricular tachycardia. *Kardiol. Pol.* **2020**, *78*, 552–558. [CrossRef]

Article

In-Hospital and One-Year Outcomes of Patients after Early and Late Resuscitated Cardiac Arrest Complicating Acute Myocardial Infarction—Data from a Nationwide Database

Robert Kowalik [1,†], Marek Gierlotka [2,†], Krzysztof Ozierański [1,*], Przemysław Trzeciak [3], Anna Fojt [1], Piotr Feusette [2], Agnieszka Tycińska [4], Grzegorz Opolski [1], Marcin Grabowski [1] and Mariusz Gąsior [3]

1. First Department of Cardiology, Medical University of Warsaw, 02-097 Warsaw, Poland; rjkowalik@wp.pl (R.K.); anna.fojt@o2.pl (A.F.); grzegorz.opolski@wum.edu.pl (G.O.); marcin.grabowski@wum.edu.pl (M.G.)
2. Department of Cardiology, Institute of Medical Sciences, University of Opole, 45-401 Opole, Poland; marek.gierlotka@gmail.com (M.G.); feusette@wp.pl (P.F.)
3. 3rd Department of Cardiology, Faculty of Medical Sciences in Zabrze, Silesian Centre for Heart Diseases in Zabrze, Medical University of Silesia in Katowice, 41-800 Zabrze, Poland; przemyslaw.t@wp.pl (P.T.); m.gasior@op.pl (M.G.)
4. Department of Cardiology, Medical University of Bialystok, 15-276 Bialystok, Poland; agnieszka.tycinska@gmail.com
* Correspondence: krzysztof.ozieranski@wum.edu.pl; Tel.: +48-22-599-2958; Fax: +48-22-599-1957
† These authors contributed equally to this work.

Abstract: The prognostic role of early (less than 48 h) resuscitated cardiac arrest (ErCA) complicating acute myocardial infarction (AMI) is still controversial. The present study aimed to analyse the short-term and one-year outcomes of patients after ErCA and late resuscitated cardiac arrest (LrCA) compared to patients without cardiac arrest (CA) complicating AMI. Data from the prospective nationwide Polish Registry of Acute Coronary Syndromes (PL-ACS) were used to assess patients with resuscitated cardiac arrest (rCA) after AMI. Baseline clinical characteristics and the predictors of all-cause death were assessed. The all-cause mortality rate, complications, performed procedures, and re-hospitalisations were assessed for the in-hospital period, 30 days after discharge, and 6- and 12-month follow-ups. Among 167,621 cases of AMI, CA occurred in 3564 (2.1%) patients, that is, 3100 (87%) and 464 (13%) patients with ErCA and LrCA, respectively. The mortality rates in the ErCA vs. LrCA and CA vs. non-CA groups were as follows: in-hospital: 32.1% vs. 59.1% ($p < 0.0001$) and 35.6% vs. 6.0% ($p < 0.0001$); 30-day: 2.2% vs. 3.2% ($p = 0.42$) and 9.9% vs. 5.2% ($p < 0.0001$); 6-month: 9.2% vs. 17.9% ($p = 0.0001$) and 12.3% vs. 21.1% ($p < 0.0001$); and 12-month: 12.3% vs. 21.1% ($p = 0.001$) and 13% vs. 7.7% ($p < 0.0001$), respectively. ErCA (hazard ratio (HR): 1.54, confidence interval (CI):1.28–1.89, $p < 0.0001$) and LrCA (HR: 2.34, CI: 1.39–3.93; $p = 0.001$) increased the risk of 12-month mortality. During the 12-month follow-up, patients after LrCA more frequently required hospitalisation due to heart failure compared to patients after ErCA. ErCA was related to a higher hospitalisation rate due to coronary-related causes and a higher rate of percutaneous coronary intervention. An episode of LrCA was associated with higher in-hospital and long-term mortality compared to ErCA. ErCA and LrCA were independent risk factors for one-year mortality.

Keywords: acute coronary syndrome; cardiac rehabilitation; sudden cardiac death; life-threatening ventricular arrhythmia; early and late cardiac arrest; secondary prevention of sudden cardiac death

1. Introduction

In recent decades, the incidence of cardiac arrest (CA) prior to hospital admission has decreased due to the fast reperfusion strategy and pharmacotherapy [1,2]. Despite this, acute myocardial infarction (AMI) is still the leading cause of life-threatening ventricular arrhythmias and CA [1,3,4]. Approximately 6–8% of patients develop hemodynamically unstable sustained ventricular tachycardia (VT) or ventricular fibrillation (VF) during the acute phase of AMI [1]. The predictors of CA differ regarding the time after AMI onset [5]. The in-hospital mortality rate of AMI is 10.5%, and it depends mainly on age and baseline clinical presentation (e.g., signs of heart failure, completeness of coronary revascularisation, and the occurrence of CA) [6]. CA requires an early introduction of guideline-recommended therapy and qualification for an implantable cardioverter–defibrillator (ICD) for the secondary prevention of sudden cardiac death (SCD), usually in patients presenting with CA occurring 48 h after AMI onset [1]. The available data suggest that patients after resuscitated CA (rCA) during hospitalisation for AMI are at a higher risk of in-hospital and post-discharge adverse events [7]. However, the prognostic role of early rCA (ErCA) (less than 48 h from the onset of AMI), particularly in long-term observations, is still controversial, and new biomarkers could improve risk stratification [8]. It is postulated that early CA is related to possible reversible causes of CA, such as acute ischemia, acute heart failure, and/or electrolyte disturbances, inducing malignant ventricular arrhythmia, and it has no impact on long-term prognosis, similar to patients without a CA episode [9].

Further data on the significance of ErCA are warranted for better early and long-term risk stratification. The present study aimed to compare the short-term and 12-month outcomes of patients after ErCA and late rCA (LrCA) to patients without CA complicating AMI.

2. Methods

2.1. Study Design

Data from the prospective nationwide Polish Registry of Acute Coronary Syndromes (PL-ACS) from 2005 to 2014 were used for the analysis. The registry was designed to gather comprehensive data on the management and long-term outcomes of AMI patients in Poland. A detailed description of the database and the methods used have been previously published [10]. In brief, the ongoing registry is linked to the government and National Health Fund data, which is the only public healthcare insurer in Poland. Data were collected using questionnaires, including demographics, medical history, clinical condition on admission, type of AMI, related procedures, and treatment. The all-cause mortality rate was assessed for the in-hospital period, 30 days after discharge, and 6-month and 12-month follow-ups. At the one-year follow-up, data on re-hospitalisations (e.g., heart failure, recurrent AMI or CA, stroke), procedures (e.g., coronary angiography, percutaneous coronary intervention (PCI), coronary artery bypass grafting (CABG), ablation, cardiac device implantation), and cardiac rehabilitation were gathered. For one-year outcome analyses, only patients with CA after AMI, who survived the index hospitalisation, were included. All analyses were performed for patients with CA (ErCA and LrCA), as well as for patients without CA complicating AMI.

The present study is a retrospective analysis of the prospective Polish Registry of Acute Coronary Syndromes (PL-ACS), which is a nationwide official government registry within the Polish health system: https://isap.sejm.gov.pl/isap.nsf/DocDetails.xsp?id=WDU20180001063 (accessed on 2 December 2021). Therefore, official approval of the study was not required from the Ethics Committee.

2.2. Definitions

ErCA patients were defined as those with CA within the first 48 h of AMI onset, regardless of whether the CA appeared during the pre-hospital or in-hospital phase. LrCA patients were defined as those with CA after the first 48 h of the onset of AMI.

2.3. Statistical Analysis

Continuous variables were presented as means (SD) or median values and interquartile ranges (IQRs) and compared between the groups by means of a Student's t-test or Mann–Whitney U test according to data distribution, respectively. Categorical data were presented as numbers of patients and percentages and compared with the use of the χ^2 test with

Pearson modification. Logistic regression was used to define predictors of in-hospital mortality and rCA occurrence during AMI among survivors.

The associations between the analysed groups and follow-up outcomes were analysed using the unadjusted and adjusted Kaplan–Meier method for multiple group comparisons. Adjusted survival and hazard ratios were calculated using the inverse probability method. A p value of less than 0.05 was considered statistically significant. All reported p values are two-sided. Analyses were performed with the use of Statistica version 13 (TIBCO Software Inc., Palo Alto, CA, USA (2017)) and R version 4.0.3 (R Foundation for Statistical Computing, Vienna, Austria).

3. Results

3.1. Study Population

The study included 167,621 cases of AMI from the 2009–2014 period. CA occurred in 3564 (2.1%) patients, that is, 3100 (87%) and 464 (13%) patients with ErCA and LrCA, respectively. Compared to the non-CA group, patients with an rCA episode were younger, more predominantly male, smokers, and more likely to have a diagnosis of STEMI, and they had more intra-hospital complications. In addition, compared to the non-CA group, patients after rCA were more likely to have a history of stroke, ischemic heart disease, and heart failure chronic obstructive pulmonary disease. Patients with rCA less frequently had a history of hypertension, hypercholesterolemia, and a previous AMI compared to the non-CA group (Table S1).

From the ErCA group and the LrCA group, 2106 patients and 190 patients, respectively, survived until discharge from the hospital. There was no difference between the groups regarding gender. The LrCA patients were older (67.9 ($\pm$12.3) vs. 63.1 ($\pm$11.5) years old ($p < 0.001$)), had a lower left ventricular ejection fraction (38 ($\pm$13) vs. 44 ($\pm$12)%), and a longer hospital stay, and they more often required implantation of a pacemaker or ICD during the index hospitalisation compared to the ErCA patients. In the ErCA group, myocardial infarction with ST-segment elevation was more frequent, while in the LrCA group, myocardial infarction without ST-segment elevation was more frequent. The ErCA patients were more likely to have Killip–Kimball class 4 during hospitalisation, as well as coronary angiography. Additionally, the LrCA group had a pulmonary oedema, recurrent AMI, and massive bleeding with blood transfusion episodes more often during the index hospitalisation. Both groups received optimal guideline-recommended therapy. There was no difference in pharmacotherapy at discharge, except for diuretics, vitamin K antagonists, and antidiabetic medications, which were more commonly prescribed in the LrCA group. The detailed clinical characteristics of both groups are presented in Tables 1–4.

Table 1. Baseline clinical characteristics of patients without cardiac arrest and with ErCA and LrCA after acute myocardial infarction (only patients who were discharged after index hospitalisation).

Variable	Non-CA N = 154,266	rCA N = 2296	p Value	ErCA N = 2106	LrCA N = 190	p Value
Age, years, mean (SD)	65.8 (11.9)	63.5 (11.7)	<0.0001	63.1 (11.5)	67.9 (12.3)	<0.0001
Age $\geq$ 65 years	80,187 (52%)	990 (43.1%)	<0.0001	875 (41.6%)	115 (60.5%)	<0.0001
Age $\geq$ 75 years	41,892 (27.2%)	476 (20.7%)	<0.0001	413 (19.6%)	63 (33.2%)	<0.0001
Age $\geq$ 85 years	7548 (4.9%)	68 (3%)	<0.0001	52 (2.5%)	16 (8.4%)	<0.0001
Male gender	98,794 (64.1%)	1578 (68.9%)	<0.0001	1449 (68.9%)	129 (67.9%)	0.77
From home admission	88,130 (57.2%)	1461 (63.7%)	<0.0001	1344 (63.9%)	117 (61.6%)	0.53
Transfer from other hospital	66,041 (42.8%)	834 (36.3%)	<0.0001	761 (36.2%)	73 (38.4%)	0.53
Hipercholesterolemia	64,577 (41.9%)	879 (38.3%)	0.0006	798 (37.9%)	81 (42.6%)	0.2
Hypertension	112,427 (72.9%)	1440 (62.7%)	<0.0001	1311 (62.3%)	129 (67.9%)	0.12
Obesity	31,882 (20.7%)	445 (19.4%)	0.13	402 (19.1%)	43 (22.6%)	0.24
Diabetes mellitus	38,799 (25.9%)	474 (21.5%)	<0.0001	406 (20.1%)	68 (37%)	<0.0001
Smoking (current or past)	91,654 (59.4%)	1480 (64.5%)	<0.0001	1371 (65.1%)	109 (57.4%)	0.033
Current smoker	45,942 (29.8%)	800 (34.8%)	<0.0001	761 (36.1%)	39 (20.5%)	<0.0001

Table 1. Cont.

Variable	Non-CA N = 154,266	rCA N = 2296	p Value	ErCA N = 2106	LrCA N = 190	p Value
Ischemic heart disease diagnosed before AMI	21,800 (14.1%)	394 (17.2%)	<0.0001	347 (16.5%)	47 (24.7%)	0.004
Family history of CAD	17,452 (11.3%)	266 (11.6%)	0.68	239 (11.4%)	27 (14.2%)	0.24
History of heart failure	11,821 (7.7%)	215 (9.4%)	0.002	182 (8.6%)	33 (17.4%)	<0.0001
History of stroke	5689 (3.7%)	114 (5%)	0.001	104 (4.9%)	10 (5.3%)	0.84
Chronic kidney disease	9256 (6%)	149 (6.5%)	0.33	122 (5.8%)	27 (14.2%)	<0.0001
Peripheral artery disease	7026 (4.6%)	122 (5.3%)	0.084	111 (5.3%)	11 (5.8%)	0.76
Chronic obstructive pulmonary disease	6031 (3.9%)	120 (5.2%)	0.0013	107 (5.1%)	13 (6.8%)	0.3
Prior myocardial infarction	19,708 (12.8%)	259 (11.3%)	0.036	364 (17.3%)	39 (20.5%)	0.26
Prior PCI	27,128 (17.6%)	403 (17.6%)	0.97	232 (11%)	27 (14.2%)	0.18
Prior CABG	5090 (3.3%)	80 (3.5%)	0.62	72 (3.4%)	8 (4.2%)	0.57
NSTEMI	83,073 (53.9%)	721 (31.4%)	<0.0001	645 (30.6%)	76 (40%)	0.008
STEMI	71,194 (46.1%)	1575 (68.6%)	<0.0001	1461 (69.4%)	114 (60%)	0.008
CA before admission	0 (0%)	1169 (50.9%)	<0.0001	1160 (55.1%)	9 (4.7%)	<0.0001
ECG heart rate, bpm, mean (SD)	79.1 (24.3)	846 (27.7)	<0.0001	84.3 (27.7)	88 (28.1)	0.078
Sinus rhythm	140,391 (91.6%)	1918 (83.6%)	<0.0001	1775 (84.4%)	143 (75.3%)	0.0012
Atrial fibrillation	8692 (5.7%)	197 (8.6%)	<0.0001	167 (7.9%)	30 (15.8%)	0.0002
Other rhythm	2421 (1.6%)	147 (6.4%)	<0.0001	136 (6.5%)	11 (5.8%)	0.72
Normal QRS	127,755 (83.5%)	1765 (77.4%)	0.0012	1625 (77.7%)	140 (74.1%)	0.25
LBBB	5843 (3.8%)	117 (5.1%)	0.057	106 (5.1%)	11 (5.8%)	0.65
RBBB	5255 (3.4%)	95 (4.2%)	<0.0001	81 (3.9%)	14 (7.4%)	0.02
Other QRS abnormalities	14,184 (9.3%)	303 (13.3%)	<0.0001	279 (13.3%)	24 (12.7%)	0.8
Normal ST segment	12,279 (8%)	79 (3.4%)	<0.0001	66 (3.1%)	13 (6.8%)	0.007
ST-segment elevation	69,412 (45.2%)	1526 (66.5%)	<0.0001	1422 (67.6%)	104 (54.7%)	0.0003
ST-segment depression	36,818 (24%)	359 (15.6%)	<0.0001	320 (15.2%)	39 (20.5%)	0.053
Negative T waves	14,164 (9.2%)	87 (3.8%)	<0.0001	77 (3.7%)	10 (5.3%)	0.27
Other ST-segment abnormalities	19,835 (12.9%)	233 (10.2%)	<0.0001	209 (9.9%)	24 (12.6%)	0.24
Systolic BP, mmHg, median (IQR)	140 (120–155)	120 (100–140)	<0.0001	120 (100–140)	130 (110–142)	0.11
Killip class 1	12,1579 (79.3%)	1217 (53.1%)	<0.0001	1107 (52.6%)	110 (57.9%)	0.16
Killip class 2	20,415 (13.3%)	501 (21.8%)	<0.0001	451 (21.4%)	50 (26.3%)	0.12
Killip class 3	3728 (2.4%)	118 (5.1%)	<0.0001	106 (5%)	12 (6.3%)	0.45
Killip class 4	1988 (1.3%)	370 (16.1%)	<0.0001	361 (17.2%)	9 (4.7%)	<0.0001

Abbreviations: ACE-I—angiotensin-converting enzyme inhibitor; AMI—acute myocardial infarction; ARB—angiotensin receptor blocker; CA—cardiac arrest; CABG—coronary artery bypass grafting; CAD—coronary artery disease; ErCA—early resuscitated cardiac arrest; CRT-D—cardiac resynchronisation therapy defibrillator; CRT-P—cardiac resynchronisation therapy pacemaker; Cx—circumflex artery; IABP—intra-aortic balloon pump; ICD—implantable cardioverter–defibrillator; ECG—electrocardiogram; IQR—interquartile range; LAD—left anterior descending; LBBB—left bundle branch block; LM—left main; LMWH—low-molecular-weight heparin; LrCA—late resuscitated cardiac arrest; NSTEMI—nonST-segment myocardial infarction; PCI—percutaneous coronary intervention; RCA—right coronary artery; RBBB—right bundle branch block; rCA—resuscitated cardiac arrest; SD—standard deviation; STEMI—ST-segment myocardial infarction; TIMI—the thrombolysis in myocardial infarction risk score; VSD—ventricular septal defect.

Table 2. In-hospital treatment and procedures of patients without cardiac arrest and with ErCA and LrCA after acute myocardial infarction (only patients who were discharged after index hospitalisation).

Variable	Non-CA N = 154,266	rCA N = 2296	p Value	ErCA N = 2106	LrCA N = 190	p Value
Thrombolysis	521 (0.4%)	23 (11%)	<0.0001	20 (1%)	3 (1.7%)	0.39
Glycoprotein IIb/IIIa inhibitors	33,532 (21.7%)	881 (38.4%)	0.0032	814 (38.7%)	67 (35.3%)	0.36
Anticoagulation (not associated with PCI)	79,366 (51.8%)	1259 (54.9%)	0.013	1147 (54.5%)	112 (59%)	0.24
Coronary angiography	141,438 (91.7%)	2137 (93.2%)	0.7	1967 (93.5%)	170 (89.5%)	0.036
Infarct-related artery—RCA	42,924 (30.3%)	759 (35.5%)	<0.0001	708 (36%)	51 (30%)	0.2
Infarct-related artery—LM	2877 (2%)	74 (3.5%)	0.00031	63 (3.2%)	11 (6.5%)	0.025
Infarct-related artery—LAD	48,046 (34%)	806 (37.7%)	<0.0001	730 (37.1%)	76 (44.7%)	0.049

Table 2. Cont.

Variable	Non-CA N = 154,266	rCA N = 2296	p Value	ErCA N = 2106	LrCA N = 190	p Value
Infarct-related artery—Cx	27,891 (19.7%)	342 (16%)	0.29	321 (16.3%)	21 (12.4%)	0.18
Infarct-related artery—bypass	1530 (1.1%)	18 (0.8%)	<0.0001	16 (0.8%)	2 (1.2%)	0.62
PCI	118,119 (76.6%)	1956 (85.2%)	<0.0001	1802 (85.6%)	154 (81.1%)	0.096
TIMI 1 before PCI	72,425 (63.1%)	1450 (77.7%)	<0.0001	1344 (78.5%)	106 (68.8%)	0.006
TIMI 3 after PCI	107,885 (93.6%)	1704 (91.3%)	0.044	1569 (91.6%)	135 (87.7%)	0.098
CABG	4297 (2.8%)	48 (2.1%)	<0.0001	46 (2.2%)	2 (1.1%)	0.44
Pacemaker	810 (0.5%)	36 (1.6%)	<0.0001	28 (1.3%)	8 (4.2%)	0.0022
ICD	243 (0.2%)	60 (2.6%)	<0.0001	34 (1.6%)	26 (13.7%)	<0.0001
CRT-D	25 (0%)	7 (0.3%)	<0.0001	6 (0.3%)	1 (0.5%)	0.91
ICD or CRT-D	268 (0.2%)	67 (2.9%)	<0.0001	40 (1.9%)	27 (14.2%)	<0.0001
Blood transfusion	4912 (3.2%)	213 (9.3%)	<0.0001	171 (8.1%)	42 (22.1%)	<0.0001
Ablation	24 (0%)	4 (0.2%)	0.28	4 (0.2%)	0 (0%)	0.76
Heart valve surgery	286 (0.2%)	2 (0.1%)	<0.0001	2 (0.1%)	0 (0%)	0.39
IABP	1382 (0.9%)	167 (7.3%)	<0.0001	150 (7.1%)	17 (9%)	0.35

For abbreviations, see Table 1.

Table 3. In-hospital complications of patients without cardiac arrest and with ErCA and LrCA after acute myocardial infarction (only patients who were discharged after index hospitalisation).

Variable	Non-CA N = 154,266	rCA N = 2296	p Value	ErCA N = 2106	LrCA N = 190	p Value
Massive bleeding	1638 (1.1%)	114 (5%)	<0.0001	93 (4.4%)	21 (11.1%)	<0.0001
Recurrent myocardial infarction	274 (0.2%)	28 (1.2%)	<0.0001	19 (0.9%)	9 (4.7%)	<0.0001
Stroke	241 (0.2%)	31 (1.4%)	<0.0001	29 (1.4%)	2 (1.1%)	0.97
Pulmonary edema	1088 (0.7%)	102 (4.4%)	<0.0001	87 (4.1%)	15 (7.9%)	0.016
Cardiogenic shock	661 (0.4%)	227 (9.9%)	<0.0001	204 (9.7%)	23 (12.1%)	0.28
Hospital CA	0 (0%)	1216 (53.0%)	<0.0001	1026 (48.7%)	190 (100%)	<0.0001
Mechanical complication: heart rupture	28 (0%)	5 (0.2%)	0.0037	4 (0.2%)	1 (0.5%)	0.89
Mechanical complication: mitral regurgitation	42 (0%)	3 (0.1%)	0.54	3 (0.1%)	0 (0%)	0.6
Mechanical complication: VSD	25 (0%)	0 (0%)	<0.0001	0 (0%)	0 (0%)	1.00
Mechanical complication: heart rupture or VSD	51 (0%)	5 (0.2%)	<0.0001	4 (0.2%)	1 (0.5%)	0.89
Mechanical complications (all)	92 (0.1%)	8 (0.4%)	<0.0001	7 (0.3%)	1 (0.5%)	0.84

For abbreviations, see Table 1.

Table 4. Discharge data of patients without cardiac arrest and with ErCA and LrCA after acute myocardial infarction (only patients who were discharged after index hospitalisation).

Variable	Non-CA N = 154,266	rCA N = 2296	p Value	ErCA N = 2106	LrCA N = 190	p Value
LVEF, %, mean (SD)	47.9 (10.6)	43.2 (12.0)	<0.0001	43.7 (11.8)	38.4 (12.9)	<0.0001
Hospitalisation length, days, median (IQR)	5 (3–7)	7 (4–11)	0.0031	6 (4–10)	12 (8–19)	<0.0001
Aspirin at discharge	141,512 (91.7%)	2069 (90.1%)	0.0052	1893 (89.9%)	176 (92.6%)	0.22
P2Y12 inhibitor at discharge	130,658 (84.7%)	1955 (85.2%)	0.55	1786 (84.8%)	169 (89%)	0.12
Acenocoumarol/warfarin at discharge	3727 (2.4%)	68 (3%)	0.091	57 (2.7%)	11 (5.8%)	0.016
Beta-blocker at discharge	128,332 (83.2%)	1822 (79.4%)	<0.0001	1665 (79.1%)	157 (82.6%)	0.24
LMWH at discharge	7399 (4.8%)	197 (8.6%)	<0.0001	176 (8.4%)	21 (11.1%)	0.2

Table 4. Cont.

Variable	Non-CA N = 154,266	rCA N = 2296	p Value	ErCA N = 2106	LrCA N = 190	p Value
ACE-I at discharge	119,911 (77.7%)	1693 (73.7%)	<0.0001	1554 (73.8%)	139 (73.2%)	0.85
ARB at discharge	3765 (2.4%)	46 (2%)	0.18	41 (2%)	5 (2.6%)	0.71
Fibrate at discharge	1688 (1.1%)	18 (0.8%)	0.16	18 (0.9%)	0 (0%)	0.39
Statin at discharge	135,497 (87.8%)	1966 (85.6%)	0.0014	1803 (85.6%)	163 (85.8%)	0.95
Calcium channel blocker at discharge	14,877 (9.6%)	133 (5.8%)	<0.0001	116 (5.5%)	17 (9%)	0.052
Nitrate at discharge	17,305 (11.2%)	188 (8.2%)	<0.0001	168 (8%)	20 (10.5%)	0.22
Diuretic at discharge	38,629 (25%)	773 (33.7%)	<0.0001	675 (32.1%)	98 (51.6%)	<0.0001
Diabetes treated with insulin at discharge	13,410 (8.7%)	189 (8.2%)	0.44	161 (7.6%)	28 (14.7%)	0.0007
Diabetes treated with oral medication at discharge	14,642 (9.5%)	154 (6.7%)	<0.0001	132 (6.3%)	22 (11.6%)	0.0051

For abbreviations, see Table 1.

3.2. In-Hospital and One-Year Observation Results

The overall mortality in AMI patients was higher in the CA group than in patients without CA: 35.6% and 6.0% in hospital, 2.3% and 1.1% at 30 days, 9.9% and 5.2% at 6 months, and 13% and 7.7% at 12 months (all $p < 0.0001$), respectively. There was no statistically significant difference in 30-day mortality between the ErCA and LrCA groups (2.2% vs. 3.2%; $p = 0.42$). At the 6- and 12-month follow-up periods, all-cause mortality was higher in the LrCA patients than in the ErCA patients (17.9% vs. 9.2%; $p = 0.0001$ and 21.1% vs. 12.3%; $p = 0.001$, respectively). Detailed data on the one-year outcomes are presented in Table 5 and Supplementary Materials.

Table 5. One-year follow-up outcomes of patients without cardiac arrest and with ErCA and LrCA after acute myocardial infarction (only patients who were discharged after index hospitalisation).

Variable	Non-CA N = 154,266	rCA N = 2296	p Value	ErCA N = 2106	LrCA N = 190	p Value
Mortality after discharge						
Death: 30 days	1765 (1.1%)	53 (2.3%)	<0.0001	47 (2.2%)	6 (3.2%)	0.42
Death: 6 months	7942 (5.2%)	228 (9.9%)	<0.0001	194 (9.2%)	34 (17.9%)	0.0001
Death: 12 months	11,947 (7.7%)	299 (13.0%)	<0.0001	259 (12.3%)	40 (21.1%)	0.0006
Re-hospitalisation with main diagnosis						
All cause	88,016 (57.1%)	1348 (58.7%)	0.11	1224 (58.1%)	124 (65.3%)	0.055
Cardiovascular cause	71,290 (46.2%)	1095 (47.7%)	0.15810	1000 (47.5%)	95 (50%)	0.51
Chronic coronary syndrome	36,659 (23.8%)	557 (24.3%)	0.57925	530 (25.2%)	27 (14.2%)	0.0007
Unstable angina	19,390 (12.6%)	225 (9.8%)	0.00007	213 (10.1%)	12 (6.3%)	0.092
Myocardial infarction	8552 (5.5%)	109 (4.8%)	0.09758	96 (4.6%)	13 (6.8%)	0.16
Chronic coronary syndrome or unstable angina or myocardial infarction	55,008 (35.7%)	766 (33.4%)	0.02262	720 (34.2%)	46 (24.2%)	0.0052
Heart failure	12,491 (8.1%)	262 (11.4%)	<0.0001	228 (10.8%)	34 (17.9%)	0.0033
Stroke	2205 (1.4%)	23 (1%)	0.08595	20 (1%)	3 (1.6%)	0.65
Cardiac rehabilitation after 30 days	32,079 (20.8%)	541 (23.6%)	0.00119	511 (24.3%)	30 (15.8%)	0.0084
Cardiac rehabilitation after 6 months	35,748 (23.2%)	592 (25.8%)	0.00326	561 (26.6%)	31 (16.3%)	0.0018
Cardiac rehabilitation after 12 months	37,258 (24.2%)	614 (26.7%)	0.00401	580 (27.5%)	34 (17.9%)	0.004
Re-hospitalisation with procedure						
Coronary angiography	39,549 (25.6%)	559 (24.4%)	0.15983	528 (25.1%)	31 (16.3%)	0.0071
PCI	31,015 (20.1%)	376 (16.4%)	0.00001	361 (17.1%)	15 (7.9%)	0.001
CABG	8081 (5.2%)	112 (4.9%)	0.44160	103 (4.9%)	9 (4.7%)	0.92

Table 5. Cont.

Variable	Non-CA N = 154,266	rCA N = 2296	p Value	ErCA N = 2106	LrCA N = 190	p Value
Pacemaker implantation	1276 (0.8%)	18 (0.8%)	0.82060	17 (0.8%)	1 (0.5%)	0.99
CRT-P implantation	51 (0.03%)	0 (0%)	0.38355	0 (0%)	0 (0%)	1.00
ICD implantation	2171 (1.4%)	94 (4.1%)	<0.0001	83 (3.9%)	11 (5.8%)	0.22
CRT-D implantation	365 (0.2%)	18 (0.8%)	<0.0001	17 (0.8%)	1 (0.5%)	0.99
ICD or CRT-D implantation	2531 (1.6%)	111 (4.8%)	<0.0001	99 (4.7%)	12 (6.3%)	0.32

For abbreviations, see Table 1.

In a multivariable model adjusted for all relevant risk factors, both ErCA (HR 1.54; 1.28–1.89; $p < 0001$) and LrCA (HR 2.34; CI 1.39–3.93; $p = 0.001$) increased the risk of one-year death compared to patients without CA after AMI (Figure 1).

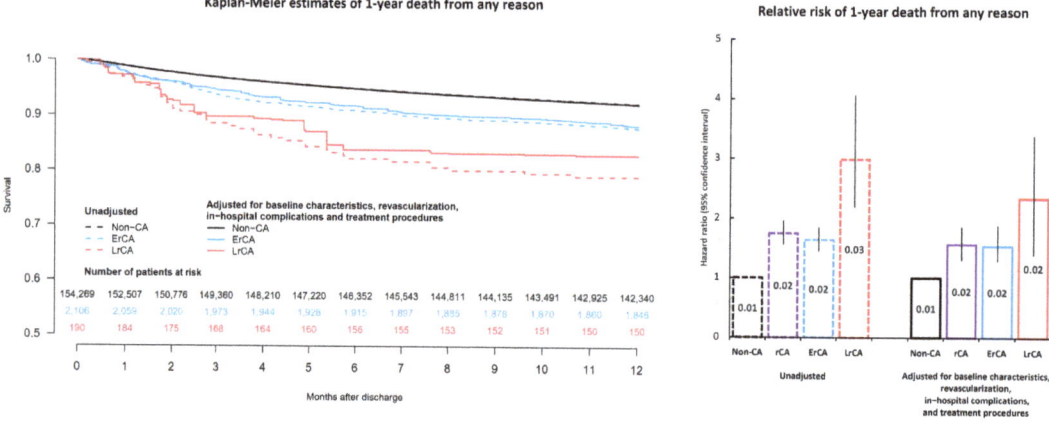

Figure 1. Central illustration. Risk of death from any reason for patients discharged home after resuscitated cardiac arrest during acute myocardial infarction.

In the multivariable analysis, the occurrence of an LrCA episode was also the second strongest factor (after Killip class 4) associated with an over 10-fold increase in the risk of in-hospital death (HR 10.30; CI 8.02–13.20; $p < 0.0001$), whereas ErCA increased the risk almost 2.5-fold (HR 2.35; CI 2.1–2.63; $p < 0.0001$) (Figure S1). The factors associated with an increased risk of CA occurrence after AMI are presented in Figure S2.

During the one-year observation, the ErCA patients were more frequently hospitalised due to chronic coronary syndrome, coronary angiography, and PCI when compared to the LrCA patients. The latter group was more likely to be hospitalised due to heart failure (17.9% vs. 10.8%; $p = 0.003$). Interestingly, only 17.9% of patients in the LrCA group underwent cardiac rehabilitation compared to 27.5% ($p = 0.004$) of the ErCA group. Figure S3 presents 1-year survival, re-hospitalisations, and procedures in AMI patients discharged home who survived cardiac arrest (early or late) compared to patients without cardiac arrest.

A comparison of the calculated relative risk of different re-hospitalisations associated with the type of CA is presented in Figure 2.

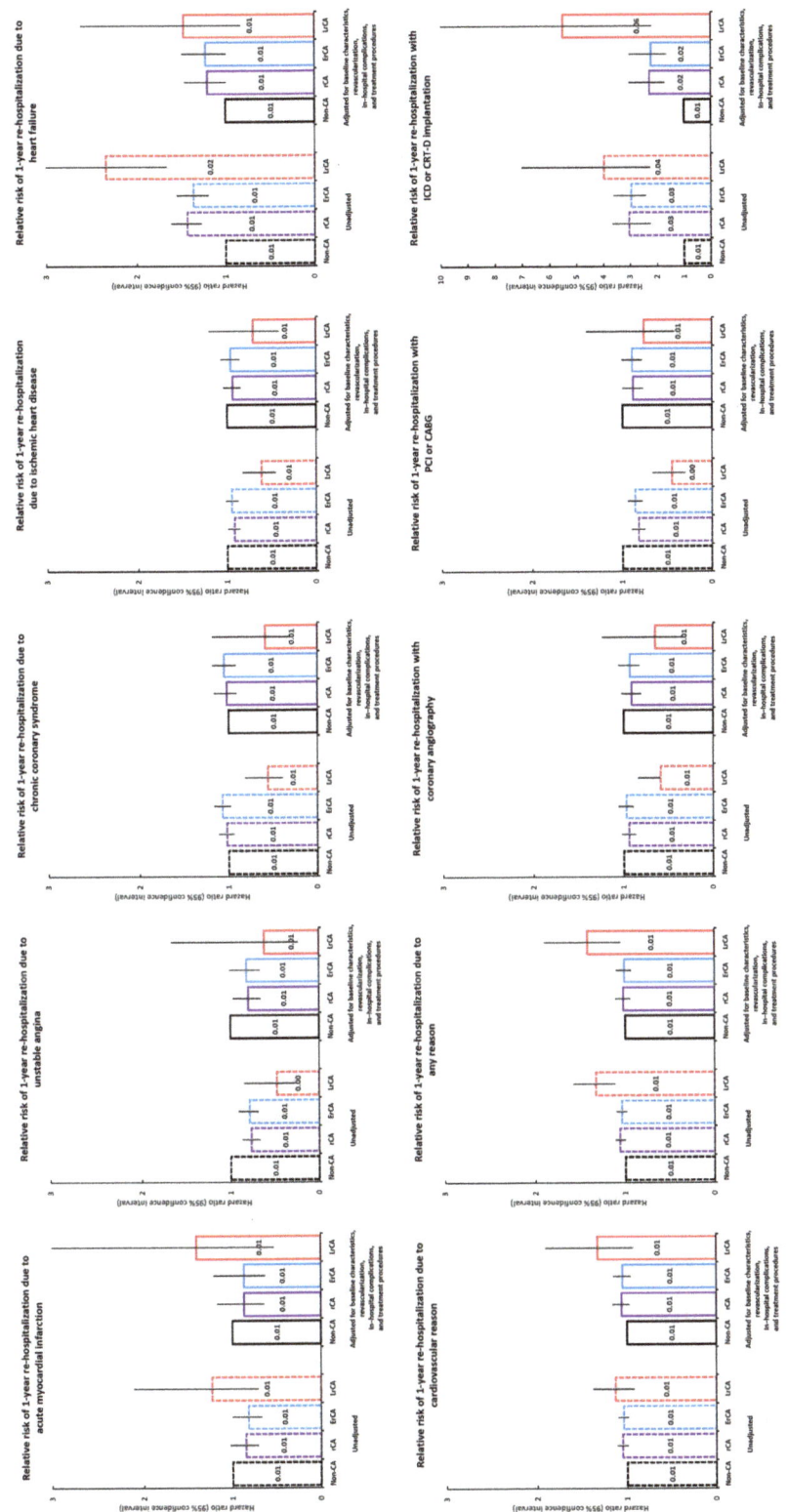

Figure 2. Relative risk of 1-year re-hospitalisation.

4. Discussion

The main observation of the present study is that ErCA, as a complication of AMI, is an independent prognostic factor of one-year mortality. ErCA, after adjustment of many factors influencing statistical significance, increases the risk of death in the 12-month follow-up (adjusted HR = 1.5).

The available data do not show a clear assessment of the impact of ErCA on the long-term prognosis of patients after AMI. Our study shows the influence of ErCA on mortality, which may be important for future recommendations for the secondary prevention of cardiac arrest.

In one of the thrombolysis-era studies based on data from the GISSI-2 database, both early and late CA episodes increased in-hospital mortality (2.5 times and 4 times, respectively), while they had no significant effect on mortality in the 6-month follow-up [11]. The results from one of the prospective cohort studies by Bougouin et al. showed that patients with AMI complicated by early ventricular fibrillation had a similar number of sudden cardiac death events during the 5-year follow-up to the group without ventricular fibrillation [12].

After an ErCA episode, which occurred within an established time of less than 48 h from the onset of AMI, the patients were classified as a non-homogeneous group with a different prognosis. This group included both patients who survived out-of-hospital CA (OHCA) and in-hospital CA (IHCA) prior to coronary reperfusion and those who had an arrhythmia during or after reperfusion. OHCA patients had by far the worst prognosis. It was demonstrated by Nair et al. that only 4% of patients from this group survived until discharge from the hospital [13].

A recent study by Podolecki et al. showed that the risk of death in long-term observation was associated with the occurrence of life-threatening ventricular arrhythmia only in the pre-reperfusion period [14]. However, this effect on long-term prognosis lost its significance after excluding patients who died within the first 30 days from admission. A similar effect of pre-reperfusion CA on long-term prognosis has also been shown in two other studies by Piccini et al. and Liang et al. [15,16]. Moreover, all three cited papers showed a significantly increased effect of early ventricular arrhythmias on in-hospital mortality [14–16].

Interestingly, the assessment of the effect of ventricular arrhythmia during revascularisation procedures gives conflicting results in terms of short-term prognosis, but most of the studies did not show an increase in mortality in the long-term follow-up [17].

Based on the current analysis, mainly LrCA, but also ErCA, is one of the strongest predictors of in-hospital and one-year mortality. LrCA increased the risk of in-hospital death by more than 10-fold (4-fold more than in the ErCA group). This observation is in line with the results of previously published papers [14,18], which showed that the occurrence of late ventricular arrhythmia is associated with a higher risk of in-hospital death by over 8-fold. In terms of the long-term prognosis, the occurrence of late ventricular arrhythmia increased the risk of death in long-term observation by nearly 3.5 times [14]. Another study by Mehta et al. showed that at any stage of follow-up, mortality in the LrCA group remained at a higher level than in the ErCA group [19]. This last observation is in line with our results. There were no differences in mortality in the 30-day observation between the ErCA and LrCA groups in our study, but the mortality was significantly higher in the LrCA group at 6- and 12-months post-hospital discharge.

We did not analyse the rhythm presentation of CA, but we collected data about the ICD and CRT-D implantation rate. In general, VF or VT is a main mechanism of CA in MI (about 80%) [9]. In our study, only 14.2% patients after LrCA, who survived until discharge from the hospital, had an implanted ICD or CRT-D, which suggests a high percentage of non-defibrillated rhythms of CA, probably due to the high percentage of severe in-hospital complications.

The next important finding from our study is the fact that ErCA episodes occur more often in younger patients. This observation was also confirmed in the study by

Sulzgruber et al. [20]. This study found an inverse correlation of patient age with the risk of developing ventricular arrhythmia in the acute phase of AMI. In addition, in this study, and in that of Piccini et al., diabetes and hypertension were found to be paradoxically protective against ventricular arrhythmias in the ErCA group [15]. This observation also coincides with the results of the present research. It could be assumed that the pharmacological treatment (beta-blockers, angiotensin-converting enzyme inhibitors, and statins) frequently used in these diseases might be responsible for such an effect.

Another important observation comes from the 12-month follow-up. The patients after ErCA were more often admitted to the hospital due to coronary events (chronic coronary syndromes, unstable angina, or recurrent AMI). They were also referred to coronary angiography and PCI more frequently than patients after LrCA. These results emphasise the importance of optimising medical care in this group.

Finally, it is worth emphasising the importance of early revascularisation strategies, which were significantly less frequently used in the LrCA group. Consequently, a significant increase in the number of repeated AMI and more frequent cardiogenic shock were observed in this study. Perhaps this observation partially explains the problem of such highly unfavourable short- and long-term prognoses of patients in older age groups treated for AMI complicated by CA.

5. Limitations

The results of the present study need to be interpreted considering some limitations. This was a retrospective analysis of an observational registry, which may result in a selection error. The ErCA group was analysed as a homogenous group without consideration of the diversity of this population, thus creating significant differences in prognosis. In the registry, we did not collect data on the rhythm presentation of CA and the timing to the return of spontaneous circulation, which are important in terms of predicting recovery from CA. To reduce the important influences of these factors, we only analysed patients who recovered after CA (resuscitated CA), and we focused on the long-term outcomes. There was a lack of data on treatment methods and the degree of neurological dysfunction of the out-of-hospital CA patients.

6. Conclusions

Both ErCA and LrCA were independent risk factors for one-year mortality. An episode of LrCA was associated with higher in-hospital and one-year mortality than ErCA. The ErCA patients were younger and had less comorbidities than LrCA patients. Further well-designed studies are required to identify clinical outcomes after ErCA (OHCA and IHCA) in long term follow-ups.

Supplementary Materials: The following supporting information can be downloaded at: https://www.mdpi.com/article/10.3390/jcm11030609/s1, Figure S1: Multivariate logistic regression model of factors affecting in-hospital mortality in the whole cohort of patients; Figure S2: Risk factors of the occurrence of resuscitated cardiac arrest (both early or late) in the cohort of patients that survived in-hospital period multivariate logistic regression model; Figure S3: 1-year survival (A), rehospitalizations (B-H) and procedures (I-K) in acute myocardial infarction patients discharged home who survived cardiac arrest (early or late) compared to patients without cardiac arrest; Table S1: Baseline clinical characteristics of patients without cardiac arrest and with ErCA and LrCA in the whole cohort of patients with acute myocardial infarction.

Author Contributions: Conceptualization, R.K., M.G. (Marek Gierlotka) and K.O.; Data curation, R.K., M.G. (Marek Gierlotka), K.O., P.T., A.F., P.F., A.T., G.O., M.G. (Marcin Grabowski) and M.G. (Mariusz Gąsior); Formal analysis, R.K., M.G. (Marek Gierlotka) and K.O.; Investigation, R.K. and M.G. (Marek Gierlotka); Methodology, R.K., M.G. (Marek Gierlotka), K.O., P.T., A.F., P.F., A.T., G.O., M.G. (Marcin Grabowski) and M.G. (Mariusz Gąsior); Project administration, R.K. and M.G. (Marek Gierlotka); Supervision, R.K. and M.G. (Marek Gierlotka); Validation, M.G. (Marek Gierlotka) and M.G. (Marcin Grabowski); Visualization, R.K., M.G. (Marek Gierlotka) and K.O.; Writing—original draft, R.K., M.G. (Marek Gierlotka) and K.O.; Writing—review & editing, R.K., M.G. (Marek Gierlotka),

K.O., P.T., A.F., P.F., A.T., G.O., M.G. (Marcin Grabowski) and M.G. (Mariusz Gąsior). All authors have read and agreed to the published version of the manuscript.

Funding: PL-ACS Registry was funded by Ministry of Health. This research received no external additional funding.

Institutional Review Board Statement: Ethical review and approval were waived for this study due to retrospective analysis of the prospective Polish Registry of Acute Coronary Syndrome.

Informed Consent Statement: Patient consent was waived due to retrospective analysis of PL-ACS Registry.

Data Availability Statement: No data available.

Conflicts of Interest: The authors declare no conflict of interest.

References

1. Ibanez, B.; James, S.; Agewall, S.; Antunes, M.J.; Bucciarelli-Ducci, C.; Bueno, H.; Widimský, P. 2017 ESC Guidelines for the management of acute myocardial infarction in patients presenting with ST-segment elevation: The Task Force for the management of acute myocardial infarction in patients presenting with ST-segment elevation of the European Society of Cardiology (ESC). *Eur. Heart J.* **2018**, *39*, 119–177. [CrossRef] [PubMed]
2. Poloński, L.; Gasior, M.; Gierlotka, M.; Kalarus, Z.; Cieśliński, A.; Dubiel, J.S.; Opolski, G. Polish Registry of Acute Coronary Syndromes (PL-ACS). Characteristics, treatments and outcomes of patients with acute coronary syndromes in Poland. *Kardiol. Pol.* **2007**, *65*, 861–872. [PubMed]
3. Nadolny, K.; Zyśko, D.; Obremska, M.; Wierzbik-Strońska, M.; Ładny, J.R.; Podgorski, M.; Gałązkowski, R. Analysis of out-of-hospital cardiac arrest in Poland in a 1-year period: Data from the POL-OHCA registry. *Kardiol. Pol.* **2020**, *78*, 404–411. [CrossRef] [PubMed]
4. Kowalik, R.J.; Fojt, A.; Ozierański, K.; Peller, M.; Andruszkiewicz, P.; Banaszewski, M.; Opolski, G. Results of targeted temperature management of patients after sudden out-of-hospital cardiac arrest: A comparison between intensive general and cardiac care units. *Kardiol. Pol.* **2020**, *78*, 30–36. [CrossRef] [PubMed]
5. Piccini, J.P.; Zhang, M.; Pieper, K.; Solomon, S.D.; Al-Khatib, S.M.; Van de Werf, F.; Pfeffer, M.A.; McMurray, J.J.; Califf, R.M.; Velazquez, E.J. Predictors of sudden cardiac death change with time after myocardial infarction: Results from the VALIANT trial. *Eur. Heart J.* **2010**, *31*, 211–221. [CrossRef] [PubMed]
6. Wojtyniak, B.; Gierlotka, M.; Opolski, G.; Rabczenko, D.; Ozierański, K.; Gąsior, M.; Zdrojewski, T. Observed and relative survival and 5-year outcomes of patients discharged after acute myocardial infarction: The nationwide AMI-PL database. *Kardiol. Pol.* **2020**, *78*, 990–998. [CrossRef] [PubMed]
7. Gorenek, B. Blomstrom Lundqvist C, European Heart Rhythm Association, Acute Cardiovascular Care Association, European Association of Percutaneous Cardiovascular Interventions. Cardiac arrhythmias in acute coronary syndromes: Position paper from the joint EHRA, ACCA, and EAPCI task force. *Europace* **2014**, *16*, 1655–1673. [PubMed]
8. Tymińska, A.; Kapłon-Cieślicka, A.; Ozierański, K.; Budnik, M.; Wancerz, A.; Sypień, P.; Filipiak, K.J. Association of galectin-3 and soluble ST2 with in-hospital and 1-year outcomes in patients with ST-segment elevation myocardial infarction treated with primary percutaneous coronary intervention. *Pol. Arch. Intern. Med.* **2019**, *129*, 770–780. [CrossRef] [PubMed]
9. Alahmar, A.E.; Nelson, C.P.; Snell, K.I.; Yuyun, M.F.; Musameh, M.D.; Timmis, A.; Samani, N.J. Resuscitated cardiac arrest and prognosis following myocardial infarction. *Heart* **2014**, *100*, 1125–1132. [CrossRef] [PubMed]
10. Gierlotka, M.; Gasior, M.; Poloński, L.; Piekarski, M.; Kamiński, M. Projekt, założenia metodyczne oraz logistyka Ogólnopolskiego Rejestru Ostrych Zespołów Wieńcowych (PL-ACS) [Project, logistics and methodology of the National Registry of Acute Coronary Syndrome (PL-ACS)]. *Kardiol. Pol.* **2005**, *62* (Suppl. 1), I13–I21. [PubMed]
11. Volpi, A.; Cavalli, A.; Santoro, L.; Negri, E.; GISSI-2 Investigators. Incidence and prognosis of early primary ventricular fibrillation in acute myocardial infarction—Results of the Gruppo Italiano per lo Studio della Sopravvivenza nell'Infarto Miocardico (GISSI-2) database. *Am. J. Cardiol.* **1998**, *82*, 265–271. [CrossRef]
12. Bougouin, W.; Marjon, E.; Puymirat, E.; Defaye, P.; Celermajer, D.S.; Le Heuzey, J.Y.; FAST-MI Registry Investigators. Incidence of sudden cardiac death after ventricular fibrillation complicating acute myocardial infarction: A 5—years cause-of-death anlysis of the FAST-AMI 2005 registry. *Eur. Heart J.* **2014**, *35*, 116–122. [CrossRef] [PubMed]
13. Nair, S.U.; Lundbye, J.B. The use of hypothermia therapy in cardiac arrest survivors. *Ther. Hypothermia Temp. Manag.* **2011**, *1*, 9–21. [CrossRef]
14. Podolecki, T.S.; Lenarczyk, R.K.; Kowalczyk, J.P.; Jedrzejczyk-Patej, E.K.; Chodor, P.K.; Mazurek, M.H.; Kalarus, Z.F. Risk stratification for complex ventricular arrhythmia complicating ST-segment elevation myocardial infarction. *Coron. Artery Dis.* **2018**, *29*, 681–686. [CrossRef] [PubMed]
15. Piccini, J.P.; Berger, J.S.; Brown, D.L. Early sustained ventricular arrhythmias complicating acute myocardial infarction. *Am. J. Med.* **2008**, *121*, 797–804. [CrossRef] [PubMed]

16. Liang, J.J.; Fender, E.A.; Cha, Y.M.; Lennon, R.J.; Prasad, A.; Barsness, G.W. Long-term outcomes in survivor of early ventricular arrhythmias after acute ST-elevation and non-ST-elevation myocardial infarction treated with percutaneous coronary interventions. *Am. J. Cardiol.* **2016**, *117*, 709–713. [CrossRef] [PubMed]
17. Mehta, R.H.; Harjai, K.J.; Grines, C.L.; Stone, G.W.; Boura, J.; Cox, D. Primary Angioplasty in Myocardial Infarction (PAMI) Investigators. Sustained ventricular tachycardia or fibrillation in the cardiac catheterization laboratory among patients receiving primary percutaneous coronary intervention: Incidence, predictors, and outcomes. *J. Am. Coll. Cardiol.* **2004**, *43*, 1765–1772. [CrossRef] [PubMed]
18. Orvin, K.; Eisen, A.; Goldenberg, I.; Gottlieb, S.; Kornowski, R.; Matetzky, S.; Haim, M. Outcome of contemporary acute coronary syndrome complicated by ventricular tachyarrhythmia. *Europace* **2016**, *18*, 219–226. [CrossRef] [PubMed]
19. Mehta, R.H.; Yu, J.; Piccini, J.P.; Tcheng, J.E.; Farkouh, M.E.; Reiffel, J.; Stone, G.W. Prognostic significance of postprocedural sustained ventricular tachycardia or fibrillation in patients undergoing primary percutaneous coronary intervention (from the HORIZONS-AMI Trial). *Am. J. Cardiol.* **2012**, *109*, 805–812. [CrossRef] [PubMed]
20. Sulzgruber, P.; Schnaubelt, S.; Koller, L.; Goliasch, G.; Niederdöckl, J.; Simon, A.; Niessner, A. Cardiac arrest as an age-dependent prognosticator for long-term mortality after acute myocardial infarction: The potential impact of infarction size. *Eur. Heart J. Acute Cardiovasc. Care* **2019**, *8*, 153–160. [CrossRef] [PubMed]

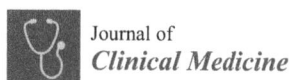

Review

Caveolin-3 and Arrhythmias: Insights into the Molecular Mechanisms

Miaomiao He [†], Jie Qiu [†], Yan Wang, Yang Bai * and Guangzhi Chen *

Division of Cardiology, Department of Internal Medicine, Tongji Hospital, Tongji Medical College, Huazhong University of Science and Technology, 1095 Jiefang Ave., Wuhan 430030, China; hemm1026@163.com (M.H.); tjqiujie@tjh.tjmu.edu.cn (J.Q.); newswangyan@tjh.tjmu.edu.cn (Y.W.)
* Correspondence: baiyang@tjh.tjmu.edu.cn (Y.B.); chengz@tjh.tjmu.edu.cn (G.C.);
  Tel./Fax: +86-27-6937-8422 (Y.B. & G.C.)
† These authors contributed equally to this work.

Abstract: Caveolin-3 is a muscle-specific protein on the membrane of myocytes correlated with a variety of cardiovascular diseases. It is now clear that the caveolin-3 plays a critical role in the cardiovascular system and a significant role in cardiac protective signaling. Mutations in the gene encoding caveolin-3 cause a broad spectrum of clinical phenotypes, ranging from persistent elevations in the serum levels of creatine kinase in asymptomatic humans to cardiomyopathy. The influence of *Caveolin-3(CAV-3)* mutations on current density parallels the effect on channel trafficking. For example, mutations in the *CAV-3* gene promote ventricular arrhythmogenesis in long QT syndrome 9 by a combined decrease in the loss of the inward rectifier current (I_{K1}) and gain of the late sodium current (I_{Na-L}). The functional significance of the caveolin-3 has proved that caveolin-3 overexpression or knockdown contributes to the occurrence and development of arrhythmias. Caveolin-3 overexpression could lead to reduced diastolic spontaneous Ca^{2+} waves, thus leading to the abnormal L-Type calcium channel current-induced ventricular arrhythmias. Moreover, *CAV-3* knockdown resulted in a shift to more negative values in the hyperpolarization-activated cyclic nucleotide channel 4 current (I_{HCN4}) activation curve and a significant decrease in I_{HCN4} whole-cell current density. Recent evidence indicates that caveolin-3 plays a significant role in adipose tissue and is related to obesity development. The role of caveolin-3 in glucose homeostasis has attracted increasing attention. This review highlights the underlining mechanisms of caveolin-3 in arrhythmia. Progress in this field may contribute to novel therapeutic approaches for patients prone to developing arrhythmia.

Keywords: caveolin-3; arrhythmias; ion channels; intercellular communication; metabolic perturbation

Citation: He, M.; Qiu, J.; Wang, Y.; Bai, Y.; Chen, G. Caveolin-3 and Arrhythmias: Insights into the Molecular Mechanisms. *J. Clin. Med.* 2022, 11, 1595. https://doi.org/10.3390/jcm11061595

Academic Editors: Paweł T. Matusik, Christian Sohns and Maciej Banach

Received: 22 January 2022
Accepted: 9 March 2022
Published: 14 March 2022

Publisher's Note: MDPI stays neutral with regard to jurisdictional claims in published maps and institutional affiliations.

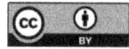

Copyright: © 2022 by the authors. Licensee MDPI, Basel, Switzerland. This article is an open access article distributed under the terms and conditions of the Creative Commons Attribution (CC BY) license (https://creativecommons.org/licenses/by/4.0/).

1. Introduction

The novel subcellular structures, named plasmalemmal vesicles, were first detected by Palade, G.E. et al. in 1953, and then renamed as caveolae intracellulares by Yamada, E. et al. due to their resemblance to 'little caves' [1]. Caveolins are the most essential proteins in caveolae, presenting in three isoforms: caveolin-1, caveolin-2, and caveolin-3. Caveolin-1 and caveolin-2 are co-expressed across many cell types, whereas caveolin-3 is specifically found in muscle tissues, such as skeletal and cardiac myocytes [2–4]. With the development of biochemical, cell biological, and genetic approaches, especially molecular markers, the molecular functions of caveolae have gradually been discovered, which involve the participation of homeostasis, most notably endocytosis, mechano-protection, and signal transduction. Composed of 151 amino acids, caveolin-3 has four major structural domains: the N-terminal domain, the scaffolding domain, the intramembrane domain, and the C-terminal domain [5–7]. Caveolin-3 exerts its effects as a scaffolding and regulatory protein for signaling molecules and moderators of ion channels and has already been linked to numerous human disease states, such as long QT syndrome, sudden infant death syndrome, myocardial hypertrophy, and diabetic cardiomyopathy [8–10] (Table 1). Furthermore, a study has demonstrated that the caveolin-3 protein can modify integrin function and mechanotransduction in the cardiac myocytes and intact heart; thus, modifications in caveolin-3 can result in the dysregulation of integrin function and predispose the heart to develop a myopathic phenotype [11]. Multiple ion channels are expressed in the caveolae in cardiomyocytes, such as the L-Type calcium channel (LTCC), T-Type calcium channel (TTCC), voltage dependent sodium channel 1.5 (Nav1.5), the voltage-dependent K channel (Kv1.5), and inward rectifier potassium channel (Kir2.x) [12–15].

Table 1. Pathogenic *CAV3* mutation associated with cardiovascular diseases.

Phenotype	CAV3 Mutation	Serum CK Concentrations	Ref.
LQTS	p.A85T	NA	Vatta, M. et al. [16]
Sudden infant death syndrome	p.V14 L	NA	Cronk, L.B. et al. [17]
Dilated cardiomyopathy	p.A46V	High	Catteruccia, M. et al. [18]
Dilated cardiomyopathy	p.T78M	High	Traverso, M. et al. [19]
Hypertrophic cardiomyopathy	p.T63S	Normal	Hayashi, T. et al. [20]
Hypertrophic cardiomyopathy	P104L	NA	Ohsawa, Y. et al. [21]
Hypercholesterolemia	p. Val44Met	High	Bruno, G. et al. [22]
Atrial standstill	p. Leu84Pro	NA	Gal, D. B. et al. [23]

NA, Not Available; LQTS, Long QT syndrome.

2. Caveolin-3 and Electrical Signal Propagation

2.1. The Sodium Current (I_{Na})

Several studies have confirmed that caveolin-3 colocalizes with the cardiac sodium channel and interacts with the dystrophin–glycoprotein complex to target multiple ion channels including *SCN5A*-encoded cardiac sodium channels (*SCN5A*, also termed Nav1.5) to the cell surface membrane [12,16,24]. *CAV-3* is a novel Long QT syndrome (LQTS)-associated gene with mutations producing a gain-of-function, LQT3-like molecular/cellular phenotype, as a pathogenic basis of sudden infant death syndrome (SIDS) [25]. It has been reported that the functional alteration of SCN5A resulting from the mutation of *CAV-3(V14L, T78M, and L79R)* is presumed to be the cause of sudden cardiac death in infants because of a significant fivefold increase in late sodium current compared with controls, just like LQT3 [16,17,26] (Table 2). Recent evidence indicates that neural nitric oxide synthase (nNOS), which mediates nitric oxide (NO) synthesis, and SCN5A form a complex with caveolin-3 in the heart, and the direct binding of caveolin-3 to nNOS suppresses the catalytic activity of nNOS [27,28]. Excessive NO synthesis and release mediated by nNOS in cardiomyocytes was shown to increase late I_{Na} [29]. It has been well documented that increased late I_{Na} caused by *CAV-3* mutation in ventricular muscle was reversed by NOS inhibitor L-NMMA, which meant that caveolin-3 was identified as an important negative regulator for cardiac late I_{Na} through a NOS-associated mechanism and contributed to both inherited arrhythmia syndromes and acquired arrhythmias in conditions [30,31]. Moreover, beta-adrenergic receptor regulation was reported to increase current densities of caveolar SCN5A through both protein kinase A (PKA)-dependent phosphorylation of sodium channels and direct G_{as} interaction with caveolin-3 which promoted the presentation of SCN5A containing caveolae to the surface membrane [32]. The roles of caveolin-3 in prolonging action potential by binding to calmodulin, which binds SCN5A and increases its slow inactivation kinetics in response to the regional increase in the concentration of calcium, have been gradually discovered. Although the above studies have confirmed the important role of caveolin-3, its specific mechanism is still unclear and may be closely related to the regulation of ion channels.

2.2. The K$^+$ Current (I_k)

The inward rectifier current (I_{K1}), dominating the terminal phases of cellular repolarization, maintains the resting membrane potential close to the potassium equilibrium potential and contributes to final phase 3 repolarization [33]. I_{k1} is mainly comprised of the rectifier potassium channel Kir2.1, which is one member of Kir2.x family in the human cardiac ventricle and is mainly encoded by KCNJ2A gene on chromosome 17 [34,35]. Kir2.x family have a unique intracellular pattern of distribution in association with specific caveolin-3 domains, which critically depends on interaction with Kir2.x- caveolin-3 binding motifs [36]. An early study demonstrated that *CAV-3* gene mutation decreased the surface expression of Kir2.1 and Kir2.2 [36,37]. Its mechanism may be closely related to the disruption in normal membrane trafficking of caveolin-3, regulating cell surface expression of Kir2.x channels, then causing decreased Kir2.x current density. Decreased Kir2.1 protein expression or function can decrease phase 3 rapid repolarization current magnitude of action potential, and prolong QT intermittent period or action potential duration, causing cardiac arrhythmia [37–40]. Moreover, a study has revealed that caveolin-3 participated in common early anterograde trafficking mechanism of the NaV1.5-Kir2.1 channelsome, which may have contributed to the potential for arrhythmias [40].

The transient outward K$^+$ current (I_{to}), responsible for rapid initial repolarization manifested as phase 1 of the AP, was partly constituted by Kv4.2 in human ventricular myocardium. Caveolin-3 is comparably co-localized with Kv4.2 channels by co-immunoprecipitation analysis. Overwhelming evidence has suggested that *CAV-3* gene mutation results in not only slower activation and recovery of $I_{Kv4.2}$, which could cause a reduction of I_{to} at physiological heart rates, but decreased $I_{Kv4.2}$, which contributes to cardiac arrhythmia [31]. It has been reported that *CAV-3* gene mutation leads to dysfunction of AngII contributing to modulate a variety of ionic currents in atrial myocytes, including I_{to}. In the heart, AngII binds two types of angiotensin receptors, namely, AngII receptor 1 (Ang1R) and AngII receptor 2 (Ang2R), with Ang1Rs mediating most of the AngII effects [41]. Ang1R is associated with caveolin-3 in mouse atrial myocytes that is required for the reduction in I_{to} by AngII [42]. There is increasing evidence that downstream signaling of Ang1R activation includes activation of protein kinase C (PKC) which catalyzes the hydrolysis of the membrane phospholipid, phosphatidylinositol biphosphate, producing diacylglycerol (DAG) [41,43–45]. Although the above studies have confirmed that the crucial role of caveolin-3 in the modulation of ionic currents, its specific mechanism is still unclear and need to be further elucidated (Figure 1).

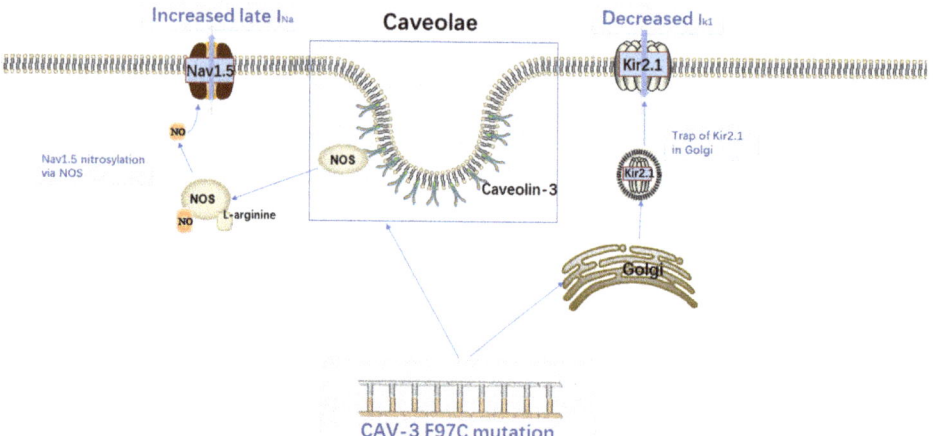

Figure 1. Cartoon illustration of arrhythmia mechanism caused by *Cav3* mutation (F97C). NOS, Nitric oxide synthase; NO, Nitric oxide.

2.3. The Ca$^+$ Current (I_{Ca})

Voltage-gated Ca^{2+} channels, including both the LTCC and TTCC, are the major handlers for the excitation-contraction coupling (ECC) and pacing activity of the heart [46–48]. TTCC have three different isoforms, CaV3.1(α1G), CaV3.2 (α1H), and CaV3.3 (α1I), which were consistently absent in human adult atrial and ventricular myocardium. In the heart, $I_{Ca,T}$ participates in Ca^{2+} entry and Ca^{2+}-dependent hormonal secretion, pacemaker activity, and arrhythmia. T-type CaV3.1 (α1G) Ca^{2+} channels play important roles in the spontaneous activity of pacemaker cells. CaV3.3 is not expressed in the heart. In the normal condition, CaV3.2 isoforms are undetectable in normal adult ventricular myocytes but are re-expressed during conditions of cardiac hypertrophy [49–51]. Considerable evidence indicates that the N terminus region of caveolin-3 closely interacts with CaV3.2 channels [52]. It has been reported that caveolin-3 could regulate protein kinase A modulation of the Ca(V)3.2 (alpha1H) T-type Ca^{2+} channels and attenuate cardiac hypertrophy via inhibition of T-type Ca^{2+} current modulated by protein kinase Cα in cardiomyocytes [52–54]. Caveolin-3 specifically inhibited the increased expression of $I_{Cav3.2}$ and suppressed the Ca^{2+}-dependent hypertrophic calcineurin-NFAT (calcineurin/nuclear factor of activated T cell) signaling pathway under pathological cardiac hypertrophy condition, thus significantly decreased the peak $I_{Cav3.2}$ current density to improve cardiac function [53].

L-type Ca channels (LTCCs) plays the vital role in cardiac ECC initiated by the action potential. Recent work has shown that caveolin-3 was associated with t-tubule formation, LTCC current to the t-tubules, and localization of LTCC regulatory proteins, such as protein kinase A (PKA) and β2-adrenoceptors [15,55–57]. In the recently reported study, global loss of caveolin-3, rather than cardiac-specific deletion of caveolin-3 protein, resulting in the pathological loss of t-tubular I_{Ca} contributes to impaired excitation-contraction coupling and thereby cardiac function in vivo [58]. Cardiac contractile performance is mainly regulated by circulating catecholamines, which bind to β-adrenergic receptors, the main catecholamine-responsive receptors on the surface of cardiac myocytes. β-adrenergic receptors(β-ARs) have two isoforms, β1-AR and β2-ARs. Multiple studies report the clustering of β2-adrenergic receptors(β2-ARs), coupled to Gs proteins and thus, inducing cAMP production, have also been shown to co-immunoprecipitate with caveoin-3 [59]. PKA is a key mediator in the molecular mechanism of the caveolin-3 affecting LTCCs by stimulating β$_2$-adrenoceptor expression [15,56].

Type 2 ryanodine receptor (RyR2), a key component of ECC in cardiomyocytes, is a cation-selective receptor channel located in the cardiac sarcoplasmic reticulum (SR) in the mammalian heart. A few Ca^{2+} ions pass through Cav1.2 to trigger a much larger Ca^{2+} release at concentration levels into the myoplasm through RyR2, thus activating action potential [60,61]. Recently, many studies have provided evidence that the RyR2 colocalized with caveolin-3 [62]. RyR2 and caveolin-3-associated dihydropyridine receptor (DHPR) forms a triple complex with HLP family which is one member of the cysteine-rich protein (Crip) [63]. The RyR2 modulates Ca^{2+} entry through caveolin-3-associated DHPR by regulating itself [15]. Caveolin-3 overexpression could lead to the reduced diastolic spontaneous Ca^{2+} waves by inhibiting the hyperphosphorylation of ryanodine receptor-2 (RyR2) at Ser2814, thus leading to the abnormal LTCC current-induced ventricular arrhythmias [64].

Striatin (STRN) is a dynamic protein that was originally purified from highly active adenylyl cyclase rich fractions and was found to bind caveolin-3 and calmodulin (CaM) in a calcium-sensitive manner [65]. Further studies attributed the role of caveolin-3 in the interaction between STRN and CaM regulating the maturation and organization of the ECC in ventricular cardiomyocytes. The expression level of STRN was inversely proportional to the interaction of caveolin-3 with the CaM/STRN complex. Thus, caveolin-3 may mediate STRN expression by producing the opposite phenotype to silence the STRN gene, but the specific mechanism needs to be further elucidated [66].

Table 2. The arrhythmia mechanism associated with change of CAV-3 expression.

CAV-3 Expression	Functional Alteration	Arrhythmia Implications	Related Mechanisms	Ref.
CAV-3 mutation (V14L, T78M, L79R)	Increased late sodium current	LQT3	NOS-dependent S-nitrosylation of SCN5A	Cheng. J. et al. [30]
	Decreased Kir2.x current density	LQT9	Downstream Ang1R signaling involves the activation of PKC	Tyan. L. et al. [42]
Caveolin-3 overexpression	Reduced diastolic spontaneous Ca^{2+} waves	Ventricular arrhythmias	Inhibition of RYR2 hyperphosphorylation	Zhang. ZH. et al. [64]
CAV-3 mutation (S141R)	Increased HCN4 current density	LQTS	NA	NA
Caveolin-3 downregulated expression	Activated $I_{Cl,\,swell}$	Atrial fibrillation	NA	NA

NOS, Nitric oxide synthase; RYR2, Ryanodine receptor-2; Ang1R, AngII receptor 1; PKC, Protein kinase C. NA, Not Available.

2.4. The Hyperpolarization-Activated Cyclic Nucleotide Channel 4 Current (I_{HCN4})

Hyperpolarization-activated cyclic nucleotide channel 4(HCN4), also named the pacemaker channel, is the dominant isoform of the sinus node region interacting with caveolin-3 [67]. HCN4 channel function is negatively modulated by caveolin-3 to modulate the channel's activity [68]. Of note, increased I_{HCN4} activity in the ventricle was shown to provoke ventricular automaticity resulting in ventricular arrhythmias [69]. Interestingly, LQTs-associated CAV-3 mutations differentially modulate HCN4 channel function indicating a pathophysiological role in clinical manifestations. One study indicated that HCN4 current properties were differentially modulated by LQTS-associated CAV-3 mutations. S141R, a CAV-3 LQTS-associated mutation, significantly increased HCN4 current density. CAV-3 KO resulted in a shift to more negative values in the I_{HCN4} activation curve and a significant decrease in I_{HCN4} whole-cell current density, which indicates that caveolin-3 mutations significantly accelerated the activation kinetics of HCN4 [68].

2.5. The Volume-Activated Cl-Channel Current ($I_{Cl,swell}$)

Atrial fibrillation (AF) is the most common sustained cardiac arrhythmia, and it has been associated with an increased risk of stroke, heart failure, and eventually, contributing to an increased risk of cardiac and total mortality. A high level of CAV-3 expression had a significant relationship with AF participants. Caveolin-3 concentrations in the serum samples were much higher in the group with persistent AF than the group with paroxysmal AF. Concentrations of caveolin-3 might be associated with the frequency and duration of AF [70]. AF associated with elevated chronic stretch is linked to a decrease in cardiomyocyte caveolae density and downregulation of the caveolin-3 [53,71].

Volume-activated Cl-channels are localized in the caveolae microdomains and can be activated on the mechanical stretch. Downregulation of caveolin-3 expression facilitates activation of $I_{Cl,swell}$ and increases sensitivity to stretch 5- to 10-fold, promoting the development of AF. Caveolin-3-mediated activation of mechanosensitive $I_{Cl,swell}$ is a critical cause of the triggering impulses that can initiate AF including AF, and this mechanism is exacerbated in the setting of chronically elevated blood pressures [72].

3. Caveolin-3 and Intercellular Communication

3.1. Caveolin-3 and ConnexIn 43

Gap junctions are collections of multiple intercellular channels comprised of connexons, to permit the rapid cell–cell transfer of action potentials, ensuring the coordinated contraction of the cardiomyocytes. ConnexIn 43 (Cx43) is the main component in cardiac gap junctions and is expressed in all atrial and ventricular myocytes. Reduced Cx43 expression can reduce function of gap junctions, resulting in promoting reentrant arrhythmias. There is extensive evidence that Cx43 plays a crucial role for rapid action potential transmission and signaling molecules that are associated with cardiac arrhythmias [73,74]. When the levels of full-length Cx43 protein are markedly reduced via an *M213L* mutation associated with an absence of GJA1-20k which is an auxiliary subunit for the trafficking of Cx43, the abnormal propagation of electrical impulse, including decrease in R wave amplitude, elongation of QRS complex duration, and increase in frequency of premature ventricular contractions (PVC), occurred in rats undergoing the loss of Cx43 gap junction that contributes to arrhythmias [75,76]. Oppositely, when Cx43 is activated by pinocembrin which is a flavonoid compound originated from propolis, Cx43 can be upregulated to alleviate ventricular arrhythmia in I/R rats [77]. Stem cell therapy in combination with enhanced protein expression of connexin-43 is a promising strategy against myocardial dysfunction, such as the post-infarction arrhythmias. More recently, data from the Rugowska, A et al. demonstrated that the increased expression of connexin-43 in human skeletal muscle-derived stem/progenitor cells reduced arrhythmogenic phenomena after their transplantation into the post-infarcted myocardium [78]. This is probably because that increased expression of Cx43 contributes to the reduction of inflammation and improvement of intercellular communication thus causing an indirect positive effect on calcium intracellular circulation.

Cx43 has been shown to interact with caveolin-3, and the mechanism of the relationship between Cx43 and caveolin-3 is still being explored. One study attributed a role of caveolin-1 in the regulation of Cx43. It maintains cardiac homeostasis by modulating cSrc activity. cSrc became activated to downregulate Cx43 without caveolin-1 expression. This process reduced ventricular conduction velocity and increased propensity for ventricular arrhythmias. Caveolin-3 regulating Cx43 function/expression may be a similar way as the Cx43 regulation of caveolin-1. However, more studies need to further confirm this hypothesis [79].

A study has shown that caveolin-3 was not only co-localized but interacts with the gap junction protein Cx43, by methods of double-hybridization and co-immunoprecipitation [80]. Moreover, the changes in caveolin-3 levels over time perfectly paralleled the pattern of changes in total Cx43 when phoneutria nigriventer spider venom (PNV) disrupt blood–brain barrier, which raise the possibility of cross-talk between Cx43 and caveolin-3 [81]. A previous study demonstrated that downregulation of caveolin-3 leads to inhibition of Cx43 gap junction communication in the lipopolysaccharide (LPS) treatment of astrocytes. Further, the specific knockout of caveolin-3 causes a downregulation of Cx43 and thus has a significant inhibitory effect on gap junctional intercellular communication (GJIC). All of those results indicated that caveolin-3 may play a crucial role in regulating Cx43 expression, but the signaling pathway between caveolin-3 and Cx43 merited further investigations [82].

3.2. Caveolin-3 and Dystrophin

The dystrophin, fundamental for muscle integrity, is a critical component of the dystrophin-glycoprotein complex that acts as a connection between the extracellular matrix and intracellular cytoskeleton [83]. Mutations in the dystrophin gene contribute to dystrophinopathies, which are mostly associated with cardiomyopathies [84]. A heart lacking functional dystrophin is mechanically weak [85]. Doyle, D.D. et al. verify that dystrophin co-localizes, co-fractionates, and co-immunoprecipitates with caveolin-3, which serves to suggest directions for further research that caveolin-3 may regulate physiological functions of dystrophin as upstream regulator [86]. Recent evidence indicates that dystrophin and its associated glycoproteins are downregulated in caveolin-3 overexpression heart, causing severe cardiac tissue degeneration, fibrosis and a reduction in cardiac functions [87]. Caveolin-3 may regulate the normal processing or stoichiometry of the dystrophin complex at the protein level [88].

3.3. Caveolin-3 and Adiponectin Receptor

Adiponectin (APN) is a benign adipokine secreted cytokine with reduced expression in obesity and diabetes [89]. The primary function of APN is to increase insulin sensitivity by sensitizing the insulin receptor signaling pathway. Adiponectin receptors are G protein-coupled receptors (GPCRs) and two receptor subtypes: AdipoR1 and AdipoR2. In both AdipoR1 and AdipoR2, the N-terminal domain exists in intracellular space and C-terminal domain presents in the external region of cells. Many studies have indicated that AdipoR1 colocalized with caveolin-3, forming AdipoR1/ caveolin-3 complex via specific caveolin-3 scaffolding domain binding motifs [90]. By interacting with AdipoR1, caveolin-3 corrals downstream molecules in close proximity with AdipoR1, thus enabling proper transmembrane signaling and cardioprotection. Recently, many studies have provided evidence that high fat diet-induced diabetes disrupted the expression of *CAV-3*, which deranged eNOS signaling in diabetic myocardium and then diminished the cardioprotective effects of APN [91–94]. Overall, caveolin-3 plays an essential role in APN-induced ceramidase recruitment and activation, although the involved detailed molecular mechanisms are still unknown.

4. Caveolin-3 and Metabolic Perturbation
4.1. Caveolin-3 and Insulin Resistance

Insulin resistance is the important defect in the pathophysiology of type 2 diabetes (T2DM). A major complication of diabetes is diabetic cardiomyopathy. The ion channel remodeling has been reported in the animal models of diabetic cardiomyopathy which could lead to a variety of arrhythmias, such as AF [95,96].

In recent years, the role of caveolin-3 in glucose homeostasis has attracted increasing attention. A previous study demonstrated that a variety of mutations were present in the *CAV-3* gene among 1–1000 patients with T2DM. A previous assessment of patients with newly developed T2DM demonstrated that K15N mutation located in the N-terminus of caveolin-3 may lead to changes in caveolin-3 secondary structure, thus causing decreased recombinant caveolin-3 expression [97]. It has been found that decreased expression and reduced localization of caveolin-3 by *CAV-3-P104L* mutation inhibited glucose uptake and glycogen synthesis [98]. The IR/PI3K/AKT/GLUT signaling pathway has been demonstrated to be a major mechanism in the development of insulin resistance [99,100]. Insulin receptor (IR) and GLUT-4 are associated with glucose metabolism, with their expression being regulated by caveolin-3 on the cell membrane. GLUT4 is one of the most important glucose transporters and is responsible for regulating and transporting 50% to 80% of body glucose. Caveolin-3 can enhance the expression of IR by stimulating IR kinase activity and activating PI3K/AKT signaling pathway. Activated AKT promoted the translocation of GLUT-4 to the plasma membrane and enhanced glucose uptake. There is evidence that increased *CAV-3* expression contributed to GLUT4 translocation and thus ameliorated high-fat-diet (HFD)-induced glucose intolerance and insulin resistance, which indicated a positive correlation between the alternation of glucose metabolism and the level of caveolin-3 [93,101]. Conversely, decreased expression levels of *CAV-3* were observed in diabetes animal models [102]. Decreased *CAV-3* expression inhibited Akt phosphorylation, and thus protein expression of GLUT4 which are molecules downstream of Akt, was significantly decreased [98]. Moreover, caveolin-3 may play a pivotal role in 17β-estradiol (E2) actions on glucose metabolism, and there is evidence that E2 intervention reduces the incidence of diabetes [92,103]. Diabetes could cause inhibition of *CAV-3* expression by regulating the activities of various enzymes and ion channels. Those changes lead to insulin resistance, inhibition of Cx43 gap junction communication and modulation of ion channel function, which contribute to susceptibility to arrhythmias.

4.2. Caveolin-3 and Adiposity

Obesity is a major concern because it is a risk factor for metabolic diseases that increase mortality rates. Recent evidence indicates that caveolin-3 plays a significant role in adipose tissue and is related to obesity development. A study has demonstrated that *CAV-3*-knockout mice increased adiposity [104]. Obesity is a complex multifactorial condition that contributes significantly to cardiovascular risk including AF. In animal models with adipose tissue, it has been found that obesity is also associated with a modest increase in QTc and QT dispersion [105,106]. Moreover, high-fat-diet-fed animals showed metabolic alterations, obesity, and insulin resistance along with the induced expression of muscle-specific caveolin-3 in retroperitoneal adipocytes and skeletal muscle in the initial phase. The mechanism was partly explained by the fact that continued exposure to the high-fat diet in the initial phase produces an increase in circulating glucose and insulin levels which could induce *CAV-3* expression [107,108]. Indeed, previous studies have reported that animals fed on a high fat diet show increased oxidative stress in muscle tissue, which also could be partly explained by the induced expression of *CAV-3* [109]. In a late phase, insulin resistance becomes apparent, accompanied by an impairment of caveolin-3 levels in skeletal muscle.

5. Perspective

Since it was discovered approximately 60 years ago, important functional roles and biochemical properties for caveolae have been identified. It is now clear that the caveolin-3 plays a critical role in the cardiovascular system and a significant role in cardiac protective signaling. *CAV-3* mutations have been linked to the LQT9, and the cause of underlying action potential duration prolongation is incompletely understood. However, there are numerous difficulties to be overcome in the process from basic laboratory research to clinical application. Caveolin-3 dysfunctions have been responsible for inherited arrhythmias. The importance of caveolin-3 changes in arrhythmias and downstream microdomain dysregulation may have important implications for arrhythmia generation.

Understanding the composition and functional roles of caveolin-3 in the heart as well as their contribution to arrhythmia syndromes is only the beginning. Many critical questions remain to be answered. Further basic science research and eventual randomized clinical trials are needed to define the precise mechanisms and therapeutic potential of caveolin-3 in patients with arrhythmias.

Author Contributions: M.H. and J.Q. performed the study and drafted the manuscript; G.C. and Y.B. organized the study and edited the manuscript; G.C. and Y.W. revised the study. All authors have read and agreed to the published version of the manuscript.

Funding: This work was supported by grants from the National Natural Science Foundation of China (No. 82070383).

Institutional Review Board Statement: Not applicable.

Informed Consent Statement: Not applicable.

Data Availability Statement: Not applicable.

Conflicts of Interest: We declare that we have no financial or personal relationships with other people or organizations that could inappropriately influence our work.

References

1. Yamada, E. The fine structure of the gall bladder epithelium of the mouse. *J. Biophys. Biochem. Cytol.* **1955**, *1*, 445–458. [CrossRef]
2. Rothberg, K.G.; Heuser, J.E.; Donzell, W.C.; Ying, Y.S.; Glenney, J.R.; Anderson, R.G. Caveolin, a protein component of caveolae membrane coats. *Cell* **1992**, *68*, 673–682. [CrossRef]
3. Song, K.S.; Scherer, P.E.; Tang, Z.; Okamoto, T.; Li, S.; Chafel, M.; Chu, C.; Kohtz, D.S.; Lisanti, M.P. Expression of caveolin-3 in skeletal, cardiac, and smooth muscle cells. Caveolin-3 is a component of the sarcolemma and co-fractionates with dystrophin and dystrophin-associated glycoproteins. *J. Biol. Chem.* **1996**, *271*, 15160–15165. [CrossRef]
4. Balijepalli, R.C.; Kamp, T.J. Caveolae, ion channels and cardiac arrhythmias. *Prog. Biophys. Mol. Biol.* **2008**, *98*, 149–160. [CrossRef]
5. Kim, J.H.; Peng, D.; Schlebach, J.P.; Hadziselimovic, A.; Sanders, C.R. Modest effects of lipid modifications on the structure of caveolin-3. *Biochemistry* **2014**, *53*, 4320–4322. [CrossRef] [PubMed]
6. Kim, J.H.; Schlebach, J.P.; Lu, Z.; Peng, D.; Reasoner, K.C.; Sanders, C.R. A pH-Mediated Topological Switch within the N-Terminal Domain of Human Caveolin-3. *Biophys. J.* **2016**, *110*, 2475–2485. [CrossRef] [PubMed]

7. Fernandez, I.; Ying, Y.; Albanesi, J.; Anderson, R.G. Mechanism of caveolin filament assembly. *Proc. Natl. Acad. Sci. USA* **2002**, *99*, 11193–11198. [CrossRef] [PubMed]
8. Koga, A.; Oka, N.; Kikuchi, T.; Miyazaki, H.; Kato, S.; Imaizumi, T. Adenovirus-mediated overexpression of caveolin-3 inhibits rat cardiomyocyte hypertrophy. *Hypertension* **2003**, *42*, 213–219. [CrossRef] [PubMed]
9. Tsutsumi, Y.M.; Horikawa, Y.T.; Jennings, M.M.; Kidd, M.W.; Niesman, I.R.; Yokoyama, U.; Head, B.P.; Hagiwara, Y.; Ishikawa, Y.; Miyanohara, A.; et al. Cardiac-specific overexpression of caveolin-3 induces endogenous cardiac protection by mimicking ischemic preconditioning. *Circulation* **2008**, *118*, 1979–1988. [CrossRef]
10. Parton, R.G. Caveolae: Structure, Function, and Relationship to Disease. *Annu. Rev. Cell Dev. Biol.* **2018**, *34*, 111–136. [CrossRef] [PubMed]
11. Israeli-Rosenberg, S.; Chen, C.; Li, R.; Deussen, D.N.; Niesman, I.R.; Okada, H.; Patel, H.H.; Roth, D.M.; Ross, R.S. Caveolin modulates integrin function and mechanical activation in the cardiomyocyte. *FASEB J. Off. Publ. Fed. Am. Soc. Exp. Biol.* **2015**, *29*, 374–384. [CrossRef]
12. Yarbrough, T.L.; Lu, T.; Lee, H.C.; Shibata, E.F. Localization of cardiac sodium channels in caveolin-rich membrane domains: Regulation of sodium current amplitude. *Circ. Res.* **2002**, *90*, 443–449. [CrossRef] [PubMed]
13. Martens, J.R.; Sakamoto, N.; Sullivan, S.A.; Grobaski, T.D.; Tamkun, M.M. Isoform-specific localization of voltage-gated K+ channels to distinct lipid raft populations. Targeting of Kv1.5 to caveolae. *J. Biol. Chem.* **2001**, *276*, 8409–8414. [CrossRef] [PubMed]
14. Bossuyt, J.; Taylor, B.E.; James-Kracke, M.; Hale, C.C. The cardiac sodium-calcium exchanger associates with caveolin-3. *Ann. N. Y. Acad. Sci.* **2002**, *976*, 197–204. [CrossRef] [PubMed]
15. Balijepalli, R.C.; Foell, J.D.; Hall, D.D.; Hell, J.W.; Kamp, T.J. Localization of cardiac L-type Ca(2+) channels to a caveolar macromolecular signaling complex is required for beta(2)-adrenergic regulation. *Proc. Natl. Acad. Sci. USA* **2006**, *103*, 7500–7505. [CrossRef] [PubMed]
16. Vatta, M.; Ackerman, M.J.; Ye, B.; Makielski, J.C.; Ughanze, E.E.; Taylor, E.W.; Tester, D.J.; Balijepalli, R.C.; Foell, J.D.; Li, Z.; et al. Mutant caveolin-3 induces persistent late sodium current and is associated with long-QT syndrome. *Circulation* **2006**, *114*, 2104–2112. [CrossRef]
17. Cronk, L.B.; Ye, B.; Kaku, T.; Tester, D.J.; Vatta, M.; Makielski, J.C.; Ackerman, M.J. Novel mechanism for sudden infant death syndrome: Persistent late sodium current secondary to mutations in caveolin-3. *Hear. Rhythm* **2007**, *4*, 161–166. [CrossRef]
18. .Catteruccia, M.; Sanna, T.; Santorelli, F.M.; Tessa, A.; Di Giacopo, R.; Sauchelli, D.; Verbo, A.; Monaco, M.L.; Servidei, S. Rippling muscle disease and cardiomyopathy associated with a mutation in the CAV3 gene. *Neuromuscul. Disord.* **2009**, *19*, 779–783. [CrossRef]
19. Traverso, M.; Gazzerro, E.; Assereto, S.; Sotgia, F.; Biancheri, R.; Stringara, S.; Giberti, L.; Pedemonte, M.; Wang, X.; Scapolan, S.; et al. Caveolin-3 T78M and T78K missense mutations lead to different phenotypes in vivo and in vitro. *Lab. Investig.* **2008**, *88*, 275–283. [CrossRef]
20. Hayashi, T.; Arimura, T.; Ueda, K.; Shibata, H.; Hohda, S.; Takahashi, M.; Hori, H.; Koga, Y.; Oka, N.; Imaizumi, T.; et al. Identification and functional analysis of a caveolin-3 mutation associated with familial hypertrophic cardiomyopathy. *Biochem. Biophys. Res. Commun.* **2004**, *313*, 178–184. [CrossRef]
21. Ohsawa, Y.; Tokoet, H.; Katsura, M.; Morimoto, K.; Yamada, H.; Ichikawa, Y.; Murakami, T.; Ohkuma, S.; Komuro, I.; Sunada, Y. Overexpression of P104L mutant caveolin-3 in mice develops hypertrophic cardiomyopathy with enhanced contractility in association with increased endothelial nitric oxide synthase activity. *Hum. Mol. Genet.* **2004**, *13*, 151–157. [CrossRef] [PubMed]
22. Bruno, G.; Puoti, G.; Oliva, M.; Colavito, D.; Allegorico, L.; Napolitano, F.; Sampaoloet, S. A novel missense mutation in CAV3 gene in an Italian family with persistent hyperCKemia, myalgia and hypercholesterolemia: Double-trouble. *Clin. Neurol. Neurosurg.* **2020**, *191*. [CrossRef] [PubMed]
23. Gal, D.B.; Wojciak, J.; Perera, J.; Tanel, R.E.; Patel, A.R. Atrial standstill in a pediatric patient with associated caveolin-3 mutation. *Hear. Case Rep.* **2017**, *3*, 513–516. [CrossRef] [PubMed]
24. Head, B.P.; Patel, H.H.; Roth, D.M.; Lai, N.C.; Niesman, I.R.; Farquhar, M.G.; Insel, P.A. G-protein-coupled receptor signaling components localize in both sarcolemmal and intracellular caveolin-3-associated microdomains in adult cardiac myocytes. *J. Biol. Chem.* **2005**, *280*, 31036–31044. [CrossRef] [PubMed]
25. Lariccia, V.; Nasti, A.A.; Alessandrini, F.; Pesaresi, M.; Gratteri, S.; Tagliabracci, A.; Amoroso, S. Identification and functional analysis of a new putative caveolin-3 variant found in a patient with sudden unexplained death. *J. Biomed. Sci.* **2014**, *21*, 58. [CrossRef] [PubMed]
26. Ackerman, M.J.; Siu, B.L.; Sturner, W.Q.; Tester, D.J.; Valdivia, C.R.; Makielski, J.C.; Towbin, J.A. Postmortem molecular analysis of SCN5A defects in sudden infant death syndrome. *JAMA* **2001**, *286*, 2264–2269. [CrossRef] [PubMed]
27. Ahern, G.P.; Hsu, S.F.; Klyachko, V.A.; Jackson, M.B. Induction of persistent sodium current by exogenous and endogenous nitric oxide. *J. Biol. Chem.* **2000**, *275*, 28810–28815. [CrossRef] [PubMed]
28. Venema, V.J.; Ju, H.; Zou, R.; Venema, R.C. Interaction of neuronal nitric-oxide synthase with caveolin-3 in skeletal muscle. Identification of a novel caveolin scaffolding/inhibitory domain. *J. Biol. Chem.* **1997**, *272*, 28187–28190. [CrossRef] [PubMed]
29. Tan, B.H.; Pundi, K.N.; Van Norstrand, D.W.; Valdivia, C.R.; Tester, D.J.; Medeiros-Domingo, A.; Makielski, J.C.; Ackerman, M.J. Sudden infant death syndrome-associated mutations in the sodium channel beta subunits. *Heart Rhythm* **2010**, *7*, 771–778. [CrossRef] [PubMed]

30. Cheng, J.; Valdivia, C.R.; Vaidyanathan, R.; Balijepalli, R.C.; Ackerman, M.J.; Makielski, J.C. Caveolin-3 suppresses late sodium current by inhibiting nNOS-dependent S-nitrosylation of SCN5A. *J. Mol. Cell. Cardiol.* **2013**, *61*, 102–110. [CrossRef] [PubMed]
31. Tyan, L.; Foell, J.D.; Vincent, K.P.; Woon, M.T.; Mesquitta, W.T.; Lang, D.; Best, J.M.; Ackerman, M.J.; McCulloch, A.D.; Glukhov, A.V.; et al. Long QT syndrome caveolin-3 mutations differentially modulate K(v) 4 and Ca(v) 1.2 channels to contribute to action potential prolongation. *J. Physiol.* **2019**, *597*, 1531–1551. [CrossRef] [PubMed]
32. Palygin, O.A.; Pettus, J.M.; Shibata, E.F. Regulation of caveolar cardiac sodium current by a single Gsalpha histidine residue. *Am. J. Physiology. Heart Circ. Physiol.* **2008**, *294*, H1693–H1699. [CrossRef] [PubMed]
33. Miake, J.; Marbán, E.; Nuss, H.B. Functional role of inward rectifier current in heart probed by Kir2.1 overexpression and dominant-negative suppression. *J. Clin. Investig.* **2003**, *111*, 1529–1536. [CrossRef]
34. Liu, G.X.; Derst, C.; Schlichthörl, G.; Heinen, S.; Seebohm, G.; Brüggemann, A.; Kummer, W.; Veh, R.W.; Daut, J.; Preisig-Müller, R. Comparison of cloned Kir2 channels with native inward rectifier K+ channels from guinea-pig cardiomyocytes. *J. Physiol.* **2001**, *532*, 115–126. [CrossRef] [PubMed]
35. Anumonwo, J.M.; Lopatin, A.N. Cardiac strong inward rectifier potassium channels. *J. Mol. Cell. Cardiol.* **2010**, *48*, 45–54. [CrossRef] [PubMed]
36. Vaidyanathan, R.; Van Ert, H.; Haq, K.T.; Morotti, S.; Esch, S.; McCune, E.C.; Grandi, E.; Eckhardt, L.L. Inward Rectifier Potassium Channels (Kir2.x) and Caveolin-3 Domain-Specific Interaction: Implications for Purkinje Cell-Dependent Ventricular Arrhythmias. *Circ. Arrhythmia Electrophysiol.* **2018**, *11*, e005800. [CrossRef] [PubMed]
37. Vaidyanathan, R.; Vega, A.L.; Song, C.; Zhou, Q.; Tan, B.H.; Berger, S.; Makielski, J.C.; Eckhardt, L.L. The interaction of caveolin 3 protein with the potassium inward rectifier channel Kir2.1: Physiology and pathology related to long qt syndrome 9 (LQT9). *J. Biol. Chem.* **2013**, *288*, 17472–17480. [CrossRef] [PubMed]
38. Chang, Y.; Yu, T.; Yang, H.; Peng, Z. Exhaustive exercise-induced cardiac conduction system injury and changes of cTnT and Cx43. *Int. J. Sports Med.* **2015**, *36*, 1–8. [CrossRef] [PubMed]
39. Vaidyanathan, R.; Reilly, L.; Eckhardt, L.L. Caveolin-3 Microdomain: Arrhythmia Implications for Potassium Inward Rectifier and Cardiac Sodium Channel. *Front. Physiol.* **2018**, *9*, 1548. [CrossRef] [PubMed]
40. Ponce-Balbuena, D.; Guerrero-Serna, G.; Valdivia, C.R.; Caballero, R.; Diez-Guerra, F.J.; Jiménez-Vázquez, E.N.; Ramírez, R.J.; Monteiro da Rocha, A.; Herron, T.J.; Campbell, K.F.; et al. Cardiac Kir2.1 and Na(V)1.5 Channels Traffic Together to the Sarcolemma to Control Excitability. *Circ. Res.* **2018**, *122*, 1501–1516. [CrossRef] [PubMed]
41. Nguyen Dinh Cat, A.; Touyz, R.M. A new look at the renin-angiotensin system–focusing on the vascular system. *Peptides* **2011**, *32*, 2141–2150. [CrossRef]
42. Tyan, L.; Turner, D.; Komp, K.R.; Medvedev, R.Y.; Lim, E.; Glukhov, A.V. Caveolin-3 is required for regulation of transient outward potassium current by angiotensin II in mouse atrial myocytes. *Am. J. Physiol. Heart Circ. Physiol.* **2021**, *320*, H787–H797. [CrossRef] [PubMed]
43. Rogers, T.B.; Lokuta, A.J. Angiotensin II signal transduction pathways in the cardiovascular system. *Trends Cardiovasc. Med.* **1994**, *4*, 110–116. [CrossRef]
44. Scholz, E.P.; Welke, F.; Joss, N.; Seyler, C.; Zhang, W.; Scherer, D.; Völkers, M.; Bloehs, R.; Thomas, D.; Katus, H.A.; et al. Central role of PKCα in isoenzyme-selective regulation of cardiac transient outward current Ito and Kv4.3 channels. *J. Mol. Cell. Cardiol.* **2011**, *51*, 722–729. [CrossRef] [PubMed]
45. Jansen, H.J.; Mackasey, M.; Moghtadaei, M.; Belke, D.D.; Egom, E.E.; Tuomi, J.M.; Rafferty, S.A.; Kirkby, A.W.; Rose, R.A. Distinct patterns of atrial electrical and structural remodeling in angiotensin II mediated atrial fibrillation. *J. Mol. Cell. Cardiol.* **2018**, *124*, 12–25. [CrossRef] [PubMed]
46. Kawai, M.; Hussain, M.; Orchard, C.H. Excitation-contraction coupling in rat ventricular myocytes after formamide-induced detubulation. *Am. J. Physiol.* **1999**, *277*, H603–H609. [CrossRef]
47. Shan, J.; Xie, W.; Betzenhauser, M.; Reiken, S.; Chen, B.X.; Wronska, A.; Marks, A.R. Calcium leak through ryanodine receptors leads to atrial fibrillation in 3 mouse models of catecholaminergic polymorphic ventricular tachycardia. *Circ. Res.* **2012**, *111*, 708–717. [CrossRef] [PubMed]
48. Nikolaev, V.O.; Moshkov, A.; Lyon, A.R.; Miragoli, M.; Novak, P.; Paur, H.; Lohse, M.J.; Korchev, Y.E.; Harding, S.E.; Gorelik, J. Beta2-adrenergic receptor redistribution in heart failure changes cAMP compartmentation. *Science* **2010**, *327*, 1653–1657. [CrossRef] [PubMed]
49. Beuckelmann, D.J.; Näbauer, M.; Erdmann, E. Characteristics of calcium-current in isolated human ventricular myocytes from patients with terminal heart failure. *J. Mol. Cell. Cardiol.* **1991**, *23*, 929–937. [CrossRef]
50. Ouadid, H.; Séguin, J.; Richard, S.; Chaptal, P.A.; Nargeot, J. Properties and Modulation of Ca channels in adult human atrial cells. *J. Mol. Cell. Cardiol.* **1991**, *23*, 41–54. [CrossRef]
51. Li, G.R.; Nattel, S. Properties of human atrial ICa at physiological temperatures and relevance to action potential. *Am. J. Physiol.* **1997**, *272*, H227–H235. [CrossRef] [PubMed]
52. Markandeya, Y.S.; Fahey, J.M.; Pluteanu, F.; Cribbs, L.L.; Balijepalli, R.C. Caveolin-3 regulates protein kinase A modulation of the Ca(V)3.2 (alpha1H) T-type Ca2+ channels. *J. Biol. Chem.* **2011**, *286*, 2433–2444. [CrossRef] [PubMed]
53. Markandeya, Y.S.; Phelan, L.J.; Woon, M.T.; Keefe, A.M.; Reynolds, C.R.; August, B.K.; Hacker, T.A.; Roth, D.M.; Patel, H.H.; Balijepalli, R.C. Caveolin-3 Overexpression Attenuates Cardiac Hypertrophy via Inhibition of T-type Ca^{2+} Current Modulated by Protein Kinase Cα in Cardiomyocytes. *J. Biol. Chem.* **2015**, *290*, 22085–22100. [CrossRef] [PubMed]

54. Chemin, J.; Taiakina, V.; Monteil, A.; Piazza, M.; Guan, W.; Stephens, R.F.; Kitmitto, A.; Pang, Z.P.; Dolphin, A.C.; Perez-Reyes, E.; et al. Calmodulin regulates Ca(v)3 T-type channels at their gating brake. *J. Biol. Chem.* **2017**, *292*, 20010–20031. [CrossRef]
55. Parton, R.G.; Way, M.; Zorzi, N.; Stang, E. Caveolin-3 associates with developing T-tubules during muscle differentiation. *J. Cell Biol.* **1997**, *136*, 137–154. [CrossRef] [PubMed]
56. Bryant, S.; Kimura, T.E.; Kong, C.H.; Watson, J.J.; Chase, A.; Suleiman, M.S.; James, A.F.; Orchard, C.H. Stimulation of ICa by basal PKA activity is facilitated by Caveolin-3 in cardiac ventricular myocytes. *J. Mol. Cell. Cardiol.* **2014**, *68*, 47–55. [CrossRef] [PubMed]
57. Galbiati, F.; Engelman, J.A.; Volonte, D.; Zhang, X.L.; Minetti, C.; Li, M.; Hou, H., Jr.; Kneitz, B.; Edelmann, W.; Lisanti, M.P. Caveolin-3 null mice show a loss of caveolae, changes in the microdomain distribution of the dystrophin-glycoprotein complex, and t-tubule abnormalities. *J. Biol. Chem.* **2001**, *276*, 21425–21433. [CrossRef]
58. Bryant, S.M.; Kong, C.H.T.; Watson, J.J.; Gadeberg, H.C.; James, A.F.; Cannell, M.B.; Orchard, C.H. Caveolin 3-dependent loss of t-tubular I(Ca) during hypertrophy and heart failure in mice. *Exp. Physiol.* **2018**, *103*, 652–665. [CrossRef] [PubMed]
59. Bhogal, N.K.; Hasan, A.; Gorelik, J. The Development of Compartmentation of cAMP Signaling in Cardiomyocytes: The Role of T-Tubules and Caveolae Microdomains. *J. Cardiovasc. Dev. Dis.* **2018**, *5*, 25. [CrossRef] [PubMed]
60. Asghari, P.; Scriven, D.R.; Hoskins, J.; Fameli, N.; van Breemen, C.; Moore, E.D. The structure and functioning of the couplon in the mammalian cardiomyocyte. *Protoplasma* **2012**, *249* (Suppl. 1), S31–S38. [CrossRef] [PubMed]
61. Fill, M.; Copello, J.A. Ryanodine receptor calcium release channels. *Physiol. Rev.* **2002**, *82*, 893–922. [CrossRef]
62. Wong, J.; Baddeley, D.; Bushong, E.A.; Yu, Z.; Ellisman, M.H.; Hoshijima, M.; Soeller, C. Nanoscale distribution of ryanodine receptors and caveolin-3 in mouse ventricular myocytes: Dilation of t-tubules near junctions. *Biophys. J.* **2013**, *104*, L22-24. [CrossRef] [PubMed]
63. Song, D.W.; Lee, K.E.; Ryu, J.Y.; Jeon, H.; Kim, D.H. The molecular interaction of heart LIM protein (HLP) with RyR2 and caveolin-3 is essential for Ca(2+)-induced Ca(2+) release in the heart. *Biochem. Biophys. Res. Commun.* **2015**, *463*, 975–981. [CrossRef] [PubMed]
64. Zhang, Z.; Fang, Q.; Du, T.; Chen, G.; Wang, Y.; Wang, D.W. Cardiac-Specific Caveolin-3 Overexpression Prevents Post-Myocardial Infarction Ventricular Arrhythmias by Inhibiting Ryanodine Receptor-2 Hyperphosphorylation. *Cardiology* **2020**, *145*, 136–147. [CrossRef]
65. Castets, F.; Rakitina, T.; Gaillard, S.; Moqrich, A.; Mattei, M.G.; Monneron, A. Zinedin, SG2NA, and striatin are calmodulin-binding, WD repeat proteins principally expressed in the brain. *J. Biol. Chem.* **2000**, *275*, 19970–19977. [CrossRef] [PubMed]
66. Nader, M.; Alotaibi, S.; Alsolme, E.; Khalil, B.; Abu-Zaid, A.; Alsomali, R.; Bakheet, D.; Dzimiri, N. Cardiac striatin interacts with caveolin-3 and calmodulin in a calcium sensitive manner and regulates cardiomyocyte spontaneous contraction rate. *Can. J. Physiol. Pharmacol.* **2017**, *95*, 1306–1312. [CrossRef] [PubMed]
67. Barbuti, A.; Terragni, B.; Brioschi, C.; DiFrancesco, D. Localization of f-channels to caveolae mediates specific beta2-adrenergic receptor modulation of rate in sinoatrial myocytes. *J. Mol. Cell. Cardiol.* **2007**, *42*, 71–78. [CrossRef]
68. Motloch, L.J.; Larbig, R.; Darabi, T.; Reda, S.; Motloch, K.A.; Wernly, B.; Lichtenauer, M.; Gebing, T.; Schwaiger, A.; Zagidullin, N.; et al. Long-QT syndrome-associated Caveolin-3 mutations differentially regulate the hyperpolarization-activated cyclic nucleotide gated channel 4. *Physiol. Int.* **2017**, *104*, 130–138. [CrossRef]
69. Kuwabara, Y.; Kuwahara, K.; Takano, M.; Kinoshita, H.; Arai, Y.; Yasuno, S.; Nakagawa, Y.; Igata, S.; Usami, S.; Minami, T.; et al. Increased expression of HCN channels in the ventricular myocardium contributes to enhanced arrhythmicity in mouse failing hearts. *J. Am. Heart Assoc.* **2013**, *2*, e000150. [CrossRef] [PubMed]
70. Sun, L.Y.; Qu, X.; Chen, L.Z.; Zheng, G.S.; Wu, X.L.; Chen, X.X.; Huang, W.J.; Zhou, H. Potential Roles of Serum Caveolin-3 Levels in Patients with Atrial Fibrillation. *Front. Aging Neurosci.* **2017**, *9*, 90. [CrossRef]
71. Reilly, S.N.; Liu, X.; Carnicer, R.; Recalde, A.; Muszkiewicz, A.; Jayaram, R.; Carena, M.C.; Wijesurendra, R.; Stefanini, M.; Surdo, N.C.; et al. Up-regulation of miR-31 in human atrial fibrillation begets the arrhythmia by depleting dystrophin and neuronal nitric oxide synthase. *Sci. Transl. Med.* **2016**, *8*, 340ra374. [CrossRef] [PubMed]
72. Egorov, Y.V.; Lang, D.; Tyan, L.; Turner, D.; Lim, E.; Piro, Z.D.; Hernandez, J.J.; Lodin, R.; Wang, R.; Schmuck, E.G.; et al. Caveolae-Mediated Activation of Mechanosensitive Chloride Channels in Pulmonary Veins Triggers Atrial Arrhythmogenesis. *J. Am. Heart Assoc.* **2019**, *8*, e012748. [CrossRef] [PubMed]
73. Andelova, K.; Egan Benova, T.; Szeiffova Bacova, B.; Sykora, M.; Prado, N.J.; Diez, E.R.; Hlivak, P.; Tribulova, N. Cardiac Connexin-43 Hemichannels and Pannexin1 Channels: Provocative Antiarrhythmic Targets. *Int. J. Mol. Sci.* **2020**, *22*, 260. [CrossRef] [PubMed]
74. Xue, J.; Yan, X.; Yang, Y.; Chen, M.; Wu, L.; Gou, Z.; Sun, Z.; Talabieke, S.; Zheng, Y.; Luo, D. Connexin 43 dephosphorylation contributes to arrhythmias and cardiomyocyte apoptosis in ischemia/reperfusion hearts. *Basic Res. Cardiol.* **2019**, *114*, 40. [CrossRef]
75. Saffitz, J.E. Arrhythmogenic cardiomyopathy and abnormalities of cell-to-cell coupling. *Heart Rhythm* **2009**, *6*, S62–S65. [CrossRef] [PubMed]
76. Xiao, S.; Shimura, D.; Baum, R.; Hernandez, D.M.; Agvanian, S.; Nagaoka, Y.; Katsumata, M.; Lampe, P.D.; Kleber, A.G.; Hong, T.; et al. Auxiliary trafficking subunit GJA1-20k protects connexin-43 from degradation and limits ventricular arrhythmias. *J. Clin. Investig.* **2020**, *130*, 4858–4870. [CrossRef] [PubMed]

77. Zhang, P.; Xu, J.; Hu, W.; Yu, D.; Bai, X. Effects of Pinocembrin Pretreatment on Connexin 43 (Cx43) Protein Expression After Rat Myocardial Ischemia-Reperfusion and Cardiac Arrhythmia. *Med. Sci. Monit. Int. Med. J. Exp. Clin. Res.* **2018**, *24*, 5008–5014. [CrossRef]
78. Rugowska, A.; Wiernicki, B.; Maczewski, M.; Mackiewicz, U.; Chojnacka, K.; Bednarek-Rajewska, K.; Kluk, M.; Majewski, P.; Kolanowski, T.; Malcher, A.; et al. Human skeletal muscle-derived stem/progenitor cells modified with connexin-43 prevent arrhythmia in rat post-infarction hearts and influence gene expression in the myocardium. *J. Physiol. Pharmacol. Off. J. Pol. Physiol. Soc.* **2019**, *70*. [CrossRef]
79. Yang, K.C.; Rutledge, C.A.; Mao, M.; Bakhshi, F.R.; Xie, A.; Liu, H.; Bonini, M.G.; Patel, H.H.; Minshall, R.D.; Dudley, S.C., Jr. Caveolin-1 modulates cardiac gap junction homeostasis and arrhythmogenicity by regulating cSrc tyrosine kinase. *Circ. Arrhythmia Electrophysiol.* **2014**, *7*, 701–710. [CrossRef]
80. Liu, L.; Li, Y.; Lin, J.; Liang, Q.; Sheng, X.; Wu, J.; Huang, R.; Liu, S.; Li, Y. Connexin43 interacts with Caveolin-3 in the heart. *Mol. Biol. Rep.* **2010**, *37*, 1685–1691. [CrossRef] [PubMed]
81. Soares, E.S.; Mendonça, M.C.; Rocha, T.; Kalapothakis, E.; da Cruz-Höfling, M.A. Are Synchronized Changes in Connexin-43 and Caveolin-3 a Bystander Effect in a Phoneutria nigriventer Venom Model of Blood-Brain Barrier Breakdown? *J. Mol. Neurosci. MN* **2016**, *59*, 452–463. [CrossRef] [PubMed]
82. Liao, C.K.; Wang, S.M.; Chen, Y.L.; Wang, H.S.; Wu, J.C. Lipopolysaccharide-induced inhibition of connexin43 gap junction communication in astrocytes is mediated by downregulation of caveolin-3. *Int. J. Biochem. Cell Biol.* **2010**, *42*, 762–770. [CrossRef]
83. Valera, I.C.; Wacker, A.L.; Hwang, H.S.; Holmes, C.; Laitano, O.; Landstrom, A.P.; Parvatiyar, M.S. Essential roles of the dystrophin-glycoprotein complex in different cardiac pathologies. *Adv. Med. Sci.* **2021**, *66*, 52–71. [CrossRef] [PubMed]
84. Sinagra, G.; Dal Ferro, M.; Gigli, M. The heart of dystrophinopathies. *Eur. J. Heart Fail.* **2021**, *23*, 1287–1289. [CrossRef]
85. Kamdar, F.; Garry, D.J. Dystrophin-Deficient Cardiomyopathy. *J. Am. Coll. Cardiol.* **2016**, *67*, 2533–2546. [CrossRef] [PubMed]
86. Doyle, D.D.; Goings, G.; Upshaw-Earley, J.; Ambler, S.K.; Mondul, A.; Palfrey, H.C.; Page, E. Dystrophin associates with caveolae of rat cardiac myocytes: Relationship to dystroglycan. *Circ. Res.* **2000**, *87*, 480–488. [CrossRef] [PubMed]
87. Aravamudan, B.; Volonte, D.; Ramani, R.; Gursoy, E.; Lisanti, M.P.; London, B.; Galbiati, F. Transgenic overexpression of caveolin-3 in the heart induces a cardiomyopathic phenotype. *Hum. Mol. Genet.* **2003**, *12*, 2777–2788. [CrossRef]
88. Sotgia, F.; Lee, J.K.; Das, K.; Bedford, M.; Petrucci, T.C.; Macioce, P.; Sargiacomo, M.; Bricarelli, F.D.; Minetti, C.; Sudol, M.; et al. Caveolin-3 directly interacts with the C-terminal tail of beta-dystroglycan. Identification of a central WW-like domain within caveolin family members. *J. Biol. Chem.* **2000**, *275*, 38048–38058. [CrossRef] [PubMed]
89. Fang, H.; Judd, R.L. Adiponectin Regulation and Function. *Compr. Physiol.* **2018**, *8*, 1031–1063. [CrossRef] [PubMed]
90. Wang, Y.; Wang, X.; Jasmin, J.F.; Lau, W.B.; Li, R.; Yuan, Y.; Yi, W.; Chuprun, K.; Lisanti, M.P.; Koch, W.J.; et al. Essential role of caveolin-3 in adiponectin signalsome formation and adiponectin cardioprotection. *Arterioscler. Thromb. Vasc. Biol.* **2012**, *32*, 934–942. [CrossRef] [PubMed]
91. Yi, W.; Sun, Y.; Gao, E.; Wei, X.; Lau, W.B.; Zheng, Q.; Wang, Y.; Yuan, Y.; Wang, X.; Tao, L.; et al. Reduced cardioprotective action of adiponectin in high-fat diet-induced type II diabetic mice and its underlying mechanisms. *Antioxid. Redox Signal.* **2011**, *15*, 1779–1788. [CrossRef] [PubMed]
92. Lei, S.; Li, H.; Xu, J.; Liu, Y.; Gao, X.; Wang, J.; Ng, K.F.; Lau, W.B.; Ma, X.L.; Rodrigues, B.; et al. Hyperglycemia-induced protein kinase C β2 activation induces diastolic cardiac dysfunction in diabetic rats by impairing caveolin-3 expression and Akt/eNOS signaling. *Diabetes* **2013**, *62*, 2318–2328. [CrossRef] [PubMed]
93. Tan, Z.; Zhou, L.J.; Mu, P.W.; Liu, S.P.; Chen, S.J.; Fu, X.D.; Wang, T.H. Caveolin-3 is involved in the protection of resveratrol against high-fat-diet-induced insulin resistance by promoting GLUT4 translocation to the plasma membrane in skeletal muscle of ovariectomized rats. *J. Nutr. Biochem.* **2012**, *23*, 1716–1724. [CrossRef] [PubMed]
94. Li, H.; Yao, W.; Liu, Z.; Xu, A.; Huang, Y.; Ma, X.L.; Irwin, M.G.; Xia, Z. Hyperglycemia Abrogates Ischemic Postconditioning Cardioprotection by Impairing AdipoR1/Caveolin-3/STAT3 Signaling in Diabetic Rats. *Diabetes* **2016**, *65*, 942–955. [CrossRef] [PubMed]
95. Hegyi, B.; Bers, D.M.; Bossuyt, J. CaMKII signaling in heart diseases: Emerging role in diabetic cardiomyopathy. *J. Mol. Cell. Cardiol.* **2019**, *127*, 246–259. [CrossRef]
96. Lau, D.H.; Nattel, S.; Kalman, J.M.; Sanders, P. Modifiable Risk Factors and Atrial Fibrillation. *Circulation* **2017**, *136*, 583–596. [CrossRef]
97. Huang, Y.; Deng, Y.; Shang, L.; Yang, L.; Huang, J.; Ma, J.; Liao, X.; Zhou, H.; Xian, J.; Liang, G.; et al. Effect of type 2 diabetes mellitus caveolin-3 K15N mutation on glycometabolism. *Exp. Ther. Med.* **2019**, *18*, 2531–2539. [CrossRef] [PubMed]
98. Shang, L.; Chen, T.; Xian, J.; Deng, Y.; Huang, Y.; Zhao, Q.; Liang, G.; Liang, Z.; Lian, F.; Wei, H.; et al. The caveolin-3 P104L mutation in LGMD-1C patients inhibits non-insulin-stimulated glucose metabolism and growth but promotes myocyte proliferation. *Cell Biol. Int.* **2019**, *43*, 669–677. [CrossRef] [PubMed]
99. Gao, Y.; Zhang, M.; Wu, T.; Xu, M.; Cai, H.; Zhang, Z. Effects of D-Pinitol on Insulin Resistance through the PI3K/Akt Signaling Pathway in Type 2 Diabetes Mellitus Rats. *J. Agric. Food Chem.* **2015**, *63*, 6019–6026. [CrossRef]
100. Yang, M.; Ren, Y.; Lin, Z.; Tang, C.; Jia, Y.; Lai, Y.; Zhou, Y.; Wu, S.; Liu, H.; Yang, G.; et al. Krüppel-like factor 14 increases insulin sensitivity through activation of PI3K/Akt signal pathway. *Cell. Signal.* **2015**, *27*, 2201–2208. [CrossRef]
101. Mu, P.; Tan, Z.; Cui, Y.; Liu, H.; Xu, X.; Huang, Q.; Zeng, L.; Wang, T. 17β-Estradiol attenuates diet-induced insulin resistance and glucose intolerance through up-regulation of caveolin-3. *Ir. J. Med. Sci.* **2011**, *180*, 221–227. [CrossRef] [PubMed]

102. Lei, S.; Su, W.; Xia, Z.Y.; Wang, Y.; Zhou, L.; Qiao, S.; Zhao, B.; Xia, Z.; Irwin, M.G. Hyperglycemia-Induced Oxidative Stress Abrogates Remifentanil Preconditioning-Mediated Cardioprotection in Diabetic Rats by Impairing Caveolin-3-Modulated PI3K/Akt and JAK2/STAT3 Signaling. *Oxidative Med. Cell. Longev.* **2019**, *2019*, 9836302. [CrossRef] [PubMed]
103. Margolis, K.L.; Bonds, D.E.; Rodabough, R.J.; Tinker, L.; Phillips, L.S.; Allen, C.; Bassford, T.; Burke, G.; Torrens, J.; Howard, B.V. Effect of oestrogen plus progestin on the incidence of diabetes in postmenopausal women: Results from the Women's Health Initiative Hormone Trial. *Diabetologia* **2004**, *47*, 1175–1187. [CrossRef] [PubMed]
104. Capozza, F.; Combs, T.P.; Cohen, A.W.; Cho, Y.R.; Park, S.Y.; Schubert, W.; Williams, T.M.; Brasaemle, D.L.; Jelicks, L.A.; Scherer, P.E.; et al. Caveolin-3 knockout mice show increased adiposity and whole body insulin resistance, with ligand-induced insulin receptor instability in skeletal muscle. *Am. J. Physiology. Cell Physiol.* **2005**, *288*, C1317–C1331. [CrossRef] [PubMed]
105. Lin, Y.K.; Chen, Y.C.; Chen, J.H.; Chen, S.A.; Chen, Y.J. Adipocytes modulate the electrophysiology of atrial myocytes: Implications in obesity-induced atrial fibrillation. *Basic Res. Cardiol.* **2012**, *107*, 293. [CrossRef] [PubMed]
106. Omran, J.; Bostick, B.P.; Chan, A.K.; Alpert, M.A. Obesity and Ventricular Repolarization: A Comprehensive Review. *Prog. Cardiovasc. Dis.* **2018**, *61*, 124–135. [CrossRef] [PubMed]
107. Gómez-Ruiz, A.; Milagro, F.I.; Campión, J.; Martínez, J.A.; de Miguel, C. Caveolin expression and activation in retroperitoneal and subcutaneous adipocytes: Influence of a high-fat diet. *J. Cell. Physiol.* **2010**, *225*, 206–213. [CrossRef] [PubMed]
108. Gómez-Ruiz, A.; Milagro, F.I.; Campión, J.; Martínez, J.A.; de Miguel, C. High-fat diet feeding alters metabolic response to fasting/non fasting conditions. Effect on caveolin expression and insulin signalling. *Lipids Health Dis.* **2011**, *10*, 55. [CrossRef]
109. Feillet-Coudray, C.; Sutra, T.; Fouret, G.; Ramos, J.; Wrutniak-Cabello, C.; Cabello, G.; Cristol, J.P.; Coudray, C. Oxidative stress in rats fed a high-fat high-sucrose diet and preventive effect of polyphenols: Involvement of mitochondrial and NAD(P)H oxidase systems. *Free Radic. Biol. Med.* **2009**, *46*, 624–632. [CrossRef] [PubMed]

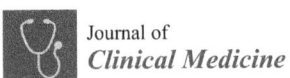

Review

Pathogenesis and Management of Brugada Syndrome: Recent Advances and Protocol for Umbrella Reviews of Meta-Analyses in Major Arrhythmic Events Risk Stratification

Hasina Masha Aziz [1], Michał P. Zarzecki [2], Sebastian Garcia-Zamora [3], Min Seo Kim [4], Piotr Bijak [5], Gary Tse [6,7,8], Hong-Hee Won [9] and Paweł T. Matusik [10,11,*]

1. Faculty of Medicine, Jagiellonian University Medical College, 31-530 Kraków, Poland; masha.aziz@student.uj.edu.pl
2. Department of Anatomy, Jagiellonian University Medical College, 31-034 Kraków, Poland; michal.zarzecki@uj.edu.pl
3. Cardiology Department, Delta Clinic, Rosario S2000, Argentina; szamora@sanatoriodelta.com.ar
4. Samsung Advanced Institute for Health Sciences & Technology (SAIHST), Sungkyunkwan University, Samsung Medical Center, Seoul 06351, Korea; minseolike@korea.ac.kr
5. John Paul II Hospital, 31-202 Kraków, Poland; p.bijak@szpitaljp2.krakow.pl
6. Cardiac Electrophysiology Unit, Cardiovascular Analytics Group, Hong Kong, China; gary.tse@kmms.ac.uk
7. Tianjin Key Laboratory of Ionic-Molecular Function of Cardiovascular Disease, Department of Cardiology, Tianjin Institute of Cardiology, Second Hospital of Tianjin Medical University, Tianjin 300070, China
8. Kent and Medway Medical School, University of Kent and Canterbury Christ Church University, Canterbury CT2 7FS, UK
9. Samsung Advanced Institute for Health Sciences & Technology (SAIHST), Samsung Genome Institute, Samsung Medical Center, Seoul 06351, Korea; wonhh@skku.edu
10. Department of Electrocardiology, Institute of Cardiology, Faculty of Medicine, Jagiellonian University Medical College, 31-202 Kraków, Poland
11. Department of Electrocardiology, The John Paul II Hospital, 31-202 Kraków, Poland
* Correspondence: pawel.matusik@uj.edu.pl

Abstract: Brugada syndrome (BrS) is a primary electrical disease associated with life-threatening arrhythmias. It is estimated to cause at least 20% of sudden cardiac deaths (SCDs) in patients with normal cardiac anatomy. In this review paper, we discuss recent advances in complex BrS pathogenesis, diagnostics, and current standard approaches to major arrhythmic events (MAEs) risk stratification. Additionally, we describe a protocol for umbrella reviews to systematically investigate clinical, electrocardiographic, electrophysiological study, programmed ventricular stimulation, and genetic factors associated with BrS, and the risk of MAEs. Our evaluation will include MAEs such as sustained ventricular tachycardia, ventricular fibrillation, appropriate implantable cardioverter–defibrillator therapy, sudden cardiac arrest, and SCDs from previous meta-analytical studies. The protocol was written following the Preferred Reporting Items for Systematic review and Meta-Analysis Protocols (PRISMA-P) guidelines. We plan to extensively search PubMed, Embase, and Scopus databases for meta-analyses concerning risk-stratification in BrS. Data will be synthesized integratively with transparency and accuracy. Heterogeneity patterns across studies will be reported. The Joanna Briggs Institute (JBI) methodology, A MeaSurement Tool to Assess systematic Reviews 2 (AMSTAR 2), and the Grading of Recommendations, Assessment, Development and Evaluation (GRADE) are planned to be applied for design and execution of our evidence-based research. To the best of our knowledge, these will be the first umbrella reviews to critically evaluate the current state of knowledge in BrS risk stratification for life-threatening ventricular arrhythmias, and will potentially contribute towards evidence-based guidance to enhance clinical decisions.

Keywords: Brugada syndrome; pathogenesis; management; primary electrical disease; arrhythmic events; sudden cardiac arrest; sudden cardiac death; risk stratification; review; protocol

Citation: Aziz, H.M.; Zarzecki, M.P.; Garcia-Zamora, S.; Kim, M.S.; Bijak, P.; Tse, G.; Won, H.-H.; Matusik, P.T. Pathogenesis and Management of Brugada Syndrome: Recent Advances and Protocol for Umbrella Reviews of Meta-Analyses in Major Arrhythmic Events Risk Stratification. *J. Clin. Med.* **2022**, *11*, 1912. https://doi.org/10.3390/jcm11071912

Academic Editors: Emmanuel Andrès and Massimo Iacoviello

Received: 7 February 2022
Accepted: 25 March 2022
Published: 30 March 2022

Publisher's Note: MDPI stays neutral with regard to jurisdictional claims in published maps and institutional affiliations.

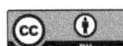

Copyright: © 2022 by the authors. Licensee MDPI, Basel, Switzerland. This article is an open access article distributed under the terms and conditions of the Creative Commons Attribution (CC BY) license (https://creativecommons.org/licenses/by/4.0/).

1. Introduction

Brugada syndrome (BrS) is a primary electrical disease associated with arrhythmias and an elevated risk of sudden cardiac death (SCD) [1,2]. It was described by Pedro and Josep Brugada in 1992 as a syndrome comprised of "right bundle branch block, persistent ST segment elevation and SCD" [3]. However, the description of the electrocardiographic (ECG) changes considered today as type 1 BrS ECG pattern was first published in 1953 [4]. The prevalence of individuals with the Brugada ECG patterns differs largely among various regions and populations of the world [5] and is more common than BrS. Pooled worldwide prevalence of BrS is 0.5 per 1000 [6] based on ECG patterns, with highest prevalence in Southeast Asia of 3.7 per 1000, reaching up to 17.7 per 1000 in Thailand [6,7]. BrS is approximately nine times more common in males [8,9], and is one of the leading causes of SCD in males below age 40 in southeast Asia [10]. Patients with BrS are considered symptomatic if they have a history of aborted SCD, ventricular fibrillation (VF), sustained ventricular tachycardia (VT), or syncope [11,12].

BrS usually presents during the third or fourth decade of life, and about 63% of patients are asymptomatic at diagnosis [7,11]. However, syncope or major arrhythmic events (MAE) can occur at any age, or SCD may even present as the first event [11]. BrS contributes towards sudden infant death syndrome, SCD in children, and estimated to cause at least 20% of all SCDs in individuals with anatomically normal cardiac structures [9,11,13,14].

2. Pathogenesis of BrS

BrS was previously described as an autosomal-dominant inherited disorder with incomplete penetrance, and absent or benign structural heart abnormalities [1,11]. The lack of significant structural heart disease in BrS patients may be visualized by echocardiography, angiography, or ventriculography [14,15]. However, magnetic resonance imaging in subgroups of patients with BrS revealed enlarged right ventricular (RV) volumes, increased RV outflow tract (RVOT) area, or mild RV wall motion abnormalities [16]. The pathomechanism observed in BrS patients involves depolarization and repolarization abnormalities, inflammation of myocytes, and fibrosis in RVOT and/or RV [9,12]. A recent study performed on whole hearts from deceased patients, whose SCD was accounted to BrS, showed biventricular myocardial fibrosis, especially in the epicardium of the RVOT [17]. RV myocardium in a number of patients with BrS type 1 ECG pattern have showed histological changes comparable to arrhythmogenic RV cardiomyopathy (ARVC), and indicate possible autoimmune causes of myocardial inflammation in BrS patients [9].

Genetic etiology, identified in about 14–34% cases, is primarily associated with sodium voltage-gated channel alpha subunit 5 (SCN5A) gene mutation affecting cardiac channels [9,18,19]. SCN5A gene encodes for the α-subunit of the sodium channels in the heart and mutations in the gene lead to reduced expression of Nav1.5 α-subunit proteins, loss of functional sodium channels, and impaired phase 0 action potential [11]. At present, other genes have been identified as susceptibility genes for BrS, and BrS is now considered an oligogenic or polygenic disease [9,20].

Currently, potassium, chloride, and calcium ion channels involved in the cardiac depolarization and repolarization process have also been described as associated with channelopathies caused by the dysfunction of regulatory proteins [21]. For example, excess outflow of potassium current during early repolarization or reduced inward current via calcium channels may contribute to BrS pathophysiology [21]. The reduced inward current flow of sodium in BrS patients may result in prolonged PR (PQ) interval, first degree atrioventricular block [22], slow cardiac conduction (intraventricular and His–Purkinje), phase 2 reentry and premature repolarization [21], low-amplitude and high-frequency electrical activity in RVOT epicardium (late potentials), and ventricular arrhythmias [12,23].

A recent study identified autoantibodies in the myocardium of BrS patients against cardiac proteins (α-actin, skeletal α-actin, connexin-43, keratin) and observed abnormal expression of Nav1.5 α-subunit proteins [9]. Another study reported distinct elevation (apolipoprotein E, clusterin, prothrombin, vitamin-D-binding protein, complement-factor H, voltage-dependent anion-selective channel protein 3, vitronectin) or reduction (alpha-1-antitrypsin, angiotensinogen, fibrinogen) in plasma proteome of BrS patients and relatives with SCN5A^{Q1118X} gene mutation compared to their healthy family members without the gene mutation, as well as antithrombin-III post-translational modifications [24]. Figure 1 displays an overview of the pathomechanism processes in BrS.

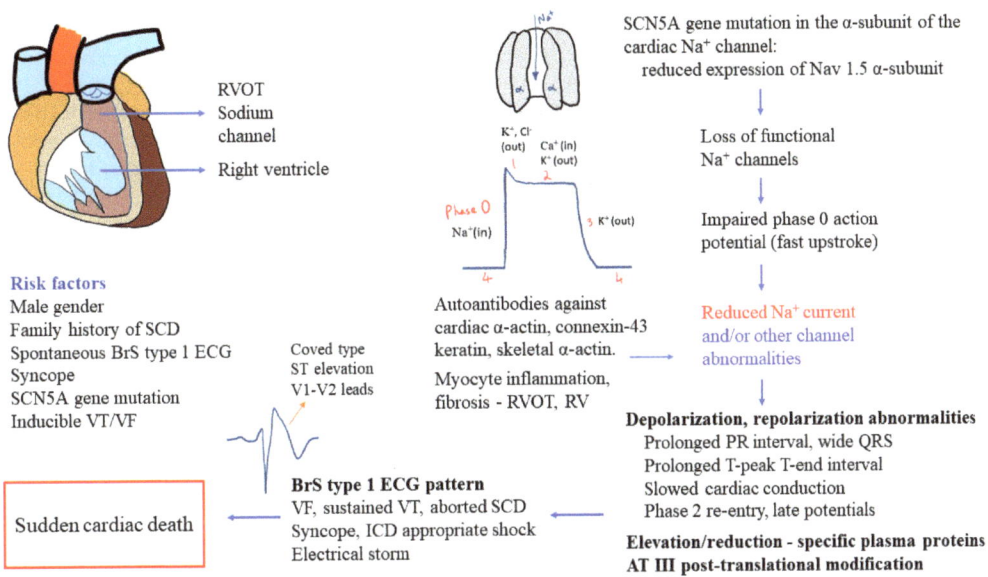

Figure 1. Overview of pathomechanisms involved in Brugada syndrome [9–12,21,22,24–27]. Abbreviations: AT—antithrombin; BrS—Brugada syndrome; Ca^{2+}—calcium; ECG—electrocardiogram; K$^+$—potassium; ICD—implantable cardioverter–defibrillator; Na$^+$—sodium; SCD—sudden cardiac death; SCN5A—sodium voltage-gated channel alpha subunit 5; RV—right ventricle; RVOT—right ventricular outflow tract; VF—ventricular fibrillation; VT—ventricular tachycardia.

3. Diagnostics and Risk Stratification

The definitions of BrS can vary depending on the guidelines used. The European Society of Cardiology (ESC) guidelines proposes that any subject with spontaneous or drug-induced type 1 Brugada ECG pattern be classified as BrS [28]. However, some investigators suggest that this may lead to overdiagnosis, and specific symptoms or clinical data are required to confirm diagnosis [29,30]. Clinical, ECG, and laboratory markers have been found to be useful in diagnostics and risk stratification in diverse groups of patients [31–41]. Despite progress in SCD prevention, the optimal diagnostics and risk stratification in BrS are a major clinical challenge [42–44].

3.1. Diagnostics in BrS

The ESC definition of BrS diagnosis states that patients must display BrS ECG pattern with ST-segment elevation ≥ 2 mm in at least one lead (V1-V2) placed in the second, third, or fourth intercostal spaces [28]. This may appear spontaneously or following intravenous drug provocation with class Ia (ajmaline or procainamide) or class Ic (flecainide or pilsicainide) sodium channel blockers [28]. The BrS type 1 ECG pattern may also be induced by fever and exercise tests [8–11,45]. The unique ECG pattern is often short-lasting, and only depending on standard 12-lead ECG may lead to underdiagnosis of 65% patients, especially those who need modified high leads or drug provocation [9]. Therefore, prolonged cardiac monitoring might be highly valuable for diagnostic process [46]. When the Brugada ECG pattern is present without life-threatening arrhythmias or SCD, after exclusion of BrS, it is known as Brugada phenocopy [8].

The Shanghai scoring system for BrS diagnosis is based on ECG, family history, clinical symptoms, and genetics, and assigns a score of ≥3.5 for probable and/or definitive BrS (type 1 BrS ECG pattern–spontaneous or drug-induced), a score from 2 to 3 for possible BrS, and a score of <2 is nondiagnostic [9,47,48]. Additionally, a score of 3 was for fever-induced BrS type 1 ECG, a score of 2 for convertible drug-induced type 2 or 3 BrS ECG pattern, a score of 2 for definite BrS in family (first-/second-degree relative), a score of 0.5 for atrial fibrillation (AF) or atrial flutter in patients younger than age 30 (no alternative etiology), and a score of 0.5 for probable pathologic genetic mutation which may lead to BrS [9]. SCN5A gene-mutation type and a BrS genetic risk score is associated with BrS phenotype in patients with spontaneous type 1 BrS ECG pattern or family members with SCN5A mutations [49]. Importantly, MRI studies have shown a correlation between maximal ECG ST segment elevation and maximal RVOT area in the presence of BrS type 1 ECG pattern [50].

3.2. Risk Stratification in BrS

ESC guidelines on ventricular arrhythmias and the prevention of SCD [28] recommend focusing on risk stratification and clinical decisions in the presence of previous SCA or documented spontaneous sustained VT, spontaneous diagnostic type 1 BrS ECG pattern, syncopal episodes, and inducible VF during programmed ventricular stimulation (PVS) (using two–three extrastimuli at two sites). According to the American Heart Association, the American College of Cardiology, and the Heart Rhythm Society (AHA/ACC/HRS) recommendations, for additional risk stratification in asymptomatic BrS patients and in patients with spontaneous type 1 BrS ECG pattern, electrophysiological study (EPS) with PVS (using single and double extrastimuli) may be beneficial [51]. Wakamiya et al. evaluated the emphasis of arrhythmic syncope history or unexplained syncope and VF inducibility by ≤two extrastimuli during PVS according to new guidelines of the Japanese Circulation Society to help determine ICD indication in patients with BrS [52]. The research studied 234 BrS patients where 20% had VF history, 43% had syncope history, and 37% were asymptomatic at diagnosis [52]. Patients underwent PVS at RV apex or RVOT (1–3 extrastimuli) and mean follow-up was 6.9 ± 5.2 years [52]. The study underlined a less aggressive approach for PVS in BrS risk stratification.

Spontaneous type 1 BrS ECG pattern and syncopal episode history, fragmented QRS (fQRS), and ventricular effective refractory period (VRP) <200 milliseconds have been independently associated with ventricular arrhythmic events in BrS [53]. Moreover, prominent R wave (≥0.3 mV or R/q ≥ 0.75) in lead aVR (aVR sign) was identified to be associated with arrhythmic events in BrS [54]. Fever may precipitate both Brugada type 1 and 2 ECG patterns in patients who have normal baseline ECG [8], and predispose to the development of life-threatening ventricular arrhythmias and SCD [10]. However, a recent study indicated that asymptomatic patients with fever-induced type 1 BrS ECG pattern, negative family history of sudden death, and without spontaneous type 1 BrS ECG pattern are at low risk for future arrhythmic events [55].

Prolonged QRS complex duration, >120 milliseconds on standard 12-lead ECG due to slowed depolarization, was more pronounced in BrS patients expressing symptoms and may predict future MAE [12]. Moreover, T-peak to T-end (Tpe) intervals were identified as novel ECG markers in BrS patients for MAE prediction. High-risk BrS patients had longer Tpe interval in lead V1 and Tpeak-Tend/QT ratio compared to low-risk BrS patients [25]. Recently, based on 12-lead ECG data extracted from automated measurements in BrS patients, novel markers (i.e., ST slope) in predicting arrhythmic events in BrS were identified [27]. The authors stated that, using a weighted scoring system determined from QRS frontal axis, QRS duration, S wave duration and ST slope in lead I, as well as R wave duration in lead III, spontaneous VT/VF incidence may be predicted [27].

A new research performed on patients with drug-induced type 1 BrS ECG pattern who underwent PVS showed that a novel ECG marker dST-Tiso interval (the longest interval from V1-2 in the second, third, or fourth intercostal space) following ajmaline injection to be a significant predictor for the inducibility of ventricular arrhythmias (sustained or hemodynamically significant polymorphic VT of VF requiring direct current shock) [56]. The dST-Tiso interval lies in between the initiation and termination (at the isoelectric line) of the elevated coved ST-segment [56]. The dST-Tiso interval displayed adjusted OR 1.03 (95% CI: 1.01–1.04, $p < 0.001$) for ventricular arrhythmias inducibility. At the same time, dST-Tiso interval > 300 ms displayed 92.0% sensitivity, 90.2% specificity, 82.1% positive predictive value, and 95.8% negative predictive value for VT/VF inducibility prediction [56].

SCN5A gene variants may be important predictors of fatal events in BrS and valuable in risk stratification [57]. Loss-of-function SCN5A mutations have shown association with prolonged ECG conduction parameters (P wave or QRS durations) and increased occurrence of lethal arrhythmic events compared to the non-loss-of-function SCN5A mutations or SCN5A(−) BrS patients [57].

In BrS individuals, the presence of structural anomalies in the epicardium of the RVOT may contribute to arrhythmias [38]. Endocardial unipolar electroanatomical mapping technology may identify RVOT electrical abnormalities with VF inducibility during PVS and assist in BrS risk stratification [38,58]. Endocardial high-density electroanatomical mapping may permit BrS risk stratification in asymptomatic patients (referred for PVS) [38].

Published studies have discussed clinical risk score models in patients with BrS and were reviewed recently in detail [59]. Briefly, the Shanghai Brugada scoring system was predictive for malignant arrhythmic events among patients evaluated for BrS who were asymptomatic ($n = 271$), experienced syncopal episodes ($n = 99$), or had previous VF ($n = 23$) [47]. Importantly, there were no malignant arrhythmic events in patients with a score of 3 or less (possible or nondiagnostic BrS) [47]. In a multicentric study of 1613 BrS patients, 20% symptomatic (after aborted SCA or syncope) at diagnosis, researchers evaluated the Shanghai score of all patients and Sieira score of 461 patients (mean follow-up 6.5 ± 4.7 years) [60]. While both scoring systems identified arrhythmic events risk in patients with significantly elevated or reduced scores, risk stratification was challenging in intermediate-risk patients, e.g., Sieira score 2–4 [60]. Another multicenter international study of 1110 BrS patients developed a risk-score model for SCD or ventricular arrhythmias, and studied 16 proposed ECG/clinical markers for risk stratification and ICD therapy indication [61]. In a median follow-up of 5.33 years, 10.3% of patients had SCD or ventricular arrhythmias, and increased risk was associated with four factors: spontaneous type-1 BrS ECG pattern (14 points), possible arrhythmic syncope or early repolarization in peripheral leads (each 12 points), and type-1 BrS ECG pattern in peripheral leads (9 points) [61].

4. Treatment of Patients with BrS

According to the ESC guidelines, implantable cardioverter–defibrillator (ICD) placement is recommended for the management of BrS patients with aborted SCD or documented spontaneous sustained VT, and should be considered in patients with spontaneous BrS type 1 ECG and previous syncope history [28]. Decision on ICD implantation and approaches for the timeline of treatment in BrS patients should involve evaluation of the risk of ventricular arrhythmias, possible complications and adverse events such as inappropriate ICD shocks, and the impact on the patients' quality of life [62,63]. Pharmacotherapy with quinidine or isoproterenol should be considered in BrS individuals for the treatment of recurrent VT/VF, such as in electrical storms [28,62]. Quinidine may also be an alternate treatment option for supraventricular arrhythmias or in patients with contraindications to ICD placement [28,62].

A relatively novel and promising approach to treatment in BrS patients is catheter ablation. Epicardial catheter ablation of the RVOT may be considered in patients with repetition of appropriate ICD shocks or previous electrical storms [28,64]. In a study of BrS patients with inducible VT/VF, catheter ablation of the epicardium of RVOT resulted in ventricular arrhythmias that were noninducible in majority of the patients, normalization of the BrS type 1 ECG pattern, and no recurrence of VT/VF in the long term follow-up [65]. In BrS individuals, lifestyle choices such as avoiding consumption of excessive alcohols or heavy meals, avoiding drugs or medications which may induce arrhythmias (http://www.brugadadrugs.org, 26 March 2022), and immediate antipyretic treatment of fevers are of great clinical value [28].

Some of the published data on MAE risk stratification in BrS seems to be inconclusive or based on limited patient groups. In addition, conflicting evidence is present for the value of PVS during EPS in risk stratification [53,66]. Therefore, we propose a series of extensive umbrella reviews to investigate previous meta-analyses on BrS and evaluate current risk stratification options such as genetic testing, ECG, and PVS for MAE risk stratification, and clinical management guidance.

5. Protocol for Umbrella Reviews of Meta-Analyses in MAE Risk Stratification in BrS

The protocol for our umbrella reviews follows the Preferred Reporting Items for Systematic review and Meta-Analysis Protocols (PRISMA-P) [67] guidelines. Modifications to the protocol will be reported in our final publications. Figure 2 displays an outline of our planned umbrella reviews.

5.1. Major Questions of Umbrella Reviews

- What is the association between MAE and clinical factors such as positive family history of SCD in BrS individuals based on an integrative evaluation of previous meta-analyses?
- How can ECG changes such as QRS complexes prolongation, fQRS, AV conduction delay, T-peak to T-end (Tpe) interval, and prolonged QTc interval be used to predict life-threatening ventricular arrhythmias in patients with BrS?
- What role does EPS, PVS, genetic studies, and features of sodium channel blocker challenge have on predicting MAE and sudden fatalities in BrS?

5.2. Aims of Umbrella Reviews

The planned umbrella reviews of meta-analyses aim to provide a critical meta-evaluation of MAE risk stratification in BrS, focusing on clinical, ECG, EPS, PVS, and genetic factors. This will significantly advance our understanding of BrS MAE risk stratification and facilitate evidence-based diagnosis and treatment approaches in clinical practice. Our research may potentially alleviate the risk of sudden death and improve the quality of life in BrS patients and their families.

5.3. Type and Method of Review

Umbrella review, systematic review, meta-evaluation of meta-analyses.

5.4. Search Strategy and Study Selection

Extensive searches of major databases PubMed, Embase, and Scopus will be performed by at least two researchers independently including the following keywords: Brugada syndrome; sudden unexpected nocturnal death syndrome; Brugada ECG; Brugada electrocardiographic; major arrhythmic event; ventricular tachycardia; ventricular fibrillation; appropriate implantable cardioverter–defibrillator therapy; sudden cardiac arrest; sudden cardiac death; prognosis; risk; and meta-analysis. Initial search queries for the databases are shown in Supplementary Materials. Timeline of the search will be until 31 March 2022, and no restrictions will be applied based on language or study publication year. From the search results, after initial screening of titles and abstracts, meta-analyses concerning BrS patients and their relevant outcomes (i.e., MAE—including SCA and SCD) will be considered for our analysis. Reference search of selected studies will be performed to identify additional meta-analyses on BrS and patients with BrS ECG patterns. Relevant abstracts (of nonpublished articles) will be entered into a supplemental table for further review and discussion.

We will evaluate the quality of obtained publications using A MeaSurement Tool to Assess systematic Reviews 2 (AMSTAR 2) [68]. It includes 16 questions to critically appraise and score studies on a scale from high to critically low. Seven domains (2,4,7,9,11,13,15) are most crucial for a systematic review. Two authors will independently apply AMSTAR 2 for each meta-analysis, and variance in evaluation will be resolved by discussion and final consensus among authors.

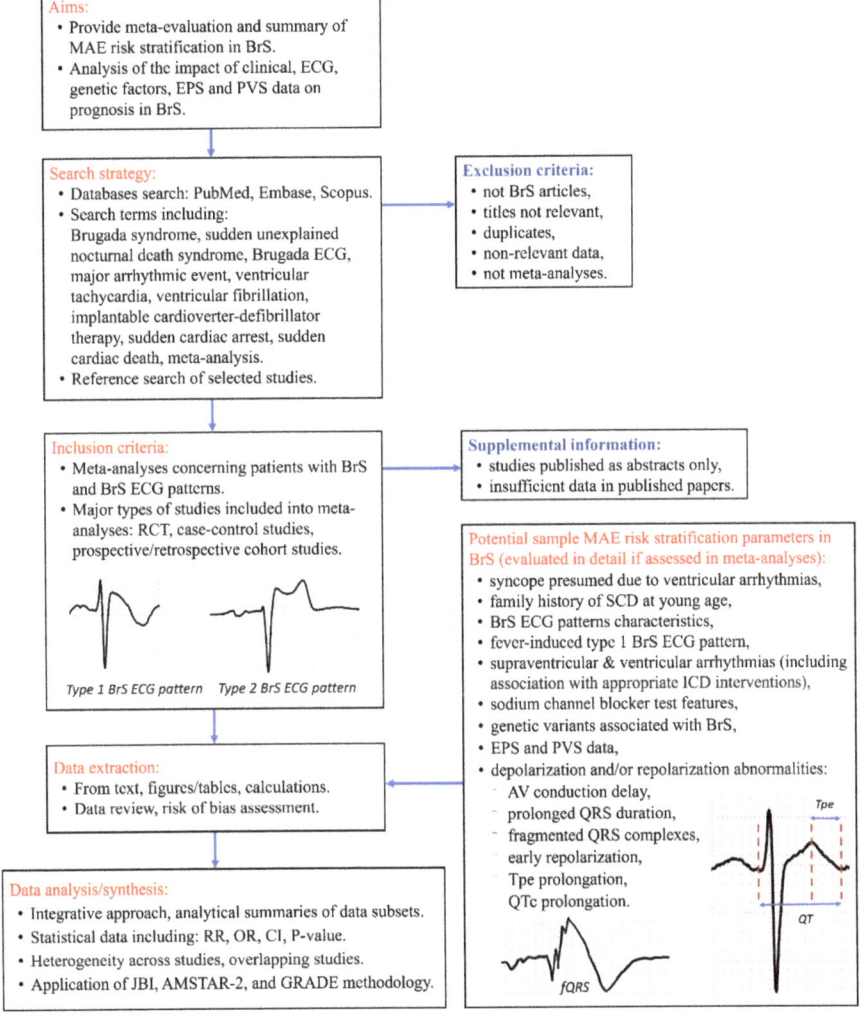

Figure 2. Flow diagram for umbrella reviews on Brugada syndrome risk stratification for major arrhythmic events. Abbreviations: AMSTAR-2—A MeaSurement Tool to Assess systematic Reviews 2; AV—atrioventricular; BrS—Brugada syndrome; CI—confidence interval; ECG—electrocardiograph; EPS—electrophysiology study; fQRS—fragmented QRS; GRADE—Grading of Recommendations, Assessment, Development and Evaluation; ICD—implantable cardioverter defibrillator; JBI—Joanna Briggs Institute; MAE—major arrhythmic events; OR—odds ratio; PVS—programmed ventricular stimulation; QT—QT interval; QTc—corrected QT; RCT—randomized controlled trial; RR—risk ratio; SCD—sudden cardiac death; Tpe—T-peak to T-end interval.

5.5. Inclusion Criteria

Meta-analyses on BrS patients concerning MAE, including sustained VT, VF, appropriate ICD therapy (antitachycardia pacing or shock), SCA, and SCD [28,69] risk stratification. Preferentially, the European Society of Cardiology (ESC) definition of BrS diagnosis will be used [28]. However, to ensure the comprehensiveness of our study, other BrS definitions used before the publication of 2015 ESC guidelines will be included, especially in terms of earlier meta-analyses. Additionally, studies on patients with BrS ECG patterns will be analyzed and considered for inclusion [70].

5.6. Exclusion Criteria

We will exclude studies with nonrelevant data, non-BrS articles, and publications that are not meta-analyses (e.g., case reports), unless required for statistical evaluation. During our search process, if we encounter abstracts with relevant meta-analytic data for BrS, and the full-text article of this work was not published, we will add the data into a supplemental table for review as it may be of clinical importance. To avoid duplication of the data, we will exclude:

- older versions of updated meta-analyses;
- publications which included smaller number of studies or smaller number of patients on the same risk stratification tool [71].

5.7. Participants/Population

Patients diagnosed with BrS, patients with BrS ECG patterns, and controls (if applicable).

5.8. Types of Interventions or Exposures

Our objective is to use an integrative approach to evaluate quantitative data from selected meta-analytic studies in BrS patients (Figure 2):

- clinical factors such as fever-induced BrS ECG pattern, syncope, and positive SCD family history;
- spontaneous and drug-induced type-1 BrS ECG pattern;
- supraventricular and ventricular arrhythmias—including appropriate ICD therapy,
- depolarization and/or repolarization abnormalities due to factors such as atrioventricular conduction delay, prolonged QRS duration, fQRS, early repolarization, late potentials, and Tpe interval prolongation;
- abnormal EPS and/or PVS;
- genetic variants associated with BrS.

5.9. Planned Umbrella Reviews Include

- Analysis of clinical (i.e., previous syncope) and ECG factors, including ECG parameters such as prolonged QRS duration, atrioventricular conduction delay, Tpe, fQRS, QTc prolongation, late potentials, arrhythmias, fever-induced type 1 BrS ECG pattern, and the impact of sodium channel blocker challenge features for MAE risk stratification in BrS.
- Evaluation of the influence of genetic factors, and family history of BrS or SCD at young age, on life-threatening ventricular arrhythmias.
- Analysis of EPS and PVS for MAE risk stratification in BrS.

5.10. Context

Our umbrella reviews will seek to investigate the impact of clinical factors, data from additional diagnostics or testing, and exposures experienced in BrS patients. We will analyze potential preventive measures, treatments, and the risk of MAE in patients with BrS and BrS ECG patterns. There are no restrictions to context. However, due to the extent of the context, we will consider writing more than one umbrella review on this topic.

5.11. Types of Studies

Studies considered for evaluation include meta-analyses of all study designs such as randomized controlled trials, prospective and retrospective cohort studies, and case-control studies.

5.12. Condition or Domain Being Studied

Clinical and ECG factors, genetic testing, family history of SCD or BrS, and EPS/PVS for MAE risk stratification or assessment in BrS patients and their families.

5.13. Main Outcomes

- Evaluation of association between multiple potential MAE risk stratification parameters and MAE in individuals with BrS (e.g., listed in Figure 2).
- Application of meta-evaluation results to facilitate evidence-based diagnosis and treatment approaches in order to mitigate the risk of SCD and improve the quality of life in BrS patients and their relatives.

5.14. Planned Measures of Effect

For each clinical and ECG factors, genetic testing, and EPS/PVS reviewed across meta-analytic studies, we plan to evaluate and compare available data for the relative risk (RR), odds ratio (OR), mean difference (MD), weighted mean difference (WMD), and risk difference (RD), as applicable. Statistical significance will be analyzed in terms of p-value <0.05 and 95% confidence intervals (CI). We plan to assess heterogeneity by analyzing Q statistics and I^2 values reported in the studies.

5.15. Data Extraction (Selection and Coding)

Full-text articles and abstracts retrieved from the search strategy and additional sources will be screened based on the eligibility criteria specified above. Data from each study will be extracted into a standardized data extraction template which will include first author name, publication year, inclusion criteria, type of studies, number of studies, databases searched, time period of the search, number of patients included, follow-up information, patient characteristics, and major research findings. Calculations and data extraction from figures and tables will be performed as needed to obtain the data of interest from each study. A comprehensive data review by at least two authors will ensure data quality and completeness of the systematic review. Discrepancies and concerns will be resolved through discussions among authors.

5.16. Risk of Bias (Quality) Assessment

At least two authors will perform the search procedure, comprehensive data extraction, and review for quality assessment. Discrepancies about quality of the articles or specific data items will be resolved by discussion and consensus between reviewers. Notes regarding all sources of data and any potential inconsistencies will be discussed.

The Grading of Recommendations, Assessment, Development and Evaluation (GRADE) will be used for evaluating the quality of evidence and presenting clinical management suggestions from our selected studies [72]. The evidence quality will be assessed on a scale from high to very low based on the indication of likely effect and the probability of the effect being different [72]. The GRADE specifications provide guidance for forming questions, selecting and scoring data of interest, analyzing evidence, assessing biases, and handling imprecision and inconsistencies in the results [72].

5.17. Strategy for Data Analysis/Synthesis

We will incorporate the Joanna Briggs Institute (JBI) Critical Appraisal Checklist for Systematic Reviews and Research Syntheses for our umbrella reviews [73]. Data will be synthesized using an integrative approach from each study for each category to provide evidence-based analysis for usage in clinical practice.

Data will be reported with transparency, accuracy, and completeness in tabular format. All sources of evidence and calculations will be reported with precision and integrity. Analytic summaries of subsets of data and our research outcome will be described in text, figures, and/or tables. In case of overlapping studies in multiple meta-analyses, inconsistency in data will be reviewed and addressed. The GRADE methodology will be applied for evaluating the quality of the evidence retrieved from our selected studies [72].

For statistical evaluation and comparison of variables from different studies, we plan to include OR, CI, risk ratio, MD, WMD, and RD based on the available data. We will consider reporting frequencies and percentages, and consider the conversion of all the common effect sizes for all factors analyzed to equivalent ORs, if applicable. We plan to determine the heterogeneity across studies according to the variance between the studies (Tau-squared, I^2). We will consider $I^2 > 50\%$ to reflect significant statistical heterogeneity. For $I^2 < 50\%$, the fixed-effects model will be used; otherwise, the random-effects model using the inverse variance heterogeneity method will be used. To identify the source of heterogeneity, sensitivity analysis using the leave-one-out method will be considered. To assess possible publication bias, we plan to perform funnel plots, Begg's, and Egger's test, if applicable. We plan to calculate sensitivity, specificity, and likelihood ratios of the different risk markers according to the available data. Finally, if the included studies vary substantially in their methodological quality, we will consider a sensitivity analysis including only those studies with a low risk of bias. We plan to use STATA 13 from StataCorp (StataCorp. 2013. Stata Statistical Software: Release 13. College Station, TX, USA: StataCorp LP.) and R software (RStudio Team (2020). RStudio: Integrated Development for R. RStudio, PBC, Boston, MA, USA) for statistical analysis.

6. Discussion

Advancement in MAE risk stratification is important for patients with cardiovascular diseases, including arrhythmogenic and conduction disorders and rare arrhythmias [74–77], which include patients with BrS and their family members. Several problems should be highlighted in diagnosis and risk stratification in patients with BrS. The initial step should be associated with detailed ECG assessment and the exclusion of Brugada phenocopy, where the Brugada ECG pattern is observed during metabolic abnormalities, ischemia, or other causes and is no longer noticed when these conditions resolve [70]. PVS may assist in evaluating the risk of arrhythmias in subgroups of patients such as BrS patients with drug-induced type 1 ECG pattern and experiencing unexplained syncope or patients without symptoms with spontaneous type 1 ECG pattern [78].

Guidelines from both ESC and AHA/ACC/HRS underlined that, at the time of their publication, genetic testing did not influence prognosis in BrS patients [28,51]. However, genetic testing and counseling may be valuable in first-degree relatives of SCD victims as it may help identify inherited BrS [51]. Progress in genetics, including genome-wide association studies and clinical research are promising in BrS patient management. We hope our research outcome will shed new light on potential new or combined factors for SCD risk stratification in BrS, and facilitate future clinical decisions and practice guidelines based on the quality of present evidence.

Our research outcome will hopefully advance our understanding of BrS risk stratification for efficient diagnosis and treatment approaches, and potentially reduce SCD risk by timely interventions such as ICD placement [63] or epicardial catheter ablation of the RVOT [64]. Our umbrella reviews may promote early detection, prevention, and counselling of patients with BrS, who might be susceptible to MAE events triggered by alcohol, fever, heavy meals, specific types of exercise, cocaine, and selected drugs [9,11,45]. Our proposed umbrella reviews will provide a valuable summary of and supplement to meta-analytical research in the scientific community for clinical practice. Further, we may consider specific ethnic and geographical factors for MAE risk stratification in BrS [6]. While highest prevalence of BrS is in Southeast Asia, the prevalence in the United States reaches about 0.012%, and the prevalence in North Africa seems to be the lowest [6,7]. When considering diverse ethnicities, BrS is 9 times more common in Asians than in Caucasians, and 36 times more common in Asians compared to Hispanics based on population-based ECG studies [6].

Our umbrella reviews will pertain to typical limitations of umbrella reviews and will be restricted to analysis of data reviewed and reported by published meta-analyses, and by any limitations of these studies. We would like to invite clinicians and researchers to send us comments on the planned umbrella reviews based on current meta-analyses. We are open to collaboration.

7. Conclusions

Our review underlines the complexity of BrS with multiple factors influencing pathogenesis, diagnostics, and risk stratification. To the best of our knowledge, the planned systematic reviews and evaluations of meta-analyses will be the first umbrella reviews to summarize the current state of knowledge in BrS meta-analyses for MAE risk stratification. Our research may contribute valuable evidence-based guidance in clinical decisions, alleviate the burden of SCD, and improve the quality of life in patients with BrS.

Supplementary Materials: The following supporting information can be downloaded at: https://www.mdpi.com/article/10.3390/jcm11071912/s1: Initial search queries for databases.

Author Contributions: Conceptualization, P.T.M. and H.M.A.; validation, all authors—H.M.A., P.T.M., G.T., M.P.Z., S.G.-Z., M.S.K., H.-H.W. and P.B.; formal analysis, all authors—H.M.A., P.T.M., G.T., M.P.Z., S.G.-Z., M.S.K., H.-H.W. and P.B.; writing original draft preparation, H.M.A.; figures for visualization, H.M.A.; writing review and editing, all authors—H.M.A., P.T.M., G.T., M.P.Z., S.G.-Z., M.S.K., H.-H.W. and P.B.; supervision, P.T.M. All authors have read and agreed to the published version of the manuscript.

Funding: This research received no external funding.

Institutional Review Board Statement: Not applicable.

Informed Consent Statement: Not applicable.

Data Availability Statement: Not applicable.

Acknowledgments: P.T.M. was supported by the Ministry of Science and Higher Education scholarship for outstanding young scientists and Jagiellonian University Medical College grant (N41/DBS/000517). The authors want to thank Angela Hardi, MLIS, AHIP for valuable help in preparation of the search strategies for planned umbrella reviews.

Conflicts of Interest: The authors declare no conflict of interest.

References

1. Sieira, J.; Brugada, P. The definition of the Brugada syndrome. *Eur. Heart J.* **2017**, *38*, 3029–3034. [CrossRef] [PubMed]
2. Matusik, P.T. Insights into channelopathies: Progress in clinical practice and research. *J. Electrocardiol.* **2017**, *50*, 534–535. [CrossRef] [PubMed]
3. Brugada, P.; Brugada, J. Right bundle branch block, persistent ST segment elevation and sudden cardiac death: A distinct clinical and electrocardiographic syndrome: A multicenter report. *J. Am. Coll. Cardiol.* **1992**, *20*, 1391–1396. [CrossRef]
4. Havakuk, O.; Viskin, S. A tale of 2 diseases: The history of long-QT syndrome and Brugada syndrome. *J. Am. Coll. Cardiol.* **2016**, *67*, 100–108. [CrossRef]
5. Matusik, P.T.; Pudło, J.; Rydlewska, A.; Podolec, J.; Lelakowski, J.; Podolec, P. Brugada syndrome: Current diagnostics, epidemiology, genetic data and novel mechanisms (RCD code: V-1A.1). *J. Rare Cardiovasc. Dis.* **2017**, *3*, 73–80. [CrossRef]
6. Vutthikraivit, W.; Rattanawong, P.; Putthapiban, P.; Sukhumthammarat, W.; Vathesatogkit, P.; Ngarmukos, T.; Thakkinstian, A. Worldwide prevalence of Brugada syndrome: A systematic review and meta-analysis. *Acta Cardiol. Sin.* **2018**, *34*, 267–277. [CrossRef]
7. Rattanawong, P.; Kewcharoen, J.; Kanitsoraphan, C.; Vutthikraivit, W.; Putthapiban, P.; Prasitlumkum, N.; Mekraksakit, P.; Mekritthikrai, R.; Chung, E.H. The utility of drug challenge testing in Brugada syndrome: A systematic review and meta-analysis. *J. Cardiovasc. Electrophysiol.* **2020**, *31*, 2474–2483. [CrossRef]
8. Bernardo, M.; Tiyyagura, S.R. A case of type I and II Brugada phenocopy unmasked in a patient with normal baseline electrocardiogram (ECG). *Am. J. Case Rep.* **2018**, *19*, 21–24. [CrossRef]

9. Chatterjee, D.; Pieroni, M.; Fatah, M.; Charpentier, F.; Cunningham, K.S.; Spears, D.A.; Chatterjee, D.; Suna, G.; Bos, J.M.; Ackerman, M.J.; et al. An autoantibody profile detects Brugada syndrome and identifies abnormally expressed myocardial proteins. *Eur. Heart J.* **2020**, *41*, 2878A–2890A. [CrossRef]
10. Roterberg, G.; El-Battrawy, I.; Veith, M.; Liebe, V.; Ansari, U.; Lang, S.; Zhou, X.; Akin, I.; Borggrefe, M. Arrhythmic events in Brugada syndrome patients induced by fever. *Ann. Noninvasive Electrocardiol.* **2019**, *25*, 135–140. [CrossRef]
11. Mizusawa, Y.; Wilde, A.A.M. Brugada syndrome. *Circ. Arrhythm Electrophysiol.* **2012**, *5*, 606–616. [CrossRef] [PubMed]
12. Rattanawong, P.; Kewcharoen, J.; Techorueangwiwat, C.; Kanitsoraphan, C.; Mekritthikrai, R.; Prasitlumkum, N.; Puttapiban, P.; Mekraksakit, P.; Vutthikraivit, W.; Sorajja, D. Wide QRS complex and the risk of major arrhythmic events in Brugada syndrome patients: A systematic review and meta-analysis. *J. Arrhythmia* **2019**, *36*, 143–152. [CrossRef] [PubMed]
13. Wu, W.; Tian, L.; Ke, J.; Sun, Y.; Wu, R.; Zhu, J.; Ke, Q. Risk factors for cardiac events in patients with Brugada syndrome: A PRISMA-compliant meta-analysis and systematic review. *Medicine* **2016**, *95*, e4214. [CrossRef] [PubMed]
14. Antzelevitch, C.; Brugada, P.; Borggrefe, M.; Brugada, J.; Brugada, R.; Corrado, D.; Gussak, I.; LeMarec, H.; Nademanee, K.; Riera, A.R.P.; et al. Brugada syndrome: Report of the second consensus conference. *Circulation* **2005**, *111*, 659–670. [CrossRef]
15. Alings, M.; Wilde, A. "Brugada" syndrome. clinical data and suggested pathophysiological mechanism. *Circulation* **1999**, *99*, 666–673. [CrossRef] [PubMed]
16. Matusik, P.T.; Rydlewska, A.; Pudło, J.; Podolec, J.; Lelakowski, J.; Podolec, P. Brugada syndrome: New concepts and algorithms in management (RCD code: V 1A.1). *J. Rare Cardiovasc. Dis.* **2018**, *3*, 151–160. [CrossRef]
17. Miles, C.; Asimaki, A.; Ster, I.C.; Papadakis, M.; Gray, B.; Westaby, J.; Finocchiaro, G.; Bueno-Beti, C.; Ensam, B.; Basu, J.; et al. Biventricular myocardial fibrosis and sudden death in patients with Brugada syndrome. *J. Am. Coll. Cardiol.* **2021**, *78*, 1511–1521. [CrossRef]
18. Zhang, Z.-H.; Barajas-Martínez, H.; Xia, H.; Li, B.; Capra, J.A.; Clatot, J.; Chen, G.-X.; Chen, X.; Yang, B.; Jiang, H.; et al. Distinct features of probands with early repolarization and Brugada syndromes carrying SCN5A pathogenic variants. *J. Am. Coll. Cardiol.* **2021**, *78*, 1603–1617. [CrossRef]
19. Tse, G.; Lee, S.; Liu, T.; Yuen, H.C.; Wong, I.C.K.; Mak, C.; Mok, N.S.; Wong, W.T. Identification of novel SCN5A single nucleotide variants in Brugada syndrome: A territory-wide study from Hong Kong. *Front. Physiol.* **2020**, *11*, 574590. [CrossRef]
20. Barc, J.; Tadros, R.; Glinge, C.; Chiang, D.Y.; Jouni, M.; Simonet, F.; Jurgens, S.J.; Baudic, M.; Nicastro, M.; Potet, F.; et al. Genome-wide association analyses identify new Brugada syndrome risk loci and highlight a new mechanism of sodium channel regulation in disease susceptibility. *Nat. Genet.* **2022**, *54*, 232–239. [CrossRef]
21. Garcia-Elias, A.; Benito, B. Ion Channel Disorders and Sudden Cardiac Death. *Int. J. Mol. Sci.* **2018**, *19*, 692. [CrossRef] [PubMed]
22. Pranata, R.; Yonas, E.; Chintya, V.; Deka, H.; Raharjo, S.B. Association between PR Interval, First-degree atrioventricular block and major arrhythmic events in patients with Brugada syndrome—Systematic review and meta-analysis. *J. Arrhythmia* **2019**, *35*, 584–590. [CrossRef] [PubMed]
23. Saha, S.A.; Krishnan, K.; Madias, C.; Trohman, R.G. Combined right ventricular outflow tract epicardial and endocardial late potential ablation for treatment of Brugada storm: A case report and review of the literature. *Cardiol. Ther.* **2016**, *5*, 229–243. [CrossRef] [PubMed]
24. Di Domenico, M.; Cuda, G.; Scumaci, D.; Grasso, S.; Gaspari, M.; Curcio, A.; Oliva, A.; Ausania, F.; Di Nunzio, C.; Ricciardi, C.; et al. Biomarker discovery by plasma proteomics in familial Brugada Syndrome. *Front. Biosci.* **2013**, *18*, 564–571. [CrossRef]
25. Zumhagen, S.; Zeidler, E.M.; Stallmeyer, B.; Ernsting, M.; Eckardt, L.; Schulze-Bahr, E. Tpeak–Tendinterval and Tpeak–Tend/QT ratio in patients with Brugada syndrome. *Europace* **2016**, *18*, 1866–1872. [CrossRef] [PubMed]
26. Tse, G.; Gong, M.; Li, C.K.H.; Leung, K.S.K.; Georgopoulos, S.; Bazoukis, G.; Letsas, K.P.; Sawant, A.C.; Mugnai, G.; Wong, M.C.S.; et al. T peak -T end, T peak -T end /QT ratio and T peak -T end dispersion for risk stratification in Brugada syndrome: A systematic review and meta-analysis. *J. Arrhythmia* **2018**, *34*, 587–597. [CrossRef]
27. Tse, G.; Lee, S.; Li, A.; Chang, D.; Li, G.; Zhou, J.; Liu, T.; Zhang, Q. Automated electrocardiogram analysis identifies novel predictors of ventricular arrhythmias in Brugada syndrome. *Front. Cardiovasc. Med.* **2021**, *7*, 399. [CrossRef]
28. Priori, S.G.; Blomström-Lundqvist, C.; Mazzanti, A.; Blom, N.; Borggrefe, M.; Camm, J.; Elliott, P.M.; Fitzsimons, D.; Hatala, R.; Hindricks, G.; et al. 2015 ESC Guidelines for the management of patients with ventricular arrhythmias and the prevention of sudden cardiac death: The task force for the management of patients with ventricular arrhythmias and the prevention of sudden cardiac death of the european society of cardiology (ESC). Endorsed by: Association for European paediatric and congenital cardiology (AEPC). *Eur. Heart J.* **2015**, *36*, 2793–2867. [CrossRef]
29. Pappone, C.; Santinelli, V. Brugada syndrome: Progress in diagnosis and management. *Arrhythmia Electrophysiol. Rev.* **2019**, *8*, 13–18. [CrossRef]
30. Antzelevitch, C.; Yan, G.-X.; Ackerman, M.J.; Borggrefe, M.; Corrado, D.; Guo, J.; Gussak, I.; Hasdemir, C.; Horie, M.; Huikuri, H.; et al. J-Wave syndromes expert consensus conference report: Emerging concepts and gaps in knowledge. *Hear. Rhythm* **2016**, *13*, e295–e324. [CrossRef]
31. Matusik, P.S.; Bryll, A.; Matusik, P.T.; Pac, A.; Popiela, T.J. Electrocardiography and cardiac magnetic resonance imaging in the detection of left ventricular hypertrophy: The impact of indexing methods. *Kardiol. Pol.* **2020**, *78*, 889–898. [CrossRef] [PubMed]
32. Kucharz, A.; Kułakowski, P. Fragmented QRS and arrhythmic events in patients with implantable cardioverter-defibrillators. *Kardiol. Pol.* **2020**, *78*, 1107–1114. [CrossRef] [PubMed]

33. Matusik, P.T. Biomarkers and cardiovascular risk stratification. *Eur. Heart J.* **2019**, *40*, 1483–1485. [CrossRef]
34. Matusik, P.T.; Małecka, B.; Lelakowski, J.; Undas, A. Association of NT-proBNP and GDF-15 with markers of a prothrombotic state in patients with atrial fibrillation off anticoagulation. *Clin. Res. Cardiol.* **2020**, *109*, 426–434. [CrossRef] [PubMed]
35. Asvestas, D.; Tse, G.; Baranchuk, A.; Bazoukis, G.; Liu, T.; Saplaouras, A.; Korantzopoulos, P.; Goga, C.; Efremidis, M.; Sideris, A.; et al. High risk electrocardiographic markers in Brugada syndrome. *Int. J. Cardiol. Heart Vasc.* **2018**, *18*, 58–64. [CrossRef]
36. Okólska, M.; Łach, J.; Matusik, P.T.; Pająk, J.; Mroczek, T.; Podolec, P.; Tomkiewicz-Pająk, L. Heart Rate variability and its associations with organ complications in adults after fontan operation. *J. Clin. Med.* **2021**, *10*, 4492. [CrossRef] [PubMed]
37. Pruszczyk, P.; Skowrońska, M.; Ciurzyński, M.; Kurnicka, K.; Lankei, M.; Konstantinides, S. Assessment of pulmonary embolism severity and the risk of early death. *Pol. Arch. Intern. Med.* **2021**, *131*. [CrossRef] [PubMed]
38. Letsas, K.P.; Vlachos, K.; Conte, G.; Efremidis, M.; Nakashima, T.; Duchateau, J.; Bazoukis, G.; Frontera, A.; Mililis, P.; Tse, G.; et al. Right ventricular outflow tract electroanatomical abnormalities in asymptomatic and high-risk symptomatic patients with Brugada syndrome: Evidence for a new risk stratification tool? *J. Cardiovasc. Electrophysiol.* **2021**, *32*, 2997–3007. [CrossRef]
39. Lee, S.; Zhou, J.; Li, K.H.C.; Leung, K.S.K.; Lakhani, I.; Liu, T.; Wong, I.C.K.; Mok, N.S.; Mak, C.; Jeevaratnam, K.; et al. Territory-wide cohort study of Brugada syndrome in Hong Kong: Predictors of long-term outcomes using random survival forests and non-negative matrix factorisation. *Open Heart* **2021**, *8*, e001505. [CrossRef]
40. Lee, S.; Wong, W.T.; Wong, I.C.K.; Mak, C.; Mok, N.S.; Liu, T.; Tse, G. Ventricular Tachyarrhythmia Risk in Paediatric/Young vs. Adult Brugada Syndrome Patients: A Territory-Wide Study. *Front. Cardiovasc. Med.* **2021**, *8*, 671666. [CrossRef]
41. Tse, G.; Zhou, J.; Lee, S.; Liu, T.; Bazoukis, G.; Mililis, P.; Wong, I.C.K.; Chen, C.; Xia, Y.; Kamakura, T.; et al. Incorporating latent variables using nonnegative matrix factorization improves risk stratification in Brugada syndrome. *J. Am. Heart Assoc.* **2020**, *9*, e012714. [CrossRef] [PubMed]
42. Letsas, K.P.; Asvestas, D.; Baranchuk, A.; Liu, T.; Georgopoulos, S.; Efremidis, M.; Korantzopoulos, P.; Bazoukis, G.; Tse, G.; Sideris, A.; et al. Prognosis, risk stratification, and management of asymptomatic individuals with Brugada syndrome: A systematic review. *Pacing Clin. Electrophysiol.* **2017**, *40*, 1332–1345. [CrossRef] [PubMed]
43. Marsman, E.M.J.; Postema, P.G.; Remme, C.A. Brugada syndrome: Update and future perspectives. *Heart* **2021**, *2020*, 318258. [CrossRef]
44. Honarbakhsh, S.; Providência, R.; Lambiase, P.D.; Centre, S.B.H.B.H. Risk stratification in Brugada syndrome: Current status and emerging approaches. *Arrhythmia Electrophysiol. Rev.* **2018**, *7*, 79–83. [CrossRef]
45. Matusik, P.T.; Komar, M.; Podolec, J.; Karkowski, G.; Lelakowski, J.; Podolec, P. Exercise ECG unmasked Brugada sign: Manifestation of the risk of sports-associated sudden cardiac arrest (RCD code: V-1A.1). *J. Rare Cardiovasc. Dis.* **2017**, *3*, 92–97. [CrossRef]
46. Abe, A.; Kobayashi, K.; Yuzawa, H.; Sato, H.; Fukunaga, S.; Fujino, T.; Okano, Y.; Yamazaki, J.; Miwa, Y.; Yoshino, H.; et al. Comparison of late potentials for 24 hours between Brugada syndrome and arrhythmogenic right ventricular cardiomyopathy using a novel signal-averaging system based on holter ECG. *Circ. Arrhythmia Electrophysiol.* **2012**, *5*, 789–795. [CrossRef]
47. Kawada, S.; Morita, H.; Antzelevitch, C.; Morimoto, Y.; Nakagawa, K.; Watanabe, A.; Nishii, N.; Nakamura, K.; Ito, H. Shanghai Score system for diagnosis of brugada syndrome: Validation of the score system and system and reclassification of the patients. *JACC Clin. Electrophysiol.* **2018**, *4*, 724–730. [CrossRef]
48. Wilde, A.A.M. The Shanghai score system in Brugada syndrome: Using it beyond a diagnostic score. *JACC Clin. Electrophysiol.* **2018**, *4*, 731–732. [CrossRef]
49. Wijeyeratne, Y.D.; Tanck, M.W.; Mizusawa, Y.; Batchvarov, V.; Barc, J.; Crotti, L.; Bos, J.M.; Tester, D.J.; Muir, A.; Veltmann, C.; et al. SCN5A Mutation Type and a Genetic Risk Score Associate Variably with Brugada Syndrome Phenotype in SCN5A Families. *Circ. Genom. Precis. Med.* **2020**, *13*, e002911. [CrossRef]
50. Veltmann, C.; Papavassiliu, T.; Konrad, T.; Doesch, C.; Kuschyk, J.; Streitner, F.; Haghi, D.; Michaely, H.; Schoenberg, S.; Borggrefe, M.; et al. Insights into the location of type I ECG in patients with Brugada syndrome: Correlation of ECG and cardiovascular magnetic resonance imaging. *Heart Rhythm* **2012**, *9*, 414–421. [CrossRef]
51. Al-Khatib, S.M.; Stevenson, W.G.; Ackerman, M.J.; Bryant, W.J.; Callans, D.J.; Curtis, A.B.; Deal, B.J.; Dickfeld, T.; Field, M.E.; Fonarow, G.C.; et al. 2017 AHA/ACC/HRS Guideline for management of patients with ventricular arrhythmias and the prevention of sudden cardiac death: A report of the American college of cardiology/American Heart association task force on clinical practice guidelines and the heart rhythm society. *J. Am. Coll. Cardiol.* **2018**, *72*, e91–e220. [CrossRef] [PubMed]
52. Wakamiya, A.; Kamakura, T.; Shinohara, T.; Yodogawa, K.; Murakoshi, N.; Morita, H.; Takahashi, N.; Inden, Y.; Shimizu, W.; Nogami, A.; et al. Improved risk stratification of patients with Brugada syndrome by the new Japanese circulation society guideline—A multicenter validation study. *Circ. J.* **2020**, *84*, 2158–2165. [CrossRef] [PubMed]
53. Priori, S.G.; Gasparini, M.; Napolitano, C.; Della Bella, P.; Ottonelli, A.G.; Sassone, B.; Giordano, U.; Pappone, C.; Mascioli, G.; Rossetti, G.; et al. Risk stratification in Brugada syndrome: Results of the PRELUDE (PRogrammed ELectrical stimUlation preDictive valuE) registry. *J. Am. Coll. Cardiol.* **2012**, *59*, 37–45. [CrossRef] [PubMed]
54. Bigi, M.A.B.; Aslani, A.; Shahrzad, S. aVR sign as a risk factor for life-threatening arrhythmic events in patients with Brugada syndrome. *Heart Rhythm* **2007**, *4*, 1009–1012. [CrossRef]
55. Tsai, C.-F.; Chuang, Y.-T.; Huang, J.-Y.; Ueng, K.-C. Long-term prognosis of febrile individuals with right precordial coved-type ST-segment elevation Brugada pattern: A 10-year prospective follow-up study. *J. Clin. Med.* **2021**, *10*, 4997. [CrossRef]

56. Iacopino, S.; Chierchia, G.-B.; Sorrenti, P.; Pesce, F.; Colella, J.; Fabiano, G.; Campagna, G.; Petretta, A.; Placentino, F.; Filannino, P.; et al. dST-Tiso Interval, a novel electrocardiographic marker of ventricular arrhythmia inducibility in individuals with ajmaline-induced Brugada type I pattern. *Am. J. Cardiol.* **2021**, *159*, 94–99. [CrossRef]
57. Ishikawa, T.; Kimoto, H.; Mishima, H.; Yamagata, K.; Ogata, S.; Aizawa, Y.; Hayashi, K.; Morita, H.; Nakajima, T.; Nakano, Y.; et al. Functionally validated SCN5A variants allow interpretation of pathogenicity and prediction of lethal events in Brugada syndrome. *Eur. Heart J.* **2021**, *42*, 2854–2863. [CrossRef]
58. Letsas, K.P.; Vlachos, K.; Efremidis, M.; Dragasis, S.; Korantzopoulos, P.; Tse, G.; Liu, T.; Bazoukis, G.; Niarchou, P.; Prappa, E.; et al. Right ventricular outflow tract endocardial unipolar substrate mapping: Implications in risk stratification of Brugada syndrome. *Rev. Cardiovasc. Med.* **2022**, *23*, 044. [CrossRef]
59. Chung, C.T.; Bazoukis, G.; Radford, D.; Coakley-Youngs, E.; Rajan, R.; Matusik, P.T.; Liu, T.; Letsas, K.P.; Lee, S.; Tse, G. Predictive risk models for forecasting arrhythmic outcomes in Brugada syndrome: A focused review. *J. Electrocardiol.* **2022**, *72*, 28–34. [CrossRef]
60. Probst, V.; Goronflot, T.; Anys, S.; Tixier, R.; Briand, J.; Berthome, P.; Geoffroy, O.; Clementy, N.; Mansourati, J.; Jesel, L.; et al. Robustness and relevance of predictive score in sudden cardiac death for patients with Brugada syndrome. *Eur. Heart J.* **2021**, *42*, 1687–1695. [CrossRef]
61. Honarbakhsh, S.; Providencia, R.; Garcia-Hernandez, J.; Martin, C.A.; Hunter, R.J.; Lim, W.Y.; Kirkby, C.; Graham, A.J.; Sharifzadehgan, A.; Waldmann, V.; et al. A primary prevention clinical risk score model for patients with Brugada syndrome (BRUGADA-RISK). *JACC: Clin. Electrophysiol.* **2021**, *7*, 210–222. [CrossRef] [PubMed]
62. Letsas, K.P.; Georgopoulos, S.; Vlachos, K. Brugada syndrome:risk stratification and management corresponding author. *J. Atr. Fibrillation* **2016**, *7*, 79–83.
63. Dereci, A.; Yap, S.C.; Schinkel, A.F.L. Meta-Analysis of clinical outcome after implantable cardioverter-defibrillator implantation in patients with Brugada syndrome. *JACC Clin. Electrophysiol.* **2019**, *5*, 141–148. [CrossRef] [PubMed]
64. Fernandes, G.C.; Fernandes, A.; Cardoso, R.; Nasi, G.; Rivera, M.; Mitrani, R.D.; Goldberger, J.J. Ablation strategies for the management of symptomatic Brugada syndrome: A systematic review. *Heart Rhythm* **2018**, *15*, 1140–1147. [CrossRef] [PubMed]
65. Nademanee, K.; Veerakul, G.; Chandanamattha, P.; Chaothawee, L.; Ariyachaipanich, A.; Jirasirirojanakorn, K.; Likittanasombat, K.; Bhuripanyo, K.; Ngarmukos, T. Arrhythmia/electrophysiology prevention of ventricular fibrillation episodes in Brugada syndrome by catheter ablation over the anterior right ventricular outflow tract epicardium. *Circulation* **2011**, *123*, 1270–1279. [CrossRef]
66. Asada, S.; Morita, H.; Watanabe, A.; Nakagawa, K.; Nagase, S.; Miyamoto, M.; Morimoto, Y.; Kawada, S.; Nishii, N.; Ito, H. Indication and prognostic significance of programmed ventricular stimulation in asymptomatic patients with Brugada syndrome. *Europace* **2020**, *22*, 972–979. [CrossRef]
67. Kamioka, H. Preferred reporting items for systematic review and meta-analysis protocols (prisma-p) 2015 statement. *Jpn. Pharmacol. Ther.* **2019**, *47*, 1177–1185.
68. Shea, B.J.; Reeves, B.C.; Wells, G.; Thuku, M.; Hamel, C.; Moran, J.; Moher, D.; Tugwell, P.; Welch, V.; Kristjansson, E.; et al. AMSTAR 2: A critical appraisal tool for systematic reviews that include randomised or non-randomised studies of healthcare interventions, or both. *BMJ* **2017**, *358*, j4008. [CrossRef]
69. Kewcharoen, J.; Rattanawong, P.; Kanitsoraphan, C.; Mekritthikrai, R.; Prasitlumkum, N.; Putthapiban, P.; Mekraksakit, P.; Pattison, R.J.; Vutthikraivit, W. Atrial fibrillation and risk of major arrhythmic events in Brugada syndrome: A meta-analysis. *Ann. Noninvasive Electrocardiol.* **2019**, *24*, e12676. [CrossRef]
70. de Luna, A.B.; Brugada, J.; Baranchuk, A.; Borggrefe, M.; Breithardt, G.; Goldwasser, D.; Lambiase, P.; Riera, A.P.; Garcia-Niebla, J.; Pastore, C.; et al. Current electrocardiographic criteria for diagnosis of Brugada pattern: A consensus report. *J. Electrocardiol.* **2012**, *45*, 433–442. [CrossRef]
71. Fusar-Poli, P.; Radua, J. Ten simple rules for conducting umbrella reviews. *Evid. -Based Ment. Health* **2018**, *21*, 95–100. [CrossRef] [PubMed]
72. Dijkers, M. Introducing GRADE: A systematic approach to rating evidence in systematic reviews and to guideline development. *KT Update* **2013**, *1*, 1–9.
73. Briggs, J. *Checklist for Systematic Reviews and Research Syntheses*; The Joanna Briggs Institute: Adelaide, Australia, 2017.
74. Sheppard, M.N. Sudden Death in congenital heart disease: The role of the autopsy in determining the actual cause. *J. Cardiovasc. Dev. Dis.* **2020**, *7*, 58. [CrossRef]
75. Podolec, P.; Matusik, P.T. New clinical classification of rare cardiovascular diseases and disorders: Relevance for cardiovascular research. *Cardiovasc. Res.* **2019**, *115*, e77–e79. [CrossRef]
76. Podolec, P.; Baranchuk, A.; Brugada, J.; Kukla, P.; Lelakowski, J.; Kopeć, G.; Rubiś, P.; Stępniewski, J.; Podolec, J.; Komar, M.; et al. Clinical classification of rare cardiac arrhythmogenic and conduction disorders, and rare arrhythmias. *Pol. Arch. Intern. Med.* **2019**, *129*, 154–159. [CrossRef]
77. Stevens, T.L.; Wallace, M.J.; el Refaey, M.; Roberts, J.D.; Koenig, S.N.; Mohler, P.J. Arrhythmogenic cardiomyopathy: Molecular insights for improved therapeutic design. *J. Cardiovasc. Dev. Dis.* **2020**, *7*, 21. [CrossRef]
78. Fauchier, L.; Isorni, M.A.; Clementy, N.; Pierre, B.; Simeon, E.; Babuty, D. Prognostic value of programmed ventricular stimulation in Brugada syndrome according to clinical presentation: An updated meta-analysis of worldwide published data. *Int. J. Cardiol.* **2013**, *168*, 3027–3029. [CrossRef]

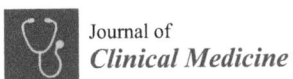

Article

Prevalence of Arrhythmia in Adults after Fontan Operation

Magdalena Okólska [1], Grzegorz Karkowski [2], Marcin Kuniewicz [2,3], Jacek Bednarek [2], Jacek Pająk [4], Beata Róg [1], Jacek Łach [5], Jacek Legutko [6,7] and Lidia Tomkiewicz-Pająk [5,*]

1. Cardiological Outpatient Clinic, Department of Cardiovascular Diseases, John Paul II Hospital, 31-202 Krakow, Poland; magdaokolska@gmail.com (M.O.); beatarog@interia.pl (B.R.)
2. Department of Electrocardiology, Institute of Cardiology, Faculty of Medicine, Jagiellonian University Medical College, John Paul II Hospital, 31-202 Krakow, Poland; gkarkowski@interia.pl (G.K.); kuniewiczm@gmail.com (M.K.); bednarekj1@gmail.com (J.B.)
3. Department of Anatomy, Jagiellonian University Medical College, 31-008 Krakow, Poland
4. Institute of Medical Sciences, Department of Surgery, Medical College of Rzeszow University, 35-959 Rzeszow, Poland; jacekpajak@poczta.onet.pl
5. Department of Cardiac and Vascular Diseases, Institute of Cardiology, Jagiellonian University Medical College, John Paul II Hospital, 31-202 Krakow, Poland; djholter@interia.pl
6. Clinical Department of Interventional Cardiology, John Paul II Hospital, 31-202 Krakow, Poland; jacek.legutko@uj.edu.pl
7. Department of Interventional Cardiology, Faculty of Medicine, Institute of Cardiology, Jagiellonian University Medical College, 31-008 Krakow, Poland
* Correspondence: ltom@wp.pl; Tel.: +48-12-614-35-15

Abstract: Structural, hemodynamic, and morphological cardiac changes following Fontan operation (FO) can contribute to the development of arrhythmias and conduction disorders. Sinus node dysfunction, junction rhythms, tachyarrhythmias, and ventricular arrhythmias (VAs) are some of the commonly reported arrhythmias. Only a few studies have analyzed this condition in adults after FO. This study aimed to determine the type and prevalence of arrhythmias and conduction disorders among patients who underwent FO and were under the medical surveillance of the John Paul II Hospital in Krakow. Data for the study were obtained from 50 FO patients (mean age 24 ± 5.7 years; 28 men (56%)). The median follow-up time was 4 (2–9) years. Each patient received a physical examination, an echocardiographic assessment, and a 24 h electrocardiogram assessment. Bradyarrhythmia was diagnosed in 22 patients (44%), supraventricular tachyarrhythmias in 14 patients (28%), and VAs in 6 patients (12%). Six patients required pacemaker implantation, and three required radiofrequency catheter ablation (6%). Arrythmias is a widespread clinical problem in adults after FO. It can lead to serious haemodynamic impairment, and therefore requires early diagnosis and effective treatment with the use of modern approaches, including electrotherapy methods.

Keywords: single ventricle; Fontan operation; cardiac arrhythmias; catheter ablation

Citation: Okólska, M.; Karkowski, G.; Kuniewicz, M.; Bednarek, J.; Pająk, J.; Róg, B.; Łach, J.; Legutko, J.; Tomkiewicz-Pająk, L. Prevalence of Arrhythmia in Adults after Fontan Operation. *J. Clin. Med.* 2022, 11, 1968. https://doi.org/10.3390/jcm11071968

Academic Editor: Adrian Covic

Received: 4 March 2022
Accepted: 28 March 2022
Published: 1 April 2022

Publisher's Note: MDPI stays neutral with regard to jurisdictional claims in published maps and institutional affiliations.

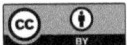

Copyright: © 2022 by the authors. Licensee MDPI, Basel, Switzerland. This article is an open access article distributed under the terms and conditions of the Creative Commons Attribution (CC BY) license (https://creativecommons.org/licenses/by/4.0/).

1. Introduction

Patients with congenital heart disease with single ventricle physiology constitute a heterogeneous and difficult-to-treat group, both in terms of hemodynamic changes and rhythm and conduction disorders. Currently, the preferred therapy for this patient population is the Fontan operation (FO), which aims at separating pulmonary and systemic circulation in order to achieve normal or near-normal blood oxygenation [1]. Over the last 50 years, the methods and techniques used for the surgical treatment of univentricular heart defects have undergone numerous changes [2]. Initially, FO was performed in a single stage, connecting the right atrium with the pulmonary artery (known as atriopulmonary connection (APC)) either directly or using a vascular prosthesis. However, this approach was eventually abandoned due to the high mortality rate and high number of complications. APC has now been replaced with the total cavopulmonary connection (TCPC), which includes an intracardiac or extracardiac conduit (ECC) between inferior vena cava and pulmonary artery, with bidirectional Glenn connection (superior vena cava–pulmonary artery) [1,2]. Some patients undergo fenestration, which allows unsaturated blood to be shunted to the systemic circulation at the atrium level, increasing cardiac output at the cost of cyanosis [3]. However, surgical traumatization, remodeling due to enhanced atrioventricular regurgitation, and increased stress and fibrogenesis of atrium and ventricle walls leads to the formation of areas of nonhomogeneous electric activity which in turn contributes to the development of arrhythmia and conduction defects [4].

Arrhythmias commonly observed in patients who, following FO, include sinus node and atrio-ventricular dysfunction, atrial tachycardia (ranging from focal arrhythmia to macro-reentry involving conduit as well as systemic atrium), atrial flutter (AFL), atrial fibrillation (AF) and ventricular arrhythmias (VAs) [1]. Thus far, only a few studies have analyzed the incidence of arrhythmic events in patients following FO. According to the literature, the incidence of sinus node dysfunction ranges from 9 to 60% [5–10]. In a study on a group of pediatric patients, Stephenson et al. [11] observed that 9.4% of children had supraventricular tachycardia (SVT) and 3.5% had VA after 8.6 years of FO. A Danish study conducted among adults >20 years of age reported that the incidence of arrhythmias in population following FO was 32% [12].

Treatment of the arrythmias in this group of patients due to complex anatomy, multiple surgical scars, and hypertrophied atrium could be very challenging. Pharmacotherapy is often ineffective and may lead to significant bradycardia. Catheter ablation can be safe and effective in reducing arrythmia burden after FO but require experienced electro-physiologist and well-equipped medical facilities [13].

The occurrence of arrhythmias significantly increases the risk of developing heart failure and sudden cardiac death (SCD) [1]. Therefore, early identification of patients who are at the highest risk of death due to arrhythmias (or atrial arrhythmias with rapid conduction to ventricles) following FO is important.

In this study, we aimed to determine the type and prevalence of rhythm and conduction abnormalities and present our own experience in treating patients following FO who were under the medical supervision of the Congenital Heart Disease Team of the John Paul II Hospital in Krakow.

2. Materials and Methods

2.1. Study Participants

This retrospective study included 50 adult patients aged over 18 years. All patients underwent FO following the diagnosis of a functionally single ventricular heart and were under the care of the John Paul II Hospital. The main exclusion criteria included diabetes, current infection, inflammation, neoplastic disease, major trauma, pregnancy, and history of alcohol abuse. The median (Q1–Q3) follow-up time was 4 (2–9) years. During regular visits in our institution, each patient went through all required examinations and procedures. Depending on their results, specific therapeutic decisions were made. The demographic, anatomic, and clinical data of the patients were obtained from their medical records. Each patient was subjected to a physical examination and an assessment of the body mass index (BMI), systemic ventricle ejection fraction, and arterial oxygen saturation. BMI was calculated by dividing the weight of the patient (kg) by height (m^2).

2.2. Echocardiography

Ejection fraction of the single ventricle was assessed using Simpson's method. Valvular competence was also evaluated in the patients by two experienced, independent cardiologists using echocardiography (Vivid 7, GE Medical Systems, Milwaukee, WI, USA) as previously described [14].

2.3. Ambulatory 24-h Electrocardiogram

Standard 24-h electrocardiographic monitoring was performed using commercially available Holter systems in all patients during their daily activities. All Holters were reviewed by two experienced observers. Recordings were analyzed using a PC-based Holter system, and those shorter than 21 h were excluded from the assessment. The predominant rhythm was defined as the one present for >50% of the time during the Holter recording.

2.4. Arrhythmia

The following groups of rhythm abnormalities were defined as tachyarrhythmias: (1) SVT, including sustained and non-sustained atrial tachycardia (AT, nsAT), supraventricular ectopic beats (Svebs), and AFL and AF; (2) VAs including sustained ventricular tachycardia (VT) and non-sustained ventricular tachycardia (nsVT), premature ventricular contraction (PVC), and ventricular fibrillation (VF). SVT and VAs were defined based on the guidelines of the European Society of Cardiology (ESC) [15–17]. Bradyarrhythmia was defined as heart rate < 60 beats per minute for a minimum of 1 min and included sinus node dysfunction and atrioventricular block (AVB) [18].

2.5. Mapping and Ablation Procedure

Patients with sustained, symptomatic atrial tachyarrhythmias, who had failed medical treatment, were recommended to undergo ablation. Catheter ablation procedures were performed under general anesthesia using the CARTO electroanatomic mapping system (Biosense Webster Inc., Diamond Bar, CA, USA). In the first case with SVT and VA ablation (2010, 2013), mapping was performed using an ablation catheter, and in the second case (2021) using a multipolar Pentaray diagnostic catheter supported with the Coherent Mapping algorithm (CARTOPRIME module). In two cases (2010, 2013), ablations were performed using 3.5 mm catheters with an open irrigated tip (Biosense Webster Navistar Thermocool), and in one case (2021) using 3.5 mm catheters with an open irrigated tip and a contact force sensor (SF, Thermocool SmartTouch®, Biosense Webster Inc., Diamond Bar, CA, USA). The parameters used for radiofrequency (RF) application were as follows: power: 35 W, flow of irrigation: 15–30 mL/min, time of application: 60 s, temperature limit: maximum 45 °C, and ablation index: posterior wall—400 and the other side—500. If arrhythmias were not present at the onset of the procedure, voltage maps (0.1–0.3 mV) were collected during sinus rhythm (Figure 1a), followed by which arrhythmias were induced with programmed atrial pacing from s 10-pole steerable diagnostic catheter located in the lateral tunnel (LT). The arrythmia mechanism was determined by high-density activation mapping and entrainment pacing (if possible) (Figure 1b). The origin of PVC was identified by activation mapping, in which the earliest endocardial potential advancing QRS was determined during PVC. Additionally, pace-mapping was applied in the earliest activation spot to confirm the localization of PVC, with a PVC compatibility of at least 95% of the complexes analyzed by an electrophysiological recording system (LABSYSTEM™ PRO, Boston Scientific, Boston, MA, USA). The SVT ablation protocol assumed initial mapping of LT followed by pulmonary atrium access if arrhythmia elimination required this. In one case of nsVT or PVC, a retrograde approach was used. The minimum follow-up period was 12 months.

Long-term efficacy was defined as the absence of SVT symptoms or arrhythmia episodes recorded in electrocardiogram (ECG) (or in 24 h electrocardiographic monitoring). In cases with VA, it was defined as a significant reduction in arrhythmia (>80% reduction in the initial amount) or the lack of VT or nsVT observation in ECG or in 24 h electrocardiographic monitoring after a healing period (after 3 months) or in repeated 24 h electrocardiographic monitoring (every 6–12 months).

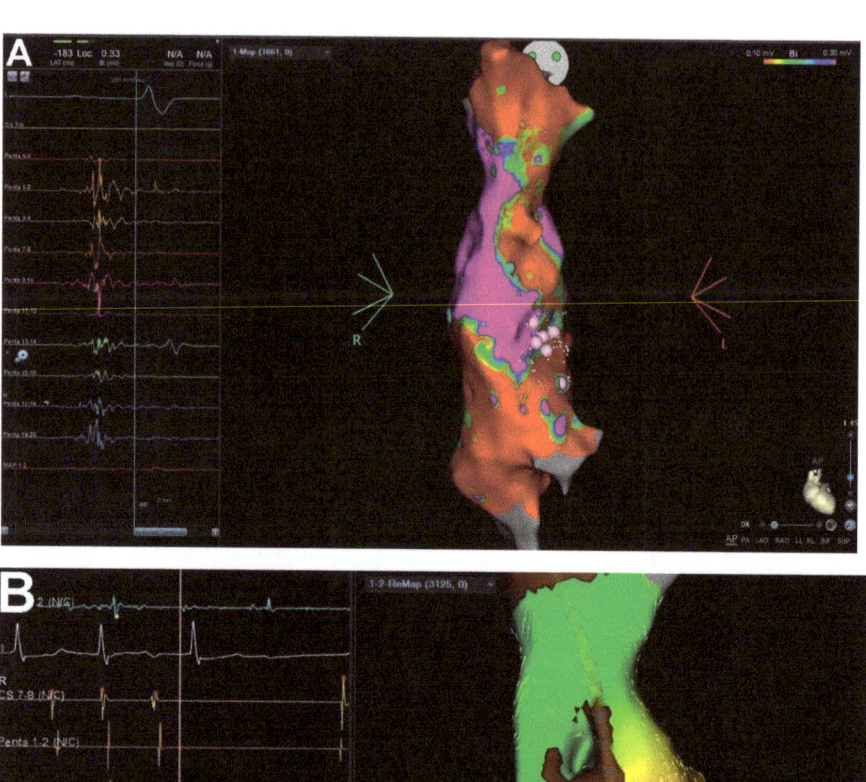
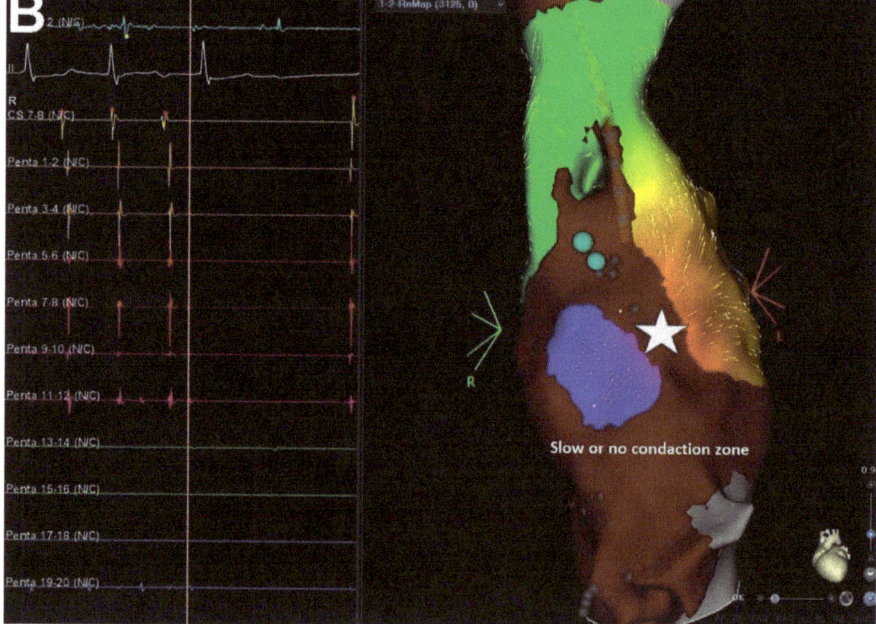

Figure 1. Procedure of supraventricular arrhythmia ablation in a patient after FO. (**A**) Fast anatomic map with a high-density voltage map (0.1–0.3 mV) of LT collected during sinus rhythm (CARTO, Biosense Webster Inc.). Extensive scaring at the anterolateral area of the tunnel with multiple double (blue dots) and fragmented potentials (white dots). Fragmented potentials recorded from Pentary diagnostic catheter are shown on the left side of the figure. (**B**) Activation map of AT (cycle length (CL): 380 ms, 80% of the CL in LT) created with a coherent mapping algorithm (CARTOPRIME, Biosense Webster Inc.). Electrocardiograms recorded from ablation and diagnostic catheters during AT termination are shown on the left side of the figure. White star—spot of AT termination during radiofrequency application.

2.6. Statistical Analysis

Data were presented as numbers and percentages for categorical variables, means with standard deviations (SDs) for normally distributed continuous variables, and medians with lower and upper quartiles (Q1–Q3) for continuous variables with a nonnormal distribution. The normality of data distribution was verified by a Kolmogorov–Smirnov test. Categorical variables were analyzed using the χ^2 test or Fisher's exact test as appropriate. All the analyses were performed in IBM SPSS Statistics for Windows, Version 25.0 (IBM Corp., Armonk, NY, USA). Statistical significance was set at $p < 0.05$.

3. Results

3.1. Patients' Characteristics

A total of 50 adult patients (mean (SD) age: 24 (5.7) years; 28 men (56%)) who underwent FO were enrolled in the study. The median (Q1–Q3) age of patients at the time of surgery was 4 (2–6) years, and the mean (SD) time after surgery was 20.5 (4.7) years. Out of 50 patients, 34 (68%) had fenestration, while 16 (32%) had no fenestration. The mean ejection fraction of the systemic ventricle was 53 ± 9.9%. The baseline characteristics of the studied patients are presented in Table 1.

Table 1. Baseline characteristics of patients after Fontan operation (FO).

Variables	Fontan Patients (n = 50)
Age, years	24 (5.7)
Female sex, n (%)	22 (44)
Height, cm	170 (8.1)
Body mass index, kg/m^2	22.6 (3.2)
Anatomic diagnosis, n (%)	
Tricuspid atresia	8 (16)
Pulmonary stenosis/TGA	15 (30)
Right ventricular hypoplasia	13 (26)
Hypoplastic left heart syndrome	6 (12)
Double-outlet right ventricle with left ventricular hypoplasia	6 (12)
Double-inflow left ventricle	1 (2)
Common atrioventricular canal	1 (2)
Systemic ventricle type, n (%)	
Left ventricle	30 (60)
Right ventricle	20 (40)
NYHA functional class, n (%)	
I	5 (10)
II	41 (82)
III	4 (8)
IV	0 (0)
Types of FO, n (%)	
Total cavopulmonary connection, 48 (96)	
Lateral tunnel	47

Table 1. *Cont.*

Variables	Fontan Patients (n = 50)
Extracardiac conduit	1
Atriopulmonary connection	2 (4)

Abbreviations: NYHA, New York Heart Association; TGA, transposition of great arteries. Continuous data are presented as means (SD), and categorical data as numbers (percentage).

3.2. Arrhythmia

Among the studied patients, bradyarrhythmia was detected in 25 (50%). The most common arrhythmia observed in patients after FO was sick sinus syndrome, which was primarily symptomatic and caused nocturnal bradycardia up to 35/min. Holter records of six patients showed pauses over 2 s. Low-atrial rhythm was recorded in five patients, and atrioventricular dissociation with substitute nodal rhythm in five. The AVB type 1 was observed in two patients, while advanced AVB (type 2 or 3) occurred in six patients and required pacemaker implantation for permanent pacing. Five devices were implanted by cardiac surgery (epicardial single (ventricle) chamber pacemaker electrode), and one was implanted intravenously (dual-chamber pacemaker) (Figure 2). After implantation, two patients developed cardiac device-related infective endocarditis requiring the removal and reimplantation of the device.

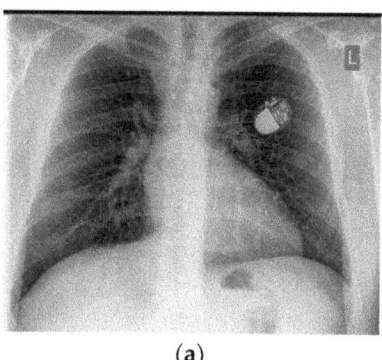
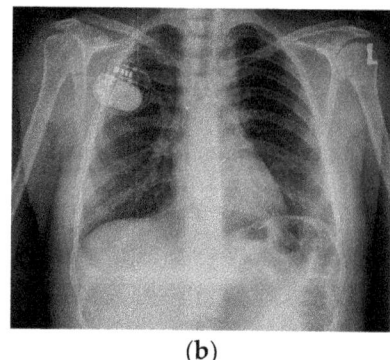

(a) (b)

Figure 2. Chest X-ray after pacemaker implantation in atriopulmonary projection after an FO procedure: (**a**) with a VVI epicardial lead after a cardiosurgery procedure and (**b**) with a DDD endocardial lead after transvenous implantation. L means left side.

Supraventricular tachyarrhythmias were noted in 14 patients (28%), of which three patients had AT (6%) and one additionally had paroxysmal AF. Permanent AF was observed in one patient. Two patients with AT (4%) required RF catheter ablation due to significant symptoms, and one had asymptomatic permanent AT with a daily average ventricular rate of about 50–55/min and remains under clinical observation. The most commonly observed arrhythmias in the SVT group were nsAT and Svebs (n = 8, 16%). From this group, three patients required medical treatment with B-blockers due to the presence of arrhythmia symptoms.

VAs were observed in six patients (12%). nsVT and PVC were recorded in all these patients. None of the patients had VT or VF. One patient required RF ablation, due to symptomatic Vas. Among the six patients, two were treated with sympathico-mimetic (salbutamol) for concomitant sinus bradycardia and one required pharmacological treatment (sotalol) due to the presence of severe VAs (nsVT) and symptoms.

Prevalence of arrhythmia identified based on Holter measurements, the number of pacemakers implanted, and ablation procedures performed in the patients after FO are presented in Table 2.

Table 2. Holter measurements, the number of pacemakers implanted, and ablation procedures performed in patients after FO.

Arrythmia Type, Catheter Ablation, Device Implanted	Fontan Patients (n = 50)
Dominant SSS with bradycardia	25 (55%)
- Pause > 2 s	6
- Low-atrial rhythm	5
- Nodal rhythm/atrioventricular dissociation	5
- AVB-1	2
- AVB-2	0
- AVB-3	6
Supraventricular tachyarrhythmias	14 (28%)
- In the form of sustained AT	3 (6%)
- In the form of nsAT, Svebs	8 (16%)
- In the form of AF/AFL	2 (4%)
VAs (in the form of nsVT and PVC)	6 (12%)
Catheter ablation	3 (6%)
- Paroxysmal AT	2 (4%)
- nsVT and PVC	1 (2%)
Device implanted (VVI/DDD)	6 (12%)
VVI—5, DDD—1, 2 devices removed because of cardiac device-related infective endocarditis	

Abbreviations: SSS, sick sinus syndrome; AVB-1, atrioventricular block type 1, AVB-2 atrioventricular block type 2; AVB-3, atrioventricular block type 3; AT, atrial tachycardia; nsAT, non-sustained atrial tachycardia; Svebs, supraventricular ectopic beats; AF, atrial fibrillation; AFL, atrial flutter; VAs, ventricular arrhythmias; nsVT, nonsustained ventricular tachycardia; PVC, premature ventricular contraction; VVI, single (ventricle) chamber pacemaker; DDD, dual-chamber pacemaker.

3.3. Catheter Ablation

Ablation was performed in three patients. Two patients had paroxysmal AT, and one had nsVT and PVC. All patients were symptomatic and resistant to pharmacological treatment. In the first case with SVT, macro-reentrant AT (cycle length: 250 ms) was eliminated from pulmonary atrium (retrograde access). In the long-term follow-up, recurrence of AT and AF was observed after 2 years, and the patient required the implantation of pacemaker (concomitant bradycardia) and intensification pharmacological treatment. In the second SVT case, two ATs were induced during ablation. The first AT was eliminated in LT, and the second was located out of LT. After failure of trans-fenestration access and additionally due to clinical character of the AT (self-terminated, not repeatable induction) trans-baffle puncture was not performed. If symptomatic arrythmia episodes recur during follow up period, redoing the procedure should be considered. During follow-up, recurrence of arrhythmia was not observed in the patients. VAs, in the form of ectopic nsVT and PVC, were located in the anterior basal side of single ventricular heart. Activation mapping and pace-mapping were carried out to determine the origin of arrhythmia. Acute success was achieved after RF application. Recurrence of arrhythmia was not observed in long-term follow-up. This patient died 6 years after ablation.

3.4. Influence of Systemic Ventricle Morphology and Fenestration on the Incidence of Rhythm Abnormalities

The presence of the right ventricle in the place of a systemic ventricle was associated with a higher risk of developing ventricular rhythm abnormalities (Table 3, Figure 3a).

Table 3. Dependency between fenestration and systemic ventricle morphology and incidence of rhythm abnormalities.

	Bradycardia				Ventricular Arrhythmia				Supraventricular Arrhythmia				Including AF/AFL			
	no		yes		no		yes		no		yes		no		yes	
Fenestration	n	%	n	%	n	%	n	%	n	%	n	%	n	%	n	%
no	10	62.50%	6	37.50%	16	100%	0	0.0%	11	68.8%	5	31.3%	14	87.5%	2	12.5%
yes	17	50.00%	17	50.00%	18	82.4%	6	17.6%	24	70.6%	10	29.4%	31	91.2%	3	8.8%
p-value	0.41				0.16				0.99				0.99			
	no		yes		no		yes		no		yes		no		yes	
Ventricular type	n	%	n	%	n	%	n	%	n	%	n	%	n	%	n	%
Right ventricle	5	50.0%	5	50.0%	7	70.0%	3	30.0%	7	70.0%	3	30.0%	9	90.0%	1	10.0%
Left ventricle	22	55.0%	18	45.0%	37	92.5%	3	7.5%	28	70.0%	12	30.0%	36	90.0%	4	10.0%
p-value	0.99				0.09				0.990				0.99			

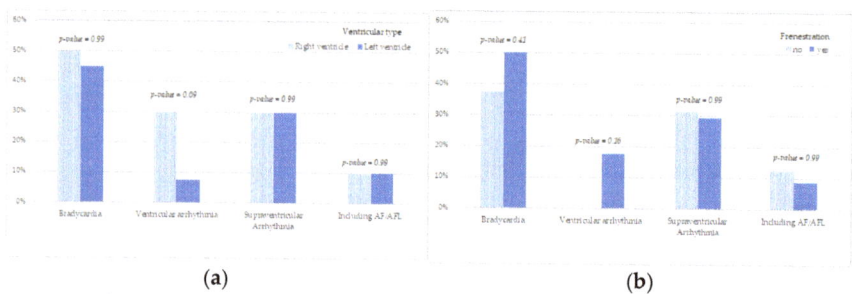

Figure 3. Dependency between ventricular type (**a**) and fenestration (**b**) and the incidence of rhythm abnormalities.

No relationship was found between the presence of fenestration and the incidence rate of rhythm and conduction abnormalities (Table 3, Figure 3b).

This study did not compare the influence of the type of surgery conducted (APC vs. TCPC) on the incidence rate and type of rhythm abnormalities as the studied population included a low number of patients who underwent APC (only 2 patients, i.e., 4%).

3.5. The Survival Assessment of Enrolled Patients

One patient, a 33-year-old man, died during the study, which is 2% of the study group and 2.9% of the patients with arrhythmias. He had undergone catheter ablation due to VAs. Recurrence of arrhythmia was not observed in the 6-year follow-up period. The reason for death was a serious hemodynamic impairment in the course of significant atrioventricular regurgitation and other extra-cardiac complications including hepatic disorders.

4. Discussion

In this study, we determined the type and prevalence of arrhythmias in the group of adult people after FO.

Among the studied patients, bradyarrhythmia was detected in 25 (50%), of which six (12%) required pacemaker implantation. Sinus node dysfunction may be caused by primary anatomical changes (occurring) in the single ventricular heart or due to direct damage to its vascular supply [19]. Previous works that compared the incidence of sinus node dysfunction in patients following LT conduit and ECC do not clearly indicate which surgical method can lower the risk of conduction abnormalities [5,7,8,20,21]. However, the latest guidelines regarding congenital heart diseases in adult patients support the use of ECC [1]. Symptomatic sinus node dysfunction requires permanent pacemaker implantation. In patients after FO, electrodes are located on the epicardium. Thus, every single decision regarding implantation, particularly in the case of young patients, should be made with caution, taking into account the possible complications in follow-up observation [22].

In the present study, supraventricular arrythmias were observed in 14 patients (28%). These data are comparable with an available study which reported that supraventricular tachyarrhythmias (including typical intra-atrial reentrant tachycardia, AFL, AF, and focal AT) were observed in approximately 20% of patients after 10 years of FO [23]. The incidence rate of arrhythmias was lower after TCPC than after APC and also lower after ECC than after intracardiac connection (LT) [1]. Studies in the literature have described several independent predictors of SVT, including the condition following APC, preoperative SVT, elderly age at the time of FO and observation period, thromboembolic episode, pacemaker implantation, moderate/serious atrioventricular valve regurgitation, and atrial enlargement [12,23]. Supraventricular arrhythmias, along with rapid conduction to ventricles, may aggravate hemodynamics in Fontan circulation and lead to heart failure over a short period of time and, in the worst cases, SCD [24]. Patients with supraventricular arrhythmias should be referred for electrophysiological assessment as soon as possible, and ablation should be performed if possible [1,25]. According to the literature, the efficacy rate of ablation is 50–70% [26]. In the present study, ablation was performed in two patients (4%). In the long-term follow-up, in the first patient recurrence of AT and AF was observed after 2 years and the patient required the implantation of a pacemaker (concomitant bradycardia) and intensification pharmacological treatment.

In the second patient, no recurrence of SVT was observed in the 8-month observation period.

Ventricular rhythm abnormalities were recorded in six of the studied patients (12%). In our studied patients the only form of VAs was ns VT and PVC and none of the patients developed sustained VT or VF. In a study by Stephenson et al. [11], the incidence of VA after 8.6 years of FO was 3.5% of patients. In a study on the combined pediatric and adult population by Rychik et al. [27], the incidence rate of ventricular rhythm abnormalities, including SCD, was assessed at 2–10%. The mechanism contributing to the formation of VAs in the population of patients following FO remains unknown. It is assumed that VAs may form from a ventriculotomy scar which allows for reentry circulation, enlargement of the defect in the interventricular septum, increase in myocardial fibrosis, and ventricular dilatation. These are especially dangerous for patients with anatomical right systemic ventricle and single-ventricle dysfunction [11]. In this study, we observed that patients with anatomical right systemic ventricle were more likely to have an increased incidence of ventricular rhythm abnormalities.

Episodes of nsVTs were recorded in six patients. One of these patients, a 27-year-old man, who was ineffectively treated with antiarrhythmic drugs, was qualified for and received RF ablation, the effect of which was sustained in the 6-year follow-up period. In recent years, novel treatment methods for arrhythmias have been developed, including ablation, and electrophysiologists and cardiologists cooperate better in treating patients with congenital heart defects. Furthermore, the development of electrophysiological mapping systems has increased the possibilities of mapping and enabled the ablation of complex atrial arrhythmias [28].

Malignant VAs may lead to SCD. Khairy et al. [29] stated that the incidence of SCD in distant time from FO is 0.15% and in most of the cases reported annually, SCD is caused by arrhythmias, although it is difficult to identify the possible prognostic factors. The treatment of VAs using an implantable cardioverter defibrillator (ICD) in patients after FO is a major challenge for electrocardiologists. The available studies in the literature have described only single patients who required treatment with ICD after FO [30–33]. In the present study, there were no cases in the patient group that would require ICD implantation.

With the extension of follow-up time, the number of arrhythmias and conduction disorders may increase significantly. Thus, the differences in the frequency of their occurrence described in the literature may result from the length of the observation time.

5. Conclusions

Early diagnosis of arrhythmia in the patients who underwent FO is important as arrhythmias may contribute to heart failure, embolization, and SCD. These patients should be treated in multidisciplinary centers by experienced specialists with the use of modern methods, such as ablation, which is a safe and effective method for treating both supraventricular arrhythmias and VAs. The treatment of this patient group with ICD still remains a huge challenge for electrocardiologists.

Further analyses on larger groups of patients are necessary to create multi-center registries. The experience exchange between centers is required for the development of guidelines for treating this complex group of patients.

Limitation of the Study

The limitation of this retrospective study is that the number of patients in the study group was small and the population was relatively mixed. As the Fontan procedure was introduced into clinical practice relatively recently, we can expect that single centers at this stage of medical development may have fewer patients under medical supervision. Thus, the limitation in the number of patients in the study group applies to most of the individual centers in the world caring for this patient population.

Author Contributions: Conceptualization, M.O. and L.T.-P.; methodology, M.O., G.K., M.K. and L.T.-P.; software, M.O., B.R. and J.Ł.; validation, M.O. and L.T.-P.; formal analysis, M.O., G.K., M.K., B.R. and J.Ł.; investigation, M.O., L.T.-P, G.K. and M.K.; resources, M.O., L.T.-P, G.K., M.K. and J.B.; data curation, M.O., J.Ł., G.K. and M.K.; writing—original draft preparation, M.O., G.K. and M.K.; writing—review and editing, L.T.-P. and J.P.; visualization, M.O., G.K. and M.K.; supervision, L.T.-P., J.L. and J.P.; project administration, L.T.-P.; funding acquisition, L.T.-P. All authors have read and agreed to the published version of the manuscript.

Funding: This work was supported by a grant of the National Science Center (2017/27/B/NZ5/02186) to L.T.-P.

Institutional Review Board Statement: This study was conducted in accordance with the guidelines of Declaration of Helsinki and approved by Bioethical Commission at the District Medical Chamber in Krakow (no. 1072.6120.11.2017).

Informed Consent Statement: All patients provided written informed consent.

Data Availability Statement: The data presented in this study are not publicly available due to upcoming publications but are available on request from the corresponding author.

Conflicts of Interest: The authors declare no conflict of interest. The sponsors had no role in the design, execution, interpretation, or writing of the study.

References

1. Baumagartner, H.; De Backer, J.; Babu-Narayan, S.V.; Budts, W.; Chessa, M.; Diller, G.-P.; Lung, B.; Kluin, J.; Lang, I.M.; Meijboom, F.; et al. 2020 ESC Guidelines for the management of adult congenital heart disease. *Eur. Heart J.* **2021**, *42*, 563–645. [CrossRef] [PubMed]
2. de Leval, M.R.; Kilner, P.; Gewillig, M.; Bull, C. Total cavopulmonary connection: A logical alternative to atriopulmonary connection for complex Fontan operations. Experimental studies and early clinical experience. *J. Thorac. Cardiovasc. Surg.* **1988**, *96*, 682–695. [CrossRef]
3. Kim, S.J.; Kim, W.H.; Lim, H.G.; Lee, J.Y. Outcome of 200 patients after an extracardiac Fontan procedure. *J. Thorac. Cardiovasc. Surg.* **2008**, *136*, 108–116. [CrossRef] [PubMed]
4. Malec, E.; Zając, A.; Pająk, J. The results of one-stage and two-stage Fontan operation in children with single ventricle. *Kardiol. Pol.* **1998**, *48*, 23–30.
5. Bae, E.J.; Lee, J.Y.; Noh, C.I.; Kim, W.H.; Kim, Y.J. Sinus node dysfunction after Fontan modifications—Influence of surgical method. *Int. J. Cardiol.* **2003**, *88*, 285–291. [CrossRef]

6. Blaufox, A.D.; Sleeper, L.A.; Bradley, D.J.; Breitbart, R.E.; Hordof, A.; Kanter, R.J.; Stephenson, E.A.; Vetter, V.L.; Saul, J.P.; Pediatric Heart Network Investigators; et al. Functional status, heart rate, and rhythm abnormalities in 521 Fontan patients 6 to 18 years of age. *J. Thorac. Cardiovasc. Surg.* **2008**, *136*, 100–107.e1. [CrossRef] [PubMed]
7. Dilawar, M.; Bradley, S.M.; Saul, J.P.; Stroud, M.R.; Balaji, S. Sinus node dysfunction after intraatrial lateral tunnel and extracardiac conduit Fontan procedures. *Pediatr. Cardiol.* **2003**, *24*, 284–288. [CrossRef] [PubMed]
8. Kumar, S.P.; Rubinstein, C.S.; Simsic, J.M.; Taylor, A.B.; Saul, J.P.; Bradley, S.M. Lateral tunnel versus extracardiac conduit Fontan procedure: A concurrent comparison. *Ann. Thorac. Surg.* **2003**, *76*, 1389–1396; discussion 96–97. [CrossRef]
9. Nurnberg, J.H.; Ovroutski, S.; Alexi-Meskishvili, V.; Ewert, P.; Hetzer, R.; Lange, P.E. New onset arrhythmias after the extracardiac conduit Fontan operation compared with the intraatrial lateral tunnel procedure: Early and midterm results. *Ann. Thorac. Surg.* **2004**, *78*, 1979–1988. [CrossRef] [PubMed]
10. Ovroutski, S.; Dahnert, I.; Alexi-Meskishvili, V.; Nurnberg, J.H.; Hetzer, R.; Lange, P.E. Preliminary analysis of arrhythmias after the Fontan operation with extracardiac conduit compared with intra-atrial lateral tunnel. *J. Thorac. Cardiovasc. Surg.* **2001**, *49*, 334–337. [CrossRef]
11. Stephenson, E.A.; Lu, M.; Berul, C.I.; Etheridge, S.P.; Idriss, S.F.; Margossian, R.; Sleeper, L.A.; Vetter, V.L.; Blaufox, A.D.; Pediatric Heart Network Investigators; et al. Arrhythmias in a contemporary Fontan cohort: Prevalence and clinical associations in a multicenter cross sectional study. *J. Am. Coll. Cardiol.* **2010**, *56*, 890–896. [CrossRef] [PubMed]
12. Idorn, L.; Juul, K.; Jensen, A.S.; Hanel, B.; Nielsen, K.G.; Andersen, H.; Reimers, J.I.; Sørensen, K.E.; Søndergaard, L. Arrhythmia and exercise intolerance in Fontan patients: Current status and future burden. *Int. J. Cardiol.* **2013**, *168*, 1458–1465. [CrossRef] [PubMed]
13. Moore, B.; Anderson, R.; Nisbet, A.; Kalla, M.; du Plessis, K.; d'Udekem, Y. Ablation of Atrial Arrhythmias After the Atriopulmonary Fontan Procedure. *JACC Clin. Electrophysiol.* **2018**, *10*, 1338–1346. [CrossRef]
14. Tomkiewicz-Pajak, L.; Podolec, P.; Drabik, L.; Pajak, J.; Kolcz, J.; Plazak, W. Single ventricle function and exercise tolerance in adult patients after Fontan operation. *Acta Cardiol.* **2014**, *69*, 155–160. [CrossRef] [PubMed]
15. Hindricks, G.; Potpara, T.; Dagres, N.; Arbelo, E.; Bax, J.J.; Blomström-Lundqvist, C.; Boriani, G.; Castella, M.; Dan, G.A.; Dilaveris, P.E.; et al. 2020 ESC Guidelines for the diagnosis and management of atrial fibrillation developed in collaboration with the European Association for Cardio-Thoracic Surgery (EACTS): The Task Force for the Diagnosis and Management of Atrial Fibrillation of the European Society of Cardiology (ESC) developed with the special contribution of the European Heart Rhythm Association (EHRA) of the ESC. *Eur. Heart J.* **2021**, *42*, 373–498. [CrossRef] [PubMed]
16. Brugada, J.; Katritsis, D.G.; Arbelo, E.; Arribas, F.; Bax, J.J.; Blomström-Lundqvist, C.; Calkins, H.; Corrado, D.; Deftereos, S.G.; Diller, G.P.; et al. 2019 ESC Guidelines for the management of patients with supraventricular tachycardia: The Task Force for the Management of Patients with Supraventricular Tachycardia of the European Society of Cardiology (ESC). *Eur. Heart J.* **2020**, *41*, 655–720; Erratum in *Eur. Heart J.* **2020**, *41*, 4258. [CrossRef]
17. Al-Khatib, S.M.; Stevenson, W.G.; Ackerman, M.J.; Bryant, W.J.; Callans, D.J.; Curtis, A.B.; Deal, B.J.; Dickfeld, T.; Field, M.E.; Fonarow, G.C.; et al. 2017 AHA/ACC/HRS Guideline for management of patients with ventricular arrhythmias and the prevention of sudden cardiac death: A report of the American College of Cardiology/American Heart Association Task Force on Clinical Practice Guidelines and the Heart Rhythm Society. *J. Am. Coll. Cardiol.* **2018**, *72*, e91–e220; Erratum in *J. Am. Coll. Cardiol.* **2018**, *72*, 1760. [CrossRef] [PubMed]
18. Baranowski, A.; Bieganowska, K.; Kozłowski, D.; Kukla, M.; Kurpesa, M.; Lelakowski, J.; Maciejewska, M.; Miszczak-Knecht, M.; Pierścińska, M. Zalecenia dotyczące stosowania rozpoznań elektrokardiograficznych Dokument opracowany przez Grup' Roboczą powołaną przez Zarząd Sekcji Elektrokardiologii Nieinwazyjnej i Telemedycyny Polskiego Towarzystwa Kardiologicznego Pod patronatem Polskiego Towarzystwa Kardiologicznego. *Kardiol. Pol.* **2010**, *68*, 336–389.
19. Cohen, M.; Wernovsky, G.; Vetter, V.L.; Wieand, T.S.; Gaynor, J.W.; Jacobs, M.L.; Spray, T.L.; A Rhodes, L. Sinus node function after a systematically staged Fontan procedure. *Circulation* **1998**, *98*, II352–II359.
20. Lasa, J.J.; Glatz, A.C.; Daga, A.; Shah, M. Prevalence of arrhythmias late after the Fontan operation. *Am. J. Cardiol.* **2014**, *113*, 1184–1188. [CrossRef] [PubMed]
21. Li, D.; Fan, Q.; Hirata, Y.; Ono, M.; An, Q. Arrhythmias after Fontan operation with intra-atrial lateral tunnel versus extra-cardiac conduit: A systematic review and meta-analysis. *Pediatr. Cardiol.* **2017**, *38*, 873–880. [CrossRef]
22. Okólska, M.; Łach, J.; Matusik, P.T.; Pająk, J.; Mroczek, T.; Podolec, P.; Tomkiewicz-Pająk, L. Heart rate variability and its associations with organ complications in adults after Fontan operation. *J. Clin. Med.* **2021**, *10*, 4492. [CrossRef] [PubMed]
23. Durongpisitkul, K.; Porter, C.J.; Cetta, F.; Offord, K.P.; Slezak, J.M.; Puga, F.J.; Schaff, H.V.; Danielson, G.K.; Driscoll, D.J. Predictors of early- and late-onset supraventricular tachyarrhythmias after Fontan operation. *Circulation* **1998**, *98*, 1099–1107. [CrossRef] [PubMed]
24. Tomkiewicz-Pająk, L.; Hoffman, P.; Trojnarska, O.; Bednarek, J.; Płazak, W.; Pająk, J.W.; Olszowska, M.; Komar, M.; Podolec, P.S. Long-term follow-up in adult patients after Fontan operation. *Kardiochir. Torakochirurgia Pol.* **2013**, *10*, 357–363.
25. Tomkiewicz-Pająk, L.; Lelakowski, J.; Pająk, J.; Kopeć, G.; Podolec, P.; Bednarek, J. Ablation of arrhythmias in adult patients after Fontan operation. *Pol. Arch. Med. Wewn.* **2013**, *123*, 723–725. [CrossRef] [PubMed]
26. Kibos, A.; Chang, S.L.; Lee, P.C.; Chen, S.A. Catheter ablation of an intra-atrial reentrant tachycardia in a young adult Fontan patient with complex palliated congenital heart disease. *Circ. J.* **2012**, *76*, 2494–2495. [CrossRef] [PubMed]

27. Rychik, J.; Atz, A.M.; Celermajer, D.S.; Deal, B.J.; Gatzoulis, M.A.; Gewillig, M.H.; Hsia, T.Y.; Hsu, D.T.; Kovacs, A.H.; McCrindle, B.W.; et al. Evaluation and management of the child and adult with Fontan circulation: A scientific statement from the American Heart Association. *Circulation* **2019**, *140*, e234–e284. [CrossRef]
28. Karkowski, G.; Kuniewicz, M.; Badacz, R.; Rajs, T.; Lelakowski, J.; Legutko, J. The CARTOPRIME module with the Coherent Mapping algorithm for ablation of complex (scar-related) atrial tachycardia. *Kardiol. Pol.* **2020**, *78*, 1180–1182. [CrossRef] [PubMed]
29. Khairy, P.; Fernandes, S.M.; Mayer, J.E., Jr.; Triedman, J.K.; Walsh, E.P.; Lock, J.E.; Landzberg, M.J. Long-term survival, modes of death, and predictors of mortality in patients with Fontan surgery. *Circulation* **2008**, *117*, 85–92. [CrossRef]
30. Pundi, K.N.; Pundi, K.N.; Johnson, J.N.; Dearani, J.A.; Li, Z.; Driscoll, D.J.; Wackel, P.L.; McLeod, C.J.; Cetta, F.; Cannon, B.C. Sudden cardiac death and late arrhythmias after the Fontan operation. *Congenit. Heart Dis.* **2017**, *12*, 17–23. [CrossRef] [PubMed]
31. Agir, A.A.; Celikyurt, U.; Karauzum, K.; Yilmaz, I.; Ozbudak, E.; Bozyel, S.; Kanko, M.; Vural, A.; Ural, D. Clinical ventricular tachycardia and surgical epicardial ICD implantation in a patient with a Fontan operation for double-inlet left ventricle. *Cardiovasc. J. Afr.* **2014**, *25*, e6–e10. [CrossRef] [PubMed]
32. Papakonstantinou, N.A.; Patris, V.; Samiotis, I.; Koutouzis, M.; Koutouzi, G.; Argiriou, M. Epicardial cardioverter defibrillator implantation due to post-Fontan ventricular tachycardia. *Ann. Cardiac Anaesth.* **2020**, *23*, 235–236. [CrossRef] [PubMed]
33. Padanilam, M.S.; Ahmed, A.S.; Clark, B.A.; Mozes, J.I.; Steinberg, L.A. Novel approach to intracardiac defibrillator placement in patients with atriopulmonary Fontan: Ventricular defibrillation with an atrial positioned ICD lead. *J. Cardiovasc. Electrophysiol.* **2021**, *32*, 3275–3278. [CrossRef] [PubMed]

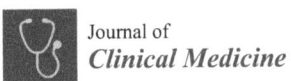

Article

Sinus Node Dysfunction after Successful Atrial Flutter Ablation during Follow-Up: Clinical Characteristics and Predictors

Guan-Yi Li [1,2], Fa-Po Chung [1,2,*], Tze-Fan Chao [1,2], Yenn-Jiang Lin [1,2], Shih-Lin Chang [1,2], Li-Wei Lo [1,2], Yu-Feng Hu [1,2], Ta-Chuan Tuan [1,2], Jo-Nan Liao [1,2], Ting-Yung Chang [1,2], Ling Kuo [1,2], Cheng-I Wu [1,2], Chih-Min Liu [1,2], Shin-Huei Liu [1,2], Wen-Han Cheng [1,2] and Shih-Ann Chen [1,2,3]

1. Division of Cardiology, Department of Medicine, Taipei Veterans General Hospital, Taipei 11217, Taiwan; lgy8065@gmail.com (G.-Y.L.); eyckeyck@gmail.com (T.-F.C.); linyennjiang@gmail.com (Y.-J.L.); ep.slchang@msa.hinet.net (S.-L.C.); gyrus1975@gmail.com (L.-W.L.); huhuhu0609@gmail.com (Y.-F.H.); duan.dachuan@gmail.com (T.-C.T.); care1980@gmail.com (J.-N.L.); tingyungchang@gmail.com (T.-Y.C.); kl19860209@gmail.com (L.K.); shawnwu64@gmail.com (C.-I.W.); sasuke9301108@hotmail.com (C.-M.L.); shinhueiliu0101@gmail.com (S.-H.L.); hill55772003@hotmail.com (W.-H.C.); epsachen@ms41.hinet.net (S.-A.C.)
2. Department of Medicine, School of Medicine, National Yang Ming Chiao Tung University, Taipei 112304, Taiwan
3. Cardiovascular Center, Taichung Veterans General Hospital, Taichung 40705, Taiwan
* Correspondence: marxtaiji@gmail.com

Abstract: Identification of sinus node dysfunction (SND) before termination of persistent AFL by catheter ablation (CA) is challenging. This study aimed to investigate the characteristics and predictors of acute and delayed SND after AFL ablation. We retrospectively enrolled 221 patients undergoing CA of persistent AFL in a tertiary referral center. Patients with SND who required a temporary pacemaker (TPM) after termination of AFL or a permanent pacemaker (PPM) during follow-up were identified. Acute SND requiring a TPM was found in 14 of 221 (6.3%) patients following successful termination of AFL. A total of 10 of the 14 patients (71.4%) recovered from acute SND. An additional 11 (5%) patients presenting with delayed SND required a PPM during follow-up, including 4 patients recovering from acute SND. Of these, 9 of these 11 patients (81.8%) underwent PPM implantation within 1 year after the ablation. In multivariable analysis, female gender and a history of hypothyroidism were associated with the requirement for a TPM following termination of persistent AFL, while older age and a history of hypothyroidism predicted PPM implantation. This study concluded that the majority of patients with acute SND still require a PPM implantation despite the initial improvement. Therefore, it is reasonable to monitor the patients closely for at least one year after AFL ablation.

Keywords: atrial flutter; catheter ablation; permanent pacemaker; sinus node dysfunction; temporary pacemaker

1. Introduction

Atrial flutter (AFL), a common atrial tachyarrhythmia, includes both typical and atypical forms. Radiofrequency catheter ablation (CA) has been implemented to terminate AFL with promising results [1]. However, sinus node dysfunction (SND) may coexist in patients with AFL. The presence of SND can become notable after termination of AFL, and a pacemaker may be required [2,3]. Detection of SND before termination of AFL is clinically challenging. At present, there are limited studies investigating the predictors or risk factors for SND following termination of AFL.

Sinus node inactivity caused by atrial tachyarrhythmias might be reversed following successful CA, and then the acute SND could recover. However, even without acute SND or after the recovery of SND following AFL ablation, sinus node function may still deteriorate in some patients during follow-up. It is a dilemma to determine the duration of observation in patients with acute SND after termination of persistent AFL and the exact time for permanent pacemaker (PPM) implantation.

Therefore, our study aimed to examine clinical characteristics and predictors of acute and delayed SND after successful elimination of persistent AFL, including typical and atypical forms.

2. Materials and Methods

2.1. Study Population

We retrospectively enrolled patients with persistent AFL, including typical and/or atypical AFL, who underwent CA at Taipei Veterans General Hospital between January 2014 and January 2020. The "persistent" AFL was defined as tachycardia lasting for more than 7 days, whilst long-standing persistent AFL was defined as sustained AFL for more than 12 months. Patients who had previously received AFL ablation or had a PPM implantation before the AFL ablation were excluded. Meanwhile, patients who had previously undergone ablation for other types of arrhythmias were still eligible. The Institutional Review Board of Taipei Veterans General Hospital approved this study in accordance with Good Clinical Practice Guidelines.

2.2. Baseline Patient Characteristics

Patients' demographics and preprocedural comorbidities are included in the database, such as age, body mass index, coronary artery disease, valvular heart disease, hypertension, diabetes mellitus, heart failure with reduced ejection fraction, chronic kidney disease, history of transient ischemic attack or stroke, hyperthyroidism, hypothyroidism, and atrial fibrillation. Additionally, the pharmacological history one year before and after the ablation, including beta-blockers, non-dihydropyridine calcium channel blockers, propafenone, and amiodarone, was documented.

The pre-procedural echocardiography was reviewed, and we recorded parameters including left atrial (LA) and right atrial (RA) diameter, LA and RA area, left ventricular ejection fraction, left ventricular hypertrophy, as well as moderate and severe mitral/tricuspid regurgitation. The minor-axis RA diameter, LA, and RA area were all measured by the 4-chamber view at end-systole according to recommendations from the American Society of Echocardiography. The 12-lead electrocardiography and ambulatory electrocardiography monitoring records within one year before the ablation were reviewed. If neither of these records revealed a sinus rhythm, the patient was classified with a "long-standing persistent AFL". Otherwise, the last recorded heart rate in sinus rhythm would be identified. Furthermore, the QRS duration prior to ablation was analyzed.

2.3. Electrophysiological Study and Catheter Ablation

Each patient signed an informed consent form. A standard electrophysiological study and CA were conducted for AFL. A decapolar catheter with an interelectrode spacing of 2-5-2 mm was inserted into the coronary sinus, with the proximal bipole located at the ostium. In our study, typical AFL was defined by the cavotricuspid isthmus (CTI) dependence and was confirmed if concealed entrainment was identified when pacing the CTI and if the difference between post-pacing interval at the CTI and flutter cycle length was within 30 ms. The other AFLs would be classified as an atypical form. Before CA, the flutter cycle length was measured at the proximal coronary sinus.

We have previously described in detail the electrophysiological study, mapping, and ablation strategies for AFL [4]. Ablation of the CTI was performed for persistent typical flutter, while linear ablation of the isthmus, which was identified by either 3D electroanatomic activation mapping or entrainment, was used for atypical flutter. Pulmonary vein isolation and/or other ablation strategies were based on patients' clinical presentation and physicians' discretion. Conduction block in both directions was confirmed simultaneously with the ablation line. In our laboratory, formal sinus node function testing was not routinely performed during AFL ablation.

2.4. Post-Ablation Follow-Up and Pacemaker Implantation

In the present study, we routinely arranged a 12-lead ECG 2 weeks after ablation at the outpatient clinic and the 24-h Holter monitoring 3 months later. If the patient was symptomatic, additional ECG, 24-h Holter monitoring, or a 7-day event recorder was arranged on a case-by-case basis to detect the recurrence of arrhythmias or post-ablation conduction system disorder.

SND is defined as a persistent condition associated with at least one of the following: (1) pronounced sinus bradycardia with a heart rate of fewer than 50 beats per minute, (2) junctional bradycardia, or (3) repeated sinus pauses longer than 3 s, (4) hemodynamic instability or symptoms related to bradycardia or sinus pause, and (5) sinus node recovery time (SNRT) > 1500 ms or corrected sinus node recovery time (CSNRT) > 550 ms.

In our study, we defined an acute SND as one that occurred following the elimination of AFL or in the same hospitalization. A new or recurrent SND during follow-up in an outpatient clinic was classified as a "delayed SND". Patients receiving either a temporary pacemaker (TPM) or a PPM implantation for SND after AFL ablation were identified. In these cases, we explored the duration of TPM back-up, the time interval between the ablation and the PPM implantation, the pacing modes of the PPM, and the averaged percentage of atrial pacing during follow-up.

2.5. Statistical Analysis

The normally distributed continuous variables are presented as means ± standard deviations, and the non-normally distributed continuous variables are presented as medians with 25 and 75% interquartile ranges (IQRs). Wilcoxon signed-rank test (Mann–Whitney U test) or Student's T-test was used to compare the differences between groups. The categorical variables are expressed as numbers and percentages and compared using the Chi-square test. A *p*-value of <0.05 was considered statistically significant. In this study, logistic regression analysis was used to determine the association between variables and acute SND that required a TPM, and Cox regression analysis was used to determine the predictors of delayed SND that required a PPM implantation after successful AFL ablation during long-term follow-up. The parameters with a *p*-value < 0.05 in the univariable regression analysis were selected for the multivariable model. A Kaplan–Meier survival curve was plotted to determine event-free survival, with the statistical significance examined using the Log-rank test. The statistical analyses were conducted using IBM Corporation's Statistical Package for the Social Sciences version 22.0 (Armonk, NY, USA).

3. Results

3.1. Patient Selection, Characteristics of Atrial Flutter, and Catheter Ablation

A total of 245 patients underwent AFL ablation in our tertiary referral center during the study period. After excluding 24 patients, 221 patients were included in the study. As shown in Supplementary Tables S1 and S2, all patients had clinically documented AFL for more than 7 days, and 104 (47.1%) patients had a long-standing persistent AFL. A total of 103 patients (46.6%) with concomitant clinically documented AF were enrolled. A total of 168 (76.0%) patients took at least 1 antiarrhythmic drug before ablation. In our electrophysiological laboratory, 177 (80.1%) patients were diagnosed with counterclockwise typical AFL, 22 (10.0%) patients with clockwise typical flutter, and 55 (24.9%) patients with atypical AFL. Regarding the ablation procedure, CTI ablation, pulmonary vein isolation, peri-superior vena cava (SVC) ablation, and bi-atrial ablation were performed in 204, 21, 5, and 23 patients, respectively. After a median follow-up period of 5.0 months (25–75% IQR: 0.7–6.5 months), AFL recurred in 19 patients (8.6%). A total of 6 patients (2.7%) received a repeat procedure of AFL ablation.

3.2. Clinical Characteristics of Sinus Node Dysfunction

Acute SND requiring a TPM was identified in 14 (6.3%) patients following termination of AFL (Figure 1). Additionally, 4 patients (28.6%) had unrecoverable SND and required implantation of a PPM 3.5 days (25–75% IQR: 0.8–4.0 days) after ablation. For the other 10 patients who recovered from the acute SND, all TPMs were removed successfully within 5 days, and in the majority (8 out of 10, 80%) within 2 days (Table 1). After a median follow-up period of 4.2 months (25–75% IQR: 3.9–8.0 months), 4 of the 14 patients (28.6%) developed delayed SND. In total, 8 of the 14 patients (57.1%) with acute SND underwent implantation of a PPM. Before catheter ablation for the 14 patients with acute SND, dizziness, fatigue, and syncope were documented in 4, 1, and 1 patient(s), respectively. Among these 6 patients, the acute SND was resolved in 4 patients. However, 2 of them developed subsequent delayed SND requiring a PPM implantation. For the remaining 207 (93.7%) patients without acute SND, delayed SND requiring a PPM was found in 7 (3.4%) patients after a median follow-up period of 4.7 months (25–75% IQR: 1.6–11.9 months) (Figure 1).

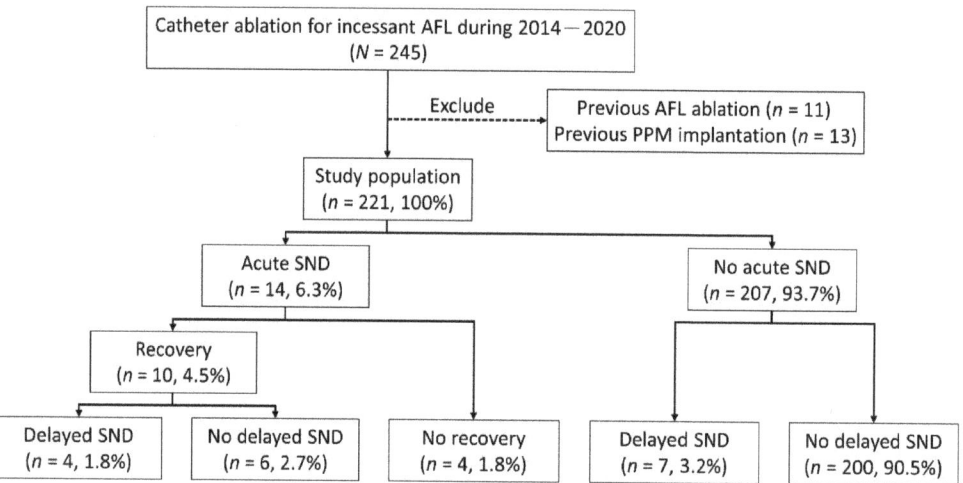

Figure 1. Flow chart of the studied patients. AFL: atrial flutter; PPM: permanent pacemaker; SND: sinus node dysfunction.

Table 1. The detailed characteristics of the patients developing acute SND after the AFL ablation.

Patient No.	Age (Year)	Gender	AFL Form	Flutter Cycle Length (ms)	Pre-Ablation Sinus Rate (bpm) †	TPM Back-Up Duration (Day)	PPM Mode
			Patients who did not recover from acute SND				
1	62	F	Typical	296	NA	3 ‡	DDD
2	64	M	Both	348	NA	4 ‡	DDD
3	43	F	Typical	294	NA	4 ‡	DDD
4	54	M	Typical	264	NA	1 ‡	DDD
			Patients who recovered from acute SND, but developed delayed SND				
5	60	F	Atypical	208	65	2	DDD
6	61	M	Typical	220	NA	1	DDD
7	78	F	Typical	244	NA	1	DDD
8	89	M	Typical	300	NA	5	DDD

Table 1. Cont.

Patient No.	Age (Year)	Gender	AFL Form	Flutter Cycle Length (ms)	Pre-Ablation Sinus Rate (bpm) [†]	TPM Back-Up Duration (Day)	PPM Mode
			Patients who recovered from acute SND, without developing delayed SND				
9	56	F	Both	288	NA	1	NA
10	68	F	Typical	309	78	3	NA
11	61	F	Typical	238	NA	2	NA
12	62	F	Typical	278	108	1	NA
13	82	F	Atypical	286	64	1	NA
14	89	M	Both	209	NA	1	NA

[†] Pre-ablation sinus rate will not be available if no documented sinus rhythm during one year before ablation; [‡] The TPMs were not removed until PPM implantation; AFL: atrial flutter; bpm: beats per minute; F: female; M: male; NA: not applicable; No.: number; PPM: permanent pacemaker; SND: sinus node dysfunction; TPM: temporary pacemaker.

In the 11 patients exhibiting delayed SND, most (9 out of 11, 81.8%) of the PPMs were implanted within one year following the ablation. Figure 2 shows the PPM-free survival curve after the ablation. After ablation, the cumulative incidence of delayed SND requiring a PPM implantation increased for several months after CA, almost reaching a plateau after 1 year. A total of 12 of the 15 patients underwent dual chamber mode (DDD) PPM implantation, while the remaining 3 underwent single chamber mode (VVI) PPM implantation. All the 8 PPMs implanted for patients with acute SND were in the DDD mode (Table 1). After the PPM implantation, 7 patients suffered from paroxysmal AF, and 3 had AFL recurrences. One patient underwent a repeat procedure for AFL ablation. For the 12 PPMs with DDD mode, after 2 weeks, 3 months, and 1 year following the implantation, the average percentage of atrial pacing was 58.2%, 56.0%, and 58.4%, respectively.

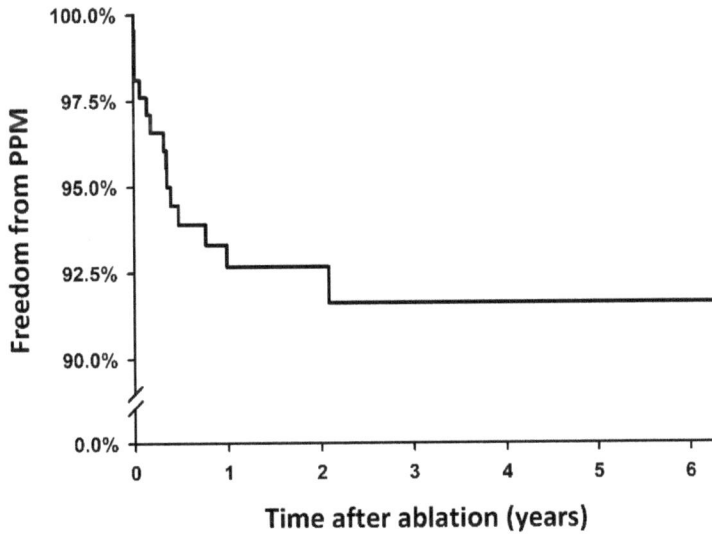

Figure 2. Kaplan–Meier estimates for the PPM implantation after ablation for persistent AFL. After ablation for persistent AFL, the cumulative incidence of delayed SND requiring a PPM implantation increased for several months, almost reaching a plateau after 1 year. AFL: atrial flutter; PPM: permanent pacemaker; SND: sinus node dysfunction.

3.3. Predictors of Sinus Node Dysfunction

The baseline characteristics of patients with and without acute SND requiring a TPM are summarized in Supplementary Table S1, and those with and without delayed SND requiring a PPM are presented in Supplementary Table S2.

Based on the univariable logistic regression analysis, a female gender, a history of hypothyroidism, and an increased LA diameter assessed by transthoracic echocardiography were found to be significant predictors of acute SND requiring a TPM implantation after termination of AFL. The multivariable stepwise models showed that female gender and hypothyroidism were the independent predictors [$p = 0.038$, OR: 3.66, 95% confidence interval (CI): 1.08–12.43; $p = 0.045$, OR: 8.80, 95% CI: 1.05–74.03, respectively] (Table 2).

Table 2. Logistic regression analysis of variables to predict acute SND requiring a TPM after AFL termination ($n = 221$).

Variables	Univariable		Multivariable	
	OR (95% CI)	p Value	OR (95% CI)	p Value
Age	1.02 (0.97–1.06)	0.504		
Female	5.10 (1.64–15.89)	0.005	3.66 (1.08–12.43)	0.038
BMI	0.96 (0.84–1.11)	0.597		
Comorbidities				
CAD	1.05 (0.32–3.49)	0.933		
MR [†]	1.22 (0.37–4.07)	0.742		
Hypertension	1.48 (0.50–4.43)	0.480		
Diabetes mellitus	1.11 (0.33–3.67)	0.870		
HFrEF	1.79 (0.57–5.60)	0.316		
Chronic kidney disease	1.56 (0.33–7.46)	0.579		
TIA/stroke	1.91 (0.22–16.48)	0.555		
Hyperthyroidism	2.49 (0.50–12.30)	0.264		
Hypothyroidism	11.33 (1.73–74.39)	0.011	8.80 (1.05–74.03)	0.045
AFL type				
CCW typical flutter	1.10 (0.30–4.14)	0.883		
CW typical flutter	1.47 (0.18–11.79)	0.718		
Atypical flutter	1.74 (0.56–5.45)	0.338		
Location of flutter circuit(s)				
Right atrium alone	1.24 (0.15–10.02)	0.841		
Left atrium alone	0.85 (0.18–3.96)	0.834		
Both atriums	0.92 (0.11–7.48)	0.936		
Ablation site(s)				
CTI	2.13 (0.44–10.43)	0.349		
PVI	1.39 (0.17–11.19)	0.757		
Biatrial ablation	1.55 (0.19–12.39)	0.682		
Flutter cycle length	1.01 (0.99–1.01)	0.210		
Concomitant AF	1.57 (0.53–4.69)	0.417		

Table 2. Cont.

Variables	Univariable		Multivariable	
	OR (95% CI)	p Value	OR (95% CI)	p Value
Pre-procedural medication				
Beta-blocker	1.75 (0.57–5.40)	0.331		
Non-DHP CCB	1.04 (0.34–3.23)	0.944		
Propafenone	0.98 (0.21–4.62)	0.983		
Amiodarone	1.92 (0.65–5.68)	0.241		
Post-procedural medication				
Beta-blocker	0.33 (0.10–1.07)	0.065		
Non-DHP CCB	1.01 (0.27–3.78)	0.988		
Propafenone	1.21 (0.32–4.56)	0.775		
Amiodarone	0.92 (0.31–2.74)	0.880		
Echocardiography				
LA diameter	1.08 (1.01–1.15)	0.031	1.07 (0.99–1.15)	0.062
LA area	1.02 (0.94–1.11)	0.685		
RA diameter	1.05 (0.99–1.13)	0.123		
RA area	1.07 (0.99–1.16)	0.093		
LVEF	0.99 (0.95–1.04)	0.739		
LVH	0.56 (0.12–2.60)	0.458		
MR [†]	1.06 (0.23–4.97)	0.942		
TR [†]	1.37 (0.36–5.19)	0.641		
Electrocardiography				
Heart rate [‡]	1.01 (0.96–1.07)	0.612		
Long-standing persistent AFL	3.01 (0.91–9.89)	0.070		
QRS duration	1.01 (0.98–1.03)	0.598		

[†] Defined as moderate to severe regurgitation; [‡] Only measured for patients with documented sinus rhythm within one year before ablation (n = 114); AAD: antiarrhythmic drugs; AF: atrial fibrillation; AFL: atrial flutter; BMI: body mass index; CAD, coronary artery disease; CCB: calcium channel blocker; CCW: counterclockwise; CTI: cavotricuspid isthmus; CW: clockwise; DHP: dihydropyridine; HFrEF: heart failure with reduced ejection fraction; LA: left atrium; LVEF: left ventricular ejection fraction; LVH: left ventricular hypertrophy; MR: mitral regurgitation; OR: odds ratio; PVI: pulmonary vein isolation; RA: right atrium; SND: sinus node dysfunction; TIA: transient ischemic stroke; TPM: temporary pacemaker; TR: tricuspid regurgitation.

Moreover, as a result of the univariable Cox proportional hazards regression analysis, older age and a history of hypothyroidism were significant predictors of delayed SND requiring a PPM implantation after AFL termination. In the stepwise multivariable model, both factors were independent predictors ($p = 0.018$, HR: 1.07, 95% CI: 1.01–1.13; $p = 0.006$, HR: 8.87, 95% CI: 1.89–41.72, respectively) (Table 3). Patients with older age and a history of hypothyroidism had higher rates of delayed SND requiring a PPM implantation during the follow-up after AFL ablation (Log-rank test, $p = 0.045$ and <0.001, respectively; Figures 3 and 4).

Table 3. Cox regression analysis of variables to predict delayed SND requiring a PPM after AFL termination (n = 221).

Variables	Univariable		Multivariable	
	HR (95% CI)	p Value	HR (95% CI)	p Value
Age	1.07 (1.01–1.12)	0.016	1.07 (1.01–1.13)	0.018
Female	1.44 (0.42–4.91)	0.564		
BMI	0.97 (0.83–1.12)	0.665		
Comorbidities				
CAD	1.52 (0.45–5.20)	0.503		
MR [†]	1.25 (0.33–4.73)	0.740		
Hypertension	1.94 (0.57–6.61)	0.292		
Diabetes mellitus	0.27 (0.03–2.10)	0.211		
HFrEF	2.89 (0.88–9.47)	0.080		
Hyperthyroidism	1.13 (0.15–8.83)	0.907		
Hypothyroidism	9.48 (2.04–44.09)	0.004	8.87 (1.89–41.72)	0.006
AFL type				
CCW typical flutter	0.41 (0.05–3.23)	0.400		
Atypical flutter	1.68 (0.49–5.73)	0.411		
Location of flutter circuit(s)				
Right atrium alone	1.00 (0.13–7.81)	0.998		
Left atrium alone	1.10 (0.24–5.09)	0.907		
Both atriums	1.18 (0.15–9.25)	0.874		
Ablation site(s)				
CTI	1.11 (0.14–8.69)	0.920		
PVI	1.07 (0.14–8.34)	0.951		
Flutter cycle length	1.00 (0.98–1.01)	0.670		
Concomitant AF	1.37 (0.42–4.49)	0.604		
Pre-procedural medication				
Beta-blocker	0.89 (0.27–2.91)	0.843		
Non-DHP CCB	0.90 (0.26–3.08)	0.868		
Propafenone	0.50 (0.06–3.92)	0.511		
Amiodarone	0.94 (0.28–3.22)	0.926		
Post-procedural medication				
Beta-blocker	0.41 (0.12–1.39)	0.151		
Non-DHP CCB	0.73 (0.16–3.38)	0.687		
Propafenone	1.38 (0.37–5.21)	0.632		
Amiodarone	0.41 (0.11–1.55)	0.190		
Echocardiography				
LA diameter	1.04 (0.96–1.13)	0.358		
LA area	1.05 (0.96–1.16)	0.294		
RA diameter	0.95 (0.87–1.05)	0.320		

Table 3. Cont.

Variables	Univariable		Multivariable	
	HR (95% CI)	p Value	HR (95% CI)	p Value
RA area	1.02 (0.91–1.14)	0.755		
LVEF	0.99 (0.93–1.05)	0.645		
LVH	1.95 (0.57–6.66)	0.287		
MR †	0.66 (0.14–3.12)	0.603		
TR †	2.39 (0.62–9.26)	0.206		
Electrocardiography				
Heart rate ‡	0.96 (0.90–1.03)	0.274		
Sinus bradycardia ‡,§	5.94 (0.99–35.57)	0.051		
Long-standing persistent AFL	1.66 (0.51–5.46)	0.401		
QRS duration	0.99 (0.97–1.02)	0.553		

† Defined as moderate to severe regurgitation; ‡ Only measured for patients with documented sinus rhythm within one year before ablation (n = 114); § Defined as sinus rate < 60 beats per minute within one year before ablation; AAD: antiarrhythmic drugs; AF: atrial fibrillation; AFL: atrial flutter; BMI: body mass index; CAD: coronary artery disease; CCB: calcium channel blocker; CCW: counterclockwise; CTI: cavotricuspid isthmus; DHP: dihydropyridine; HFrEF: heart failure with reduced ejection fraction; HR: hazard ratio; LA: left atrium; LVEF: left ventricular ejection fraction; LVH: left ventricular hypertrophy; MR: mitral regurgitation; PPM: permanent pacemaker; PVI: pulmonary vein isolation; RA: right atrium; SND: sinus node dysfunction; TR: tricuspid regurgitation.

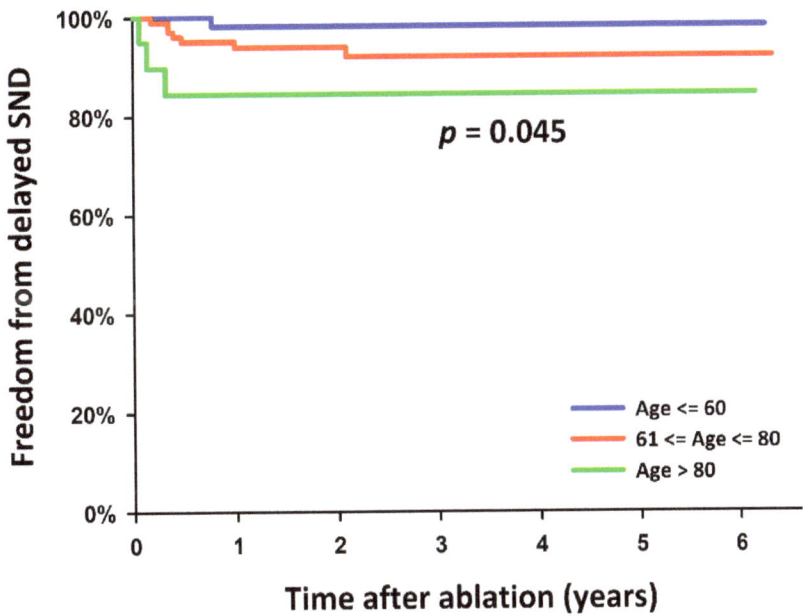

Figure 3. Kaplan–Meier estimates for the delayed SND requiring a PPM after ablation for persistent AFL among patients in the different age groups, with the statistical significance examined using the Log-rank test. AFL: atrial flutter; PPM: permanent pacemaker; SND: sinus node dysfunction.

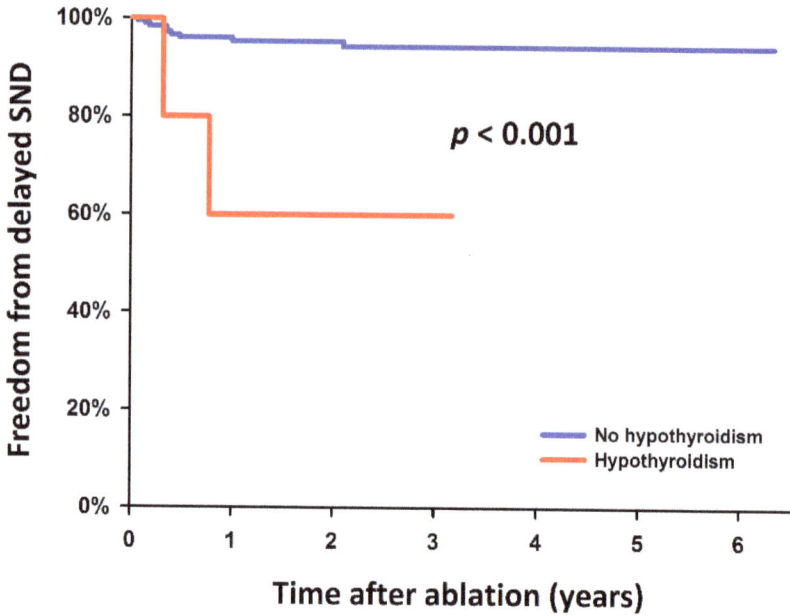

Figure 4. Kaplan–Meier estimates for the delayed SND requiring a PPM after ablation for persistent AFL among patients with and without a history of hypothyroidism, with the statistical significance examined using the Log-rank test. AFL: atrial flutter; PPM: permanent pacemaker; SND: sinus node dysfunction.

4. Discussion

4.1. Major Findings

After successful elimination of the AFL, 14 (6.3%) patients required a TPM for acute SND. It should be noted that although some of them initially recovered from acute SND, 57.1% of patients eventually required a PPM. Irrespective of the absence or recovery of acute SND, 11 (5.0%) patients developed delayed SND requiring a PPM during follow-up, mostly within 1 year after ablation (9 out of 11, 81.8%). The underlying history of hypothyroidism and older age were both predictors of delayed SND.

4.2. The Mechanism of Sinus Node Dysfunction following Atrial Flutter Elimination

SND, historically referred to as sick sinus syndrome, is commonly caused by senescence of the sinoatrial node and surrounding atrial muscle. Most frequently, it is associated with atrial arrhythmias as part of the tachycardia–bradycardia syndrome (TBS) [2,3]. The mechanisms of TBS include alterations in myocardial architecture, ion channel metabolism, and gene expression [5–7]. Over the past decade, catheter ablation has advanced significantly, enabling a high proportion of AF and AFL to be completely eliminated [8–10]. Typically, SND will become apparent after atrial arrhythmias have been eliminated.

The second possible mechanism of SND following CA is an iatrogenic injury to the sinus node. During peri-SVC ablation for AF or AFL, direct damage to the sinus node has been reported, especially along the anterolateral free wall of the SVC [11,12]. Additionally, if the sinoatrial nodal artery is the only artery that supplies the sinus node, an injury to this artery may result in SND [13]. Given the anatomic consideration, occlusion of the sinoatrial nodal artery during LA anterior line ablation of perimetral flutter may result in SND [14,15]. Ozturk et al. found that ablation near the medial or posterior aspects of the LA appendage could also damage the sinoatrial nodal artery [16].

Some other studies, however, provided contradictory results. Deshmukh et al. demonstrated that the risk of SND after ablation is similar to cardioversion in patients with AF, suggesting that causality may be due to a common electrophysiologic substrate as opposed to the ablation process itself [17]. The present study provided evidence in support of these findings by demonstrating that no ablation site for AFL could significantly predict subsequent SND (Tables 2 and 3). In addition, as shown in the supplementary Tables S1 and S2, 5 of 221 patients in our cohort underwent peri-SVC ablation, and none of them developed acute or delayed SND.

4.3. Characteristics of Acute and Delayed Sinus Node Dysfunction

SND has been reported to be reversed after the elimination of atrial tachyarrhythmias. It has been demonstrated in an animal model by Raitt MH et al. that electrical remodeling can be reversed following termination of persistent AF by cardioversion [18]. Several human studies have also demonstrated a reverse remodeling of sinus node function following CA for AF [7,19–21]. In contrast, Inada et al. found that SND progressed even after paroxysmal AF had been eliminated after a 5-year follow-up [22]. The discrepancy between these findings implies that acute SND observed after termination of AFL could recover in some patients, whereas sinus node function may still deteriorate during follow-up in patients without acute SND or after the recovery of the initial SND. Due to the variability and uncertainty of sinus node function following elimination of AFL, it is clinically challenging to determine the appropriate duration for observation and the time point for advancing to PPM implantation.

In the retrospective study by Song et al., 8% of patients developed acute SND after AFL ablation, but half of these cases were transient, and most of them improved within a day [23]. Furthermore, Semmler et al. reported that acute SND developed in 40 (3.2%) patients undergoing AF ablation. There were 37.5% of patients with acute SND of a transient nature, and all of their TPMs were removed within 2 days [24]. Similarly, in our study, 6.3% of patients had acute SND after AFL ablation. TPM was successfully removed in most of these cases within two days, except for one case on the third day and another case on the fifth day after ablation. Accordingly, for the recovery from SND, a reasonable period for observation would be around 1 week.

According to Song et al., the median time for PPM implantation after AFL ablation was 20.5 days (25–75% IQR: 15.25 to 38.25 days), although 1 patient had PPM implantation 1 year and 7 months after CA [23]. In Kim et al.'s study, 121 patients underwent CA for AF with TBS, and 11 patients (9.1%) received PPM within a median period of 21 months after CA [25]. There was a wide variation between the times of ablation and the times for PPM implantation. Moreover, we observed in the present study that most PPMs for delayed SND were implanted several months after AFL ablation and gradually plateaued after 1 year. It is a reasonable and safe policy to closely monitor for delayed SND for at least one year after AFL ablation, especially in patients with a high risk of SND.

Skjøth F et al. found that PPM was implanted more frequently following AFL ablation than AF ablation in a nationwide cohort study [26]. As indicated above, this finding appears to be consistent with a comparison of the present study with those mentioned. Furthermore, patients with AFL tend to experience a shorter interval between catheter ablation and PPM implantation than those with AF. Possible explanations for the above findings may be related to the different remodeling of the heart. Medi C et al. reported that right atrial remodeling was more advanced in patients with AFL as compared with patients with AF [27]. It may lead to a higher degree of SND and the early requirement of PPM after AFL ablation.

4.4. Predictors of Sinus Node Dysfunction following Atrial Flutter Termination

In previous studies, several risk factors or predictors of SND after termination of AF have been reported, including older age, a female gender, a low preprocedural ventricular rate, and a large left atrium [24,28–32]. The present study found that age, female gender, and the underlying history of hypothyroidism were predictive of SND after AFL ablation. SND is associated with senescence of the sinoatrial node and surrounding atrial myocardium, and this phenomenon is frequently accompanied by the process of aging. As demonstrated both in the present study as well as in previous studies, older age can serve as a predictor for SND following termination of atrial tachyarrhythmias [17,24,28]. Moreover, Sairaku et al. reported that female gender was an independent predictor of SND requiring a PPM in cases of persistent typical flutter [33], and higher rates of SND and PPM implantation have also been reported after AF ablation in female patients [17,28], which was consistent with our findings.

Thyroid hormones are both inotropic and chronotropic by multiple mechanisms, including the regulation of the sympathetic nervous system and ion channels [34]. For the comprehensive investigation of the relationship between thyroid hormone deficiency and SND, we checked the medical history and laboratory data of the 5 patients with hypothyroidism in our cohort. All these 5 patients had been under thyroxine supplements, but 2 of them developed delayed SND after recovery from acute SND (Supplementary Tables S1 and S2). The thyroid function test showed euthyroid in 1 case but still hypothyroid in the other during the peri- and post-ablation period before PPM implantation. Thyroxine deficiency might not be the only contributor to the SND in hypothyroidism, and it requires further studies to determine the reversibility of cardiac remodeling and sinus node function after thyroxine supplementation. Despite the identified risk factors, given the small number of patients with SND following AFL termination, future validation is necessary.

4.5. Strengths and Limitations

This is, to the best of our knowledge, the first analysis of the predictors, characteristics, and prognosis of acute and delayed SND following ablation for persistent AFL, including typical and atypical forms, as well as the clinical application of TPM and PPM.

Nevertheless, there are some limitations to this study. The retrospective design of this study results in some inevitable biases. Additionally, we excluded patients with severe atrioventricular nodal dysfunction, which might have confounded the primary endpoint of SND. Furthermore, the cause of SND may be multifactorial, and it is difficult to clearly clarify the etiology in most of our patients. A previous study used computed tomography to assess the post-ablation sinus nodal artery injury [13], but we did not perform it routinely for our cohort. Thus, it is difficult to evaluate the confounding effect of the causes of SND on the outcomes. Finally, the sample size was small, and the follow-up period was short. Further large-scale studies are needed to determine the long-term incidence and prognosis of SND. We, however, believe that the current findings can not only optimize the pre-procedural risk stratification but also serve as guidance for short-term and long-term management for patients with SND following ablation.

5. Conclusions

The TPM was required for acute SND in 6.3% of patients after the elimination of the AFL. Despite initially recovering from acute SND, 57.1% of patients with acute SND eventually required a PPM. It should also be noted that irrespective of the absence or recovery of acute SND, 5.0% of patients developed delayed SND requiring a PPM during follow-up, mostly within 1 year after ablation. An observation period of at least one year after AFL ablation is reasonable.

Supplementary Materials: The following supporting information can be downloaded at: https://www.mdpi.com/article/10.3390/jcm11113212/s1, Table S1: Comparison of baseline characteristics between patients with and without acute SND requiring a TPM after AFL termination; Table S2: Comparison of baseline characteristics of patients with and without delayed SND requiring a PPM after AFL termination.

Author Contributions: Conceptualization, F.-P.C. and T.-F.C.; methodology, S.-L.C.; software, Y.-F.H. and C.-M.L.; validation, S.-H.L., Y.-J.L. and W.-H.C.; formal analysis, G.-Y.L.; investigation, T.-C.T.; resources, J.-N.L.; data curation, T.-Y.C.; writing—original draft preparation, G.-Y.L.; writing—review and editing, L.K.; visualization, C.-I.W.; supervision, L.-W.L.; project administration, S.-A.C.; funding acquisition, F.-P.C. All authors have read and agreed to the published version of the manuscript.

Funding: This work was supported by the Ministry of Science and Technology (grant numbers MOST 109-2314-B-075-075-MY3, MOST 109-2314-B-010-058-MY2, MOST 109-2314-B-075-074-MY3, MOST 109-2314-B-075-076-MY3, MOST 107-2314-B-010-061-MY2, MOST 106-2314-B-075-006-MY3, MOST 106-2314-B-010-046-MY3, and MOST 106-2314-B-075-073-MY3), Research Foundation of Cardiovascular Medicine, Szu-Yuan Research Foundation of Internal Medicine, and Taipei Veterans General Hospital (grant numbers V106C-158, V106C-104, V107C-060, V107C-054, V109C-113, V110C-116, and V111C-159).

Institutional Review Board Statement: The study was conducted in accordance with the Declaration of Helsinki, and approved by the Institutional Review Board of Taipei Veterans General Hospital (2021-09-007CC, 18 September 2021).

Informed Consent Statement: Informed consent was obtained from all subjects involved in the study.

Data Availability Statement: The data presented in this study are not publicly available due to upcoming publications but are available on request from the corresponding author.

Conflicts of Interest: The authors declare no conflict of interest.

References

1. Hindricks, G.; Potpara, T.; Dagres, N.; Arbelo, E.; Bax, J.J.; Blomström-Lundqvist, C.; Boriani, G.; Castella, M.; Dan, G.-A.; Dilaveris, P.E.; et al. 2020 ESC Guidelines for the diagnosis and management of atrial fibrillation developed in collaboration with the European Association for Cardio-Thoracic Surgery (EACTS): The Task Force for the diagnosis and management of atrial fibrillation of the European Society of Cardiology (ESC) Developed with the special contribution of the European Heart Rhythm Association (EHRA) of the ESC. *Eur. Heart J.* **2021**, *42*, 373–498. [PubMed]
2. Short, D.S. The syndrome of alternating bradycardia and tachycardia. *Br. Heart J.* **1954**, *16*, 208–214. [CrossRef] [PubMed]
3. Rubenstein, J.J.; Schulman, C.L.; Yurchak, P.M.; DeSanctis, R.W. Clinical spectrum of the sick sinus syndrome. *Circulation* **1972**, *46*, 5–13. [CrossRef] [PubMed]
4. Tai, C.T.; Chen, S.A. Electrophysiological mechanisms of atrial flutter. *Indian Pacing Electrophysiol. J.* **2006**, *6*, 119–132. [CrossRef]
5. Yeh, Y.H.; Burstein, B.; Qi, X.Y.; Sakabe, M.; Chartier, D.; Comtois, P.; Wang, Z.; Kuo, C.T.; Nattel, S. Funny current downregulation and sinus node dysfunction associated with atrial tachyarrhythmia: A molecular basis for tachycardia-bradycardia syndrome. *Circulation* **2009**, *119*, 1576–1585. [CrossRef]
6. Sanders, P.; Morton, J.B.; Kistler, P.M.; Davidson, N.C.; Hussin, A.; Spence, S.J.; Lindsay, C.B.; Vohra, J.K.; Sparks, P.B.; Kalman, J.M. Electrophysiological and electroanatomic characterization of the atria in sinus node disease: Evidence of diffuse atrial remodeling. *Circulation* **2004**, *109*, 1514–1522. [CrossRef]
7. Jackson, L.R., 2nd; Rathakrishnan, B.; Campbell, K.; Thomas, K.L.; Piccini, J.P.; Bahnson, T.; Stiber, J.A.; Daubert, J.P. Sinus Node Dysfunction and Atrial Fibrillation: A Reversible Phenomenon? *Pacing Clin. Electrophysiol.* **2017**, *40*, 442–450. [CrossRef]
8. O'Neill, L.; Wielandts, J.-Y.; Gillis, K.; Hilfiker, G.; Waroux, J.-B.L.P.D.; Tavernier, R.; Duytschaever, M.; Knecht, S. Catheter Ablation in Persistent AF, the Evolution towards a More Pragmatic Strategy. *J. Clin. Med.* **2021**, *10*, 4060. [CrossRef]
9. McCarthy, P.M.; Cox, J.L.; Kislitsina, O.N.; Kruse, J.; Churyla, A.; Malaisrie, S.C.; Mehta, C.K. Surgery and Catheter Ablation for Atrial Fibrillation: History, Current Practice, and Future Directions. *J. Clin. Med.* **2021**, *11*, 210. [CrossRef]
10. Kaba, R.A.; Momin, A.; Camm, J. Persistent Atrial Fibrillation: The Role of Left Atrial Posterior Wall Isolation and Ablation Strategies. *J. Clin. Med.* **2021**, *10*, 3129. [CrossRef]
11. Chen, G.; Dong, J.Z.; Liu, X.P.; Zhang, X.Y.; Long, D.Y.; Sang, C.H.; Ning, M.; Tang, R.B.; Jiang, C.X.; Ma, C.S. Sinus node injury as a result of superior vena cava isolation during catheter ablation for atrial fibrillation and atrial flutter. *Pacing Clin. Electrophysiol.* **2011**, *34*, 163–170. [CrossRef]
12. Killu, A.M.; Fender, E.A.; Deshmukh, A.J.; Munger, T.M.; Araoz, P.; Brady, P.A.; Packer, U.L.; Friedman, P.A.; Mulpuru, S.K.; Cha, Y.-M.; et al. Acute Sinus Node Dysfunction after Atrial Ablation: Incidence, Risk Factors, and Management. *Pacing Clin. Electrophysiol.* **2016**, *39*, 1116–1125. [CrossRef] [PubMed]
13. Barra, S.; Gopalan, D.; Baran, J.; Fynn, S.; Heck, P.; Agarwal, S. Acute and sub-acute sinus node dysfunction following pulmonary vein isolation: A case series. *Eur. Heart J. Case Rep.* **2018**, *2*, ytx020. [CrossRef] [PubMed]
14. Yokokawa, M.; Sundaram, B.; Oral, H.; Morady, F.; Chugh, A. The course of the sinus node artery and its impact on achieving linear block at the left atrial roof in patients with persistent atrial fibrillation. *Heart Rhythm* **2012**, *9*, 1395–1402. [CrossRef] [PubMed]

15. Miyazaki, Y.; Ueda, N.; Otsuka, F.; Miyamoto, K.; Noguchi, T.; Kusano, K. Rescue percutaneous coronary intervention for sinus node dysfunction following left atrial flutter ablation. *Heart Rhythm Case Rep.* **2021**, *7*, 529–532. [CrossRef] [PubMed]
16. Ozturk, E.; Saglam, M.; Bozlar, U.; Sivrioglu, A.K.; Karaman, B.; Onat, L.; Basekim, C.C. Arterial supply of the sinoatrial node: A CT coronary angiographic study. *Int. J. Cardiovasc. Imaging* **2011**, *27*, 619–627. [CrossRef]
17. Deshmukh, A.J.; Yao, X.; Schilz, S.; Van Houten, H.; Sangaralingham, L.R.; Asirvatham, S.J.; Friedman, P.A.; Packer, U.L.; Noseworthy, P.A. Pacemaker implantation after catheter ablation for atrial fibrillation. *J. Interv. Card. Electrophysiol.* **2016**, *45*, 99–105. [CrossRef]
18. Raitt, M.H.; Kusumoto, W.; Giraud, G.; McAnulty, J.H. Reversal of electrical remodeling after cardioversion of persistent atrial fibrillation. *J. Cardiovasc. Electrophysiol.* **2004**, *15*, 507–512. [CrossRef]
19. Hocini, M.; Sanders, P.; Deisenhofer, I.; Jais, P.; Hsu, L.-F.; Scavée, C.; Weerasoriya, R.; Raybaud, F.; Macle, L.; Shah, D.C.; et al. Reverse remodeling of sinus node function after catheter ablation of atrial fibrillation in patients with prolonged sinus pauses. *Circulation* **2003**, *108*, 1172–1175. [CrossRef]
20. Chen, Y.W.; Bai, R.; Lin, T.; Salim, M.; Sang, C.H.; Long, D.Y.; Yu, R.H.; Tang, R.B.; Guo, X.Y.; Yan, X.L.; et al. Pacing or ablation: Which is better for paroxysmal atrial fibrillation-related tachycardia-bradycardia syndrome? *Pacing Clin. Electrophysiol.* **2014**, *37*, 403–411. [CrossRef]
21. Khaykin, Y.; Marrouche, N.F.; Martin, D.O.; Saliba, W.; Schweikert, R.; Wexman, M.; Strunk, B.; Beheiry, S.; Saad, E.; Bhargava, M.; et al. Pulmonary vein isolation for atrial fibrillation in patients with symptomatic sinus bradycardia or pauses. *J. Cardiovasc. Electrophysiol.* **2004**, *15*, 784–789. [CrossRef] [PubMed]
22. Inada, K.; Yamane, T.; Tokutake, K.-I.; Yokoyama, K.-I.; Mishima, T.; Hioki, M.; Narui, R.; Ito, K.; Tanigawa, S.-I.; Yamashita, S.; et al. The role of successful catheter ablation in patients with paroxysmal atrial fibrillation and prolonged sinus pauses: Outcome during a 5-year follow-up. *Europace* **2014**, *16*, 208–213. [CrossRef] [PubMed]
23. Song, C.; Jin, M.-N.; Lee, J.-H.; Kim, I.-S.; Uhm, J.-S.; Pak, H.-N.; Lee, M.-H.; Joung, B. Predictors of sick sinus syndrome in patients after successful radiofrequency catheter ablation of atrial flutter. *Yonsei Med. J.* **2015**, *56*, 31–37. [CrossRef] [PubMed]
24. Semmler, V.; von Krogh, F.; Haller, B.; Reents, T.; Bourier, F.; Telishevska, M.; Kottmaier, M.; Kornmayer, M.; Brooks, S.; Koch-Büttner, K.; et al. The incidence, indications and predictors of acute pacemaker implantation after ablation of persistent atrial fibrillation. *Clin. Res. Cardiol.* **2019**, *108*, 651–659. [CrossRef]
25. Kim, D.-H.; Choi, J.-I.; Lee, K.N.; Ahn, J.; Roh, S.Y.; Lee, D.I.; Shim, J.; Kim, J.S.; Lim, H.E.; Park, S.W.; et al. Long-term clinical outcomes of catheter ablation in patients with atrial fibrillation predisposing to tachycardia-bradycardia syndrome: A long pause predicts implantation of a permanent pacemaker. *BMC Cardiovasc. Disord.* **2018**, *18*, 106. [CrossRef]
26. Skjøth, F.; Vadmann, H.; Hjortshøj, S.P.; Riahi, S.; Lip, G.Y.H.; Larsen, T.B. Disease progression after ablation for atrial flutter compared with atrial fibrillation: A nationwide cohort study. *Int. J. Clin. Pract.* **2018**, *72*, e13258. [CrossRef]
27. Medi, C.; Teh, A.W.; Roberts-Thomson, K.; Morton, J.B.; Kistler, P.; Kalman, J.M. Right atrial remodeling is more advanced in patients with atrial flutter than with atrial fibrillation. *J. Cardiovasc. Electrophysiol.* **2012**, *23*, 1067–1072. [CrossRef]
28. Kawaji, T.; Shizuta, S.; Yamagami, S.; Aizawa, T.; Yoshizawa, T.; Kato, M.; Yokomatsu, T.; Miki, S.; Ono, K.; Kimura, T. Impact of Pre-Existing Bradycardia on Subsequent Need for Pacemaker Implantation After Radiofrequency Catheter Ablation for Atrial Fibrillation. *Circ. J.* **2018**, *82*, 2493–2499. [CrossRef]
29. Hada, M.; Miyazaki, S.; Kajiyama, T.; Yamaguchi, M.; Kusa, S.; Nakamura, H.; Hachiya, H.; Tada, H.; Hirao, K.; Iesaka, Y. Catheter ablation of paroxysmal atrial fibrillation in patients with sick sinus syndrome. *Heart Vessels* **2019**, *34*, 503–508. [CrossRef]
30. Sunaga, A.; Masuda, M.; Kanda, T.; Fujita, M.; Iida, O.; Okamoto, S.; Ishihara, T.; Matsuda, Y.; Watanabe, T.; Sakata, Y.; et al. A low fibrillatory wave amplitude predicts sinus node dysfunction after catheter ablation in patients with persistent atrial fibrillation. *J. Interv. Card Electrophysiol.* **2015**, *43*, 253–261. [CrossRef]
31. Kim, D.; Shim, C.Y.; Hong, G.-R.; Cho, I.J.; Lee, S.H.; Chang, H.-J.; Lee, S.; Ha, J.-W.; Chang, B.-C. Sinus node dysfunction after surgical atrial fibrillation ablation with concomitant mitral valve surgery: Determinants and clinical outcomes. *PLoS ONE* **2018**, *13*, e0203828. [CrossRef] [PubMed]
32. Masuda, M.; Inoue, K.; Iwakura, K.; Okamura, A.; Koyama, Y.; Kimura, R.; Toyoshima, Y.; Doi, A.; Sotomi, Y.; Komuro, I.; et al. Preprocedural ventricular rate predicts subsequent sick sinus syndrome after ablation for long-standing persistent atrial fibrillation. *Pacing Clin. Electrophysiol.* **2012**, *35*, 1074–1080. [CrossRef] [PubMed]
33. Sairaku, A.; Nakano, Y.; Oda, N.; Makita, Y.; Kajihara, K.; Tokuyama, T.; Motoda, C.; Fujiwara, M.; Kihara, Y. Prediction of sinus node dysfunction in patients with persistent atrial flutter using the flutter cycle length. *Europace* **2012**, *14*, 380–387. [CrossRef] [PubMed]
34. Vargas, U.H.; Bonelo, P.A.; Sierra, T. Effects of thyroid hormones on the heart. *Clin. Investig. Arterioscler.* **2014**, *26*, 296–309.

Article

Fifteen-Year Differences in Indications for Cardiac Resynchronization Therapy in International Guidelines—Insights from the Heart Failure Registries of the European Society of Cardiology

Agata Tymińska [1], Krzysztof Ozierański [1,*], Emil Brociek [1], Agnieszka Kapłon-Cieślicka [1], Paweł Balsam [1], Michał Marchel [1], Maria G. Crespo-Leiro [2], Aldo P. Maggioni [3,4], Jarosław Drożdż [5], Grzegorz Opolski [1] and Marcin Grabowski [1]

1. First Department of Cardiology, Medical University of Warsaw, 02-091 Warsaw, Poland; agata.tyminska@wum.edu.pl (A.T.); emil.brociek@gmail.com (E.B.); agnieszka.kaplon@gmail.com (A.K.-C.); pawel.balsam@wum.edu.pl (P.B.); michal.marchel@wum.edu.pl (M.M.); grzegorz.opolski@wum.edu.pl (G.O.); marcin.grabowski@wum.edu.pl (M.G.)
2. Unidad de Insuficiencia Cardiaca Avanzada y Trasplante Cardiaco, Hospital Universitario A Coruna, CIBERCV, 15006 La Coruna, Spain; marisacrespo@gmail.com
3. ANMCO Research Centre, 50121 Florence, Italy; maggioni@anmco.it
4. EURObservational Research Programme, European Society of Cardiology, Sophia-Antipolis, 06903 Valbonne, France
5. 2nd Department of Cardiology, Central University Hospital, Medical University of Lodz, 92-213 Lodz, Poland; jaroslaw.drozdz@umed.pl
* Correspondence: krzysztof.ozieranski@wum.edu.pl; Tel.: +48-22-5992958; Fax: +48-22-5991957

Abstract: Cardiac resynchronization therapy (CRT) applied to selected patients with heart failure (HF) improves their prognosis. In recent years, eligibility criteria for CRT have regularly changed. This study aimed to investigate the changes in eligibility of real-life HF patients for CRT over the past fifteen years. We reviewed European and North American guidelines from this period and applied them to HF patients from the ESC-HF Pilot and ESC-Long-Term Registries. Taking into consideration the criteria assessed in this study (including all classes of recommendations i.e., class I, IIa and IIb, as well as patients with AF and SR), the 2013 (ESC) guidelines would have qualified the most patients for CRT (266, 18.3%), while the 2015 (ESC) guidelines would have qualified the least (115, 7.9%; p-value for differences between all analyzed papers <0.0001). There were only 26 patients (1.8%) who would be eligible for CRT using the class I recommendations across all of the guidelines. These results demonstrate the variability in recommendations for CRT over the years. Moreover, this data indicates underuse of this form of pacing in HF and highlights the need for more studies in order to improve the outcomes of HF patients and further personalize their management.

Keywords: cardiac resynchronization therapy; heart failure; cardiomyopathy; left bundle branch block

1. Introduction

The incidence and morbidity of heart failure (HF) is increasing, with a high prevalence in developed countries, where it affects approximately 1–2% of adults, rising to ≥10% in those aged 70 years or over. Prognosis of HF patients remains poor, as the 5-year mortality rate after diagnosis is approximately 50% [1,2]. Although there are well established therapies for HF with reduced ejection fraction (HFrEF) further research is necessary to improve the symptoms and outcomes of patients with HF.

CRT (cardiac resynchronization therapy) is a method of treating advanced chronic HF, aiming to improve synchrony of both ventricles [1,3]. In patients who respond to the therapy ("responders"), CRT is an effective treatment for reducing HF morbidity and mortality, as well as improving patients' quality of life. However, the selection criteria for

CRT are still imperfect, and it should be noted that it is not certain that all HF patients benefit from this form of cardiac pacing.

In patients with primarily chronic HF (i.e., excluding patients with primarily high degree atrioventricular block, as this indicates that the patient will need permanent ventricular pacing), the indications for CRT have been changing in line with the publication of new international guidelines i.e., of the European Society of Cardiology (ESC) and American associations (ACC—American College of Cardiology; AHA—American Heart Association; HFSA—Heart Failure Society of America; HRS—Heart Rhythm Society). Over the years, the decisions on CRT implantation were made using, among others, numerous of the following criteria: the presence of a left bundle branch block (LBBB); left ventricular ejection fraction (LVEF); different QRS durations; different levels of severity of symptoms of HF according to the New York Heart Association (NYHA) class; left ventricular dimensions; the presence of atrial fibrillation (AF) or sinus rhythm (SR); indications for permanent conventional pacing; the presence of optimal medical therapy for HF [1,3–11]. Furthermore, successive guidelines that are published shortly after the previous ones often substantially change the profile of a patient who is eligible for CRT. Therefore, the current focus of HF therapy is shifting towards better characterization of the underlying etiology of HF and personalized management.

This study aimed to investigate the changes in eligibility for CRT of real-life patients with HF from the ESC-HF registries according to the differences in international guidelines published in the last fifteen-years, with a particular focus on the newest ESC (2021) and ACC/AHA/HFSA (2022) recommendations.

2. Patients and Methods

2.1. Study Design

The data was collected from the multi-center, prospective, observational ESC-HF Pilot and the ESC-HF Long-Term registries of the European Society of Cardiology (ESC). These registries lasted from 2009 to 2010 in 136 European cardiology centers (including 29 centers from Poland) and from 2011 to 2015 in 211 European cardiology centers (including 35 centers from Poland), respectively. The studies enrolled outpatients and inpatients with chronic, worsening or new-onset HF who were at least 18 years of age and met the diagnostic criteria for HF. There were no other specific exclusion criteria. All participating patients signed informed consent. Records collected in both registries referred to clinical characteristics, laboratory tests' results, HF management and one-year follow-up. A detailed study design was published previously [12,13]. The study protocol was approved by the local ethics committees.

The ESC-HF Pilot and the ESC-HF Long-Term registries enrolled 5118 and 12,440 patients across Europe, respectively. The current analysis consisted of 1456 (out of 2019 patients enrolled in Polish centers) both ambulatory and hospitalized, clinically stable HF patients. Only patients with available data on CRT eligibility criteria were included. Patients with a paced rhythm on ECG were excluded from the analysis. Criteria for CRT implantation in the major international (ESC and America's) guidelines from 2007 to 2022 that were considered for this study are listed in the Supplementary Table S1. The CRT eligibility criteria were assessed in the studied group. Common classification of recommendations presented in the guidelines were used: class I (indicated/recommended); class IIa (should be considered); class IIb (may be considered); class III (contraindicated/not recommended). The following parameters were considered in the aforementioned guidelines and analyzed in this study: LVEF, presence of LBBB, QRS duration, SR or AF, the NYHA class, and HF etiology (ischemic). Patients with SR or AF were analyzed separately according to the general indications for CRT. Patients' clinical status, comorbidities, expected lifetime duration and actual time of HF optimal pharmacotherapy were not considered in the analysis.

Data on patients who presented with indications for pacing, atrioventricular node (AVN) ablation or pacemaker/implantable cardioverter defibrillator (ICD) upgrade to

CRT was not available in the database and, therefore, was not considered in the analysis. Indications for CRT-pacemaker (CRT-P) or CRT-defibrillator (CRT-D) were also not the target of the analysis.

2.2. Statistical Analysis

The results were presented as median and quartiles for continuous variables, and as frequencies and percentages for ordinal variables and non-normally distributed continuous variables. The frequencies of the categorical variables were compared by Fisher's exact test. A *p*-value below 0.05 was considered significant for all tests. All tests were two-tailed. Statistical analyses were performed using SPSS software, version 22 (IBM SPSS Statistics 22, IBM, New York, NY, USA).

3. Results

3.1. Clinical Characteristics

Baseline characteristics of the studied group are presented in Table 1. Briefly, median age was 67 (58–76) years and 67% of the patients were males. Median LVEF was 37% (25–50). LVEF $\leq 35\%$ was observed in most patients (55%). Ischemic etiology of HF was present in 54%. Numerous comorbidities were highly prevalent (i.e., coronary artery disease, hypertension, peripheral artery disease, diabetes, chronic kidney disease, chronic obstructive pulmonary disease, previous stroke, or transient ischemic attack). Use of HF guideline-recommended medications was on a satisfactory level.

Table 1. Baseline characteristics of the study group.

Variable	HF Patients n = 1456
Baseline characteristics	
Age, years	66.5 (58.0–76.4)
Male	981 (67.4%)
BMI, kg/m^2	27.8 (25.0–31.4); n = 1404
LVEF, %	37 (25–50)
LBBB QRS morphology	199 (13.7%)
QRS, ms	103 (90–120)
HFrEF	798 (54.8%)
HFmrEF	288 (19.8%)
HFpEF	370 (25.4%)
Previous HF hospitalization	781 (53.9%); n = 1450
Coronary artery disease	788 (54.2%); n = 1455
Moderate or severe mitral regurgitation	623 (45.9%); n = 1358
Hypertension	935 (64.3%); n = 1453
AF	442 (30.4%)
Peripheral artery disease	170 (11.7%); n = 1455
Diabetes	470 (32.3%)
Chronic kidney disease	260 (17.9%); n = 1454
COPD	236 (16.2%); n = 1454
Prior stroke or TIA	160 (11.0%); n = 1454
Current or former smoking	835 (58.0%); n = 1440

Table 1. Cont.

Variable	HF Patients n = 1456
Clinical status	
Heart rate, bpm	70 (65–80); n = 1054
NYHA class	2 (2–3)
NYHA class I	138 (9.5%)
NYHA class II	894 (61.4%)
NYHA class III	400 (27.5%)
NYHA ambulatory class IV	24 (1.6%)
Pharmacotherapy	
ACE-I	1120 (77.0%); n = 1455
ARB	162 (11.1%); n = 1454
β-blocker	1317 (90.5%); n = 1455
Diuretic	1211 (83.2%); n = 1455
MRA	967 (66.5%); n = 1454
Statins	960 (66.0%); n = 1455
Oral Anticoagulant	606 (41.7%); n = 1454
Antiplatelets	902 (62.0%); n = 1455
Digitalis	336 (23.1%); n = 1455
Amiodarone	127 (8.7%); n = 1455
Other Antiarrhythmic	81 (5.6%); n = 1455
CCB	214 (14.7%); n = 1455

ACE-I—angiotensin-converting enzyme inhibitor; AF—atrial fibrillation; ARB—angiotensin receptor blocker; BMI—body mass index; bpm—beats per minute; CCB—calcium channel blocker; COPD—chronic obstructive pulmonary disease; LVEF—left ventricular ejection fraction; MRA—mineralocorticoid receptor antagonist; NYHA—New York Heart Association; HFmrEF—heart failure with mid-range ejection fraction; HFrEF—heart failure with reduced ejection fraction; HFpEF—heart failure with preserved ejection fraction; TIA—transient ischemic attack. Continuous variables are presented as medians and interquartile ranges.

3.2. Patients Eligible for CRT Implantation

In the study group 1014 (69.6%) patients had SR and 442 (30.4%) patients had AF. When considering patients with SR, the smallest number of patients with class I indications for CRT was 45 (4.4%) following the 2012/2013 (ACC/AHA/HRS), 2021 (ESC) and 2022 (ACC/AHA/HFSA) guidelines, while the biggest number of patients with class I indications for CRT was 137 (13.5%) following the 2010 (ESC) guidelines (p-value for differences between all groups < 0.0001). Class IIa indications were present in 17 (1.7%) and 97 patients (9.6%) based on the 2015 (ESC) and 2022 (ACC/AHA/HFSA) guidelines (p-value for differences between all groups < 0.0001), respectively. Class IIb indications were present in 28 (2.8%) and 80 patients (7.9%) using the 2015 (ESC) and 2022 (ACC/AHA/HFSA) guidelines, when compared to the 2013 (ESC) guidelines (p-value for differences between all groups < 0.0001).

Within the AF cohort, indications for CRT implantation ranged from 17 patients (3.8%) using the 2015 (ESC) and 2016 (ESC) guidelines, to 86 patients (19.5%) based on 2022 (ACC/AHA/HFSA) guidelines (p-value for differences between all groups < 0.0001).

Taking into consideration the criteria assessed in this study (including all classes of recommendations and patients with AF and SR), the highest number of patients that would have qualified for CRT was 266 (18.3%) by using the 2013 (ESC) guidelines, while the fewest was 115 (7.9%) when considering the 2015 (ESC) guidelines (p-value for differences between all groups < 0.0001). There were only 26 patients (1.8%) who would be eligible for CRT using the class I recommendations across all of the guidelines (the common criteria in these patients were: SR, LVEF ≤ 35%, LBBB, QRS ≥ 150 ms, NYHA class III or ambulatory class IV). The results are presented in Table 2.

Table 2. The changes in eligibility for CRT of real-life patients with heart failure according to differences in the last fifteen-years international guidelines.

Class *	Guidelines Listed by Year of Publication								p-Value
	2022 (ACC/ AHA/ HFSA)	2021 (ESC)	2016 (ESC)	2015 (ESC)	2013 (ESC)	2012/2013 (ACC/ AHA/ HRS)	2010 (ESC)	2007 (ESC)	
	Patients with SR (n = 1014)								
I	45 (4.4%)	45 (4.4%)	83 (8.2%)	53 (5.2%)	104 (10.3%)	45 (4.4%)	137 (13.5%)	98 (9.6%)	<0.001
IIa	97 (9.6%)	76 (7.5%)	38 (3.7%)	17 (1.7%)	35 (3.5%)	77 (7.6%)	-	-	<0.001
IIb	28 (2.8%)	33 (3.3%)	33 (3.3%)	28 (2.8%)	80 (7.9%)	48 (4.7%)	-	-	<0.001
	Patients with AF (n = 442)								
IIa	86 (19.5%)	31 (7.0%)	17 (3.8%)	17 (3.8%)	47 (10.6%)	54 (12.2%)	31 (7.0%)	47 (10.6%)	<0.001
	Total (n = 1456)								
	256 (17.6%)	185 (12.7%)	171 (11.7%)	115 (7.9%)	266 (18.3%)	224 (15.4%)	168 (11.5%)	145 (10.0%)	<0.001

ACC—American College of Cardiology; AHA—American Heart Association; AF—atrial fibrillation; ESC—European Society of Cardiology; HFSA—Heart Failure Society of America; HRS—Heart Rhythm Society; SR—sinus rhythm. * Class of recommendation: class I (indicated/recommended); class IIa (should be considered); class IIb (may be considered); class III (contraindicated/not recommended).

The differences in patients' eligibility for CRT according to the recent (ACC/AHA/HFSA (2022) and ESC (2021)) guidelines are presented in Tables 3 and 4. Among the 1456 patients in the study group, 256 (17.6%) and 185 (12.7%) patients were eligible for CRT based on the ACC/AHA/HFSA (2022) and ESC (2021) guidelines ($p < 0.001$), respectively (Table 2). The largest difference in eligibility between these guidelines were observed within patients with AF—86 (19.5%) and 31 (7.0%) would have qualified for CRT according to the ACC/AHA/HFSA (2022) and ESC (2021) guidelines ($p < 0.001$), respectively. Whereas, in terms of class I indication for CRT, 45 (4.4%) patients with SR were eligible for CRT according to both guidelines.

Table 3. Patients with heart failure and sinus rhythm eligible for CRT based on the recent ACC/AHA/HFSA (2022) and ESC (2021) guidelines.

Guidelines	SR OMT Ischemic Etiology	SR OMT LVEF ≤ 35%			
		LBBB			
	QRS ≥ 150 ms		QRS 130–149 ms		120–129 ms
	NYHA class I	NYHA class II–IV	NYHA class II	NYHA class III–IV	NYHA class II–IV
ACC/AHA/HFSA 2022	1 (0.1%)	45 (4.4%)	20 (2.0%)	18 (1.8%)	21 (2.1%)
ESC 2021	-	45 (4.4%)	20 (2.0%)	18 (1.8%)	-
	Non-LBBB				
	QRS ≥ 150 ms		QRS 130–149 ms		120–129 ms
		NYHA class II–IV	NYHA class II	NYHA class III–IV	NYHA class III–IV
ACC/AHA/HFSA 2022	-	38 (3.7%)	-	15 (1.5%)	12 (1.2%)
ESC 2021	-	38 (3.7%)	18 (1.8%)	15 (1.5%)	-

The meaning of colors: Green = class I of recommendation (indicated/recommended); Yellow = class IIa of recommendation (should be considered); Orange = class IIb of recommendation (may be considered); Red = class III of recommendation (contraindicated/not recommended); AHA—American Heart Association; ESC—European Society of Cardiology; HFSA—Heart Failure Society of America; LBBB—left bundle branch block; LVEF—left ventricular ejection fraction; NYHA—New York Heart Association; OMT—optimal medical treatment; SR—sinus rhythm.

Table 4. Patients with heart failure and atrial fibrillation eligible for CRT based on the recent ACC/AHA/HFSA (2022) and ESC (2021) guidelines.

Guidelines	ACC/AHA/HFSA 2022	ESC 2021
Eligibility criteria	AF Strategy to ensure biventricular capture LVEF ≤ 35%	
	QRS ≥ 120 ms	QRS ≥ 130 ms
	NYHA class II–IV	NYHA class III–IV
Number of patients	86 (19.5%)	31 (7.0%)

The meaning of color: Yellow = class IIa of recommendation (should be considered); AF—atrial fibrillation; AHA—American Heart Association; ESC—European Society of Cardiology; HFSA—Heart Failure Society of America; LVEF—left ventricular ejection fraction; NYHA—New York Heart Association.

4. Discussion

This study assessed the applicability of eligibility criteria of real-life patients with HF by comparing the international guidelines for CRT, with special focus on the latest 2021 ESC and 2022 AHA/ACC/HFSA papers [1,3,7]. The criteria described in the guidelines are mostly derived from randomized control trials or meta-analyses which are rigorously interpreted by the guideline task forces forming specific recommendations. In the last fifteen years, as more scientific evidence was published, further guidelines emerged. This study demonstrates areas of consistency and inconsistency in recommendations for CRT and suggests underuse of CRT in the population of HF patients.

CRT increases strength and improves the synchrony of ventricular contractions, extends left ventricular diastolic filling time, increases cardiac output and systolic blood pressure, as well as reduces functional mitral regurgitation [14]. This translates into visible clinical effects: reduction of the severity of HF symptoms, improvement of exercise tolerance, as well as a reduction of morbidity and mortality due to HF [3]. In addition to the clinical efficacy of CRT, its cost-effectiveness has been evaluated in several analyses [15–20]. After reviewing literature that describes years of experience with CRT, the optimal profile of a patient who could benefit most from CRT can be specified (Figure 1) [1,3,7,21–24]. Before evaluating the indications for CRT, the patient should receive optimal treatment of HF according to the current best medical knowledge for at least 3 months (or even 6–9 months) [1,25]. Optimizing the treatment of comorbidities and achieving the highest recommended (tolerated) doses of drugs that improve the prognosis in HF may result in the withdrawal of indications for CRT.

CRT has been shown to be clinically useful mainly for patients with LVEF ≤ 35%, who represented approximately half of the study group. Some studies considered an LVEF ≤ 30% [26,27]. This specific indication for patients with LVEF ≤ 30% was included only in 2012 and 2022 guidelines [6,7]. Interestingly, in this study only 1 patient could have qualified for CRT based on this criterion (SR, ischemic HF, NYHA class I, QRS width ≥ 150 ms and LVEF ≤ 30%).

CRT is most effective for patients with SR, although several trials have shown the benefits of its use for patients with AF [28–30]. In these patients, the success of CRT depends primarily on the proportion of achieved biventricular pacing, and for many patients, AVN ablation is required. In this study, in all but the AHA/ACC/HFSA 2022 guidelines, more patients with SR than AF met the criteria for CRT. This is probably due to the fact that in recent years there has been a visible trend towards more intensive heart rate/rhythm control with the use of pharmacotherapy, and especially using invasive methods (AF or AVN ablation) [1,7,31]. In this study, the presence of an uncontrolled heart rate in patients who are potential candidates for AF or AVN ablation were not analyzed due to the lack of specific data.

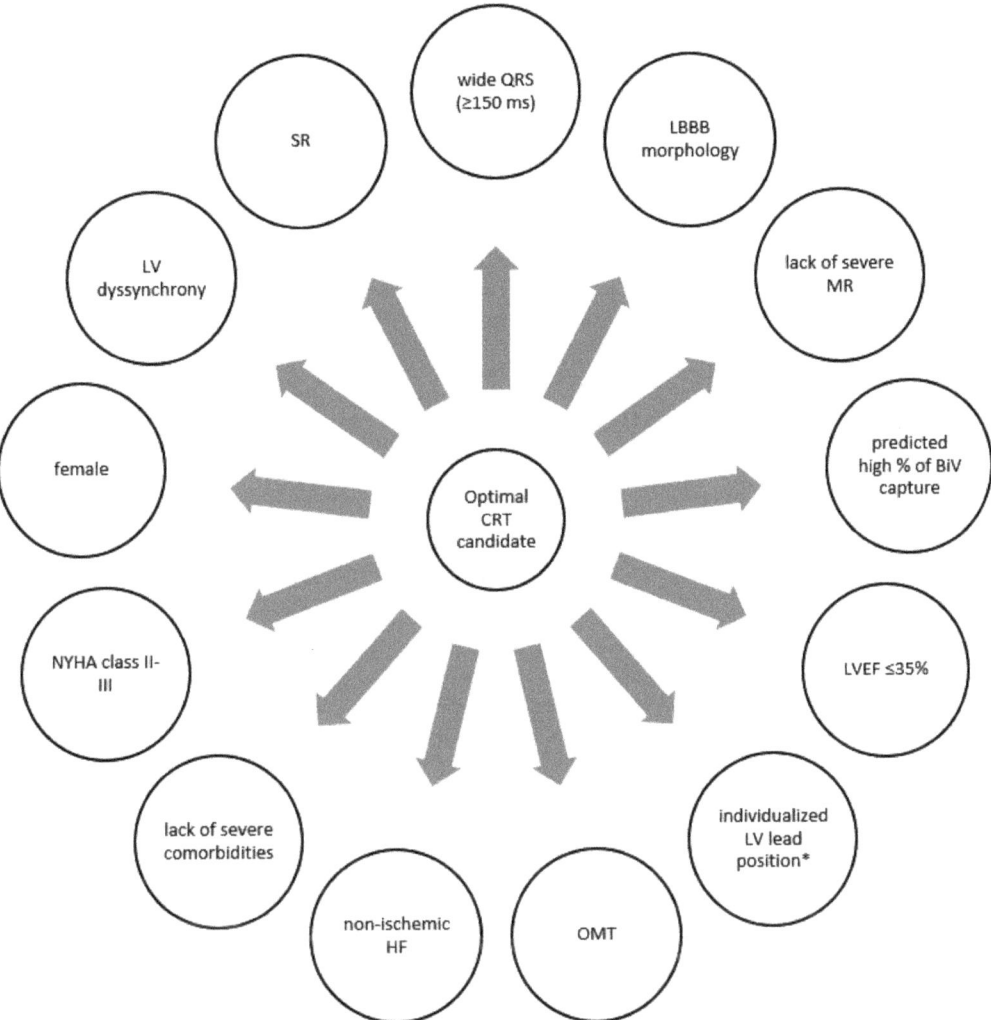

Figure 1. Selected clinical parameters associated with higher probability of favorable response to cardiac resynchronization therapy. BiV—biventricular; CRT—cardiac resynchronization therapy; HF—heart failure; LBBB—left bundle branch block; LV—left ventricle; LVEF—left ventricle ejection fraction; MR—mitral regurgitation; NYHA—New York Heart Association; OMT—optimal medical therapy; SR—sinus rhythm; %—percentage; * posterolateral lead position; correct pacing parameters; avoided scar areas.

The beneficial effects of CRT have been extensively proven in patients with NYHA class II–IV HF (over 90% of patients in our study). While one study observed a non-significant trend towards a lower risk of death from any cause in patients with NYHA class I, LBBB, and ischemic cardiomyopathy, this indication was included in the AHA/ACC/HFSA 2022 guidelines, but not in the ESC 2021 guidelines [1,3,7,32–34]. Additionally, the current ESC 2021 guidelines do not include HF etiology in the decision-making process for CRT implantation. However, it was shown that patients with ischemic heart disease are at greater risk of sudden cardiac death and, therefore, benefit more from ICD than patients with non-ischemic cardiomyopathy [1,3,35]. On the other hand, extensive myocardial scarring in patients with ischemic HF may attenuate clinical benefit from CRT, and if possible, lead placement should avoid scarred areas [1,3]. NYHA class varies with time, depending on the current condition of the patient, reported subjective symptoms, and received medications, hence it is the least objective parameter used to qualify for CRT and it is responsible for large variations in the number of patients who could receive CRT. The presence of LBBB, LVEF value, QRS width, and heart rhythm allow for greater objectivization of indications for CRT.

QRS duration predicts CRT response and was the inclusion criterion in all randomized clinical trials. Since 2016, the ESC guidelines based on the Echo-CRT trial did not recommend CRT in patients with a QRS duration < 130 ms, due to suggested possible harm from CRT in these patients [1,3,36,37]. According to the AHA/ACC/HFSA 2022 guidelines, CRT implantation is possible with a QRS duration $\geq$ 120 ms, both in LBBB and non-LBBB patients [7]. In our study, 3.2% of patients with SR and a QRS duration of 120–129 ms could have qualified for CRT following the AHA/ACC/HFSA 2022 criteria.

Several studies showed that LBBB morphology is more likely to have a favorable response to CRT when compared to non-LBBB morphology. CRT significantly reduced (36% reduction) a composite endpoint in patients with LBBB, while such benefits were not observed in patients with non-LBBB conduction abnormalities [38,39].

It should also be considered that due to the high complexity of the procedure, CRT implantation is associated with a significant risk of complications (including infectious and haemorrhagic), especially in patients with multiple comorbidities (including long-term diabetes, advanced chronic kidney disease, and cancer), in advanced age, or whose life expectancy does not significantly exceed one year. Hence, it is important to be familiarized with the currently applicable guidelines and to apply them in practice after taking into consideration the individual profile of a single patient. Current therapeutic strategies and risk assessment are imperfect as they are based in majority only on LVEF, NYHA, QRS width and LBBB presence, and do not include more specific criteria. Still more data, particularly from real-world patient studies, are necessary to improve and personalize HF management.

Real-world data suggest that even around 30% of the HFrEF population would have indications for CRT [1]. However, a recent survey from Sweden showed that of nearly 13,000 HFrEF patients, only 7% had received CRT, while 24% had an indication but had not received CRT [40]. QUALIFY (QUAlity of adherence to guideline recommendations for LIFe-saving treatment in heart failure: an international surveY) showed a low use of implantable devices in patients with HFrEF: CRT-D (6.3%) and CRT-P (1.4%) [41]. In the previous analyses of the ESC-HF Pilot and ESC-HF Long-Term, CRT was present in 1.8% and 5.9% of patients, respectively [42,43]. In our study, the biggest number of patients would be eligible for CRT according to the 2013 ESC guidelines (18.3%), whereas based on the recent ESC 2021 and AHA/ACC/HFSA 2022 guidelines, only 12.7% and 17.6% were eligible for CRT, respectively. These results indicate that there are significant differences in the eligibility criteria between the current guidelines. Regardless of the guidelines, there seems to still be potential to increase the frequency of CRT use in patients with HF, as it should be pointed out that, with regard to the criteria, more patients could in fact receive CRT.

Our study possesses some limitations. The inclusion of real-life patients with HF followed up by cardiologists is an important advantage of ESC-HF Pilot and ESC-HF-LT registries, but drawbacks include the observational character. Furthermore, only the predefined data in the Case Report Forms designed by the coordinators of the registries were available for analysis (e.g., data on indications for permanent pacing, AVN ablation, and expected survival time were lacking). The registries were not primarily focused on the indications for CRT implantation, hence analyses errors are possible. The exact number of patients that would have effectively received CRT based on the guidelines is unknown. However, this study was designed to present a general concept of the differences in eligibility for CRT in patients with HF according to the recent international guidelines.

5. Conclusions

The results of our study show that a high variability in the percentage of patients meeting the CRT eligibility criteria was observed since 2007. Across the fifteen years, the criteria overlapped entirely only in a small percentage of cases. Despite general consistency in international guideline recommendations for CRT implantation, each time the decision to qualify a patient for CRT (and the choice between CRT-P and CRT-D) requires an individual approach and a careful assessment of indications and contraindications for this form of HF therapy.

Supplementary Materials: The following supporting information can be downloaded at: https://www.mdpi.com/article/10.3390/jcm11113236/s1, Table S1: Indications for Cardiac Resynchronization Therapy in the major international guidelines.

Author Contributions: A.T., K.O., E.B. conceived the concept for the study, designed the analysis, interpreted the data, and wrote the manuscript. A.T., K.O., E.B. performed statistical analysis, A.T., K.O., P.B., A.K.-C., M.M. were responsible for data acquisition. P.B., A.K.-C., M.M., M.G.C.-L., A.P.M., J.D., G.O., M.G. interpreted the data and critically revised the manuscript. M.G.C.-L., A.P.M. designed the Registries. J.D. was a national coordinator of the Registries. All authors have read and agreed to the published version of the manuscript.

Funding: This research received no external funding.

Institutional Review Board Statement: The study protocol was approved by the local ethics committees.

Informed Consent Statement: All participating patients signed informed consent.

Data Availability Statement: The data presented in this study are available for three years following the publication on request from the corresponding author.

Conflicts of Interest: The authors declare no conflict of interest.

References

1. McDonagh, T.A.; Metra, M.; Adamo, M.; Gardner, R.S.; Baumbach, A.; Bohm, M.; Burri, H.; Butler, J.; Celutkiene, J.; Chioncel, O.; et al. 2021 ESC Guidelines for the diagnosis and treatment of acute and chronic heart failure. *Eur. Heart J.* **2021**, *42*, 3599–3726. [CrossRef]
2. Gerber, Y.; Weston, S.A.; Redfield, M.M.; Chamberlain, A.M.; Manemann, S.M.; Jiang, R.; Killian, J.M.; Roger, V.L. A contemporary appraisal of the heart failure epidemic in Olmsted County, Minnesota, 2000 to 2010. *JAMA Intern. Med.* **2015**, *175*, 996–1004. [CrossRef]
3. Glikson, M.; Nielsen, J.C.; Kronborg, M.B.; Michowitz, Y.; Auricchio, A.; Barbash, I.M.; Barrabes, J.A.; Boriani, G.; Braunschweig, F.; Brignole, M.; et al. 2021 ESC Guidelines on cardiac pacing and cardiac resynchronization therapy. *Eur. Heart J.* **2021**, *42*, 3427–3520. [CrossRef]
4. Brignole, M.; Auricchio, A.; Baron-Esquivias, G.; Bordachar, P.; Boriani, G.; Breithardt, O.A.; Cleland, J.; Deharo, J.C.; Delgado, V.; Elliott, P.M.; et al. 2013 ESC Guidelines on cardiac pacing and cardiac resynchronization therapy: The Task Force on cardiac pacing and resynchronization therapy of the European Society of Cardiology (ESC). Developed in collaboration with the European Heart Rhythm Association (EHRA). *Eur. Heart J.* **2013**, *34*, 2281–2329.
5. Dickstein, K.; Vardas, P.E.; Auricchio, A.; Daubert, J.C.; Linde, C.; McMurray, J.; Ponikowski, P.; Priori, S.G.; Sutton, R.; van Veldhuisen, D.J.; et al. 2010 Focused Update of ESC Guidelines on device therapy in heart failure: An update of the 2008 ESC Guidelines for the diagnosis and treatment of acute and chronic heart failure and the 2007 ESC guidelines for cardiac and resynchronization therapy. Developed with the special contribution of the Heart Failure Association and the European Heart Rhythm Association. *Eur. Heart J.* **2010**, *31*, 2677–2687. [PubMed]
6. Epstein, A.E.; DiMarco, J.P.; Ellenbogen, K.A.; Estes, N.A., 3rd; Freedman, R.A.; Gettes, L.S.; Gillinov, A.M.; Gregoratos, G.; Hammill, S.C.; Hayes, D.L.; et al. 2012 ACCF/AHA/HRS focused update incorporated into the ACCF/AHA/HRS 2008 guidelines for device-based therapy of cardiac rhythm abnormalities: A report of the American College of Cardiology Foundation/American Heart Association Task Force on Practice Guidelines and the Heart Rhythm Society. *Circulation* **2013**, *127*, e283–e352.
7. Heidenreich, P.A.; Bozkurt, B.; Aguilar, D.; Allen, L.A.; Byun, J.J.; Colvin, M.M.; Deswal, A.; Drazner, M.H.; Dunlay, S.M.; Evers, L.R.; et al. 2022 AHA/ACC/HFSA Guideline for the Management of Heart Failure: A Report of the American College of Cardiology/American Heart Association Joint Committee on Clinical Practice Guidelines. *Circulation* **2022**, *145*, e895–e1032. [CrossRef]
8. Ponikowski, P.; Voors, A.A.; Anker, S.D.; Bueno, H.; Cleland, J.G.F.; Coats, A.J.S.; Falk, V.; González-Juanatey, J.R.; Harjola, V.P.; Jankowska, E.A.; et al. 2016 ESC Guidelines for the diagnosis and treatment of acute and chronic heart failure: The Task Force for

the diagnosis and treatment of acute and chronic heart failure of the European Society of Cardiology (ESC)Developed with the special contribution of the Heart Failure Association (HFA) of the ESC. *Eur. Heart J.* **2016**, *37*, 2129–2200. [PubMed]
9. Priori, S.G.; Blomström-Lundqvist, C.; Mazzanti, A.; Blom, N.; Borggrefe, M.; Camm, J.; Elliott, P.M.; Fitzsimons, D.; Hatala, R.; Hindricks, G.; et al. 2015 ESC Guidelines for the management of patients with ventricular arrhythmias and the prevention of sudden cardiac death: The Task Force for the Management of Patients with Ventricular Arrhythmias and the Prevention of Sudden Cardiac Death of the European Society of Cardiology (ESC). Endorsed by: Association for European Paediatric and Congenital Cardiology (AEPC). *Eur. Heart J.* **2015**, *36*, 2793–2867.
10. Vardas, P.E.; Auricchio, A.; Blanc, J.J.; Daubert, J.C.; Drexler, H.; Ector, H.; Gasparini, M.; Linde, C.; Morgado, F.B.; Oto, A.; et al. Guidelines for cardiac pacing and cardiac resynchronization therapy: The Task Force for Cardiac Pacing and Cardiac Resynchronization Therapy of the European Society of Cardiology. Developed in collaboration with the European Heart Rhythm Association. *Eur. Heart J.* **2007**, *28*, 2256–2295.
11. Yancy, C.W.; Jessup, M.; Bozkurt, B.; Butler, J.; Casey, D.E., Jr.; Drazner, M.H.; Fonarow, G.C.; Geraci, S.A.; Horwich, T.; Januzzi, J.L.; et al. 2013 ACCF/AHA guideline for the management of heart failure: A report of the American College of Cardiology Foundation/American Heart Association Task Force on practice guidelines. *Circulation* **2013**, *128*, e240–e327. [CrossRef]
12. Crespo-Leiro, M.G.; Anker, S.D.; Maggioni, A.P.; Coats, A.J.; Filippatos, G.; Ruschitzka, F.; Ferrari, R.; Piepoli, M.F.; Delgado Jimenez, J.F.; Metra, M.; et al. European Society of Cardiology Heart Failure Long-Term Registry (ESC-HF-LT): 1-year follow-up outcomes and differences across regions. *Eur. J. Heart Fail.* **2016**, *18*, 613–625. [CrossRef]
13. Maggioni, A.P.; Dahlstrom, U.; Filippatos, G.; Chioncel, O.; Leiro, M.C.; Drozdz, J.; Fruhwald, F.; Gullestad, L.; Logeart, D.; Metra, M.; et al. EURObservational Research Programme: The Heart Failure Pilot Survey (ESC-HF Pilot). *Eur. J. Heart Fail.* **2010**, *12*, 1076–1084. [CrossRef] [PubMed]
14. Rybak, K.; Kubik, M.; Kowara, M.K.; Cudnoch-Jędrzejewska, A. Cardiac resynchronization therapy–beneficial alterations observed on molecular level—A review. *Heart Beat J.* **2020**, *5*, 10–15. [CrossRef]
15. Calvert, M.J.; Freemantle, N.; Yao, G.; Cleland, J.G.; Billingham, L.; Daubert, J.C.; Bryan, S. Cost-effectiveness of cardiac resynchronization therapy: Results from the CARE-HF trial. *Eur. Heart J.* **2005**, *26*, 2681–2688. [CrossRef]
16. Feldman, A.M.; de Lissovoy, G.; Bristow, M.R.; Saxon, L.A.; De Marco, T.; Kass, D.A.; Boehmer, J.; Singh, S.; Whellan, D.J.; Carson, P.; et al. Cost effectiveness of cardiac resynchronization therapy in the Comparison of Medical Therapy, Pacing, and Defibrillation in Heart Failure (COMPANION) trial. *J. Am. Coll. Cardiol.* **2005**, *46*, 2311–2321. [CrossRef]
17. Fox, M.; Mealing, S.; Anderson, R.; Dean, J.; Stein, K.; Price, A.; Taylor, R.S. The clinical effectiveness and cost-effectiveness of cardiac resynchronisation (biventricular pacing) for heart failure: Systematic review and economic model. *Health Technol. Assess.* **2007**, *11*, 3–4. [CrossRef]
18. Linde, C.; Mealing, S.; Hawkins, N.; Eaton, J.; Brown, B.; Daubert, J.C. Cost-effectiveness of cardiac resynchronization therapy in patients with asymptomatic to mild heart failure: Insights from the European cohort of the REVERSE (Resynchronization Reverses remodeling in Systolic Left Ventricular Dysfunction). *Eur. Heart J.* **2011**, *32*, 1631–1639. [CrossRef]
19. Noyes, K.; Veazie, P.; Hall, W.J.; Zhao, H.; Buttaccio, A.; Thevenet-Morrison, K.; Moss, A.J. Cost-effectiveness of cardiac resynchronization therapy in the MADIT-CRT trial. *J. Cardiovasc. Electrophysiol.* **2013**, *24*, 66–74. [CrossRef]
20. Phil Hider, R.W.; Hogan, S.; Bidwell, S.; Day, P.; Hall, K.; Kirk, R. Cardiac Resynchronisation Therapy for Severe Heart Failure. Available online: http://www.msac.gov.au/internet/msac/publishing.nsf/Content/9B4B8995B0E279D4CA25801000123B1D/$File/1042-One_page_summary.pdf (accessed on 27 May 2022).
21. Nakai, T.; Ikeya, Y.; Kogawa, R.; Otsuka, N.; Wakamatsu, Y.; Kurokawa, S.; Ohkubo, K.; Nagashima, K.; Okumura, Y. What Are the Expectations for Cardiac Resynchronization Therapy? A Validation of Two Response Definitions. *J. Clin. Med.* **2021**, *10*, 514. [CrossRef]
22. Ghossein, M.A.; Zanon, F.; Salden, F.; van Stipdonk, A.; Marcantoni, L.; Engels, E.; Luermans, J.; Westra, S.; Prinzen, F.; Vernooy, K. Left Ventricular Lead Placement Guided by Reduction in QRS Area. *J. Clin. Med.* **2021**, *10*, 5935. [CrossRef]
23. Wouters, P.C.; Vernooy, K.; Cramer, M.J.; Prinzen, F.W.; Meine, M. Optimizing lead placement for pacing in dyssynchronous heart failure: The patient in the lead. *Heart Rhythm* **2021**, *18*, 1024–1032. [CrossRef] [PubMed]
24. Tymińska, A.; Ozierański, K.; Balsam, P.; Maciejewski, C.; Wancerz, A.; Brociek, E.; Marchel, M.; Crespo-Leiro, M.G.; Maggioni, A.P.; Drożdż, J.; et al. Ischemic Cardiomyopathy versus Non-Ischemic Dilated Cardiomyopathy in Patients with Reduced Ejection Fraction—Clinical Characteristics and Prognosis Depending on Heart Failure Etiology (Data from European Society of Cardiology Heart Failure Registries). *Biology* **2022**, *11*, 341. [CrossRef]
25. Łasocha, D.; Tajstra, M.; Josiak, K.; Zając, D.; Dickstein, K.; Linde, C.; Normand, C.; Szumowski, Ł.J.; Sterliński, M. Methods Employed to Assess Left Ventricular Ejection Fraction in Patients Referred for Cardiac Resynchronization Therapy in Poland as Compared to other European Countries. Results from the European Cardiac Resynchronization Therapy Survey II. *Heart Beat J.* **2019**, *4*, 34–39. [CrossRef]
26. Moss, A.J.; Hall, W.J.; Cannom, D.S.; Klein, H.; Brown, M.W.; Daubert, J.P.; Estes, N.A., 3rd; Foster, E.; Greenberg, H.; Higgins, S.L.; et al. Cardiac-resynchronization therapy for the prevention of heart-failure events. *N. Engl. J. Med.* **2009**, *361*, 1329–1338. [CrossRef]
27. Tang, A.S.; Wells, G.A.; Talajic, M.; Arnold, M.O.; Sheldon, R.; Connolly, S.; Hohnloser, S.H.; Nichol, G.; Birnie, D.H.; Sapp, J.L.; et al. Cardiac-resynchronization therapy for mild-to-moderate heart failure. *N. Engl. J. Med.* **2010**, *363*, 2385–2395. [CrossRef] [PubMed]

28. Doshi, R.N.; Daoud, E.G.; Fellows, C.; Turk, K.; Duran, A.; Hamdan, M.H.; Pires, L.A.; Group, P.S. Left ventricular-based cardiac stimulation post AV nodal ablation evaluation (the PAVE study). *J. Cardiovasc. Electrophysiol.* **2005**, *16*, 1160–1165. [CrossRef]
29. Tolosana, J.M.; Hernandez Madrid, A.; Brugada, J.; Sitges, M.; Garcia Bolao, I.; Fernandez Lozano, I.; Martinez Ferrer, J.; Quesada, A.; Macias, A.; Marin, W.; et al. Comparison of benefits and mortality in cardiac resynchronization therapy in patients with atrial fibrillation versus patients in sinus rhythm (Results of the Spanish Atrial Fibrillation and Resynchronization [SPARE] Study). *Am. J. Cardiol.* **2008**, *102*, 444–449. [CrossRef]
30. Healey, J.S.; Hohnloser, S.H.; Exner, D.V.; Birnie, D.H.; Parkash, R.; Connolly, S.J.; Krahn, A.D.; Simpson, C.S.; Thibault, B.; Basta, M.; et al. Cardiac Resynchronization Therapy in Patients with Permanent Atrial Fibrillation. *Circ. Heart Fail.* **2012**, *5*, 566–570. [CrossRef]
31. Hindricks, G.; Potpara, T.; Dagres, N.; Arbelo, E.; Bax, J.J.; Blomstrom-Lundqvist, C.; Boriani, G.; Castella, M.; Dan, G.A.; Dilaveris, P.E.; et al. 2020 ESC Guidelines for the diagnosis and management of atrial fibrillation developed in collaboration with the European Association for Cardio-Thoracic Surgery (EACTS): The Task Force for the diagnosis and management of atrial fibrillation of the European Society of Cardiology (ESC) Developed with the special contribution of the European Heart Rhythm Association (EHRA) of the ESC. *Eur. Heart J.* **2021**, *42*, 373–498.
32. Al-Khatib, S.M.; Anstrom, K.J.; Eisenstein, E.L.; Peterson, E.D.; Jollis, J.G.; Mark, D.B.; Li, Y.; O'Connor, C.M.; Shaw, L.K.; Califf, R.M. Clinical and economic implications of the Multicenter Automatic Defibrillator Implantation Trial-II. *Ann. Intern. Med.* **2005**, *142*, 593–600. [CrossRef]
33. Pagourelias, E.D.; Efthimiadis, G.K.; Vassilikos, V. Survival with cardiac-resynchronization therapy. *N. Engl. J. Med.* **2014**, *371*, 477.
34. Goldenberg, I.; Kutyifa, V.; Klein, H.U.; Cannom, D.S.; Brown, M.W.; Dan, A.; Daubert, J.P.; Estes, N.A., 3rd; Foster, E.; Greenberg, H.; et al. Survival with cardiac-resynchronization therapy in mild heart failure. *N. Engl. J. Med.* **2014**, *370*, 1694–1701. [CrossRef] [PubMed]
35. Haugaa, K.H.; Tilz, R.; Boveda, S.; Dobreanu, D.; Sciaraffia, E.; Mansourati, J.; Papiashvili, G.; Dagres, N. Implantable cardioverter defibrillator use for primary prevention in ischaemic and non-ischaemic heart disease-indications in the post-DANISH trial era: Results of the European Heart Rhythm Association survey. *Europace* **2017**, *19*, 660–664. [CrossRef]
36. Ruschitzka, F.; Abraham, W.T.; Singh, J.P.; Bax, J.J.; Borer, J.S.; Brugada, J.; Dickstein, K.; Ford, I.; Gorcsan, J., 3rd; Gras, D.; et al. Cardiac-resynchronization therapy in heart failure with a narrow QRS complex. *N. Engl. J. Med.* **2013**, *369*, 1395–1405. [CrossRef]
37. Steffel, J.; Robertson, M.; Singh, J.P.; Abraham, W.T.; Bax, J.J.; Borer, J.S.; Dickstein, K.; Ford, I.; Gorcsan, J., 3rd; Gras, D.; et al. The effect of QRS duration on cardiac resynchronization therapy in patients with a narrow QRS complex: A subgroup analysis of the EchoCRT trial. *Eur. Heart J.* **2015**, *36*, 1983–1989. [CrossRef] [PubMed]
38. Sipahi, I.; Carrigan, T.P.; Rowland, D.Y.; Stambler, B.S.; Fang, J.C. Impact of QRS duration on clinical event reduction with cardiac resynchronization therapy: Meta-analysis of randomized controlled trials. *Arch. Intern. Med.* **2011**, *171*, 1454–1462. [CrossRef] [PubMed]
39. Sipahi, I.; Chou, J.C.; Hyden, M.; Rowland, D.Y.; Simon, D.I.; Fang, J.C. Effect of QRS morphology on clinical event reduction with cardiac resynchronization therapy: Meta-analysis of randomized controlled trials. *Am. Heart J.* **2012**, *163*, 260–267.e263. [CrossRef]
40. Lund, L.H.; Braunschweig, F.; Benson, L.; Ståhlberg, M.; Dahlström, U.; Linde, C. Association between demographic, organizational, clinical, and socio-economic characteristics and underutilization of cardiac resynchronization therapy: Results from the Swedish Heart Failure Registry. *Eur. J. Heart Fail.* **2017**, *19*, 1270–1279. [CrossRef]
41. Opolski, G.; Ozierański, K.; Lelonek, M.; Balsam, P.; Wilkins, A.; Ponikowski, P.; On Behalf Of The Polish Qualify, I. Adherence to the guidelines on the management of systolic heart failure in ambulatory care in Poland. Data from the international QUALIFY survey. *Pol. Arch. Intern. Med.* **2017**, *127*, 657–665.
42. Balsam, P.; Ozierański, K.; Kapłon-Cieślicka, A.; Borodzicz, S.; Tymińska, A.; Peller, M.; Marchel, M.; Crespo-Leiro, M.G.; Maggioni, A.P.; Drożdż, J.; et al. Differences in clinical characteristics and 1-year outcomes of hospitalized patients with heart failure in ESC-HF Pilot and ESC-HF-LT registries. *Pol. Arch. Intern. Med.* **2019**, *129*, 106–116.
43. Balsam, P.; Tymińska, A.; Kapłon-Cieślicka, A.; Ozierański, K.; Peller, M.; Galas, M.; Marchel, M.; Drożdż, J.; Filipiak, K.J.; Opolski, G. Predictors of one-year outcome in patients hospitalised for heart failure: Results from the Polish part of the Heart Failure Pilot Survey of the European Society of Cardiology. *Kardiol. Pol.* **2016**, *74*, 9–17. [CrossRef] [PubMed]

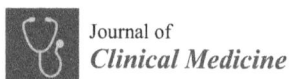

Article

Clinical Data, Chest Radiograph and Electrocardiography in the Screening for Left Ventricular Hypertrophy: The CAR$_2$E$_2$ Score

Patrycja S. Matusik [1], Amira Bryll [2], Agnieszka Pac [3], Tadeusz J. Popiela [2] and Paweł T. Matusik [4,5,*]

1. Department of Diagnostic Imaging, University Hospital, 30-688 Kraków, Poland; patrycja.s.matusik@gmail.com
2. Department of Radiology, Faculty of Medicine, Jagiellonian University Medical College, 30-688 Kraków, Poland; bryllamira@gmail.com (A.B.); msjpopie@cyf-kr.edu.pl (T.J.P.)
3. Chair of Epidemiology and Preventive Medicine, Faculty of Medicine, Jagiellonian University Medical College, 31-034 Kraków, Poland; agnieszka.pac@uj.edu.pl
4. Department of Electrocardiology, Institute of Cardiology, Faculty of Medicine, Jagiellonian University Medical College, 31-202 Kraków, Poland
5. Department of Electrocardiology, The John Paul II Hospital, 31-202 Kraków, Poland
* Correspondence: pawel.matusik@uj.edu.pl or pawel.matusik@wp.eu; Tel.: +48-12-614-2277

Citation: Matusik, P.S.; Bryll, A.; Pac, A.; Popiela, T.J.; Matusik, P.T. Clinical Data, Chest Radiograph and Electrocardiography in the Screening for Left Ventricular Hypertrophy: The CAR$_2$E$_2$ Score. *J. Clin. Med.* **2022**, *11*, 3585. https://doi.org/10.3390/jcm11133585

Academic Editor: Boyoung Joung

Received: 30 April 2022
Accepted: 16 June 2022
Published: 22 June 2022

Publisher's Note: MDPI stays neutral with regard to jurisdictional claims in published maps and institutional affiliations.

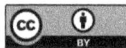

Copyright: © 2022 by the authors. Licensee MDPI, Basel, Switzerland. This article is an open access article distributed under the terms and conditions of the Creative Commons Attribution (CC BY) license (https://creativecommons.org/licenses/by/4.0/).

Abstract: Left ventricular hypertrophy (LVH) is associated with adverse clinical outcomes and implicates clinical decision-making. The aim of our study was to assess the importance of different approaches in the screening for LVH. We included patients who underwent cardiac magnetic resonance (CMR) imaging and had available chest radiograph in medical documentation. Cardiothoracic ratio (CTR), transverse cardiac diameter (TCD), clinical and selected electrocardiographic (ECG)-LVH data, including the Peguero-Lo Presti criterion, were assessed. CMR–LVH was defined based on indexed left ventricular mass-to-body surface area. Receiver operating characteristics analyses showed that both the CTR and TCD (CTR: area under the curve: [AUC] = 0.857, $p < 0.001$; TCD: AUC = 0.788, $p = 0.001$) were predictors for CMR–LVH. However, analyses have shown that diagnoses made with TCD, but not CTR, were consistent with CMR–LVH. From the analyzed ECG–LVH criteria, the Peguero-Lo Presti criterion was the best predictor of LVH. The best sensitivity for screening for LVH was observed when the presence of heart failure, ≥40 years in age (each is assigned 1 point), increased TCD and positive Peguero-Lo Presti criterion (each is assigned 2 points) were combined (CAR$_2$E$_2$ score ≥ 3 points). CAR$_2$E$_2$ score may improve prediction of LVH compared to other approaches. Therefore, it may be useful in the screening for LVH in everyday clinical practice in patients with prevalent cardiovascular diseases.

Keywords: clinical data; chest X-ray; electrocardiogram; cardiac magnetic resonance imaging; left ventricular hypertrophy; screening; diagnostics

1. Introduction

The demarcation between the normal and the pathological clinical findings is crucial. Clinical, chest radiograph and electrocardiographic (ECG) data might be helpful in this regard, especially in patients suspected of having or with cardiovascular diseases. Among others, it is important to be familiar with the abnormal appearance and dimensions of the cardiac silhouette on the chest radiograph (X-ray) before diagnosing cardiac enlargement [1]. Generally, cardiac enlargement on a chest radiograph is defined as a cardiothoracic ratio (CTR) of greater than 0.5 in posterior-anterior view [2,3]. Another indicator of cardiac enlargement is increased transverse cardiac diameter (TCD). Different TCD cut-off points have been described, while the values of 155 mm in men or 145 mm in women in posterior-anterior view are most commonly determined as increased [4]. However, there are limited data in the literature describing clinically significant abnormal chest radiograph features. It was demonstrated that CTR is sensitive and has a strong negative predictive value for

28. Doshi, R.N.; Daoud, E.G.; Fellows, C.; Turk, K.; Duran, A.; Hamdan, M.H.; Pires, L.A.; Group, P.S. Left ventricular-based cardiac stimulation post AV nodal ablation evaluation (the PAVE study). *J. Cardiovasc. Electrophysiol.* **2005**, *16*, 1160–1165. [CrossRef]
29. Tolosana, J.M.; Hernandez Madrid, A.; Brugada, J.; Sitges, M.; Garcia Bolao, I.; Fernandez Lozano, I.; Martinez Ferrer, J.; Quesada, A.; Macias, A.; Marin, W.; et al. Comparison of benefits and mortality in cardiac resynchronization therapy in patients with atrial fibrillation versus patients in sinus rhythm (Results of the Spanish Atrial Fibrillation and Resynchronization [SPARE] Study). *Am. J. Cardiol.* **2008**, *102*, 444–449. [CrossRef]
30. Healey, J.S.; Hohnloser, S.H.; Exner, D.V.; Birnie, D.H.; Parkash, R.; Connolly, S.J.; Krahn, A.D.; Simpson, C.S.; Thibault, B.; Basta, M.; et al. Cardiac Resynchronization Therapy in Patients with Permanent Atrial Fibrillation. *Circ. Heart Fail.* **2012**, *5*, 566–570. [CrossRef]
31. Hindricks, G.; Potpara, T.; Dagres, N.; Arbelo, E.; Bax, J.J.; Blomstrom-Lundqvist, C.; Boriani, G.; Castella, M.; Dan, G.A.; Dilaveris, P.E.; et al. 2020 ESC Guidelines for the diagnosis and management of atrial fibrillation developed in collaboration with the European Association for Cardio-Thoracic Surgery (EACTS): The Task Force for the diagnosis and management of atrial fibrillation of the European Society of Cardiology (ESC) Developed with the special contribution of the European Heart Rhythm Association (EHRA) of the ESC. *Eur. Heart J.* **2021**, *42*, 373–498.
32. Al-Khatib, S.M.; Anstrom, K.J.; Eisenstein, E.L.; Peterson, E.D.; Jollis, J.G.; Mark, D.B.; Li, Y.; O'Connor, C.M.; Shaw, L.K.; Califf, R.M. Clinical and economic implications of the Multicenter Automatic Defibrillator Implantation Trial-II. *Ann. Intern. Med.* **2005**, *142*, 593–600. [CrossRef]
33. Pagourelias, E.D.; Efthimiadis, G.K.; Vassilikos, V. Survival with cardiac-resynchronization therapy. *N. Engl. J. Med.* **2014**, *371*, 477.
34. Goldenberg, I.; Kutyifa, V.; Klein, H.U.; Cannom, D.S.; Brown, M.W.; Dan, A.; Daubert, J.P.; Estes, N.A., 3rd; Foster, E.; Greenberg, H.; et al. Survival with cardiac-resynchronization therapy in mild heart failure. *N. Engl. J. Med.* **2014**, *370*, 1694–1701. [CrossRef] [PubMed]
35. Haugaa, K.H.; Tilz, R.; Boveda, S.; Dobreanu, D.; Sciaraffia, E.; Mansourati, J.; Papiashvili, G.; Dagres, N. Implantable cardioverter defibrillator use for primary prevention in ischaemic and non-ischaemic heart disease-indications in the post-DANISH trial era: Results of the European Heart Rhythm Association survey. *Europace* **2017**, *19*, 660–664. [CrossRef]
36. Ruschitzka, F.; Abraham, W.T.; Singh, J.P.; Bax, J.J.; Borer, J.S.; Brugada, J.; Dickstein, K.; Ford, I.; Gorcsan, J., 3rd; Gras, D.; et al. Cardiac-resynchronization therapy in heart failure with a narrow QRS complex. *N. Engl. J. Med.* **2013**, *369*, 1395–1405. [CrossRef]
37. Steffel, J.; Robertson, M.; Singh, J.P.; Abraham, W.T.; Bax, J.J.; Borer, J.S.; Dickstein, K.; Ford, I.; Gorcsan, J., 3rd; Gras, D.; et al. The effect of QRS duration on cardiac resynchronization therapy in patients with a narrow QRS complex: A subgroup analysis of the EchoCRT trial. *Eur. Heart J.* **2015**, *36*, 1983–1989. [CrossRef] [PubMed]
38. Sipahi, I.; Carrigan, T.P.; Rowland, D.Y.; Stambler, B.S.; Fang, J.C. Impact of QRS duration on clinical event reduction with cardiac resynchronization therapy: Meta-analysis of randomized controlled trials. *Arch. Intern. Med.* **2011**, *171*, 1454–1462. [CrossRef] [PubMed]
39. Sipahi, I.; Chou, J.C.; Hyden, M.; Rowland, D.Y.; Simon, D.I.; Fang, J.C. Effect of QRS morphology on clinical event reduction with cardiac resynchronization therapy: Meta-analysis of randomized controlled trials. *Am. Heart J.* **2012**, *163*, 260–267.e263. [CrossRef]
40. Lund, L.H.; Braunschweig, F.; Benson, L.; Ståhlberg, M.; Dahlström, U.; Linde, C. Association between demographic, organizational, clinical, and socio-economic characteristics and underutilization of cardiac resynchronization therapy: Results from the Swedish Heart Failure Registry. *Eur. J. Heart Fail.* **2017**, *19*, 1270–1279. [CrossRef]
41. Opolski, G.; Ozierański, K.; Lelonek, M.; Balsam, P.; Wilkins, A.; Ponikowski, P.; On Behalf Of The Polish Qualify, I. Adherence to the guidelines on the management of systolic heart failure in ambulatory care in Poland. Data from the international QUALIFY survey. *Pol. Arch. Intern. Med.* **2017**, *127*, 657–665.
42. Balsam, P.; Ozierański, K.; Kapłon-Cieślicka, A.; Borodzicz, S.; Tymińska, A.; Peller, M.; Marchel, M.; Crespo-Leiro, M.G.; Maggioni, A.P.; Drożdż, J.; et al. Differences in clinical characteristics and 1-year outcomes of hospitalized patients with heart failure in ESC-HF Pilot and ESC-HF-LT registries. *Pol. Arch. Intern. Med.* **2019**, *129*, 106–116.
43. Balsam, P.; Tymińska, A.; Kapłon-Cieślicka, A.; Ozierański, K.; Peller, M.; Galas, M.; Marchel, M.; Drożdż, J.; Filipiak, K.J.; Opolski, G. Predictors of one-year outcome in patients hospitalised for heart failure: Results from the Polish part of the Heart Failure Pilot Survey of the European Society of Cardiology. *Kardiol. Pol.* **2016**, *74*, 9–17. [CrossRef] [PubMed]

Journal of Clinical Medicine

Article

Clinical Data, Chest Radiograph and Electrocardiography in the Screening for Left Ventricular Hypertrophy: The CAR_2E_2 Score

Patrycja S. Matusik [1], Amira Bryll [2], Agnieszka Pac [3], Tadeusz J. Popiela [2] and Paweł T. Matusik [4,5,*]

[1] Department of Diagnostic Imaging, University Hospital, 30-688 Kraków, Poland; patrycja.s.matusik@gmail.com
[2] Department of Radiology, Faculty of Medicine, Jagiellonian University Medical College, 30-688 Kraków, Poland; bryllamira@gmail.com (A.B.); msjpopie@cyf-kr.edu.pl (T.J.P.)
[3] Chair of Epidemiology and Preventive Medicine, Faculty of Medicine, Jagiellonian University Medical College, 31-034 Kraków, Poland; agnieszka.pac@uj.edu.pl
[4] Department of Electrocardiology, Institute of Cardiology, Faculty of Medicine, Jagiellonian University Medical College, 31-202 Kraków, Poland
[5] Department of Electrocardiology, The John Paul II Hospital, 31-202 Kraków, Poland
* Correspondence: pawel.matusik@uj.edu.pl or pawel.matusik@wp.eu; Tel.: +48-12-614-2277

Abstract: Left ventricular hypertrophy (LVH) is associated with adverse clinical outcomes and implicates clinical decision-making. The aim of our study was to assess the importance of different approaches in the screening for LVH. We included patients who underwent cardiac magnetic resonance (CMR) imaging and had available chest radiograph in medical documentation. Cardiothoracic ratio (CTR), transverse cardiac diameter (TCD), clinical and selected electrocardiographic (ECG)-LVH data, including the Peguero-Lo Presti criterion, were assessed. CMR–LVH was defined based on indexed left ventricular mass-to-body surface area. Receiver operating characteristics analyses showed that both the CTR and TCD (CTR: area under the curve: [AUC] = 0.857, $p < 0.001$; TCD: AUC = 0.788, $p = 0.001$) were predictors for CMR–LVH. However, analyses have shown that diagnoses made with TCD, but not CTR, were consistent with CMR–LVH. From the analyzed ECG–LVH criteria, the Peguero-Lo Presti criterion was the best predictor of LVH. The best sensitivity for screening for LVH was observed when the presence of heart failure, ≥40 years in age (each is assigned 1 point), increased TCD and positive Peguero-Lo Presti criterion (each is assigned 2 points) were combined (CAR_2E_2 score ≥ 3 points). CAR_2E_2 score may improve prediction of LVH compared to other approaches. Therefore, it may be useful in the screening for LVH in everyday clinical practice in patients with prevalent cardiovascular diseases.

Keywords: clinical data; chest X-ray; electrocardiogram; cardiac magnetic resonance imaging; left ventricular hypertrophy; screening; diagnostics

Citation: Matusik, P.S.; Bryll, A.; Pac, A.; Popiela, T.J.; Matusik, P.T. Clinical Data, Chest Radiograph and Electrocardiography in the Screening for Left Ventricular Hypertrophy: The CAR_2E_2 Score. *J. Clin. Med.* **2022**, *11*, 3585. https://doi.org/10.3390/jcm11133585

Academic Editor: Boyoung Joung

Received: 30 April 2022
Accepted: 16 June 2022
Published: 22 June 2022

Publisher's Note: MDPI stays neutral with regard to jurisdictional claims in published maps and institutional affiliations.

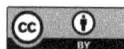

Copyright: © 2022 by the authors. Licensee MDPI, Basel, Switzerland. This article is an open access article distributed under the terms and conditions of the Creative Commons Attribution (CC BY) license (https://creativecommons.org/licenses/by/4.0/).

1. Introduction

The demarcation between the normal and the pathological clinical findings is crucial. Clinical, chest radiograph and electrocardiographic (ECG) data might be helpful in this regard, especially in patients suspected of having or with cardiovascular diseases. Among others, it is important to be familiar with the abnormal appearance and dimensions of the cardiac silhouette on the chest radiograph (X-ray) before diagnosing cardiac enlargement [1]. Generally, cardiac enlargement on a chest radiograph is defined as a cardiothoracic ratio (CTR) of greater than 0.5 in posterior-anterior view [2,3]. Another indicator of cardiac enlargement is increased transverse cardiac diameter (TCD). Different TCD cut-off points have been described, while the values of 155 mm in men or 145 mm in women in posterior-anterior view are most commonly determined as increased [4]. However, there are limited data in the literature describing clinically significant abnormal chest radiograph features. It was demonstrated that CTR is sensitive and has a strong negative predictive value for screening for left ventricular (LV) enlargement by studies performed so far [2]. TCD is a more direct measure of cardiac size and a moderate correlation between TCD and LV end-diastolic volume (LVEDV) measured by cardiac magnetic resonance (CMR) was found [1]. However, the clinical value of CTR and TCD in prediction of LV hypertrophy (LVH) is poorly known [5].

Increased LV mass (LVM) may arise from multiple molecular mechanism, is associated with adverse clinical outcomes and may implicate clinical decision-making [6,7]. CMR imaging is considered the gold standard for assessment of LVM [8]. In comparison to chest radiograph, this imaging modality is not influenced by some extracardiac factors such as extensive thoracic fat deposits or chest wall expansion. However, CMR is not always available, is more complex in assessment and is relatively expensive. Those factors limit the use of CMR as a screening tool [9]. Transthoracic echocardiography is easier to perform and cheaper, but it also has limited availability for general population screening [10]. Currently, ECG is the most frequently used as a first screening tool to identify LVH [11]. The major limitation of ECG–LVH criteria, in the screening for LVH, is low sensitivity [12–15].

The aim of our study was to assess the importance of different approaches in the screening for LVH, including clinical data, chest radiograph parameters and ECG–LVH criteria used alone and in combination.

2. Materials and Methods

2.1. Study Population

We included patients with prevalent cardiovascular diseases who underwent CMR imaging in the Department of Diagnostic Imaging, University Hospital in Kraków (Poland) between 2011 and 2015 and had available chest radiograph taken in the posterior-anterior projection in the upright position during inspiration in medical documentation. Baseline patient clinical and demographic data and medication history were obtained from a structured medical records review. The study was approved by the local ethics committee.

2.2. CMR Imaging

CMR images were obtained using a 1.5 Tesla GE Signa HDxt scanner (General Electric, Milwaukee, WI, USA). The fast imaging employing steady-state acquisition (FIESTA) cine technique and other techniques such as those reported previously were implemented [16,17]. Left ventricular ejection fraction (LVEF), left ventricular end-systolic volume (LVESV), LVEDV and LVM were assessed with the use of standard volumetric techniques and calculated with commercially available QMass® MR analysis software, version 7.6 (Medis Medical Imaging Systems bv, Leiden, The Netherlands) [16]. LVM was indexed for body surface area (BSA) and LVH diagnosed based on CMR (CMR–LVH) was defined as LVM/BSA >72 g/m^2 in men or >55 g/m^2 in women [18].

2.3. Chest Radiographs

Chest radiographs were taken in the posterior-anterior projection in the upright position during inspiration. The TCD was measured by drawing a vertical line through the vertebral bodies and calculating the sum of segments drawn perpendicular from the midline to the farthest edge of the cardiac silhouette in both directions [19,20]. CTR was calculated as a ratio of TCD to the greatest horizontal distance between the inner borders of the ribs within the chest [20,21]. Abnormal chest radiograph parameters, indicating cardiac enlargement, were determined as a CTR > 0.5 and as a TCD $\geq$ 155 mm in men or $\geq$145 mm in women [2–4].

2.4. ECG Analysis

ECG data were available for 38 patients. Standard 12-lead ECGs were recorded at 25 mm/s paper speed and calibration of 10 mm/mV and were assessed by an investigator who was primarily blinded to the patient's CMR data. We evaluated 10 different ECG criteria for the LVH, as described previously [16]. In the current analysis, we used the following ECG–LVH criteria: R wave amplitude in aVL + S wave amplitude in V3 (Cornell voltage) >2.8 mV for men or >2.0 mV for female [22], (R wave amplitude in aVL + S wave amplitude in V3) × QRS duration for men or (R wave amplitude in aVL + S wave amplitude in V3 + 0.8 mV) × QRS duration for women (Cornell (voltage-duration) product) ≥244.0 mV × ms [23], S wave amplitude in V1 + R wave amplitude in V5 or V6 (Sokolow-Lyon voltage) >3.5 mV [24], the deepest S-wave in any single lead + S wave amplitude in V4 (Peguero-Lo Presti) ≥2.3 mV for female or ≥2.8 mV for men [13], and at least one positive ECG–LVH criterion (when all 10 previously described ECG criteria were applied together) [16].

2.5. A Fortified Method to Screen for Left Ventricular Hypertrophy

We assessed the rule described by Park et al., which included combining female sex, selected cardiovascular risk factors (age ≥65 years and body mass index (BMI) ≥25 kg/m^2), chest radiograph (CTR ≥ 0.5) and the ECG–LVH criterion (Sokolow-Lyon voltage ≥3.5 mV) [5]. A score of ≥2 points indicated LVH [5].

2.6. Statistical Analysis

Continuous variables were tested with the t test or the Mann–Whitney test and were presented as means ± standard deviations (SD) or medians and interquartile ranges (IQR), when appropriate. Associations between categorical variables were assessed using the Pearson χ^2 test or Fisher exact test, and results were given as numbers and percentages. Spearman rank correlation was used to measure the degree of association between two continuous variables. Receiver operating characteristics (ROC) analysis was used to find out the best variables to discriminate between patients with and without CMR–LVH. Based on the performed analyses, we modified the score proposed by Park et al. and proposed a modified score for LVH screening. Comparison of proportions was implemented to test for differences in positive LVH diagnoses. The different method used for screening for LVH was compared using the McNemar test. The agreement between the chest radiograph, ECG–LVH and combined criteria and the diagnosis of CMR–LVH was compared using the Cohen's kappa coefficient. Additionally, specificity, sensitivity, positive predictive value, negative predictive value, accuracy and likelihood ratios were calculated for CTR, TCD, ECG–LVH criteria and combined criteria for LVH screening. Statistical significance was defined as $p < 0.05$ for all tests. Statistical analyses were carried out using IBM SPSS Statistics (version 25, IBM Corp., Armonk, NY, USA), Statistica (version 13.3, TIBCO Software Inc., Palo Alto, CA, USA) to compare areas under the curves (AUC) in analyses of receiver operating characteristics (Hanley and McNeil formula), while confidence intervals (CI) were calculated, and comparison of proportions were performed using MedCalc software (version 20.110, Medcalc Software Ltd., Ostend, Belgium) (available at: https://www.medcalc.org/, accessing date: 12 March 2022).

3. Results

3.1. Study Population

The study group consisted of 55 patients (16.4% female) with a median age of 42.0 (29.0–63.0) years. Among the studied patients, hypertension was present in 23 (41.8%), dyslipidemia in 21 (38.2%), diabetes in 8 (14.5%), atrial fibrillation in 8 (14.5%), chronic kidney disease in 6 (10.9%), coronary artery disease in 22 (40.0%) and heart failure in 35 (63.6%). Median LVEF was 42.7 (24.7–60.0)%, LVEDV was 189.6 (162.3–276.3) ml, LVESV was 94.3 (65.6–205.5) ml, while LVM was 161.0 (127.3–225.6) g. The prevalence of CMR–LVH was 72.7%. The threshold of age of ≥40 years, as a predictor of LVH, was determined based on ROC analysis (Youden index = 0.38; AUC, 0.679; 95% CI, 0.517–0.841; $p = 0.04$). Baseline characteristics of the patients with or without CMR–LVH, based on indexed LVM for BSA, is shown in Table 1.

Table 1. Characteristics of the patients with and without left ventricular hypertrophy based on left ventricular mass indexed by body surface area.

Parameters	LVH; n = 40	No LVH; n = 15	p Value
Demographic characteristics and anthropometric data			
Age (years)	51.5 (32.3–64.0)	33.0 (25.0–47.0)	0.04
Age ≥40 years	26 (65.0%)	4 (26.7%)	0.01
Age ≥65 years	11 (27.5%)	2 (13.3%)	0.48 *
Female sex, n (%)	7 (17.5%)	2 (13.3%)	1 *
BMI (kg/m^2)	25.1 (22.1–29.0)	26.8 (23.1–28.7)	0.63
BMI ≥ 25 kg/m^2, n (%)	20 (50.0%)	9 (60.0%)	0.5
BMI ≥ 30 kg/m^2, n (%)	7 (17.5%)	3 (20.0%)	1 *
Cardiovascular diseases, comorbidities and risk factors, n (%)			
Heart failure	30 (75.0%)	5 (33.3%)	0.004
CAD	18 (45.0%)	4 (26.7%)	0.22
Myocardial infarction	10 (25.0%)	2 (13.3%)	0.35
Diabetes mellitus	7 (17.5%)	1 (6.7%)	0.42 *
Hypertension	18 (45.0%)	5 (33.3%)	0.44
Dyslipidemia	17 (42.5%)	4 (26.7%)	0.28
Smoking	11 (27.5%)	2 (13.3%)	0.48
Atrial fibrillation	7 (17.5%)	1 (6.7%)	0.42 *
CKD	5 (12.5%)	1 (6.7%)	1 *
CMR parameters			
LVEF (%)	29.7 (23.4–50.5)	59.5 (50.9–66.2)	<0.001
LVM (g)	173.0 (152.9–234.0)	126.0 (114.4–134.5)	<0.001
LVEDV (mL)	228.0 (169.4–322.4)	169.5 (123.0–189.6)	0.002
LVEDV/BSA > 117 (M), >101 (F), n (%)	20 (50.0%)	0 (0.0%)	0.001
LVESV (mL)	124.6 (84.7–261.7)	65.6 (58.3–74.1)	<0.001
Chest radiograph data			
CTR	0.50 ± 0.07	0.42 ± 0.04	<0.001
CTR > 0.5, n (%)	17 (42.5%)	0 (0.0%)	0.002 *
TCD (mm)	167.7 ± 26.9	141.4 ± 16.9	0.001
TCD ≥ 155 mm (M), ≥145 mm (F), n (%)	28 (70.0%)	3 (20.0%)	0.001

Data are presented as mean ± standard deviation or median (interquartile range) or number (percentage). * Fisher exact test (exact significance, 2-sided). BMI—body mass index; BSA—body surface area; CAD—coronary artery disease; CKD—chronic kidney disease; CMR—cardiac magnetic resonance; CTR—cardiothoracic ratio; F—female; LVEDV—left ventricular end-diastolic volume; LVEF—left ventricular ejection fraction; LVESV—left ventricular end-systolic volume; LVM—left ventricular mass; M—male; TCD—transverse cardiac diameter.

3.2. Associations between Radiographic and Basic CMR Variables

Both CTR and TCD showed positive correlations with LVM (R = 0.53, $p < 0.001$; R = 0.73, $p < 0.001$, respectively). Similarly, positive correlations were observed between these radiographic parameters and LVEDV (R = 0.47, $p < 0.001$; R = 0.61, $p < 0.001$), and LVESV (R = 0.52, $p < 0.001$; R = 0.66, $p < 0.001$), while both CTR and TCD showed significant negative correlations with LVEF (R = −0.58, $p < 0.001$; R = −0.64, $p < 0.001$). Receiver operating characteristics analysis showed that both the CTR and TCD (CTR: area under curve: AUC = 0.857, $p < 0.001$; TCD: AUC = 0.788, $p = 0.001$; Figure 1) were predictors for CMR–LVH. When comparing AUC for these criteria, no significant difference between them was observed ($p = 0.14$).

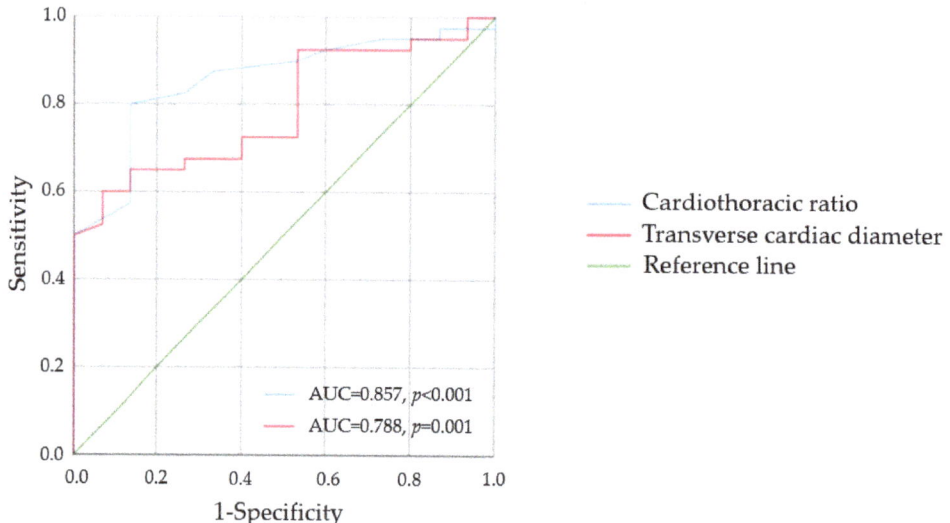

Figure 1. Area under the curve of chest radiograph criteria representing the predictive performance of left ventricular hypertrophy based on left ventricular mass indexed by body surface area. AUC—area under the curve.

3.3. Characteristics of the Patients with Normal and Increased Chest Radiograph Indicators of Cardiac Size Enlargement

Patients with CTR > 0.5 were older and had higher BMI (60.0 (40.5–69.5) vs. 36.0 (27.0–60.5) years, $p = 0.009$; 29.0 ± 5.6 vs. 24.8 ± 3.7 kg/m^2, $p = 0.002$; Table 2) when compared to patients with normal CTR. In patients with CTR > 0.5, atrial fibrillation and heart failure were more common than in the remaining patients (35.3% vs. 5.3%, $p = 0.008$ and 94.1% vs. 50.0%, $p = 0.002$, respectively). Similarly, patients with TCD ≥ 155 mm in men or ≥ 145 mm in women were older when compared to patients with normal TCD (60.0 (37.0–70.0) vs. 32.5 (27.0–44.3) years, $p < 0.001$; Table 2). However, there was no significant difference in BMI between these two groups (27.0 (24.0–30.2) vs. 23.8 (22.1–27.5) kg/m^2, $p = 0.08$). On the other hand, in patients with TCD ≥ 155 mm in men or ≥145 mm in women, cardiovascular disease risk factors and comorbidities (heart failure, hypertension and dyslipidemia) were observed more frequently when compared to the remaining patients (80.6% vs. 41.7%, $p = 0.005$; 54.8% vs. 25.0%, $p = 0.03$, 51.6% vs. 20.8%, $p = 0.03$, respectively).

Table 2. Baseline characteristics of the patients with normal and increased chest radiograph indicators of cardiac size enlargement.

Parameters	CTR > 0.5 (n = 17)	CTR ≤ 0.5 (n = 38)	p Value	TCD ≥ 155 mm (M) or ≥ 145 mm (F) (n = 31)	TCD < 155 mm (M) or < 145 mm (F) (n = 24)	p Value
\multicolumn{7}{c}{Demographic characteristics and anthropometric data}
Age (years)	60.0 (40.5–69.5)	36.0 (27.0–60.5)	0.009	60.0 (37.0–70.0)	32.5 (27.0–44.3)	<0.001
Age ≥40 years	14 (82.4%)	16 (42.1%)	0.006	23 (74.2%)	7 (29.2%)	0.001
Age ≥65 years	6 (35.3%)	7 (18.4%)	0.19 *	12 (38.7%)	1 (4.2%)	0.003
Female sex, n (%)	2 (11.8%)	7 (18.4%)	0.71 *	3 (9.7%)	6 (25.0%)	0.16 *
BMI (kg/m^2)	29.0 ± 5.6	24.8 ± 3.7	0.002	27.0 (24.0–30.2)	23.8 (22.1–27.5)	0.08
BMI ≥ 25 kg/m^2, n (%)	14 (82.4%)	15 (39.5%)	0.003	20 (64.5%)	9 (37.5%)	0.047
BMI ≥ 30 kg/m^2, n (%)	6 (35.3%)	4 (10.5%)	0.05 *	7 (22.6%)	3 (12.5%)	0.49 *
\multicolumn{7}{c}{Cardiovascular diseases, comorbidities and risk factors, n (%)}
Heart failure	16 (94.1%)	19 (50.0%)	0.002	25 (80.6%)	10 (41.7%)	0.005
CAD	10 (58.8%)	12 (31.6%)	0.06	16 (51.6%)	6 (25.0%)	0.06
Myocardial infarction	4 (23.5%)	8 (21.1%)	1 *	9 (29.0%)	3 (12.5%)	0.19
Diabetes mellitus	5 (29.4%)	3 (7.9%)	0.09 *	6 (19.4%)	2 (8.3%)	0.44 *
Hypertension	8 (47.1%)	15 (39.5%)	0.6	17 (54.8%)	6 (25.0%)	0.03
Dyslipidemia	9 (52.9%)	12 (31.6%)	0.13	16 (51.6%)	5 (20.8%)	0.03
Smoking	3 (17.6%)	10 (26.3%)	0.73 *	7 (22.6%)	6 (25.0%)	1
Atrial fibrillation	6 (35.3%)	2 (5.3%)	0.008 *	6 (19.4%)	2 (8.3%)	0.44 *
CKD	2 (11.8%)	4 (10.5%)	1 *	5 (16.1%)	1 (4.2%)	0.22 *
\multicolumn{7}{c}{CMR parameters}
LVEF (%)	25.6 ± 9.1	49.2 ± 16.7	<0.001	29.5 (21.0–46.7)	58.2 (42.7–63.0)	<0.001
LVM (g)	233.6 (181.9–271.3)	134.7 (120.9–167.0)	<0.001	201.6 ± 62.8	136.8 ± 29.1	<0.001
LVM/BSA > 72 g/m^2 (M) or >55 g/m^2 (F), n (%)	17 (100.0%)	23 (60.5%)	0.002 *	28 (90.3%)	12 (50.0%)	0.001
LVEDV (mL)	317.3 (239.7–392.0)	175.2 (140.2–199.5)	<0.001	228.8 (168.7–355.6)	173.9 (136.3–194.6)	0.005
LVEDV/BSA > 117 (M), >101 (F), n (%)	14 (82.4%)	6 (15.8%)	<0.001	17 (54.8%)	3 (12.5%)	0.002
LVESV (mL)	239.4 (152.4–313.1)	82.4 (63.3–112.4)	<0.001	173.9 (82.1–271.3)	71.7 (58.0–104.9)	0.001
\multicolumn{7}{c}{Chest radiograph data}
CTR	0.57 ± 0.05	0.44 ± 0.04	<0.001	0.53 ± 0.06	0.42 ± 0.04	<0.001
TCD (mm)	192.3 ± 17.9	146.3 ± 16.3	<0.001	171.0 (161.8–194.3)	140.7 (130.3–149.5)	<0.001
TCD ≥ 155 mm (M), ≥145 mm (F), n (%)	17 (100%)	14 (36.8%)	<0.001	17 (54.8%)	0 (0.0%)	<0.001

Data are presented as mean ± standard deviation or median (interquartile range) or number (percentage). * Fisher exact test (exact significance, 2-sided). BMI—body mass index; BSA—body surface area; CAD—coronary artery disease; CKD—chronic kidney disease; CMR—cardiac magnetic resonance; CTR—cardiothoracic ratio; F—female; LVEDV—left ventricular end-diastolic volume; LVEF—left ventricular ejection fraction; LVESV—left ventricular end-systolic volume; LVM—left ventricular mass; M—male; TCD—transverse cardiac diameter.

3.4. Radiographic and Electrocardiographic Criteria in the Screening for LVH

When comparing a group of 38 patients with available ECG data, we observed that only the Peguero-Lo Presti criterion was more frequently positive in patients with CMR–LVH (56.0% vs. 15.4%, p = 0.02). Performed analyses (the McNemar test) have shown that diagnoses of cardiac enlargement made with TCD, but not CTR, were consistent with CMR–LVH. From ECG–LVH criteria only, at least one positive ECG criterion was consistent with CMR in LVH diagnosis (Table 3).

Table 3. Radiographic and electrocardiographic criteria in the screening for left ventricular hypertrophy in patients with and without left ventricular hypertrophy based on left ventricular mass indexed by body surface area.

Parameters	LVH; n = 25		No LVH; n = 13		McNemar Test
	TP	FN	FP	TN	
	Chest radiograph indicators of cardiac size enlargement				
CTR > 0.5	7 (28.0%)	18 (72.0%)	0 (0.0%)	13 (100.0%)	<0.001
TCD ≥ 155 mm (M), ≥145 mm (F)	14 (56.0%)	11 (44.0%)	3 (23.1%)	76.9%)	0.06
	ECG-LVH criteria				
Cornell voltage	1 (4.0%)	24 (96.0%)	0 (0.0%)	13 (100.0%)	<0.001
Cornell product	2 (8.0%)	23 (92.0%)	0 (0.0%)	13 (100.0%)	<0.001
Peguero-Lo Presti criterion	14 (56.0%)	11 (44.0%)	2 (15.4%)	11 (84.6%)	0.02
Sokolow-Lyon voltage	3 (12.0%)	22 (88.0%)	1 (7.7%)	12 (92.3%)	<0.001
At least one positive ECG-LVH criterion	14 (56.0%)	11 (44.0%)	3 (23.1%)	10 (76.9%)	0.06

Data are presented as number (percentage). CTR—cardiothoracic ratio; ECG—electrocardiographic; FN—false negative; FP—false positive; LVH—left ventricular hypertrophy; TCD—transverse cardiac diameter; TN—true negative; TP—true positive. Calculations were made for 38 patients.

From chest radiograph parameters, the highest sensitivity was observed for TCD; however, specificity of this parameter was lower when compared to CTR (56.0 (34.9–75.6)% vs. 28.0 (12.1–49.4)%; 76.9 (46.2–95.0)% vs. 100.0 (75.3–100.0)%, respectively; Table 4). Moreover, the sensitivity for TCD was the same as sensitivities for the Peguero-Lo Presti criterion and at least one positive ECG-LVH criterion and higher than sensitivities for Cornell criteria and the Sokolow–Lyon voltage criterion (Table 4). The positive predictive value, negative predictive value, accuracy, positive and negative likelihood ratio of all the analyzed chest radiographs and ECG-LVH criteria are shown in Table 4.

3.5. A Novel Screening Tool for LVH

We modified the Park rule based on the results of our statistical analyses. We replaced CTR by TCD and the Sokolow–Lyon voltage criterion by other ECG–LVH criteria (at least one ECG-LVH criterion positive and Peguero-Lo Presti criterion; Model 1 and 2, respectively). Moreover, we tested whether our new score based on a point system in which 1 point is assigned for heart failure and age ≥40 years, and 2 points are assigned for chest radiograph indicating cardiac enlargement (TCD indicating cardiac enlargement) and positive Peguero-Lo Presti criterion (CAR_2E_2 score), improves prediction of LVH compared to other approaches used for LVH screening. The methodology of the CAR_2E_2 score calculation is depicted in Figure 2.

Table 4. Radiographic and electrocardiographic criteria in the screening for left ventricular hypertrophy and their sensitivity, specificity, positive predictive value, negative predictive value, accuracy, positive likelihood ratio and negative likelihood ratio. Data are shown for indexed left ventricular mass by body surface area.

Parameters	Sensitivity (%) (95% CI)	Specificity (%) (95% CI)	PPV (%) (95% CI)	NPV (%) (95% CI)	Accuracy (%) (95% CI)	PLR (95% CI)	NLR (95% CI)
		Chest radiograph indicators of cardiac size enlargement					
CTR > 0.5	28.0 (12.1–49.4)	100.0 (75.3–100.0)	100.0 *	41.9 (36.1–48.0)	52.6 (35.8–69.0)	*	0.7 (0.6–0.9)
TCD ≥ 155 mm (M), ≥145 mm (F)	56.0 (34.9–75.6)	76.9 (46.2–95.0)	82.4 (62.0–93.0)	47.6 (34.8–60.8)	63.2 (46.0–78.2)	2.4 (0.9–7.0)	0.6 (0.3–1.0)
		ECG-LVH criteria					
Cornell voltage	4.0 (0.1–20.4)	100.0 (75.3–100.0)	100.0 *	35.1 (33.3–37.0)	36.8 (21.8–54.0)	*	1.0 (0.9–1.0)
Cornell product	8.0 (1.0–26.0)	100.0 (75.3–100.0)	100.0 *	36.1 (33.5–38.8)	39.5 (24.0–56.6)	*	0.9 (0.8–1.0)
Peguero-Lo Presti criterion	56.0 (34.9–75.6)	84.6 (54.6–98.1)	87.5 (65.1–96.3)	50.0 (37.8–62.2)	65.8 (48.7–80.4)	3.6 (1.0–13.6)	0.5 (0.3–0.9)
Sokolow-Lyon voltage	12.0 (2.6–31.2)	92.3 (64.0–99.8)	75.0 (25.7–96.3)	35.3 (30.6–40.3)	39.5 (24.0–56.6)	1.6 (0.2–13.6)	1.0 (0.8–1.2)
At least one positive ECG-LVH criterion	56.0 (34.9–75.6)	76.9 (46.2–95.0)	82.4 (62.0–93.0)	47.6 (34.8–60.8)	63.2 (46.0–78.2)	2.4 (0.9–7.0)	0.6 (0.3–1.0)

Data are presented as percentage (95% CI) or number (95% CI). CI—confidence interval; CTR—cardiothoracic ratio; ECG—electrocardiographic; LVH—left ventricular hypertrophy; NLR—negative likelihood ratio; NPV—negative predictive value; PLR- positive likelihood ratio; PPV—positive predictive value; TCD—transverse cardiac diameter. Calculations were made for 38 patients. *—95% CI, PLR and/or NLR not available.

1 point is assigned for:

Congestive heart failure   **A**ge (≥ 40 years)

2 points are assigned for:

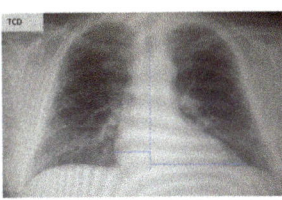

chest **R**adiograph indicating cardiac enlargement (TCD ≥ 155 mm in men or ≥ 145 mm in female)

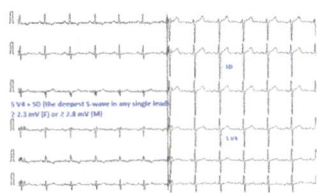

ECG-LVH criterion (Peguero-Lo Presti ≥ 2.3 mV for female or ≥ 2.8 mV for men)

Figure 2. The Congestive heart failure, Age, chest Radiograph and Electrocardiographic data (CAR_2E_2) score assessment.

3.6. Combined Criteria in the Screening for LVH

When comparing a group of 38 patients with the available ECG data, we observed that only Model 2 at the score ≥2 and CAR_2E_2 score of ≥3 were more frequently positive in patients with CMR–LVH (60.0% vs. 23.1%, p = 0.03; 72.0% vs. 23.1%, 0.004, respectively). When comparing these 2 differentiating criteria using a comparison of proportion test, there was no difference between them. Performed analyses (the McNemar test) demonstrated that Model 1 at the score ≥2, Model 2 at the score ≥2 and CAR_2E_2 score at the score ≥3 were in agreement with CMR in LVH diagnosis (Table 5). However, the strongest agreement was found for the CAR_2E_2 score, when compared to TCD, with at least one positive ECG-

LVH criterion, Model 1 at a score of ≥2 and Model 2 at a score of ≥2 (κ coefficient of 0.46 vs. 0.29; 0.29; −0.12; −0.12, respectively).

Table 5. Combined criteria in the screening of left ventricular hypertrophy in patients with and without left ventricular hypertrophy based on left ventricular mass indexed by body surface area.

Parameters	LVH; n = 25		No LVH; n = 13		McNemar Test
	TP	FN	FP	TN	
Combined Rules with Use the Clinical Risk Factors, Chest Radiograph and ECG-LVH Criteria					
Model proposed by Park et al. [5] at score ≥2 [†]	10 (40.0%)	15 (60.0%)	2 (15.4%)	11 (84.6%)	0.002
Model 1 at score ≥2 [‡]	15 (60.0%)	10 (40.0%)	4 (30.8%)	9 (69.2%)	0.18
Model 2 at score ≥2 [#]	15 (60.0%)	10 (40.0%)	3 (23.1%)	10 (76.9%)	0.09
CAR_2E_2 score ≥3 [##]	18 (72.0%)	7 (28.0%)	3 (23.1%)	10 (76.9%)	0.344

Data are presented as number (percentage). [†] Includes female sex, age ≥65 years, BMI ≥ 25 kg/m^2, Sokolow-Lyon voltage ≥3.5 mV, and CTR ≥ 0.5. [‡] Includes female sex, age ≥65 years, BMI ≥ 25 kg/m^2, at least one ECG-LVH criterion positive, and TCD ≥ 155 mm (M), ≥145 mm (F). [#] Includes female sex, age ≥65 years, BMI ≥ 25 kg/m^2, Peguero-Lo Presti criterion ≥2.3 mV (F) or ≥2.8 mV (M), and TCD ≥ 155 mm (M), ≥145 mm (F). [##] Includes congestive heart failure, age (≥40 years), Peguero-Lo Presti criterion: the deepest S-wave in any single lead + S wave amplitude in V4 ≥ 2.3 mV (F) or ≥2.8 mV (M), and TCD ≥ 155 mm (M), ≥145 mm (F). ECG—electrocardiographic; FN—false negative; FP—false positive; LVH—left ventricular hypertrophy; TN—true negative; TP—true positive. Calculations were made for 38 patients.

The rule described by Parke et al. combining the risk factors, ECG and chest radiograph criteria showed a sensitivity of 40.0 (21.1–61.3)% and specificity of 84.6 (54.6–98.1)%. After modification of this rule by replacing CTR by TCD and replacing the Sokolow–Lyon voltage by other ECG criterion (at least one ECG-LVH criterion positive and Peguero-Lo Presti criterion), we observed a sensitivity of 60.0 (38.7–78.9)% in both of cases (Table 6). The best sensitivity was observed for a CAR_2E_2 score of ≥3 (72.0 (50.6–87.9)%). The positive predictive value, negative predictive value, accuracy and positive and negative likelihood ratios of all the analyzed combined criteria are shown in Table 6.

Receiver operating characteristics analysis showed that only a CAR_2E_2 score of ≥3 (AUC = 0.763, $p < 0.001$; Figure 3) was a predictor of CMR–LVH. Additionally, in ROC analysis, a CAR_2E_2 score of <3 points was a predictor of a lack of CMR–LVH (AUC = 0.745, $p = 0.005$).

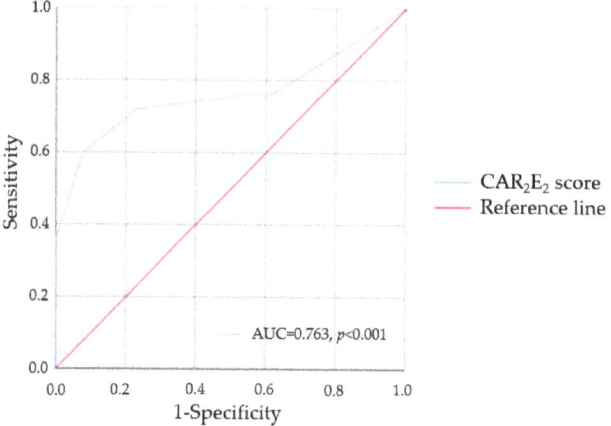

Figure 3. Area under the curve of CAR_2E_2 score representing the predictive performance of left ventricular hypertrophy based on left ventricular mass indexed by body surface area. AUC—area under the curve.

Table 6. Combined criteria for screening of left ventricular hypertrophy and their sensitivity, specificity, positive predictive value, negative predictive value, accuracy, positive likelihood ratio and negative likelihood ratio. Data are shown for indexed left ventricular mass by body surface area.

Parameters	Sensitivity (%) (95% CI)	Specificity (%) (95% CI)	PPV (%) (95% CI)	NPV (%) (95% CI)	Accuracy (%) (95% CI)	PLR (95% CI)	NLR (95% CI)
Combined Rules with Use the Clinical Risk Factors, Chest Radiograph and ECG-LVH Criteria							
Model proposed by Park et al. [5] score ≥ 2 [†]	40.0 (21.1–61.3)	84.6 (54.6–98.1)	83.3 (56.2–95.1)	42.3 (33.1–52.1)	55.3 (38.3–71.4)	2.6 (0.7–10.2)	0.7 (0.5–1.1)
Model 1 score ≥ 2 [‡]	60.0 (38.7–78.9)	69.2 (38.6–90.9)	79.0 (61.0–90.0)	47.4 (33.0–62.2)	63.2 (46.0–78.2)	2.0 (0.8–4.7)	0.6 (0.3–1.1)
Model 2 score ≥ 2 [#]	60.0 (38.7–78.9)	76.9 (46.2–95.0)	83.3 (63.8–93.4)	50.0 (36.2–63.8)	65.8 (48.7–80.4)	2.6 (0.9–77.4)	0.5 (0.3–0.9)
CAR_2E_2 score ≥ 3 [##]	72.0 (50.6–87.9)	76.9 (46.2–95.0)	85.7 (68.3–94.3)	58.8 (41.6–74.1)	73.7 (57.0–86.6)	3.1 (1.1–8.7)	0.4 (0.2–0.7)

Data are presented as percentage (95% CI) or number (95% CI). [†] Includes female sex, age $\geq$65 years, BMI ≥ 25 kg/m^2, Sokolow-Lyon voltage criterion: S wave amplitude in V1 + R wave amplitude in V5 or V6 ≥ 3.5 mV, and CTR ≥ 0.5. [‡] Includes female sex, age $\geq$65 years, BMI ≥ 25 kg/m^2, at least one ECG-LVH criterion positive, and TCD ≥ 155 mm (M), ≥ 145 mm (F). [#] Includes female sex, age $\geq$65 years, BMI ≥ 25 kg/m^2, Peguero-Lo Presti criterion: the deepest S-wave in any single lead + S wave amplitude in V4 ≥ 2.3 mV (F) or ≥ 2.8 mV (M), and TCD ≥ 155 mm (M), ≥ 145 mm (F). [##] Includes congestive heart failure, age ≥ 40 years, Peguero-Lo Presti criterion, and TCD ≥ 155 mm (M), ≥ 145 mm (F). CI—confidence interval; ECG—electrocardiographic; LVH—left ventricular hypertrophy; NLR—negative likelihood ratio; NPV—negative predictive value; PLR—positive likelihood ratio; PPV—positive predictive value. Calculations were made for 38 patients.

Importantly, when we tested the CAR_2E_2 score, and used CTR in the place of TCD (as "R_2") and all investigated ECG–LVH criteria in place of Peguero-Lo Presti criterion (as "E_2") interchangeably, there was no observed difference regarding AUC in ROC analysis in the prediction of CMR–LVH.

4. Discussion

There is increasing interest in the use of markers and risk scores as well as in testing their clinical applicability in cardiovascular medicine [25–33]. Several factors have been found to be associated with LVH assessed by different modalities [7,16]. Studies performed so far have demonstrated that there is a relationship between CTR and LVM measured by echocardiography [5,34,35]. Rayner et al. revealed that CTR (R = 0.34, $p < 0.02$) was independently correlated with LVM when evaluated with this modality [34]. Similar correlation of CTR and LVM determined by echocardiography (R = 0.43, $p < 0.01$) was found in another study performed by Buba et al. [35]. However, research investigating the association between CTR and LVM determined by CMR is lacking. Our study demonstrates that both CTR and TCD were predictors of CMR–LVH in receiver operating characteristics analyses and have shown moderate correlation not only with the LVM, but also with LVEDV, LVESV and LVEF. However, the strongest correlations were observed for TCD. Similarly to our results, Morales et al. have shown that while a good relation was found between LVEDV and TCD, this relation was less significant for the CTR [1]. These data suggest that TCD may be a better indicator than CTR of LV dimension and hypertrophy. However, it should also be remembered that CTR and TCD do not take into account changes in the size of the heart throughout the cardiac cycle.

Moreover, CTR and TCD may be influenced by several other factors, such as pericardial fat, elevation of the diaphragm either due to poor inspiration or obesity, the breathing phase or thoracic alterations (e.g., severe scoliosis, pectus excavatum) [2,36–39]. However, TCD seems to be influenced by deformities of the chest (especially affecting the transverse chest diameter) to a lesser extent than CTR. Importantly, identifying factors explaining the discrepancies between chest radiograph parameters and CMR–LVH may improve diagnostic abilities. For example, right ventricular enlargement may cause greater TCD and CTR measures [40–42]. In a study of heart failure patients, Fukuta et al. revealed that increased CTR correlated more strongly with the size of the right ventricle than LV [41]. Recently, it has also been demonstrated that CTR could play a role in predicting right ventricular enlargement in patients with suspected pulmonary embolism during COVID-19 [42]. Elevation of the diaphragm due to high BMI can place the heart in a more horizontal position leading to an increase of TCD and CTR. Our study showed that patients with and without CMR-LVH did not significantly differ in BMI. Inversely, these parameters were significantly different when compared to patients with normal and higher CTR and trended toward higher BMI values in patients with increased TCD than patients with normal TCD. This suggests that especially high BMI may be responsible for some discrepancies between chest radiograph parameters and CMR–LVH. However, verification of this hypothesis requires further investigation.

Ribeiro et al., in a study on hypertensive patients, demonstrated that CTR had a sensitivity of 16.7% and a specificity of 88.3% for identifying the LVH [43]. For comparison, for ECG criteria (Romhilt–Estes point score system) sensitivity and specificity for the detection of LVH were 12.5% and 92.2%, respectively [43]. These findings show that chest radiographs may be useful for detecting LVH in hypertensive patients. Moreover, some studies suggest that the standard CRT criterion is not a good enough indicator of cardiac enlargement and therefore consider the introduction of another cut-off point for CTR or indicate TCD assessment as a better method [44–46]. Our study performed in patients with prevalent cardiovascular diseases revealed that from chest radiograph parameters, the highest sensitivity was observed for TCD, and this sensitivity was the same as for the Peguero-Lo Presti criterion and at least one positive ECG-LVH criterion. Moreover, the sensitivity of TCD was higher than sensitivities for Cornel criteria and the Sokolow–Lyon voltage criterion. These data suggest that chest radiographs may be valuable in screening for LVH not only in hypertensive patients but also in subgroups with prevalent cardiovascular diseases.

Increased LVM may impair LV function and might predict HF in some individuals [47,48]. Studies have shown that LVH is the most frequent myocardial abnormality associated with HF with preserved EF, and its prevalence increases with age [48,49]. Interestingly, we have shown that the combination of cardiovascular risk factors (heart failure and age $\geq$40 years) with chest radiograph parameters and ECG criteria may improve screening for LVH. After modification of a model proposed by Park et al. [5] by replacing the CTR by TCD and replacing the Sokolow–Lyon voltage by another ECG criterion (at least one ECG-LVH criterion positive and Peguero-Lo Presti criterion), we observed better sensitivity than the sensitivities of ECG and chest radiograph criteria solely. However, it should be mentioned that the fortified method for screening for LVH proposed by Park et al. was previously tested only in a hypertensive Asian population [5]. Thus, further studies on this topic performed on a larger and more diversified cohort are required. Moreover, we revealed that the novel score system that we have proposed, the CAR_2E_2 score, had the best sensitivity and may be considered as a fortified method for screening for LVH in daily clinical practice. A screening tool with high sensitivity may be preferred in the context of LVH (due to, e.g., very low/no risk, low cost and high availability of transthoracic echocardiography in many clinical settings) [50]. Due to there being no difference in AUC in ROC analysis, in the prediction of CMR–LVH, when CTR was used instead of TCD and all investigated ECG–LVH criteria instead of the Peguero-Lo Presti criterion, in clinical practice both of these radiological criteria and also investigated ECG–LVH criteria, besides the Peguero-Lo Presti criterion, might be useful and potentially used interchangeably. Our study also revealed that the CAR_2E_2 score may be useful for patients with fewer than 3 points by being a predictor of a lack of CMR–LVH. However, it is important to remember that these patients with a positive ECG–LVH criterion and/or chest radiograph suggestive of cardiac enlargement should not be excluded from further diagnostic processes. Despite the strongest agreement with CMR–LVH for a CAR_2E_2 score of $\geq$3, when compared to chest radiograph parameters indicating cardiac enlargement or ECG–LVH criteria, studies have shown that ECG and chest radiograph used alone are also useful in screening for LVH [16,36].

Identifying the underlying etiology of LVH is a common, and sometimes challenging clinical problem. It is especially crucial to differentiate physiological changes in the heart, e.g., of an athlete, with pathological forms of LVH, for example, in patients with aortic stenosis or some cardiomyopathies, and examinations included in the CAR_2E_2 score might provide clinical clues. Evaluation consisting of a detailed clinical history (e.g., older age in aortic stenosis patients), chest radiograph (e.g., aortic valve calcification and widening of the ascending aorta in aortic stenosis) and ECG (e.g., physiological in black/African athletes T wave inversions in V1-V4 accompanied by convex ST segment elevation) might be useful in clinical differentiation [37,51–53]. In echocardiography, we usually observe normal contractility, as well as normal global longitudinal strain, along with usually normal LV wall thickness in athletes [54], while specific alterations are observed in patients with aortic stenosis. Additionally, CMR, especially with late gadolinium enhancement, may provide further diagnostic clues and prognostic information [54–56].

There are several limitations of our study which should be mentioned. Chest radiograph, ECG and CMR studies were not always performed on the same day. Our study has a retrospective nature and relatively small group of included patients with cardiovascular diseases. Therefore, our results may not be representative for the whole population and should be confirmed in a larger group of patients. However, even in this relatively small group, we could find differences in the tested chest radiograph parameters, ECG–LVH criteria and combined approaches for LVH detection. Finally, we did not investigate associations of the CAR_2E_2 score with major adverse cardiovascular events. This should be evaluated in further studies. However, the components of our new score have proven the relationship with unfavorable clinical outcomes [29,33,36,57,58]. Therefore, CAR_2E_2 score is most likely related to increased clinical risk.

5. Conclusions

CAR_2E_2 score may improve prediction of LVH compared to other approaches, including chest radiograph parameters used on their own and in combination with selected clinical data and ECG–LVH criteria. Therefore, it may be useful in the screening for LVH in everyday clinical practice in patients with prevalent cardiovascular diseases.

Author Contributions: Conceptualization, P.S.M., P.T.M. Methodology, P.S.M., P.T.M. Software, P.S.M. Validation, P.S.M. Formal Analysis, P.S.M., A.P. Investigation, P.S.M. Resources, P.S.M. Data Curation, P.S.M. Writing—Original Draft Preparation, P.S.M. Writing—Review and Editing, P.T.M., A.B., A.P., T.J.P. Visualization, P.S.M., P.T.M. Supervision, P.T.M., T.J.P. Project Administration, P.S.M. Funding Acquisition, P.T.M. All authors have read and agreed to the published version of the manuscript.

Funding: P.T.M. was supported by the Ministry of Science and Higher Education scholarship for outstanding young scientists, the Polish Cardiac Society 2018 Scientific Grant in cooperation with Berlin-Chemie/Menarini (sponsor of the grant: Berlin-Chemie/Menarini Poland LLC) and by Jagiellonian University Medical College grant (N41/DBS/000517).

Institutional Review Board Statement: The approval for this study from the local ethics committee was obtained (Opinion number 39/KBL/OIL/2018).

Informed Consent Statement: Not applicable. The study had retrospective character.

Data Availability Statement: Not applicable.

Conflicts of Interest: The authors declare no conflict of interest.

References

1. Morales, M.-A.; Prediletto, R.; Rossi, G.; Catapano, G.; Lombardi, M.; Rovai, D. Routine Chest X-ray: Still Valuable for the Assessment of Left Ventricular Size and Function in the Era of Super Machines? *J. Clin. Imaging Sci.* **2012**, *2*, 25. [CrossRef]
2. Loomba, R.S.; Shah, P.H.; Nijhawan, K.; Aggarwal, S.; Arora, R. Cardiothoracic ratio for prediction of left ventricular dilation: A systematic review and pooled analysis. *Futur. Cardiol.* **2015**, *11*, 171–175. [CrossRef]

3. Giamouzis, G.; Sui, X.; Love, T.E.; Butler, J.; Young, J.B.; Ahmed, A. A Propensity-Matched Study of the Association of Cardiothoracic Ratio with Morbidity and Mortality in Chronic Heart Failure. *Am. J. Cardiol.* **2008**, *101*, 343–347. [CrossRef]
4. Vogl, T.J.; Reith, W.; Rummeny, E.J. *Diagnostic and Interventional Radiology*; Springer: Berlin/Heidelberg, Germany, 2016.
5. Park, H.E.; Chon, S.-B.; Na, S.H.; Lee, H.; Choi, S.-Y. A Fortified Method to Screen and Detect Left Ventricular Hypertrophy in Asymptomatic Hypertensive Adults: A Korean Retrospective, Cross-Sectional Study. *Int. J. Hypertens.* **2018**, *2018*, 6072740. [CrossRef]
6. Sygitowicz, G.; Maciejak-Jastrzebska, A.; Sitkiewicz, D. MicroRNAs in the development of left ventricular remodeling and postmyocardial infarction heart failure. *Pol. Arch. Intern. Med.* **2020**, *130*, 59–65.
7. Xu, L.; Chen, G.; Liang, Y.; Zhou, C.; Zhang, F.; Fan, T.; Chen, X.; Zhou, H.; Yuan, W. T helpers 17 cell responses induced cardiac hypertrophy and remodeling in essential hypertension. *Pol. Arch. Intern. Med.* **2021**, *131*, 257–265. [CrossRef]
8. Armstrong, A.C.; Gjesdal, O.; Almeida, A.; Nacif, M.; Wu, C.; Bluemke, D.A.; Brumback, L.; Lima, J.A.C. Left Ventricular Mass and Hypertrophy by Echocardiography and Cardiac Magnetic Resonance: The Multi-Ethnic Study of Atherosclerosis. *Echocardiography* **2013**, *31*, 12–20. [CrossRef]
9. Bluemke, D.A.; Kronmal, R.A.; Lima, J.A.; Liu, K.; Olson, J.; Burke, G.L.; Folsom, A.R. The Relationship of Left Ventricular Mass and Geometry to Incident Cardiovascular Events: The MESA (Multi-Ethnic Study of Atherosclerosis) Study. *J. Am. Coll. Cardiol.* **2008**, *52*, 2148–2155. [CrossRef]
10. Alfakih, K.; Reid, S.; Hall, A.; Sivananthan, M.U. The assessment of left ventricular hypertrophy in hypertension. *J. Hypertens.* **2006**, *24*, 1223–1230. [CrossRef]
11. Bacharova, L.; Schocken, D.; Estes, E.H.; Strauss, D. The Role of ECG in the Diagnosis of Left Ventricular Hypertrophy. *Curr. Cardiol. Rev.* **2014**, *10*, 257–261. [CrossRef]
12. Pewsner, D.; Jüni, P.; Egger, M.; Battaglia, M.; Sundstrom, J.; Bachmann, L.M. Accuracy of electrocardiography in diagnosis of left ventricular hypertrophy in arterial hypertension: Systematic review. *BMJ* **2007**, *335*, 711. [CrossRef]
13. Peguero, J.G.; Presti, S.L.; Perez, J.; Issa, O.; Brenes, J.C.; Tolentino, A. Electrocardiographic Criteria for the Diagnosis of Left Ventricular Hypertrophy. *J. Am. Coll. Cardiol.* **2017**, *69*, 1694–1703. [CrossRef]
14. Jalanko, M.; Heliö, T.; Mustonen, P.; Kokkonen, J.; Huhtala, H.; Laine, M.; Jääskeläinen, P.; Tarkiainen, M.; Lauerma, K.; Sipola, P.; et al. Novel electrocardiographic features in carriers of hypertrophic cardiomyopathy causing sarcomeric mutations. *J. Electrocardiol.* **2018**, *51*, 983–989. [CrossRef]
15. Lim, D.Y.; Sng, G.; Ho, W.H.; Hankun, W.; Sia, C.-H.; Lee, J.S.; Shen, X.; Tan, B.Y.; Lee, E.C.; Dalakoti, M.; et al. Machine learning versus classic electrocardiographic criteria for the detection of echocardiographic left ventricular hypertrophy in a pre-participation cohort. *Kardiologia Polska* **2021**, *79*, 654–661. [CrossRef]
16. Matusik, P.S.; Bryll, A.; Matusik, P.T.; Pac, A.; Popiela, T.J. Electrocardiography and cardiac magnetic resonance imaging in the detection of left ventricular hypertrophy: The impact of indexing methods. *Kardiol. Pol.* **2020**, *78*, 889–898. [CrossRef]
17. Matusik, P.S.; Bryll, A.; Matusik, P.T.; Pac, A.; Popiela, T.J. Ischemic and non-ischemic patterns of late gadolinium enhancement in heart failure with reduced ejection fraction. *Cardiol. J.* **2021**, *28*, 67–76. [CrossRef]
18. Petersen, S.E.; Aung, N.; Sanghvi, M.; Zemrak, F.; Fung, K.; Paiva, J.M.; Francis, J.M.; Khanji, M.Y.; Lukaschuk, E.; Lee, A.; et al. Reference ranges for cardiac structure and function using cardiovascular magnetic resonance (CMR) in Caucasians from the UK Biobank population cohort. *J. Cardiovasc. Magn. Reson.* **2017**, *19*, 18. [CrossRef]
19. Zhu, Y.; Xu, H.; Zhu, X.; Wei, Y.; Yang, G.; Tang, L.; Xu, Y. Which can predict left ventricular size and systolic function: Cardiothoracic ratio or transverse cardiac diameter. *J. X-ray Sci. Technol.* **2015**, *23*, 557–565. [CrossRef]
20. Chana, H.S.; Martin, C.A.; Cakebread, H.E.; Adjei, F.D.; Gajendragadkar, P.R. Diagnostic accuracy of cardiothoracic ratio on admission chest radiography to detect left or right ventricular systolic dysfunction: A retrospective study. *J. R. Soc. Med.* **2015**, *108*, 317–324. [CrossRef]
21. Esmail, H.; Oni, T.; Thienemann, F.; Omar-Davies, N.; Wilkinson, R.; Ntsekhe, M. Cardio-Thoracic Ratio Is Stable, Reproducible and Has Potential as a Screening Tool for HIV-1 Related Cardiac Disorders in Resource Poor Settings. *PLoS ONE* **2016**, *11*, e0163490. [CrossRef]
22. Baranowski, R.; Wojciechowski, D.; Kozłowski, D.; Kukla, P.; Kurpesa, M.; Lelakowski, J.; Maciejewska, M.; Średniawa, B.; Wranicz, J.K. Compendium for performing and describing the resting electrocardiogram. Diagnostic criteria describe rhythm, electrical axis of the heart, QRS voltage, automaticity and conduction disorders. Experts' group statement of the Working Group on Noninvasive Ele. *Kardiol. Pol.* **2016**, *74*, 493–500. [CrossRef]
23. Buchner, S.; Debl, K.; Haimerl, J.; Djavidani, B.; Poschenrieder, F.; Feuerbach, S.; Riegger, G.A.; Luchner, A. Electrocardiographic diagnosis of left ventricular hypertrophy in aortic valve disease: Evaluation of ECG criteria by cardiovascular magnetic resonance. *J. Cardiovasc. Magn. Reson.* **2009**, *11*, 18. [CrossRef]
24. Baranowski, R.; Wojciechowski, D.; Kozłowski, D.; Kukla, P.; Kurpesa, M.; Lelakowski, J.; Maciejewska, M.; Średniawa, B.; Wranicz, J.K. [Electrocardiographic criteria for diagnosis of the heart chamber enlargement, necrosis and repolarisation abnormalities including acute coronary syndromes. Experts' group statement of the Working Group on Noninvasive Electrocardiology and Telemedicine of]. *Kardiol. Pol.* **2016**, *74*, 812–819. [CrossRef]
25. Uygur, B.; Celik, O.; Demir, A.R.; Sahin, A.A.; Guner, A.; Avci, Y.; Bulut, U.; Tasbulak, O.; Demirci, G.; Uzun, F.; et al. A simplified acute kidney injury predictor following transcatheter aortic valve implantation: The ACEF score. *Kardiologia Polska* **2021**, *79*, 662–668. [CrossRef]

26. Canepa, M.; Palmisano, P.; Dell'Era, G.; Ziacchi, M.; Ammendola, E.; Accogli, M.; Occhetta, E.; Biffi, M.; Nigro, G.; Ameri, P.; et al. Usefulness of the MAGGIC Score in Predicting the Competing Risk of Non-Sudden Death in Heart Failure Patients Receiving an Implantable Cardioverter-Defibrillator: A Sub-Analysis of the OBSERVO-ICD Registry. *J. Clin. Med.* **2021**, *11*, 121. [CrossRef]
27. Yamada, S.; Kaneshiro, T.; Yoshihisa, A.; Nodera, M.; Amami, K.; Nehashi, T.; Takeishi, Y. Albumin-Bilirubin Score for Prediction of Outcomes in Heart Failure Patients Treated with Cardiac Resynchronization Therapy. *J. Clin. Med.* **2021**, *10*, 5378. [CrossRef]
28. Özdemir, E.; Esen, Ş.; Emren, S.V.; Karaca, M.; Nazlı, C. Association between Intermountain Risk Score and long-term mortality with the transcatheter aortic valve implantation procedure. *Kardiologia Polska* **2021**, *79*, 1215–1222. [CrossRef]
29. Matusik, P.T. Biomarkers and Cardiovascular Risk Stratification. *Eur. Heart J.* **2019**, *40*, 1483–1485. [CrossRef]
30. Okólska, M.; Skubera, M.; Matusik, P.; Płazak, W.; Pająk, J.; Róg, B.; Podolec, P.; Tomkiewicz-Pająk, L. Chronotropic incompetence causes multiple organ complications in adults after the Fontan procedure. *Kardiologia Polska* **2021**, *79*, 410–417. [CrossRef]
31. Okólska, M.; Łach, J.; Matusik, P.T.; Pająk, J.; Mroczek, T.; Podolec, P.; Tomkiewicz-Pająk, L. Heart Rate Variability and Its Associations with Organ Complications in Adults after Fontan Operation. *J. Clin. Med.* **2021**, *10*, 4492. [CrossRef]
32. Tsai, C.-F.; Chuang, Y.-T.; Huang, J.-Y.; Ueng, K.-C. Long-Term Prognosis of Febrile Individuals with Right Precordial Coved-Type ST-Segment Elevation Brugada Pattern: A 10-Year Prospective Follow-Up Study. *J. Clin. Med.* **2021**, *10*, 4997. [CrossRef] [PubMed]
33. Matusik, P.T.; Leśniak, W.J.; Heleniak, Z.; Undas, A. Thromboembolism and bleeding in patients with atrial fibrillation and stage 4 chronic kidney disease: Impact of biomarkers. *Kardiologia Polska* **2021**, *79*, 1086–1092. [CrossRef] [PubMed]
34. Rayner, B.L.; Goodman, H.; Opie, L.H. The chest radiographA useful investigation in the evaluation of hypertensive patients. *Am. J. Hypertens.* **2004**, *17*, 507–510. [CrossRef]
35. Buba, F.; Okeahialam, B.; Anjorin, C. The Value of Chest Radiogram and Electrocardiogram in the Assessment of Left Ventricular Hypertrophy among Adult Hypertensives. *J. Med. Sci.* **2008**, *8*, 298–301. [CrossRef]
36. Truszkiewicz, K.; Poręba, R.; Gać, P. Radiological Cardiothoracic Ratio in Evidence-Based Medicine. *J. Clin. Med.* **2021**, *10*, 2016. [CrossRef] [PubMed]
37. Libby, P.; Bonow, R.O.; Mann, D.L.; Tomaselli, G.F.; Bhatt, D.; Solomon, S.D.; Braunwald, E. Braunwald's Heart Disease. In *A Textbook of Cardiovascular Medicine*; Elsevier: Philadelphia, PA, USA, 2021.
38. Okute, Y.; Shoji, T.; Hayashi, T.; Kuwamura, Y.; Sonoda, M.; Mori, K.; Shioi, A.; Tsujimoto, Y.; Tabata, T.; Emoto, M.; et al. Cardiothoracic Ratio as a Predictor of Cardiovascular Events in a Cohort of Hemodialysis Patients. *J. Atheroscler. Thromb.* **2017**, *24*, 412–421. [CrossRef]
39. Perez, A.A.; Ribeiro, A.L.P.; Barros, M.V.L.; De Sousa, M.R.; Bittencourt, R.J.; Machado, F.S.; Rocha, M.O.C. Value of the radiological study of the thorax for diagnosing left ventricular dysfunction in Chagas' disease. *Arq. Bras. de Cardiol.* **2003**, *80*, 208–213. [CrossRef]
40. Grotenhuis, H.B.; Zhou, C.; Tomlinson, G.; Isaac, K.V.; Seed, M.; Grosse-Wortmann, L.; Yoo, S.-H. Cardiothoracic ratio on chest radiograph in pediatric heart disease: How does it correlate with heart volumes at magnetic resonance imaging? *Pediatr. Radiol.* **2015**, *45*, 1616–1623. [CrossRef]
41. Fukuta, H.; Little, W.C. Contribution of Systolic and Diastolic Abnormalities to Heart Failure with a Normal and a Reduced Ejection Fraction. *Prog. Cardiovasc. Dis.* **2007**, *49*, 229–240. [CrossRef]
42. Truszkiewicz, K.; Poręba, M.; Poręba, R.; Gać, P. Radiological Cardiothoracic Ratio as a Potential Predictor of Right Ventricular Enlargement in Patients with Suspected Pulmonary Embolism Due to COVID-19. *J. Clin. Med.* **2021**, *10*, 5703. [CrossRef]
43. Ribeiro, S.M.; Morceli, J.; Gonçalves, R.S.; da Silva Franco, R.J.; Habermann, F.; Meira, D.A.; Matsubara, B.B. Accuracy of chest radiography plus electrocardiogram in diagnosis of hypertrophy in hypertension. *Arq. Bras. Cardiol.* **2012**, *99*, 825–833. [CrossRef] [PubMed]
44. Screaton, N. The cardiothoracic ratio—An inaccurate and outdated measurement: New data from CT. *Eur. Radiol.* **2010**, *20*, 1597–1598. [CrossRef] [PubMed]
45. Simkus, P.; Gimeno, M.G.; Banisauskaite, A.; Noreikaite, J.; McCreavy, D.; Penha, D.; Arzanauskaite, M. Limitations of cardiothoracic ratio derived from chest radiographs to predict real heart size: Comparison with magnetic resonance imaging. *Insights Imaging* **2021**, *12*, 158. [CrossRef] [PubMed]
46. Schlett, C.L.; Kwait, D.C.; Mahabadi, A.A.; Bamberg, F.; O'Donnell, C.J.; Fox, C.S.; Hoffmann, U. Simple area-based measurement for multidetector computed tomography to predict left ventricular size. *Eur. Radiol.* **2010**, *20*, 1590–1596. [CrossRef] [PubMed]
47. Gradman, A.H.; Alfayoumi, F. From Left Ventricular Hypertrophy to Congestive Heart Failure: Management of Hypertensive Heart Disease. *Prog. Cardiovasc. Dis.* **2006**, *48*, 326–341. [CrossRef] [PubMed]
48. Heinzel, F.R.; Hohendanner, F.; Jin, G.; Sedej, S.; Edelmann, F. Myocardial hypertrophy and its role in heart failure with preserved ejection fraction. *J. Appl. Physiol.* **2015**, *119*, 1233–1242. [CrossRef] [PubMed]
49. Cuspidi, C.; Meani, S.; Sala, C.; Valerio, C.; Negri, F.; Mancia, G. Age related prevalence of severe left ventricular hypertrophy in essential hypertension: Echocardiographic findings from the ETODH study. *Blood Press.* **2012**, *21*, 139–145. [CrossRef]
50. Herman, C. What makes a screening exam "good"? *Virtual Mentor* **2006**, *8*, 34–37.
51. Papadakis, M.; Carre, F.; Kervio, G.; Rawlins, J.; Panoulas, V.F.; Chandra, N.; Basavarajaiah, S.; Carby, L.; Fonseca, T.; Sharma, S. The prevalence, distribution, and clinical outcomes of electrocardiographic repolarization patterns in male athletes of African/Afro-Caribbean origin. *Eur. Heart J.* **2011**, *32*, 2304–2313. [CrossRef]
52. Kwon, J.; Lee, S.Y.; Jeon, K.; Lee, Y.; Kim, K.; Park, J.; Oh, B.; Lee, M. Deep Learning–Based Algorithm for Detecting Aortic Stenosis Using Electrocardiography. *J. Am. Heart Assoc.* **2020**, *9*, e014717. [CrossRef]

53. Mont, L.; Pelliccia, A.; Sharma, S.; Biffi, A.; Borjesson, M.; Terradellas, J.B.; Carré, F.; Guasch, E.; Heidbuchel, H.; La Gerche, A.; et al. Pre-participation cardiovascular evaluation for athletic participants to prevent sudden death: Position paper from the EHRA and the EACPR, branches of the ESC. Endorsed by APHRS, HRS, and SOLAECE. *Eur. J. Prev. Cardiol.* **2016**, *24*, 41–69. [CrossRef] [PubMed]
54. Augustine, D.X.; Howard, L. Left Ventricular Hypertrophy in Athletes: Differentiating Physiology from Pathology. *Curr. Treat. Options Cardiovasc. Med.* **2018**, *20*, 96. [CrossRef] [PubMed]
55. Petersen, S.E.; Selvanayagam, J.B.; Francis, J.M.; Myerson, S.G.; Wiesmann, F.; Robson, M.D.; Östman-Smith, I.; Casadei, B.; Watkins, H.; Neubauer, S. Differentiation of athlete's heart from pathological forms of cardiac hypertrophy by means of geometric indices derived from cardiovascular magnetic resonance. *J. Cardiovasc. Magn. Reson.* **2005**, *7*, 551–558. [CrossRef] [PubMed]
56. Dweck, M.; Joshi, S.; Murigu, T.; Alpendurada, F.; Jabbour, A.; Melina, G.; Banya, W.; Gulati, A.; Roussin, I.; Raza, S.; et al. Midwall Fibrosis Is an Independent Predictor of Mortality in Patients with Aortic Stenosis. *J. Am. Coll. Cardiol.* **2011**, *58*, 1271–1279. [CrossRef] [PubMed]
57. Tanaka, K.; Tanaka, F.; Onoda, T.; Tanno, K.; Ohsawa, M.; Sakata, K.; Omama, S.; Ogasawara, K.; Ishibashi, Y.; Itai, K.; et al. Prognostic Value of Electrocardiographic Left Ventricular Hypertrophy on Cardiovascular Risk in a Non-Hypertensive Community-Based Population. *Am. J. Hypertens.* **2018**, *31*, 895–901. [CrossRef]
58. D'Agostino Sr, R.B.; Vasan, R.S.; Pencina, M.J.; Wolf, P.A.; Cobain, M.; Massaro, J.M.; Kannel, W.B. General cardiovascular risk profile for use in primary care: The Framingham Heart Study. *Circulation* **2008**, *117*, 743–753. [CrossRef]

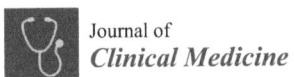

Article

Combined Effects of Age and Comorbidities on Electrocardiographic Parameters in a Large Non-Selected Population

Paolo Giovanardi [1,2,*], Cecilia Vernia [3], Enrico Tincani [4], Claudio Giberti [5], Federico Silipo [6] and Andrea Fabbo [7]

1. Cardiology Service, Department of Primary Care, Health Authority and Services of Modena, 41124 Modena, Italy
2. Cardiology Unit, Ospedale S. Agostino–Estense, Azienda Ospedaliero-Universitaria Modena, 41126 Baggiovara, Italy
3. Department of Physics, Informatic and Mathematics, University of Modena and Reggio Emilia, 41125 Modena, Italy; cecilia.vernia@unimore.it
4. Internal Medicine Division, Ospedale S. Agostino–Estense, Azienda Ospedaliero-Universitaria Modena, 41126 Baggiovara, Italy; tincani.enrico@aou.mo.it
5. Department of Sciences and Methods for Engineering, University of Modena and Reggio Emilia, 42122 Reggio Emilia, Italy; claudio.giberti@unimore.it
6. Department of Clinical Engineering, Health Authority and Services and Azienda Ospedaliero-Universitaria Modena, 41124 Modena, Italy; f.silipo@ausl.mo.it
7. Geriatric Service—Cognitive Disorders and Dementia, Department of Primary Care, Health Authority and Services of Modena, 41124 Modena, Italy; a.fabbo@ausl.mo.it
* Correspondence: p.giovanardi@ausl.mo.it; Tel.: +39-059-437411 or +39-059-3961111; Fax: +39-0536-886684

Citation: Giovanardi, P.; Vernia, C.; Tincani, E.; Giberti, C.; Silipo, F.; Fabbo, A. Combined Effects of Age and Comorbidities on Electrocardiographic Parameters in a Large Non-Selected Population. *J. Clin. Med.* **2022**, *11*, 3737. https://doi.org/10.3390/jcm11133737

Academic Editors: Christian Sohns and Paweł T. Matusik

Received: 29 April 2022
Accepted: 24 June 2022
Published: 28 June 2022

Publisher's Note: MDPI stays neutral with regard to jurisdictional claims in published maps and institutional affiliations.

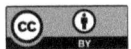

Copyright: © 2022 by the authors. Licensee MDPI, Basel, Switzerland. This article is an open access article distributed under the terms and conditions of the Creative Commons Attribution (CC BY) license (https://creativecommons.org/licenses/by/4.0/).

Abstract: Background: Previous studies have evaluated average electrocardiographic (ECG) values in healthy subjects or specific subpopulations. However, none have evaluated ECG average values in not selected populations, so we examined ECG changes with respect to age and sex in a large primary population. Methods: From digitized ECG stored from 2008 to 2021 in the Modena province, 130,471 patients were enrolled. Heart rate, P, QRS and T wave axis, P, QRS and T wave duration, PR interval, QTc, and frontal QRS-T angle were evaluated. Results: All ECG parameters showed a dependence on age, but only some of them with a straight-line correlation: QRS axis ($p < 0.001$, $R^2 = 0.991$, $r = 0.996$), PR interval ($p < 0.001$, $R^2 = 0.978$, $r = 0.989$), QTc ($p < 0.001$, $R^2 = 0.935$, $r = 0.967$), and, in over 51.5 years old, QRS-T angle ($p < 0.001$, $R^2 = 0.979$, $r = 0.956$). Differences between females and males and in different clinical settings were observed. Conclusions: ECG changes with ageing are explainable by intrinsic modifications of the heart and thorax and with the appearance of cardiovascular diseases and comorbidities. Age-related reference values were computed and applicable in clinical practice. Significant deviations from mean values and from Z-scores should be investigated.

Keywords: electrocardiogram; ECG; electrocardiography; Z scores; ageing; reference values; QRS-T angle; PR interval; QT corrected; heart axis

1. Introduction

The Electrocardiogram (ECG) is an inexpensive and non-invasive diagnostic technique used worldwide for the management of acute and chronic cardiovascular and not cardiovascular diseases; ECG is considered an outdated investigation but nowadays many clinical decisions are still based on ECG interpretation.

Many years ago, normal ECG values were established [1], and previous studies have evaluated average ECG values in specific subpopulations, such as healthy subjects [2], athletes [3], females [4], young [5] and elderly people [6], showing that ECG values should be corrected for age [7] and ethnicity [8,9]. To our knowledge, none of the previous studies have evaluated ECG average values in a large non-selected population with cardiovascular diseases and with comorbidities.

Moreover, the use of digitized programs for automated ECG interpretation has demonstrated a good accuracy and a favorable cost–benefit analysis.

Therefore, this cross-sectional observational study was designed to analyze the effect of age and sex on an extensive set of ECG parameters (heart axis, waves duration, times of conduction and repolarization, frontal QRS-T angle) in a large contemporary primary population.

2. Material and Methods

2.1. Study Design

A retrospective review of digitized ECGs recorded was made within the province of Modena from January 2008 to September 2021, together with retrospective clinical data collection. The study was performed in accordance with the Ethical Standards of the 1975 Helsinki Declaration revised in 2013 and was approved by the local Ethic Committee of Modena (AVEN) with protocol number 2605/2021, date of approval 21 September 2021.

2.2. Study Population

The province of Modena, located in central Emilia-Romagna, Italy, has a population of 702,549 people (www.provincia.modena.it, accessed on 30 September 2021) spread across 47 municipalities.

National health general practitioners refer their patients to national health system core facilities for clinical tests; ECGs are recorded in Emergency Departments, surgical and medical Hospital Units, and in- and out-of-hospital Ambulatories.

All patients with a digitized ECG archived in any facility within the Province of Modena were eligible.

2.3. ECG Recording and Inclusion–Exclusion Criteria

ECGs were recorded at rest in the supine position using a standard 12-lead tracing at 25 mm/s speed, 10 mm/mV amplitude, with a sampling rate of at least 500 Hz and were archived into a "MUSE®" electronic archive (GE Marquette Healthcare, Milwaukee, WI, USA).

Automated analysis was performed through a digitized multi-channel computer-assisted program (GE 12SL ECG Analysis), which uses validated algorithms for ECG parameters measurement. ECG diagnoses were confirmed by trained cardiologists.

ECGs were discarded when incomplete or had a bad signal quality, waveform recognition errors, or electrode interchanges. ECGs were also discarded in patients with pacemaker or implantable cardioverter-defibrillator, with complete or incomplete left or right bundle-branch block, with atrial fibrillation or atrial flutter, with supraventricular tachycardia, Wolff–Parkinson–White syndrome and second- or third-degree atrioventricular block. ECGs of pediatric patients (up to 15 years of age) and of very old people (more than 90 years of age) were also excluded.

In the case of patients with multiple ECGs archived in the dataset, only the first one was included. ECGs were then separated into three groups according to the facility where they were recorded.

2.4. Clinical Data

For the enrolled patients, age, sex, demographic data, cardiovascular risk factors, and comorbidities were retrospectively collected from in- and out-of-hospital databases. Diabetes was defined as a group of metabolic disorders characterized by hyperglycemia resulting from defects in insulin secretion, insulin action, or both. Systemic arterial hypertension was defined as the increase of systolic blood pressure equal to or above 140 mmHg and/or a diastolic blood pressure equal to or above 90 mmHg. Dyslipidemia was defined as a disorder in lipoprotein metabolism resulting in elevation of the blood concentration of cholesterol and/or triglycerides and tobacco smoke as the active exposure to tobacco products. Heart failure was defined as a syndrome with symptoms and or signs caused by structural and/or functional cardiac abnormalities. Coronary artery diseases were defined as a group of diseases characterized by the reduction of blood flow to the heart muscle because of a partial or complete blockage of the coronary arteries. Stroke was defined as a neurological deficit of cerebrovascular cause. Chronic obstructive pulmonary disease was defined as a chronic inflammatory lung disease that causes obstructed airflow. Dementia was defined as the chronic deterioration in cognitive function not expected from the usual consequences of biological aging. Cancer was defined as a large group of diseases starting in any organ or tissue of the body when abnormal cells grow uncontrollably and can invade other parts of the body. Chronic kidney disease was defined as a kidney damage or glomerular filtration rate <60 mL/min/1.73 m^2 for more than three months.

2.5. ECG Parameters

The following parameters were extracted from the MUSE® electronic archive [10,11]:
- Heart rate.
- P, QRS, and T wave axes were recorded from peak amplitudes in the extremity leads.
- P and T wave durations were calculated through the mean of the 12 ECG leads.
- PR interval was defined as the time between the beginning of atrial depolarization to the onset of ventricular depolarization and was measured through the mean of the 12 ECG leads. Prolonged PR interval, or first-degree atrioventricular block, was defined by an interval greater than 212 milliseconds (ms) [10].
- QRS complex duration was established through the mean of the 12 ECG leads.
- QT interval was defined as the time between the beginning of ventricular depolarization and the end of ventricular repolarization measuring the mean of the 12 leads. QT corrected (QTc) was established through Bazett's correction and a prolonged QTc was defined by an interval greater than 457 ms [10].
- Frontal QRS-T angle was calculated as the absolute difference in value between the frontal plane QRS and T wave axes. If the difference between the QRS and T wave axes was greater than 180 degrees (deg) the resultant QRS-T angle would be calculated as 360 deg minus the absolute angle to obtain a value between 0 deg and 180 deg [12,13].

ECG data were transferred into an Excel file and statistical analysis was performed.

2.6. Statistical Analysis

Continuous variables are displayed as mean ± standard deviation, while categorical data are displayed as frequencies. A two-tailed p-value ≤ 0.05 was considered statistically significant, with a 95% confidence interval.

The mean values ± standard deviation of the ECG parameters together with -2 and $+2$ Z-scores in the whole population and in the three groups (Emergency Departments, Hospital Units, and in- and out-of-hospital Ambulatories) were computed. The ANOVA test to check the hypothesis that the three groups came from populations with the same mean against the alternative hypothesis that the population means were not all the same was performed. T-test (or Wilcoxon test in the case of not-normal data) was used to check the same null hypothesis for pairs of subgroup data.

The difference of means between males and females in the whole population was analyzed through the t-test.

To investigate the null hypothesis of independence of ECG parameters from age, a chi-square test was performed. Regression analysis was used to assess the linear dependence of ECG parameters on age and the coefficient of determination R^2 was used to determine the best linear fit. Pearson's correlation coefficient (r) values were also given.

For the significant parameters at linear regression analysis, mean values and -2 and $+2$ Z-scores (corresponding to 2.3rd and 97.7th percentiles) were tabulated according to 15 age categories (5 years each, from 15 to 90 years old). The moving mean values over a sliding 5-year window, together with the standard deviations over the same moving windows, were calculated. Analyses were performed with MATLAB (R 2021 b).

3. Results

3.1. Population Data

From January 2008 to September 2021, 309,405 ECGs were archived in the MUSE® electronic archive in the national health system facilities of Modena. Of these, after exclusions, 130,471 patients were enrolled. The Emergency Department group was composed of 29,560 patients, the Hospital Units group of 85,239 patients, and the Ambulatory group of 15,672 patients (baseline characteristics of the study population and exclusion criteria are shown in Table 1). The database comprised 1,565,652 data points.

Table 1. Baseline characteristics of the study population and exclusion criteria.

Clinical Characteristics of the Enrolled Patients:		Exclusion Criteria:	
Enrolled patients §	130,471	Incorrect or incomplete ECG §	2826
Men §	63,261 (48.5%)	Bad signals qualities ECG §	26,659
Women §	67,210 (51.5%)	Young and very old people §	12,902
Mean age at enrollment date (years) *	56.8 ± 19.4	Multiple ECG §	89,870
Emergency Departments group §	29,560	Atrial fibrillation §	10,245
Men §	14,658 (49.6%)	Atrial flutter §	1957
Women §	14,902 (50.4%)	Supraventricular tachycardia §	3721
Surgical/Medical Units group §	85,239	Wolff-Parkinson-White §	434
Men §	41,519 (48.7%)	Bundle branch block §	19,660
Women §	43,720 (51.3%)	Pacemaker or implantable cardioverter-defibrillator §	8670
Ambulatory group §	15,672	Second-degree AV block §	1698
Men §	7084 (45.2%)	Third-degree AV block §	292
Women §	8588 (54.8%)	Excluded patients §	178,934

§ Number of patients, % percent of patients, * Mean ± standard deviation.

The prevalence of cardiovascular risk factors in the study population according to age (15–54 years vs. 55–90 years) were: diabetes 3.3% vs. 16.3%, hypertension 9.6% vs. 38.2%, dyslipidemia 17.6% vs. 36.4%, and tobacco smoke 18.1% vs. 3.9%, respectively.

The prevalence of cardiovascular diseases and comorbidities in the study population according to age (15–54 years vs. 55–90 years) were: cardiovascular diseases 3.3% vs. 18.2%, cerebrovascular diseases 0.9% vs. 9.4%, chronic obstructive pulmonary diseases 7.5% vs. 15.9%, dementia 0.3% vs. 5.1%, cancer 4.9% vs. 19%, and chronic kidney disease 0.8% vs. 8.2%, respectively.

Figure 1 shows the age distribution of the enrolled patients, while Table 2 shows average ECG values and Z-scores in the whole population and in the Emergency Department, Hospital Units, and in- and out-of-hospital Ambulatories groups.

3.2. ECG Analysis

The effects of age, sex, and of the different facilities on the considered ECG parameters were:

- Heart rate significantly increased with ageing, without a linear correlation ($p < 0.001$, $R^2 = 0.06$, r= -0.246, Figure 2a). Females had greater heart rate than males (74.6 ± 14.3 beats per minute (bpm) vs. 70.9 ± 14.6 bpm, respectively, $p < 0.001$, Figure 3a). Heart rate was greater in the Emergency Department group (Table 2).

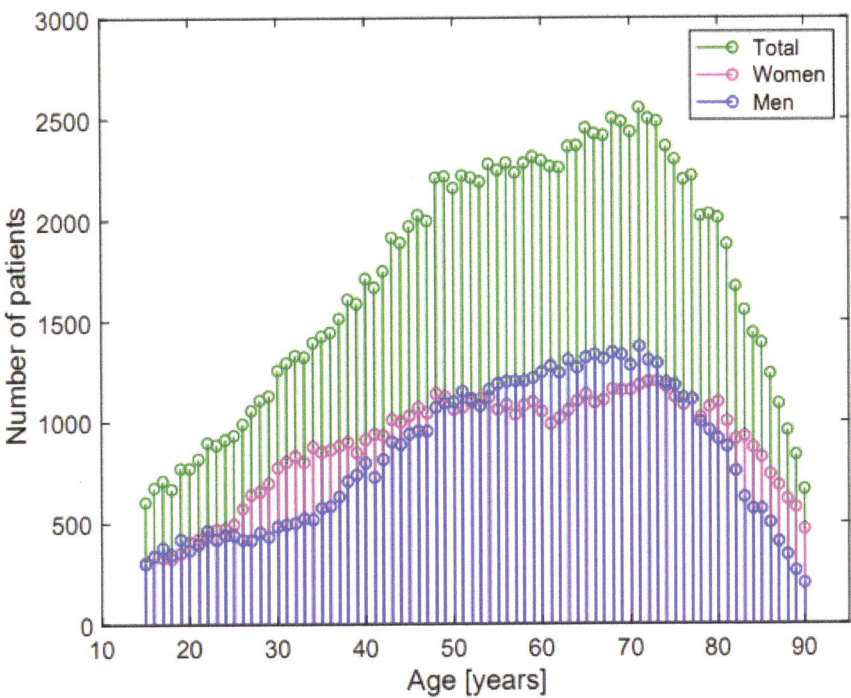

Figure 1. Age-distribution of the study population.

Table 2. Mean ECG values and Z-scores −2 and +2 in the study population and in the three groups.

	Study Population 130,471 Patients		Emergency Department Group 29,560 Patients		Hospital Units Group 85,239 Patients		Ambulatory Group 15,672 Patients		
	Mean ± sd *		Mean ± sd *		Mean ± sd *		Mean ± sd *		
	Z Scores −2	Z Scores +2	Z Scores −2	Z Scores +2	Z Scores −2	Z Scores +2	Z Scores −2	Z Scores +2	p-Value
Heart rate (bpm °)	72.8 ± 14.5		76.9 ± 16.7		72.1 ± 13.8		69.0 ± 12.0		<0.001
	50	108	50	116	50	105	49	97	
P wave axis (deg ˆ)	50.2 ± 22.4		53.8 ± 22.0		49.4 ± 22.5		48.2 ± 22.1		<0.001
	−2	85	2	86	−3	85	−2	82	
QRS axis (deg ˆ)	27.8 ± 39.3		34.5 ± 41.0		25.0 ± 39.2		30.1 ± 35.2		0.033
	−51	89	−52	93	−51	88	−43	86	
T wave axis (deg ˆ)	41.9 ± 31.8		45.7 ± 32.4		41.4 ± 32.9		37.7 ± 23.0		<0.001
	−14	110	−14.6	111	−15	116	−5	77	
P wave duration (ms #)	98.3 ± 19.6		100.0 ± 19.9		98.1 ± 19.7		96.6 ± 18.0		<0.001
	52	130	52	132	52	128	54	126	
QRS duration (ms #)	89.5 ± 13.3		90.1 ± 13.5		89.6 ± 13.5		87.7 ± 11.6		<0.001
	70	118	70	120	70	120	68	112	
T wave duration (ms #)	189.1 ± 40.0		187.9 ± 41.3		189.1 ± 40.7		191.4 ± 32.7		<0.001
	58	246	58	250	54	248	92	238	
PR interval (ms #)	155.7 ± 27.6		156.6 ± 28.1		156.1 ± 27.9		152.2 ± 24.8		0.302
	112	220	114	222	112	222	112	208	
QTc interval (ms #)	430.1 ± 29.0		435.7 ± 29.0		429.8 ± 29.4		421.0 ± 23.8		<0.001
	379	492	384	496	379	494	374	468	
Frontal QRS-T angle (deg ˆ)	32.1 ± 31.9		32.6 ± 33.1		33.0 ± 32.6		26.4 ± 24.2		0.073
	1	131	1	135	1	135	1	94	

* mean ± standard deviation, ° beats per minute, ˆ degrees, # millisecond.

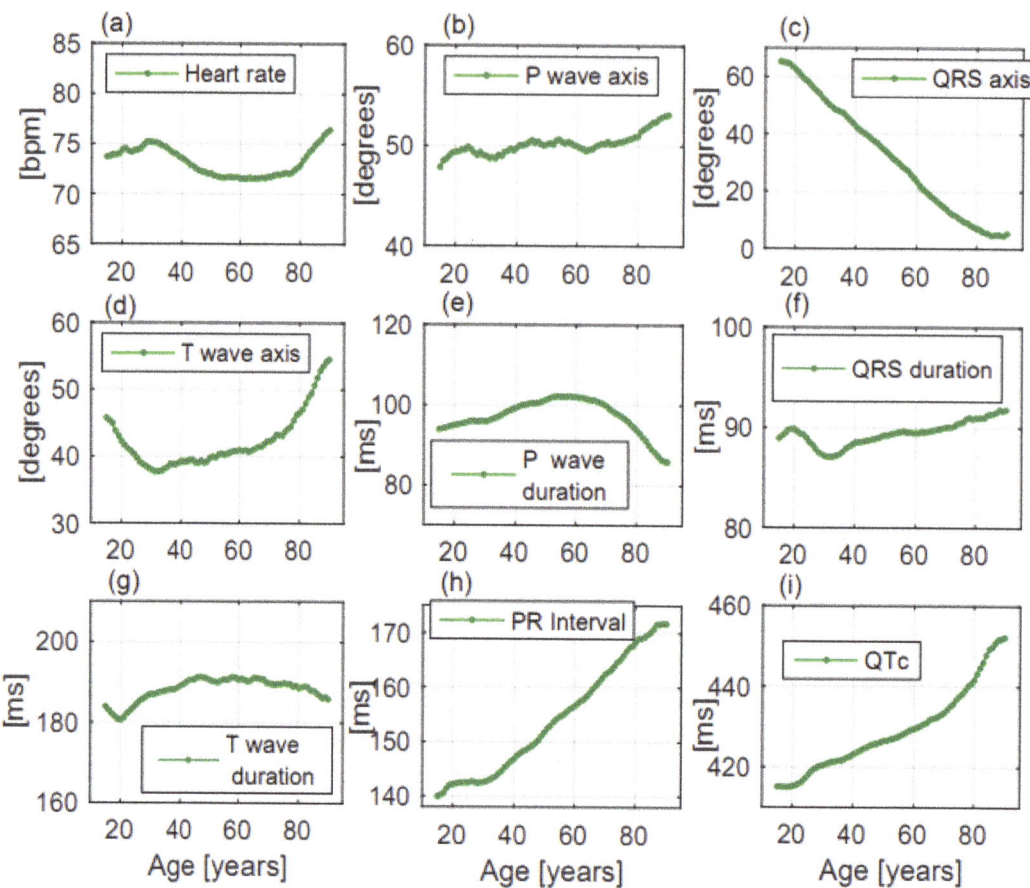

Figure 2. ECG changes with ageing of the considered parameters in the enrolled population. All the parameters (**a**–**i**) changed with ageing but only QRS axis (**c**), PR interval (**h**), and QTc (**i**) presented a linear change with increasing age.

- P wave axis slightly but significantly turned to the right, without a linear correlation ($p < 0.001$, $R^2 = 0.692$, $r = 0.832$, Figure 2b). Females had greater values than males (50.8 ± 22.2 deg vs. 49.6 ± 22.6 deg, respectively, $p = 0.014$, Figure 3b). P wave axis turned to the right mainly in the Emergency Department facility (Table 2).
- QRS axis with a straight-line correlation turned to the left ($p < 0.001$, $R^2 = 0.991$, $r = -0.996$, Figure 2c). Differences between females and males were not statistically significant (30.8 ± 37.1 deg vs. 24.5 ± 41.3 deg, respectively, $p = 0.177$, Figure 3c). A greater shift to the left was evident in the Hospital Units group (Table 2).
- T wave axis significantly turned to the right ($p < 0.001$, $R^2 = 0.419$, $r = 0.648$, Figure 2d), but without a linear correlation. No significant differences between females and males were observed (42.6 ± 31.1 deg vs. 41.2 ± 32.6 deg, respectively, $p = 0.819$, Figure 3d). T wave shifted to the right mainly in the Emergency Department group (Table 2).

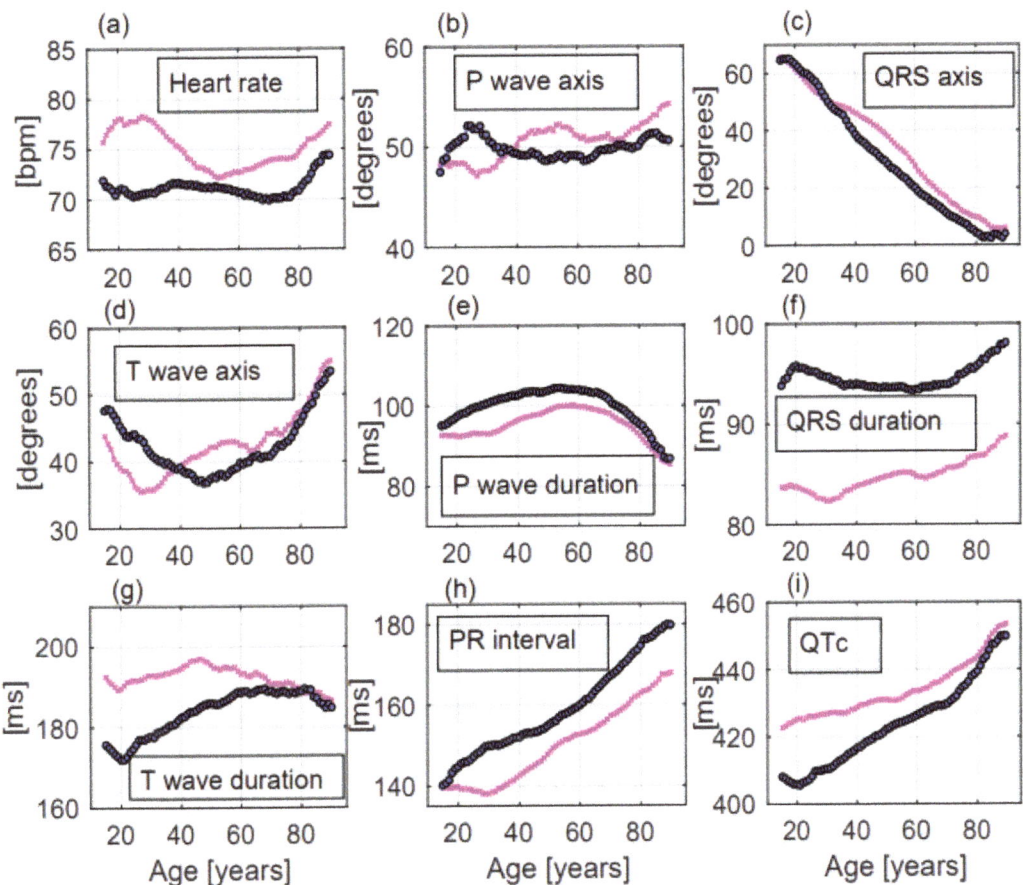

Figure 3. ECG changes with ageing of the considered parameters in females—and in males—Significant differences between females and males were observed for most of the ECG parameters (**a–i**). Especially heart rate and QTc were significantly greater in females (**a,i**) while QRS duration and PR interval were significantly greater in males (**f,h**).

- P wave duration increased with ageing without a linear correlation ($p < 0.001$, $R^2 = 0.051$, $r = -0.227$, Figure 2e). p duration was lower in females with respect to males (95.9 ± 19.1 ms vs. 100.9 ± 19.8 ms, respectively, $p < 0.001$, Figure 3e). Greater P waves were observed in the Emergency Department group (Table 2).
- QRS duration significantly increased with ageing ($p = 0.001$, $R^2 = 0.608$, $r = 0.78$, Figure 2f), but without a linear correlation. QRS was shorter in females than in males along all ages (84.9 ± 11.4 ms vs. 94.3 ± 13.5 ms, respectively, $p < 0.001$, Figure 3f). Greater QRS values were recorded in the Emergency Department group (Table 2).
- T wave duration significantly changed with ageing, without a linear correlation ($p < 0.001$, $R^2 = 0.302$, $r = 0.55$, Figure 2g). T wave duration was greater in females with respect to males (192.6 ± 43.9 ms vs. 185.5 ± 35.0 ms, respectively, $p < 0.001$, Figure 3g). Greater T waves were observed in the Ambulatory group (Table 2).
- PR interval increased with a straight-line correlation with ageing ($p < 0.001$, $R^2 = 0.978$, $r = 0.989$, Figure 2h). PR was shorter in females with respect to males along all ages (151.1 ± 25.9 ms vs. 160.5 ± 28.6 ms, respectively, $p < 0.001$, Figure 3h). No significant differences among the three groups were observed (Table 2).

- QTc increased with a straight-line correlation ($p < 0.001$, $R^2 = 0.935$, $r = 0.967$, Figure 2i). Females had longer QTc values with respect to males (434.6 ± 27.7 ms vs. 425.4 ± 29.5 ms, respectively, $p < 0.001$, Figure 3i) but with increasing age the differences became null. QTc values were greater in the Emergency Department group (Table 2).
- Frontal QRS-T angle increased without a linear correlation ($p < 0.001$, $R^2 = 0.717$, $r = 0.847$, Figure 4a) but when the analysis was performed including only patients older than 51.5 years, QRS-T angle revealed a straight-line correlation with ageing ($p < 0.001$, $R^2 = 0.979$, $r = 0.956$, Figure 4b). No significant differences between females and males (30.8 ± 30.6 deg vs. 33.5 ± 33.1 deg, respectively, $p = 0.203$, Figure 4c) and between the three groups were observed (Table 2). The proportion of patients with a QRS-T angle greater than 90 deg rapidly increased among patients older than 51.5 years (Figure 4d).

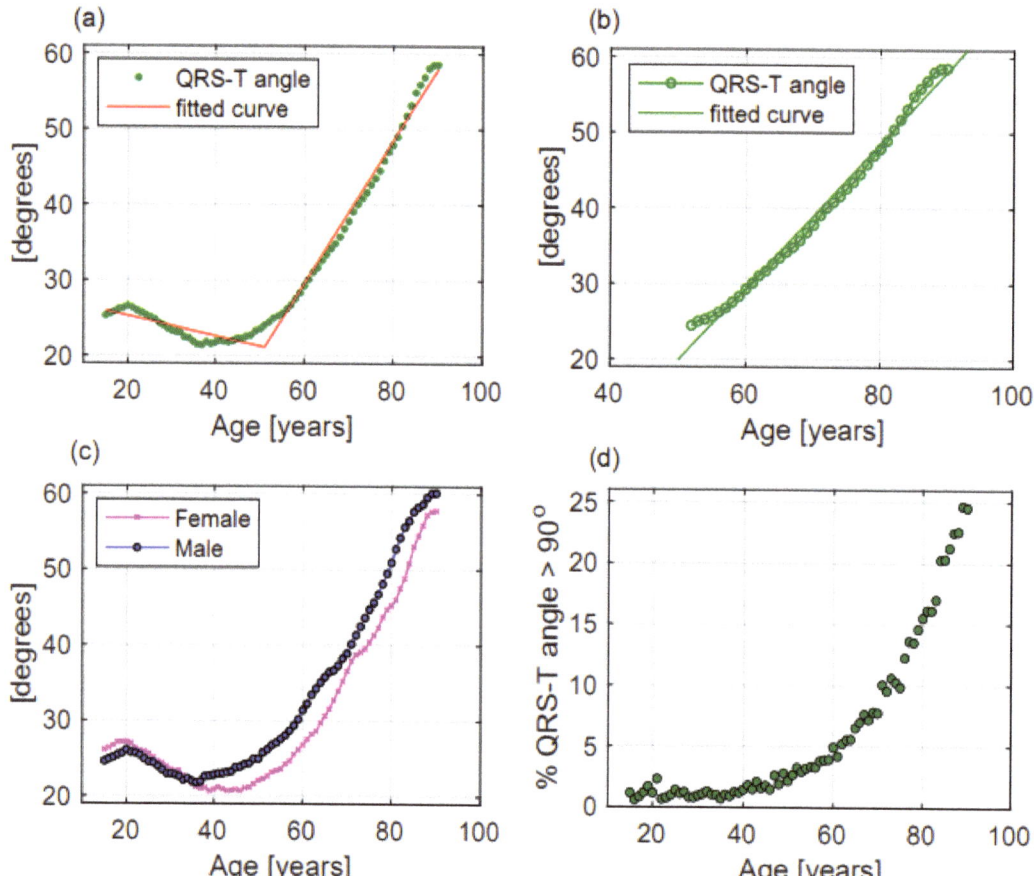

Figure 4. QRS-T angle modifications with ageing in the whole population (**a**), in patients older than 51.5 years (**b**), in females and males (**c**); and (**d**) percentage of patients with QRS-T angle greater than 90 deg according to age. In panels (**a**–**c**) dots represent mean values of QRS-T angle while in panel (**d**) green dots represent the percentage of patients with a QRS-T angle greater than 90 deg. In panels (**a**,**b**) lines represent the fitted curve.

Tables 3 and 4. show, respectively, the mean values ± standard deviation and Z-scores −2 and +2 (computed in 15 age categories of 5 years each) of parameters with a linear correlation with ageing and of frontal QRS-T angle in the whole population, in males and females.

Table 3. Mean ECG values, computed in 15 age categories of 5 years each, of the parameters with a straight-line correlation with age and mean QRS-T angle values. For each age category, in the upper line, means ± standard deviation in the whole population; in the bottom line, means ± standard deviation in males and females.

Age (Years)	QRS Axis * (deg ˆ)		PR Interval * (ms #)		QTc Interval * (ms #)		QRS-T Angle * (deg ˆ)	
	Men *	Women *	Men *	Women *	Men *	Women *	Men *	Women *
15–19	64.9 ± 24.7		140.7 ± 20.8		415.1 ± 26.2		25.9 ± 19.4	
	65.2 ± 26.2	64.6 ± 23.0	141.7 ± 20.0	139.5 ± 21.6	406.7 ± 25.3	424.0 ± 24.4	25.1 ± 18.9	26.7 ± 19.8
20–24	60.1 ± 26.7		142.5 ± 20.4		416.0 ± 26.1		26.0 ± 20.0	
	61.1 ± 28.4	59.2 ± 25.0	145.9 ± 20.8	139.3 ± 19.6	406.4 ± 26.0	425.1 ± 22.9	25.7 ± 20.1	26.3 ± 19.9
25–29	54.9 ± 27.5		142.6 ± 20.6		419.6 ± 25.0		24.3 ± 19.1	
	57.0 ± 28.9	53.4 ± 26.4	148.4 ± 21.2	138.6 ± 19.2	409.9 ± 24.9	426.5 ± 22.6	23.9 ± 18.9	24.6 ± 19.2
30–34	49.5 ± 28.7		143.1 ± 21.1		421.1 ± 24.6		23.1 ± 19.3	
	48.7 ± 31.3	49.9 ± 27.1	150.2 ± 20.7	138.7 ± 20.1	411.3 ± 24.5	427.2 ± 22.6	22.6 ± 20.1	23.3 ± 18.8
35–39	45.9 ± 29.7		145.5 ± 21.4		422.0 ± 24.0		21.4 ± 18.8	
	43.2 ± 32.0	47.9 ± 27.8	151.3 ± 21.6	141.1 ± 20.2	414.8 ± 24.6	427.4 ± 22.0	21.9 ± 20.1	21.0 ± 17.6
40–44	40.9 ± 32.0		148.0 ± 20.4		424.1 ± 26.0		21.9 ± 21.5	
	36.3 ± 33.4	44.8 ± 30.2	152.9 ± 20.4	143.8 ± 19.5	417.7 ± 25.0	429.6 ± 25.5	23.0 ± 23.4	20.9 ± 19.7
45–49	37.0 ± 33.5		149.9 ± 21.2		425.8 ± 25.4		22.6 ± 22.8	
	32.0 ± 35.1	41.5 ± 31.3	153.9 ± 20.8	146.2 ± 20.8	420.3 ± 25.5	430.9 ± 24.1	24.2 ± 24.8	21.1 ± 20.6
50–54	31.6 ± 33.8		153.0 ± 21.6		427.0 ± 25.3		24.4 ± 24.6	
	26.9 ± 34.8	36.5 ± 32.1	156.0 ± 21.4	150.0 ± 21.5	423.2 ± 26.0	430.8 ± 24.1	26.2 ± 26.1	22.6 ± 22.9
55–59	27.2 ± 35.1		155.4 ± 22.8		428.5 ± 26.1		26.8 ± 26.9	
	23.1 ± 36.4	31.9 ± 33.0	158.5 ± 23.4	151.9 ± 21.4	424.9 ± 26.6	432.6 ± 24.9	28.7 ± 28.4	24.6 ± 24.8
60–64	20.9 ± 35.6		157.6 ± 24.7		430.3 ± 26.7		31.1 ± 30.3	
	17.7 ± 37.4	24.7 ± 32.9	161.3 ± 25.6	153.1 ± 22.7	427.1 ± 26.9	434.1 ± 25.9	33.5 ± 32.5	28.2 ± 27.2
65–69	16.4 ± 37.3		160.5 ± 26.8		432.3 ± 27.1		34.9 ± 32.8	
	13.9 ± 39.6	19.3 ± 34.2	164.9 ± 28.0	155.3 ± 24.2	429.1 ± 28.3	436.1 ± 25.1	36.7 ± 34.0	32.7 ± 31.2
70–74	12.1 ± 38.4		163.3 ± 29.4		435.1 ± 29.3		40.1 ± 35.5	
	9.8 ± 40.8	14.5 ± 35.5	168.2 ± 31.3	157.9 ± 26.0	431.2 ± 29.5	439.4 ± 28.5	41.3 ± 36.6	38.7 ± 34.2
75–79	9.2 ± 40.8		166.7 ± 32.9		439.1 ± 30.5		44.5 ± 38.7	
	7.2 ± 44.0	11.3 ± 37.2	172.2 ± 35.0	161.2 ± 29.6	436.1 ± 30.8	442.1 ± 29.9	46.8 ± 40.2	42.3 ± 37.0
80–84	6.2 ± 42.3		169.0 ± 35.2		444.4 ± 33.6		50.5 ± 42.4	
	2.8 ± 46.2	8.8 ± 38.9	176.1 ± 38.0	163.5 ± 31.9	442.4 ± 33.0	445.9 ± 33.9	54.2 ± 43.8	47.6 ± 41.0
85–90	4.9 ± 45.4		171.3 ± 37.8		451.0 ± 36.0		57.5 ± 45.9	
	3.3 ± 49.5	5.9 ± 42.9	178.5 ± 40.9	167.1 ± 35.2	448.5 ± 36.1	452.4 ± 35.8	59.3 ± 46.4	56.4 ± 45.6

* Mean ± standard deviation, ˆ degrees, # milliseconds.

Table 4. Z-scores −2 and +2, computed in 15 age categories of 5 years each, of the three parameters with a straight-line correlation with age and of QRS-T angle. On each cell Z-scores −2 (on the left) and +2 (on the right). For each age category, in the upper line, −2 and + 2 Z-scores in the whole population; in the bottom line, −2 and + 2 Z-scores in males and females.

Age (Years)	QRS Axis (deg ˆ) Z Scores −2 and + 2				PR Interval (ms #) Z Scores −2 and + 2				QTc Interval (ms #) Z Scores −2 and + 2				QRS-T angle (deg ˆ) Z Scores −2 and + 2			
	Men		Women		Men		Women		Men		Women		Men		Women	
15–19		3		98		104		185		364.5		466		1		77
	−0.49	102	9	96	106	185	104	185.1	360	459	376	470	1	74	1	82
20–24		−5		96		108		186		366		464		1		75
	−7	97.5	−3	94	108	190	106	184	361	455	378	467	1	73	1	75.8
25–29		−6		93		108		190		372		467		1		71.5
	−7.9	96	−4	91	114	196	108	184	364	462	384	470	1	72.9	1	71
30–34		−14		92		108		190		373.2		469		1		74
	−18.7	93	−9	91.5	116	197.5	104	182	364	461	383.5	471	1	77	1	71.5
35–39		18		91		110		192		375		469		1		69
	−24	93	−11	89	116	198	106.6	186	369	467	385	470.7	1	77	1	65

Table 4. Cont.

Age (Years)	QRS Axis (deg°) Z Scores −2 and +2		PR Interval (ms#) Z Scores −2 and +2		QTc Interval (ms#) Z Scores −2 and +2		QRS-T angle (deg°) Z Scores −2 and +2	
	Men	Women	Men	Women	Men	Women	Men	Women
40–44	−27 / −33, 89	89 / −20, 89	116, 198	112 / 108, 186	371, 468.6	192 / 377, 474 / 385.7, 477	1, 87.6	1 / 80.4 / 1, 72.3
45–49	−31 / −38, 88	88 / −24, 88	116, 200	112 / 110, 192	373, 473	196 / 378, 477 / 386.7, 480	1, 96.2	1 / 88 / 1, 79.3
50–54	−36 / −40, 85.9	86 / −30, 87	118, 204	116 / 112, 196	378, 479	200 / 381, 479 / 386, 480	1, 105	1 / 97.4 / 1, 91
55–59	−42.5 / −48, 84	85 / −33, 86	118, 210	116 / 114, 200	378, 481.6	206 / 382, 483 / 388, 484.4	1, 114.6	1 / 107 / 1, 97
60–64	−47 / −51, 83	82 / −41, 81	118, 218	116 / 114, 204	381, 486	214 / 384, 487 / 388, 488	1, 135	1 / 122 / 1, 106.7
65–69	−53 / −56, 84	82 / −47, 80	120, 230	116 / 114, 210	381, 492	222 / 384, 491 / 390, 490	1, 138	1 / 132 / 1, 124
70–74	−57 / −61, 83	81 / −51, 80	118, 240	116 / 116, 218	383.5, 497	230 / 386, 498 / 392.2, 498	1, 147.5	1 / 142 / 1, 136
75–79	−61 / −64, 90	84 / −53, 81	119.4, 256	118 / 116, 230	384, 508	244 / 388, 510 / 393, 513.3	1, 154	1 / 153 / 1, 151
80–84	−63 / −67.5, 90	86 / −58, 83	120, 268	118 / 114, 236	390, 525	254 / 391, 525 / 392, 525	1, 164	1 / 161 / 1, 160
85–90	−64 / −67, 132.6	99.6 / −61, 90.8	116, 280	116 / 116, 254	390, 539.3	266 / 392, 536 / 395.2, 535	2, 170	2 / 169 / 2, 168

° degrees, # milliseconds.

4. Discussion

In this large non-selected population, ageing and comorbidities influenced the considered ECG parameters, but a straight-line correlation was found only for QRS wave axis, PR, and QTc intervals. Secondarily, significant differences between females and males were found. Lastly, different mean values for some ECG parameters were registered mainly in the Emergency Department group.

Ageing produces structural and functional changes in the cardiovascular system, which involves the appearance of cardiovascular diseases and comorbidities [14]. The consequences of these conditions are the appearance of vascular stiffness, fibrosis, hypertrophy, and the involution of muscular tissue, valves, and arteries [15]. Moreover, with increasing age, heart position into the thorax changes, thoracic impedance grows, the use of heart conduction-modifying drugs increases, and the exposure to environmental factors rises [16,17].

Jorgensen and coll. already demonstrated that ECG changes with ageing were associated with the appearance of cardiovascular risk factors [18], while in a large population of Latinos Silva and coll. observed a greater prevalence of ECG abnormalities in old males [19].

We found that the straight-line changing parameters were an expression of the leftward deviation of the ventricular axis (QRS axis), of the slowdown conduction between atria and ventricles (PR interval), and of the prolongation of ventricular repolarization (QTc interval). Linear correlations were not found for P, QRS, and T waves duration and for P and T waves axes.

In healthy population studies, Van der Ende and coll. previously observed that increasing age was associated with a linear increase of PR and QT intervals and with a weak increase of P and QRS waves duration [2]. Rijnbeek and coll. in a smaller population observed the same results, excluding the stability of QRS duration [14], while Palhares and coll. in a large healthy Brazilian population evaluated mean ECG values also at extreme ages, observing smaller changes with increasing age [9].

We claim that our results are similar, but more applicable to clinical practice, having been obtained in a large non-selected population with cardiovascular risk factors and acute and chronic diseases that had been excluded from previous healthy population studies.

Heart rate: the increase in heart rate is a well-known risk factor for mortality [20]. In this study, it was higher in young patients, mildly decreased in the middle-aged population, and then increased again in old people, and overall, was higher in females. Previous healthy population studies showed fewer fluctuations in heart rate with increasing age [2,9,10,14]. We claim that in our study heart rate changes in old subjects were mainly attributable to the enrolled patients with acute diseases.

P, QRS, and T wave axes: changes in the cardiac axis have been associated with an increased risk of death [21]. In this study, P and T wave axes weakly turned to the right while QRS axis turned to the left with a straight-line correlation. Previous healthy population studies have observed smaller changes in the heart axis with increasing age [2,9,10,14]. Regardless of the QRS axis, our results could be explained by the appearance of hypertension and diabetes and especially by changes in heart position and in thoracic impedance.

P, QRS, and T wave duration: in this study mean P and T wave duration had small changes with increasing age, while QRS duration slightly increased without a linear correlation. P and QRS duration were greater in males, while T duration was greater in females. Additionally, previous studies have observed the same results [2,9,10,14], and our work confirmed that increasing age was not strictly associated with the increase in times of contraction.

PR interval: PR duration has been associated with the appearance of atrial fibrillation and with cardiovascular death [22]. Like previous studies, our work confirmed that the PR interval—greater in males—increased with a straight-line correlation in the entire population and in the three groups.

QTc interval: QTc is a globally utilized parameter influenced by many factors, associated with an increased arrhythmic risk, and calculable with various methods (Framingham, Hodges, Fredericia, Bazett, Rautaharju) [23]. Like previous studies, we observed a linear increase of QTc with increasing age utilizing Bazett's correction but differences between males and females became null with ageing. This behavior could be attributable to sexual hormones: in males, QTc is related to testosterone levels, causing a hormone effect on cardiac ion channels [24,25]. QTc assessment before and during the use of heart conduction-modifying drugs, for their association with an increased risk of sudden cardiac death, is strongly recommended [26].

Frontal QRS-T angle: QRS-T angle could be determined through vectorcardiography (spatial QRS-T angle) and through standard ECG recording (frontal QRS-T angle) [27]; it represents the disjunction between left ventricular depolarization and repolarization and is a strong predictor of cardiovascular death and of coronary artery diseases [28,29].

Aro and coll. showed that a frontal QRS-T angle greater than 100 deg was associated with a high risk of sudden cardiac death [30]. Except for the short report of Marcolino and coll. in a population of Latinos [31], to our knowledge, previous studies have not investigated QRS-T angle changes with ageing.

In this study, the QRS-T angle remained stable until middle age, and then rapidly increased with a straight-line correlation. QRS-T angle better reflected the appearance of cardiovascular diseases and comorbidities than the changes in heart position and thoracic impedance. The evidence of an abnormal QRS-T angle especially in young and middle-aged subjects should be explained and the underlying presence of coronary artery diseases be excluded.

Most of the considered parameters have a clinical significance and a prognostic role with respect to the appearance of atrial fibrillation, sudden cardiovascular death, and major cardiovascular events [32–34], so their precise characterization is crucial. This work demonstrated, in a large contemporary primary population, that ECG is influenced by ageing, sex, cardiovascular diseases, and comorbidities but is difficult to be defined the weight of each of these conditions.

The study provided mean and Z-score reference values for the ECG parameters with a straight-line correlation with age and sex. The detection of abnormal ECG values should be investigated by clinicians excluding the presence of cardiomyopathies, congenital and arrhythmogenic heart diseases, subtle hypertension, or ischemic heart diseases.

Moreover, clinicians should consider the effects of many drugs and of acute diseases, particularly infectious diseases, on ECG. A recent example is represented by SARS-CoV−2, which is able to cause ECG abnormalities and arrhythmias due to its ability to alter ion and especially calcium homeostasis [35–37].

For many years, ECG reporting has been considered a simple and subjective procedure, but a new era is coming. News ECG parameters are disposable and the use of algorithms such as "heart age" [38] or "age gap" [39] could increase the diagnostic and prognostic power. Moreover, the use of artificial intelligence can allow us to identify the presence of many conditions such as left ventricular systolic dysfunction, coronary artery diseases, accessory pathways, aortic stenosis, and hypertrophic cardiomyopathy [40–42]. At present, these new technological opportunities are not widely available, but the simple use of reference values and Z-scores could give an additional value to ECG interpretation.

5. Limitations

This study has limitations, mainly due to its retrospective nature, such as the unknown prevalence of patients utilizing cardiotoxic drugs or heart conduction-modifying drugs, the unknown exposure to environmental factors, and the unknown prevalence of pulmonary hypertension or left ventricular hypertrophy [43]. Despite these limitations, we claim that these unknown factors did not skew the results, because the sample size is strong and the straight-line correlations started from a young age and continued up to very old age.

6. Conclusions

The results of our study, obtained in a large primary population, are more applicable in clinical practice than those of previous healthy population studies conducted in order to maximize the effects of age, sex, and co-pathologies on ECG.

Most of the considered ECG parameters changed with increasing age but only a few of them with a linear correlation.

ECG modifications were also influenced by sex and comorbidities and were usually greater in the Emergency Department group.

Reference values expressed by means of and Z-scores were computed for linearly changing parameters; their use could improve the diagnostic and prognostic ability of clinicians in ECG interpretation.

Significant deviations from mean values and from Z-scores should be investigated by clinicians, and the evaluation of the QRS-T angle especially in young and middle-aged patients could be improved.

The expression of ECG values as Z-scores may provide additional information. Therefore, ECG could increasingly become a prognostic tool more than a diagnostic test.

Author Contributions: Conceptualization: P.G., E.T. and C.V.; Methodology: P.G., E.T., F.S. and C.V.; Statistical analysis: C.V., C.G. and E.T.; Software: F.S. and C.V.; Validation: C.V. and C.G.; Formal analysis and investigation: P.G., E.T. and A.F.; Data curation: F.S., C.V. and P.G.; Writing—original draft preparation: P.G., E.T., C.G., C.V., F.S. and A.F.; Writing-review: P.G., E.T., C.G., C.V., F.S. and A.F., Editing: P.G., E.T., C.G., C.V., F.S. and A.F.; Visualization: P.G., E.T., C.G., C.V., F.S. and A.F.; Supervision: P.G. and C.V.; Project administration: P.G., C.V. and F.S. All authors have read and agreed to the published version of the manuscript.

Funding: This research received no external funding.

Institutional Review Board Statement: This study was performed in accordance with the Ethical Standards of the 1975 Helsinki Declaration revised in 2013 and was approved by the local Ethics Committee of Modena (AVEN) with protocol number 2605/2021, date of approval 21 September 2021.

Informed Consent Statement: For this retrospective study informed consent was not collected causing of the anonymous collection of electrocardiographic, demographic, and clinical data from electronic archives.

Data Availability Statement: The data presented in this study were extracted from a "MUSE®" GE Marquette Healthcare electronic archive and are deposited in the Department of Clinical Engineering.

Data are available on request from the corresponding author with prior authorization from the Health Authority and Services of Modena.

Acknowledgments: In loving memory of Rita Vandelli. Thanks to Ben Turner and to Eleonora Barbieri for their English revision.

Conflicts of Interest: The authors declare no conflict of interest.

References

1. Simonson, E.; Keys, A. The spatial QRS and T vector in 178 normal middle-aged men; body weight, height, relationship of QRS and T and preliminary standards. *Circulation* **1954**, *9*, 105–114. [CrossRef] [PubMed]
2. Van Der Ende, M.Y.; Siland, J.E.; Snieder, H.; Van Der Harst, P.; Rienstra, M. Population-based values and abnormalities of the electrocardiogram in the general Dutch population: The LifeLines Cohort Study. *Clin. Cardiol.* **2017**, *40*, 865–872. [CrossRef] [PubMed]
3. Marek, J.; Bufalino, V.; Davis, J.; Marek, K.; Gami, A.; Stephan, W.; Zimmerman, F. Feasibility and findings of large-scale electrocardiographic screening in young adults: Data from 32,561 subjects. *Heart Rhythm* **2011**, *8*, 1555–1559. [CrossRef] [PubMed]
4. Rautaharju, P.M.; Zhang, Z.-M.; Gregg, R.E.; Haisty, W.K.; Vitolins, M.Z.; Curtis, A.B.; Warren, J.; Horaček, M.B.; Zhou, S.H.; Soliman, E.Z. Normal standards for computer-ECG programs for prognostically and diagnostically important ECG variables derived from a large ethnically diverse female cohort: The Women's Health Initiative (WHI). *J. Electrocardiol.* **2013**, *46*, 707–716. [CrossRef]
5. Bratincsák, A.; Kimata, C.; Limm-Chan, B.N.; Vincent, K.P.; Williams, M.R.; Perry, J.C. Electrocardiogram Standards for Children and Young Adults Using Z-Scores. *Circ. Arrhythmia Electrophysiol.* **2020**, *13*, e008253. [CrossRef]
6. Vicent, L.; Martínez-Sellés, M. Electrocardiogeriatrics: ECG in advanced age. *J. Electrocardiol.* **2017**, *50*, 698–700. [CrossRef]
7. Khane, R.S.; Surdi, A.D.; Bhatkar, R.S. Changes in ECG pattern with advancing age. *J. Basic Clin. Physiol. Pharmacol.* **2011**, *22*, 97–101. [CrossRef]
8. Friedman, A.; Chudow, J.; Merritt, Z.; Shulman, E.; Fisher, J.; Ferrick, K.; Krumerman, A. Electrocardiogram abnormalities in older individuals by race and ethnicity. *J. Electrocardiol.* **2020**, *63*, 91–93. [CrossRef]
9. Palhares, D.M.F.; Marcolino, M.S.; Santos, T.M.M.; Da Silva, J.L.P.; Gomes, P.R.; Ribeiro, L.B.; Macfarlane, P.W.; Ribeiro, A.L.P. Normal limits of the electrocardiogram derived from a large database of Brazilian primary care patients. *BMC Cardiovasc. Disord.* **2017**, *17*, 152. [CrossRef]
10. Mason, J.W.; Ramseth, D.J.; Chanter, D.O.; Moon, T.E.; Goodman, D.B.; Mendzelevski, B. Electrocardiographic reference ranges derived from 79,743 ambulatory subjects. *J. Electrocardiol.* **2007**, *40*, 228–234.e8. [CrossRef]
11. Sharma, S.; Drezner, J.A.; Baggish, A.; Papadakis, M.; Wilson, M.G.; Prutkin, J.M.; La Gerche, A.; Ackerman, M.J.; Börjesson, M.; Salerno, J.C.; et al. International recommendations for electrocardiographic interpretation in athletes. *Eur. Heart J.* **2018**, *39*, 1466–1480. [CrossRef] [PubMed]
12. Macfarlane, P.W. The frontal plane QRS-T angle. *Europace* **2012**, *14*, 773–775. [CrossRef] [PubMed]
13. Chua, K.C.; Teodorescu, C.; Reinier, K.; Uy-Evanado, A.; Aro, A.L.; Nair, S.G.; Chugh, H.; Jui, J.; Chugh, S.S. Wide QRS-T Angle on the 12-Lead ECG as a Predictor of Sudden Death Beyond the LV Ejection Fraction. *J. Cardiovasc. Electrophysiol.* **2016**, *27*, 833–839. [CrossRef] [PubMed]
14. Rijnbeek, P.R.; van Herpen, G.; Bots, M.L.; Man, S.; Verweij, N.; Hofman, A.; Hillege, H.; Numans, M.E.; Swenne, C.A.; Witteman, J.C.; et al. Normal values of the electrocardiogram for ages 16–90 years. *J. Electrocardiol.* **2014**, *47*, 914–921. [CrossRef] [PubMed]
15. Inoue, Y.Y.; Ambale-Venkatesh, B.; Mewton, N.; Volpe, G.J.; Ohyama, Y.; Sharma, R.K.; Wu, C.O.; Liu, C.-Y.; Bluemke, D.A.; Soliman, E.Z.; et al. Electrocardiographic Impact of Myocardial Diffuse Fibrosis and Scar: MESA (Multi-Ethnic Study of Atherosclerosis). *Radiology* **2017**, *282*, 690–698. [CrossRef] [PubMed]
16. Rabkin, S.W. Aging effects on QT interval: Implications for cardiac safety of antipsychotic drugs. *J. Geriatr. Cardiol.* **2014**, *11*, 20–25. [CrossRef]
17. Mehta, A.J.; Kloog, I.; Zanobetti, A.; Coull, B.A.; Sparrow, D.; Vokonas, P.; Schwartz, J. Associations between Changes in City and Address Specific Temperature and QT Interval—The VA Normative Aging Study. *PLoS ONE* **2014**, *9*, e106258. [CrossRef]
18. Jørgensen, P.G.; Jensen, J.S.; Marott, J.L.; Jensen, G.B.; Appleyard, M.; Mogelvang, R. Electrocardiographic Changes Improve Risk Prediction in Asymptomatic Persons Age 65 Years or Above Without Cardiovascular Disease. *J. Am. Coll. Cardiol.* **2014**, *64*, 898–906. [CrossRef]
19. Silva, M.; Palhares, D.; Ribeiro, L.; Gomes, P.; Macfarlane, P.; Ribeiro, A.; Marcolino, M. Prevalence of major and minor electrocardiographic abnormalities in one million primary care Latinos. *J. Electrocardiol.* **2020**, *64*, 36–41. [CrossRef]
20. Jensen, M.T.; Suadicani, P.; Hein, H.O.; Gyntelberg, F. Elevated resting heart rate, physical fitness and all-cause mortality: A 16-year follow-up in the Copenhagen Male Study. *Heart* **2013**, *99*, 882–887. [CrossRef]
21. Li, Y.; Shah, A.J.; Soliman, E.Z. Effect of Electrocardiographic P-Wave Axis on Mortality. *Am. J. Cardiol.* **2014**, *113*, 372–376. [CrossRef] [PubMed]
22. Cheng, S. Long-term Outcomes in Individuals with Prolonged PR Interval or First-Degree Atrioventricular Block. *JAMA* **2009**, *301*, 2571–2577. [CrossRef] [PubMed]

23. Vandenberk, B.; Vandael, E.; Robyns, T.; Vandenberghe, J.; Garweg, C.; Foulon, V.; Ector, J.; Willems, R. Which QT Correction Formulae to Use for QT Monitoring? *J. Am. Heart Assoc.* **2016**, *5*, e003264. [CrossRef]
24. Zhang, Y.; Ouyang, P.; Post, W.S.; Dalal, D.; Vaidya, D.; Blasco-Colmenares, E.; Soliman, E.Z.; Tomaselli, G.F.; Guallar, E. Sex-Steroid Hormones and Electrocardiographic QT-Interval Duration: Findings From the Third National Health and Nutrition Examination Survey and the Multi-Ethnic Study of Atherosclerosis. *Am. J. Epidemiol.* **2011**, *174*, 403–411. [CrossRef] [PubMed]
25. Charbit, B.; Christin-Maître, S.; Démolis, J.-L.; Soustre, E.; Young, J.; Funck-Brentano, C. Effects of Testosterone on Ventricular Repolarization in Hypogonadic Men. *Am. J. Cardiol.* **2009**, *103*, 887–890. [CrossRef]
26. Ray, W.A.; Chung, C.P.; Murray, K.T.; Hall, K.; Stein, C.M. Atypical Antipsychotic Drugs and the Risk of Sudden Cardiac Death. *N. Engl. J. Med.* **2009**, *360*, 225–235. [CrossRef]
27. Oehler, A.; Feldman, T.; Henrikson, C.A.; Tereshchenko, L. QRS-T Angle: A Review. *Ann. Noninvasive Electrocardiol.* **2014**, *19*, 534–542. [CrossRef]
28. Zhang, Z.-M.; Prineas, R.J.; Case, D.; Soliman, E.; Rautaharju, P.M. Comparison of the Prognostic Significance of the Electrocardiographic QRS/T Angles in Predicting Incident Coronary Heart Disease and Total Mortality (from the Atherosclerosis Risk in Communities Study). *Am. J. Cardiol.* **2007**, *100*, 844–849. [CrossRef]
29. Hnatkova, K.; Seegers, J.; Barthel, P.; Novotny, T.; Smetana, P.; Zabel, M.; Schmidt, G.; Malik, M. Clinical value of different QRS-T angle expressions. *Europace* **2017**, *20*, 1352–1361. [CrossRef]
30. Aro, A.L.; Huikuri, H.V.; Tikkanen, J.T.; Junttila, M.J.; Rissanen, H.A.; Reunanen, A.; Anttonen, O. QRS-T angle as a predictor of sudden cardiac death in a middle-aged general population. *Europace* **2011**, *14*, 872–876. [CrossRef]
31. Marcolino, M.S.; Carvalho, E.A.; Santos, T.M.; Palhares, D.M.; Ribeiro, A.L. Frontal QRS-T angle: Normal range for Latinos and association of an abnormal angle with comorbidities. *Circulation* **2016**, *134*, A15966.
32. Alonso, A.; Chen, L.Y. PR interval, P-wave duration, and mortality: New insights, additional questions. *Heart Rhythm* **2014**, *11*, 99–100. [CrossRef] [PubMed]
33. Aeschbacher, S.; O'Neal, W.T.; Krisai, P.; Loehr, L.; Chen, L.Y.; Alonso, A.; Soliman, E.Z.; Conen, D. Relationship between QRS duration and incident atrial fibrillation. *Int. J. Cardiol.* **2018**, *266*, 84–88. [CrossRef] [PubMed]
34. Tikkanen, J.T.; Kenttä, T.; Porthan, K.; Huikuri, H.V.; Junttila, M.J. Electrocardiographic T Wave Abnormalities and the Risk of Sudden Cardiac Death: The Finnish Perspective. *Ann. Noninvasive Electrocardiol.* **2015**, *20*, 526–533. [CrossRef]
35. De Vita, A.; Ravenna, S.E.; Covino, M.; Lanza, O.; Franceschi, F.; Crea, F.; Lanza, G.A. Electrocardiographic Findings and Clinical Outcome in Patients with COVID-19 or Other Acute Infectious Respiratory Diseases. *J. Clin. Med.* **2020**, *9*, 3647. [CrossRef]
36. Farré, N.; Mojón, D.; Llagostera, M.; Belarte-Tornero, L.C.; Calvo-Fernández, A.; Vallés, E.; Negrete, A.; García-Guimaraes, M.; Bartolomé, Y.; Fernández, C.; et al. Prolonged QT Interval in SARS-CoV-2 Infection: Prevalence and Prognosis. *J. Clin. Med.* **2020**, *9*, 2712. [CrossRef]
37. Giovanardi, P.; Manni, B.; Vaccina, A.; Cavazzuti, L.; Salvia, C.; Latronico, M.; Fabbo, A. Early COVID-19 infection: The wide spectrum of extrapulmonary symptoms in elderly patients. *Aging Med.* **2020**, *3*, 276–277. [CrossRef]
38. Ball, R.L.; Feiveson, A.H.; Schlegel, T.T.; Starc, V.; Dabney, A.R. Predicting "Heart Age" Using Electrocardiography. *J. Pers. Med.* **2014**, *4*, 65–78. [CrossRef]
39. Ladejobi, A.O.; Medina-Inojosa, J.R.; Cohen, M.S.; Attia, Z.I.; Scott, C.G.; LeBrasseur, N.K.; Gersh, B.J.; Noseworthy, P.A.; Friedman, P.A.; Kapa, S.; et al. The 12-lead electrocardiogram as a biomarker of biological age. *Eur. Heart J.-Digit. Health* **2021**, *2*, 379–389. [CrossRef]
40. Noseworthy, P.A.; Attia, Z.I.; Brewer, L.C.; Hayes, S.N.; Yao, X.; Kapa, S.; Friedman, P.A.; Lopez-Jimenez, F. Assessing and Mitigating Bias in Medical Artificial Intelligence. *Circ. Arrhythmia Electrophysiol.* **2020**, *13*, e007988. [CrossRef]
41. Senoner, T.; Pfeifer, B.; Barbieri, F.; Adukauskaite, A.; Dichtl, W.; Bauer, A.; Hintringer, F. Identifying the Location of an Accessory Pathway in Pre-Excitation Syndromes Using an Artificial Intelligence-Based Algorithm. *J. Clin. Med.* **2021**, *10*, 4394. [CrossRef] [PubMed]
42. Siontis, K.C.; Noseworthy, P.A.; Attia, Z.I.; Friedman, P.A. Artificial intelligence-enhanced electrocardiography in cardiovascular disease management. *Nat. Rev. Cardiol.* **2021**, *18*, 465–478. [CrossRef] [PubMed]
43. Chlabicz, M.; Jamiołkowski, J.; Paniczko, M.; Sowa, P.; Szpakowicz, M.; Łapińska, M.; Jurczuk, N.; Kondraciuk, M.; Ptaszyńska-Kopczyńska, K.; Raczkowski, A.; et al. ECG Indices Poorly Predict Left Ventricular Hypertrophy and Are Applicable Only in Individuals with Low Cardiovascular Risk. *J. Clin. Med.* **2020**, *9*, 1364. [CrossRef] [PubMed]

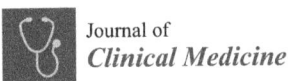

Article

Using Minimum Redundancy Maximum Relevance Algorithm to Select Minimal Sets of Heart Rate Variability Parameters for Atrial Fibrillation Detection

Szymon Buś [1,*], Konrad Jędrzejewski [1] and Przemysław Guzik [2]

[1] Institute of Electronic Systems, Faculty of Electronics and Information Technology, Warsaw University of Technology, Nowowiejska 15/19, 00-665 Warsaw, Poland; konrad.jedrzejewski@pw.edu.pl
[2] Department of Cardiology-Intensive Therapy and Internal Disease, Poznan University of Medical Sciences, 60-355 Poznan, Poland; pguzik@ptkardio.pl
* Correspondence: szymon.bus.dokt@pw.edu.pl; Tel.: +48-22-2345883

Abstract: Heart rate is quite regular during sinus (normal) rhythm (SR) originating from the sinus node. In contrast, heart rate is usually irregular during atrial fibrillation (AF). Complete atrioventricular block with an escape rhythm, ventricular pacing, or ventricular tachycardia are the most common exceptions when heart rate may be regular in AF. Heart rate variability (HRV) is the variation in the duration of consecutive cardiac cycles (RR intervals). We investigated the utility of HRV parameters for automated detection of AF with machine learning (ML) classifiers. The minimum redundancy maximum relevance (MRMR) algorithm, one of the most effective algorithms for feature selection, helped select the HRV parameters (including five original), best suited for distinguishing AF from SR in a database of over 53,000 60 s separate electrocardiogram (ECG) segments cut from longer (up to 24 h) ECG recordings. HRV parameters entered the ML-based classifiers as features. Seven different, commonly used classifiers were trained with one to six HRV-based features with the highest scores resulting from the MRMR algorithm and tested using the 5-fold cross-validation and blindfold validation. The best ML classifier in the blindfold validation achieved an accuracy of 97.2% and diagnostic odds ratio of 1566. From all studied HRV features, the top three HRV parameters distinguishing AF from SR were: the percentage of successive RR intervals differing by at least 50 ms (pRR50), the ratio of standard deviations of points along and across the identity line of the Poincare plots, respectively (SD2/SD1), and coefficient of variation—standard deviation of RR intervals divided by their mean duration (CV). The proposed methodology and the presented results of the selection of HRV parameters have the potential to develop practical solutions and devices for automatic AF detection with minimal sets of simple HRV parameters. Using straightforward ML classifiers and the extremely small sets of simple HRV features, always with pRR50 included, the differentiation of AF from sinus rhythms in the 60 s ECGs is very effective.

Keywords: electrocardiogram; ECG; atrial fibrillation; machine learning; feature selection; minimum redundancy maximum relevance; MRMR

Citation: Buś, S.; Jędrzejewski, K.; Guzik, P. Using Minimum Redundancy Maximum Relevance Algorithm to Select Minimal Sets of Heart Rate Variability Parameters for Atrial Fibrillation Detection. *J. Clin. Med.* **2022**, *11*, 4004. https://doi.org/10.3390/jcm11144004

Academic Editors: Christian Sohns and Paweł T. Matusik

Received: 30 April 2022
Accepted: 9 July 2022
Published: 11 July 2022

Publisher's Note: MDPI stays neutral with regard to jurisdictional claims in published maps and institutional affiliations.

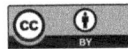

Copyright: © 2022 by the authors. Licensee MDPI, Basel, Switzerland. This article is an open access article distributed under the terms and conditions of the Creative Commons Attribution (CC BY) license (https://creativecommons.org/licenses/by/4.0/).

1. Introduction

Atrial fibrillation (AF) is characterized by the less organized and nearly random electrical activity of both atria accompanied by an irregular ventricular rhythm. [1–3]. AF can be either asymptomatic in many patients unaware of its existence or entirely symptomatic with paroxysmal or persistent palpitations, dyspnea, angina, worsened exercise tolerance, and occasional syncope [2,3]. This arrhythmia is associated with a significantly increased risk of heart failure, cognitive decline due to vascular dementia, ischemic stroke, and premature death [2,3].

AF is the most common sustained cardiac arrhythmia, particularly in older people and those with cardiovascular risk factors such as hypertension, diabetes, smoking, coronary artery disease, or obesity [2–4]. It is usually a consequence of structural and/or functional changes in the left atrium or both atria [2–4]. However, AF is not a rare finding in structurally and functionally normal left atria, e.g., in hyperthyroid disease, after alcohol consumption, or if autonomic dysregulation is present [5,6]. The estimated lifetime risk of AF is about 30%, meaning that one in three adult individuals of European ancestry may develop it in the future [2–4].

Signal processing and machine learning (ML) techniques enable automatic detection of AF [2,3]. According to the most recent guidelines of the European Society of Cardiology, AF can be diagnosed using an electrocardiogram (ECG) if: (1) it is present in the entire 12-lead ECG or (2) if fewer ECG leads are available, it lasts for at least 30 s. However, in many cases of transient, paroxysmal AF, long-term ECG monitoring is required to diagnose it [2,3]. Mobile ECG monitors with built-in signal processing and ML capabilities are a promising tool for this task [2,3]. However, such devices' computational capacity and memory are limited, and real-time performance is required. It poses additional requirements on ECG processing and classification algorithms, which have to be simultaneously time- and memory-efficient and provide sufficient performance quality.

Several approaches are used in the automated detection of AF from an ECG. Some methods analyze the electrical activity of atria because no P-wave is present on the ECG during AF. QRS cancellation methods, such as average beat subtraction [7], principal component analysis (PCA) [8], independent component analysis (ICA) [9], and singular value decomposition (SVD) [10,11], are used for atrial electrical activity extraction. The processing of atrial waveform may include time-frequency analysis to determine the presence of P-waves or f-waves (fibrillatory waves) on an ECG.

However, atrial activity-based AF detection methods are sensitive to poor signal quality. Atrial waveforms on an ECG have much lower amplitude than ventricular waveforms, are less defined at the beginning and end, and may overlap with U or T waves, particularly at higher heart rates. Technical artifacts resulting from electromagnetic noise, body movements, or poor electrical skin properties also severely impact the signal. Additionally, the methods of atrial activity extraction are computationally expensive and may not be suitable for real-time use, e.g., in mobile ECG monitors.

One commonly used approach to AF detection is the analysis of heart rate variability (HRV), defined by the variation in the duration of consecutive cardiac cycles. In contrast to AF, sinus rhythm (SR) is a normal cardiac rhythm and usually is quite regular within a specific time. Measures of beat-to-beat changes in cardiac cycle duration during SR are used for physiological and clinical purposes (mainly prediction) but also in sports and psychology studies [12–15]. In general, although some variation in the duration of cardiac cycles exists in SR, its extent is much larger in AF. HRV-based methods rely on the significant and strong irregularity of the duration of the cardiac cycles in AF. The distance between R-waves of consecutive QRS complexes corresponding to the electrical activity of the right and left ventricles of the heart can be used as the length of the cardiac cycle. R-wave detection is well established, precise, and computationally efficient. The analysis of RR intervals (differences between consecutive R-wave peaks on an ECG) enables the detection of irregularity in heart rhythm. Dozens of HRV parameters [12] are derived from RR-interval time series and can be used as input features for ML algorithms.

Using too many features in ML algorithms may bring redundant information, leading to an insignificant increase in their performance with an increasing feature set or even to deterioration of the results. The same issue applies to adding HRV features in ML algorithms for AF detection since substantial overlap exists between many HRV parameters, and some may contribute similar information. Feature selection in AF detection has been studied. In a study conducted by Michel et al. [16], several approaches, including γ-metric, mean decrease in accuracy (MDA), mean decrease in Gini (MDG), and area under the curve (AUC), were used to select the most relevant HRV features from a 60 s ECG. AUC was also employed for the feature selection in [17]. Boon et al. [18] used a genetic algorithm to optimize both the selection of the classifier metaparameters and the selection of the HRV feature set from a 15 min ECG. Mustaqeem et al. [19] selected the best features for classifying 16 different cardiac rhythms using a wrapper algorithm around a random forest. In a study conducted by de Chazal et al. [20], the best features in four groups were identified using linear discriminant analysis (LDA). In the PhysioNet/Computing in Cardiology Challenge 2017 [21], where four different rhythms (AF/SR/noisy/another rhythm) had to be identified in short ECG recordings, several participants incorporated feature selection [22–24]. The approaches to selecting feature sets (some of which included HRV) ranged from maximal information coefficient (MIC) and maximum redundancy maximum relevance (MRMR) [22], backward elimination [23], to the reduction of the entropy [24]. Unfortunately, the detailed results of selecting features were not included in these papers. In a study conducted by Krasteva et al. (2020), signals from the PhysioNet/CinC Challenge 2017 database were classified using features from HRV, morphology analysis, heartbeat classification, principal component analysis (PCA) of PQRST and TQ, P-wave analysis, TQ-segment analysis and noise correction [25]. The HRV parameters included the percentage of successive RR intervals differing by at least 50 ms (pRR50) and the ratio of standard deviations of points across (SD1) and along the identity line (SD2) of the Poincare plots, i.e., SD1/SD2. Relative feature importance (separately in four rhythms) was investigated based on the weights of the activated neurons in a neural network. Christov et al. [26] used forward stepwise selection with the linear discrimination analysis (LDA) classifier to select the most important features in three HR ranges (<50, 50–100, >100 beats per minute (bpm)) for differentiating four rhythms (AF/SR/noisy/other) of the PhysioNet/CinC Challenge 2017 database. The features were derived from HRV, average beat morphology, and analysis of atrial f-waves. pRR50 was ranked highest in the two upper HR ranges and SD1/SD2 was second in the 50–100 bpm range. Shao et al. [27] proposed a system for AF detection in wearable devices. Thirty-one features (including some based on RR interval series) were ranked by their importance obtained from the CatBoost model. The impact of the number of features in the ML model on the Matthews correlation coefficient (MCC) scores was presented. Parsi et al. [28] used established and new HRV parameters to predict the onset of paroxysmal AF. MRMR, infinite latent feature selection (ILFS), and least absolute shrinkage and selection operator (LASSO) were used for feature selection. The accuracy in 10-fold CV (by a patient) was 97.7%. Biton et al. [29] extracted the following features from a 7–10 s 12-lead ECG: deep neural network features, morphology, HRV, and electronic medical record system (EMR) metadata. A subset of features was selected using MRMR to predict AF occurring within 5 years (59.6% sensitivity, 96.3% specificity in the test set). Zhu et al. [30] used a combined approach with MRMR, Fisher, and correlation criteria for the selection of HRV parameters for AF detection in a database containing several types of cardiac rhythms. They also studied the impact of the number of neurons in the hidden layer of the neural network on classification performance. In a thesis by Kotynia [31], MRMR was used for ranking 24 morphology and HRV features (including SDRR, pRR50, SD1, SD2, and SD1/SD2) in 10, 15, 30, and 60 s ECGs in AF/SR and AF/non-AF classification. In 10 s and 15 s segments, pRR50 had the highest MRMR rank in AF/SR classification. However, the database was relatively small (from 324 60 s segments to 5504 10 s segments). Jiang et al. [32] studied AF detection in a 24 s ballistocardiogram using several ML classifiers. They used MRMR to select the most relevant among several novel nonlinear persistent homology features and studied the impact of the number of features on classification performance. Ballistocardiogram measures rhythmic motions of the whole body caused by heart contractions and blood propelling into the aorta. The signal quality is far from optimal, not even closely comparable to an ECG. The readings and measurements are not as reliable as an ECG. However, we found the proposed methodology useful and adapted it to conduct a similar analysis for HRV parameters from an ECG [32]. Parsi et al. [33] used HRV features from 1 min and 5 min ECG segments for the prediction of ventricular fibrillation (VF) and ventricular tachycardia (VT). First, a Student's t-test was used to eliminate features with the lowest discriminatory properties. The remaining features were ranked using MRMR and ILFS. Three classifiers were applied to predict the VT-VF event using an optimal number of features from each method (determined in the learning phase). In 1 min and 5 min segments, the best classification results in the test set were obtained using feature sets selected by MRMR (6 features in both cases) [33].

Several ML methods (classifiers) are suitable for automatic AF detection, regardless of which feature extraction method (such as HRV analysis or time-frequency analysis) is used. A threshold for a single parameter can be used for AF/SR discrimination [34]. Support vector machine (SVM) [35–38] is widely used due to its ability to fit relatively complex datasets. Artificial neural networks (ANN) [39], including deep convolutional neural networks (CNN) [40], and recurrent neural networks (RNN) [41], are also used for the detection of AF. Training the ANN classifier can take significantly longer than SVM, depending on a neural network's size, architecture, and different metaparameters. However, deeper neural networks can fit more complex datasets. Another classification algorithm is the decision tree [38,42]. It is easily interpretable and fast to train, but its usefulness in complex classification problems is limited. The sensitivity and specificity in AF detection reported in the literature vary depending on the dataset and the methods used. We included the results from selected studies on automated AF detection in Table 1.

Table 1. Atrial fibrillation detection results from the literature.

Reference	Dataset	Accuracy [%]	Sensitivity [%]	Specificity [%]	Classifier	Notes
Parsi et al., 2021 [28]	Physionet Atrial Fibrillation Prediction Database	97.7	98.8	96.7	SVM (also MLP, RF, KNN)	5 min ECG segments, established and new HRV parameters, the distinction between SR and rhythm just before the onset of AF. 10-fold cross-validation (by the patient).
Biton et al., 2021 [29]	Telehealth Network of Minas Gerais (TNMG) database	-	59.6	95.3	RF	DNN features from a raw 12-lead ECG (7–10 s), morphology, HRV, EMR metadata. Prediction of developing AF within 5 years.
Zhu et al., 2021 [30]	13,354 short-term ECG segments	90.46	94.04	86.74	ANN	10 s ECG, seven classes (rhythms). Feature selection: correlation with label, MRMR, Fisher criterion.
Jiang et al., 2022 [32]	Own BCG database	94.50	96.70	92.62	SVM (also KNB, LR, RF, BT)	24 s BCG signal, MRMR feature selection, 10-fold CV
Oster et al., 2013 [34]	AFDB	-	92.7	94.2	RR entropy threshold	Length: 12 RR intervals, features: coefficient of sample entropy.
Mohebbi et al., 2008 [35]	MIT-BIH Arrhythmia Database	-	99.07	100	SVM	HRV from 32 RR, feature selection with LDA
Sepulveda-Suescun et al., 2017 [36]	AFDB	97.8	97.9	97.8	SVM	Poincare plot-based HRV. Only 226 AF and 264 SR segments.
Nguyen et al., 2018 [37]	2017 PhysioNet/Computers in Cardiology Challenge Database	95.15	-	-	SVM	30–60 s recordings, HRV
Mei et al., 2018 [38]	2017 PhysioNet/Computers in Cardiology Challenge Database	96.6	83.2	98.6	BT	30–60 s recordings, HRV, and frequency analysis
Pourbabaee et al., 2018 [40]	Physionet PAF prediction challenge database	91	-	-	KNN (and other classifiers)	Neural network-extracted features.
Faust et al., 2018 [41]	AFDB	99.77	99.87	99.61	RNN	Sequence of 100 RR intervals
Ma et al., 2020 [43]	MIT-BIH Arrhythmia Database	98.3	97.4	99.3	Shallow ANN	RR interval series as features, not specified how long.

Table 1. Cont.

Reference	Dataset	Accuracy [%]	Sensitivity [%]	Specificity [%]	Classifier	Notes
Marsili et al., 2016 [44]	AFDB	98.44	97.33	98.67	Symbolic dynamics, threshold	Beat-by-beat classification based on RR intervals (symbolic dynamics).
Erdenebayar et al., 2019 [45]	AFDB, MIT-BIH Normal Sinus Rhythm Database	98.7	98.7	98.6	CNN	30 s segments, CNN features from raw ECG, training/test division not specified.
Mousavi et al., 2020 [46]	AFDB	82.41	90.53	79.54	Bidirectional RNN	5 s RR interval sequence
Faust el al., 2020 [47]	AFDB, LTAFDB	94			RNN	100 RR sequence, blindfold validation on LTAFDB

AF—atrial fibrillation, AFDB—MIT-BIH Atrial Fibrillation Database, ANN—artificial neural network, BCG—ballistocardiogram, BT—bagging tree, CNN—convolutional neural network, DNN—deep neural network, ECG—electrocardiogram, EMR—electronic medical record, HRV—heart rate variability, KNB—kernel naive Bayes, KNN—K nearest neighbors, LDA—linear discrimination analysis, LR—linear regression, LTAFDB—Long-Term Atrial Fibrillation Database, MLP—multilayer perceptron, MRMR—minimum redundancy maximum relevance, PAF—paroxysmal atrial fibrillation, RF—random forest, RNN—recurrent neural network, RR—distance between peaks of consecutive R-waves, SR—sinus rhythm, SVM—support vector machine.

We aimed to study the impact of the selection of HRV parameters (features in terms of ML) employed as inputs in ML algorithms for distinguishing AF from SR. Some HRV features have been rarely or never used for this purpose.

2. Materials and Methods

We used one of the most effective filter-based algorithms for feature selection, i.e., MRMR [48], which has recently been relatively widely used in ML [22,29–33,49]. The MRMR algorithm maximizes the relevance (ability) of the set of features for correct classification and minimizes the redundancy between the features. To determine the relevance and redundancy, the mutual information between the features and between individual features and the classification output are calculated, respectively.

We identified minimal sets of one to six of the selected HRV features, allowing us to achieve the best performance of automatic AF detection. We decided to use several different, relatively simple classifiers and compare their performance to check if the effectiveness of the MRMR-based feature selection is classifier-dependent. For feature sets containing from one to six features with the highest MRMR scores, each classifier was tuned in the 5-fold cross-validation in the training set to obtain the highest accuracy. The tuned classifiers were then trained on the entire training set and validated on the whole test set. For the small sets of HRV features, we determined statistical and diagnostic measures for the automatic AF detection algorithms. To our knowledge, such research results have never been reported.

In all models, pRR50 was the most relevant HRV feature and thus was always present. To study the effects of minimal sets composed of other HRV features, we have post-hoc defined an additional study aim to explore the diagnostic properties of ML algorithms for separating SR from AF ECGs using HRV features after exclusion of pRR50. Therefore, the entire process (feature selection, metaparameter tuning, training, and validation) was then repeated after excluding pRR50 to evaluate how much it would negatively impact the performance of classifiers.

The potential application of our findings in miniature devices determines the number of HRV features and the choice of relatively simple ML algorithms for AF detection. Devices such as bio-patches, wearables, or implantable devices are critically limited by the available computational resources and the acceptable energy consumption.

2.1. Data Used in the Study

Two open databases were used in the study: the MIT-BIH Atrial Fibrillation Database (AFDB) [50,51] and the Long Term AF Database (LTAFDB) [51,52]. Both databases contain ECG signals, annotations of detected QRS locations, and annotations of rhythm type.

Distances between two consecutive QRS complexes, i.e., RR intervals, correspond to each cardiac cycle's duration. Each QRS complex was annotated as one of the following beats: sinus, supraventricular or ventricular, and an artifact if the noise was present instead of a QRS complex. RR intervals were annotated with the type of beat corresponding to the QRS complex at the beginning of each cardiac cycle. The AFDB database contained 23 ECG recordings with a mean duration of 10 h. In the LTAFDB database, 84 ECG recordings lasted, on average, 24 h.

2.2. Software Tools

We used Python programming language (version 3.9, Python Software Foundation, Wilmington, DE, USA) for all the analyses except for the MRMR algorithm, for which we used the implementation from the Statistics and Machine Learning Toolbox in Matlab (version 2021a, Mathworks, Natick, MA, USA). For classification, we used the scikit-learn Python library (version 0.24.2).

2.3. Splitting Data into the Training Set and Test Set

Several different methods are used to assess classification performance [53,54]. Both k-fold cross-validation and blindfold validation were performed in this study to evaluate potential data leakage problems. Data leakage occurs when random samples for training and test datasets result in very similar data, e.g., from the same patient, present in both sets, leading to an over-optimistic estimation of classification performance [55]. In many publications, recordings from the same patients as in the training set or even different segments of the same recordings are present in the validation set [35,36,43,44], which leads to very good but unreliable results. This issue is rarely discussed in publications on ML-based arrhythmia detection. It was addressed in the context of AF detection in [46], where its impact on classification metrics was demonstrated.

In [41], data from 20 out of 23 patients in AFDB were used for the training part. The 10-fold cross-validation of the model was performed on the training set, and the data from the three remaining patients were used for the blindfold validation. The reported blindfold validation performance was even higher than in the 10-fold validation (accuracy 99.77% vs. 98.51%), which can be due to the small size of the validation set. In [47], the classifier from [41] was validated on a different database (LTAFDB) than the training set (AFDB), achieving 94% accuracy. Other results can be found in [46], where the classifier was trained on RR intervals from 5 s ECG segments from AFDB and tested on the PhysioNet Computing in Cardiology Challenge 2017, achieving 96.98% accuracy.

We argue that data leakage should not be ignored as it can lead to overfitting the dataset and decrease performance when new data is introduced. Properly dividing data into a training set and a test set is crucial for reliable estimation of classification performance. We randomly selected 2/3 AFDB patients and 2/3 LTAFDB as the training set and the remaining 1/3 of the patients from each database as the test set. This way, we aimed to achieve two things: 1. data from no patient is simultaneously present in both sets, and 2. training and test sets are both large and varied. Classification metrics from the blindfold validation on the test set were compared with the 5-fold cross-validation on the training set. The test set differed from the set used for training the ML classifiers, with no patients present in both sets in the blindfold validation. Such an approach is closer to real-life ECG monitoring when the data from the tested person was not previously used for training the AF detection algorithm.

2.4. Data Preprocessing

Uninterrupted, non-overlapping 60 s fragments of ECG with either AF or SR were chosen for analysis, and segments containing other rhythms were discarded. We used the QRS annotations from the databases to calculate the RR intervals. ECG fragments containing both AF and SR were also excluded to limit the scope of the study to the differentiation between pure AF and pure SR. RR intervals shorter than 240 ms or longer than 3000 ms were removed to limit the impact of potentially unnoticed technical artifacts on the analysis. ECG segments in which the removed RRs lasted at least 10% (6 s) of the total segment duration (60 s) were also discarded from the study. The number of studied AF and SR segments (before and after removing some segments with artifacts) are summarized in Table 2.

Table 2. The number of electrocardiogram segments with atrial fibrillation (AF) and sinus rhythm (SR) in training and test sets before and after discarding the segments with artifacts.

Dataset	AF Total	AF Filtered	SR Total	SR Filtered
Training	27,630	26,464	27,823	27,311
Test	11,191	11,167	25,461	14,294

2.5. Feature Extraction

In the HRV analysis [12,56], many signal parameters can be computed using RR intervals time series. In AF, lengths of RR intervals usually alter more than in SR. For this study, we calculated the HRV parameters from several groups. The measures reflecting differences between consecutive RR intervals or RR intervals variance include:

- pRR50 (percentage of successive differences between RR intervals greater or equal to 50 ms)—it is an example of counting statistics in which the rate of a specific event (in this case, the difference between two consecutive RR intervals of at least 50 ms) is counted;
- SD1 (standard deviation of points in the Poincare plot across the identity line)—it reflects the short-term RR variability from the Poincare plot;
- SD2 (standard deviation of points in the Poincare plot along the identity line)—it shows the long-term RR variability from the Poincare plot;
- SDRR (standard deviation of RR intervals)—it reflects the total HRV;
- RRdif = mean($|RR_{n+1} - RR_n|$) (mean of absolute differences between successive RR) − it summarizes the averaged range of differences between two consecutive RR intervals.

The relative measures of RR-interval-derived difference or variance include:

- CV = SDRR/(mean RR) (coefficient of variance)—it reflects the dispersion of the total variance around the mean;
- SD2/SD1 [57]—describes how much the long-term variance changes with the short-term variance. Another interpretation is how much the dispersions of points along and across the identity line change when compared to another. If SD2/SD1 is over 1, then the long-term HRV is larger than the short-term HRV, and vice versa;
- relRRdif = RRdif/(mean RR) (relative RRdif)—it shows the average rate of the absolute differences between successive RR normalized to the mean of all RR intervals.

The measures of relative changes between two consecutive RR intervals:

- meanSuccRat = mean(RR_{n+1}/RR_n) (mean ratio of successive RR), the interpretation of this parameter is as follows: what is the average relative change between two consecutive RR intervals in a specific ECG segment;
- SDSuccRat = SD (RR_{n+1}/RR_n) (standard deviation of ratios of successive RR), the interpretation of this parameter is as follows: what is the variability of the relative changes between two consecutive RR intervals in a specific ECG segment.

The absolute descriptors of the RR interval distribution:

- mean RR (mean of RR intervals);
- RRrange = max(RR) − min(RR).

The relative descriptor of the RR interval distribution:

- relRRrange = RRrange/(mean RR) (relative RRrange), the interpretation of this parameter is as follows: how much the range between the shortest and the longest RR interval in a specific ECG segment is larger than the mean of all RR intervals in the same ECG segment.

Some of these parameters (mean RR, SDRR, SD1, SD2, and pRR50) are widely used in the HRV analysis of long-term ECG recordings, mainly for predictive purposes [12,58]. In [59], several of these parameters (mean RR, SDRR, SD1, SD2, pRR50, CV) were listed among typical HRV features for AF detection. The computation of these parameters is straightforward and thus potentially suitable for mobile devices. In the remaining part of the paper, we refer to analyzed ECG signal segments as samples and to the HRV parameters representing them as features. Such terminology is common in ML and might help avoid confusion between the metaparameters of classifiers and HRV parameters.

2.6. Feature Selection

Feature selection was conducted solely on the training set. One approach is selecting the features with the highest area under the receiver operating characteristic (ROC) curve (AUC). The AUCs of specific features are presented in Figure 1. pRR50 has the highest AUC, followed by relRRdif, RRdif, CV and relRRrange. However, selecting feature sets based only on AUC is not well suited when the features are correlated and carry redundant information.

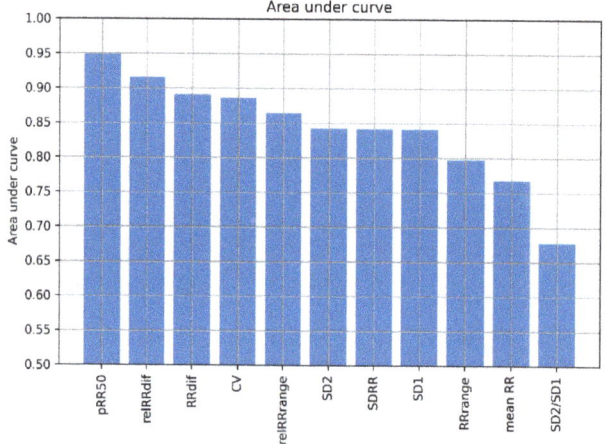

Figure 1. Area under receiver operating characteristic curve (AUC) of heart rate variability features. pRR50—percentage of successive differences between RR intervals greater or equal to 50 ms; SD1 and SD2—standard deviation of points in the Poincare plot across and along the identity line, respectively; SDRR—standard deviation of RR intervals; RRdif—mean of absolute differences between successive RR; CV—coefficient of variance; relRRdif = RRdif/(mean RR); mean RR—mean of RR intervals; RRrange = max(RR) − min(RR); relRRrange = RRrange/(mean RR) (relative RRrange).

For this reason, we decided to use the MRMR algorithm to select the best feature sets for AF detection for ML algorithms. It is a filter-based feature selection algorithm [60], which orders the most relevant features providing minimal redundancy between subsequent features simultaneously. MRMR scores obtained for 60 s ECG recordings are presented in Figure 2.

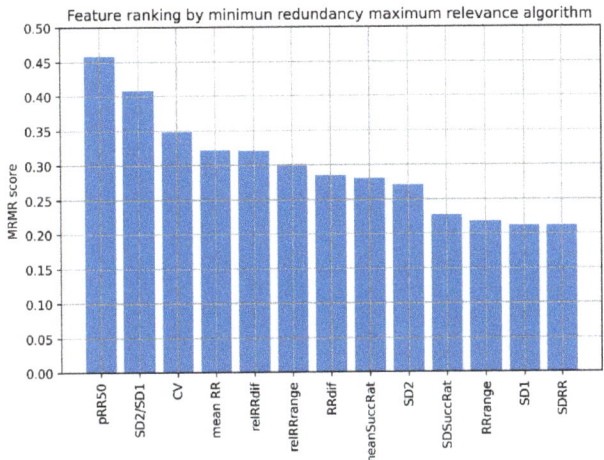

Figure 2. Ranking of heart rate variability features by minimum redundancy maximum relevance (MRMR) algorithm. pRR50—percentage of successive differences between RR intervals greater or equal to 50 ms; SD1 and SD2—standard deviation of points in the Poincare plot across and along the identity line, respectively; mean RR—mean of RR intervals; SDRR—standard deviation of RR intervals; RRdif—mean of absolute differences between successive RR; CV—coefficient of variance; relRRdif = RRdif/(mean RR); meanSuccRat—mean ratio of successive RR; SDSuccRat—standard deviation of ratios of successive RR; RRrange = max(RR) − min(RR); relRRrange = RRrange/(mean RR) (relative RRrange).

The results show that the highest MRMR scores are obtained subsequently for pRR50, SD2/SD1, and CV, followed by mean RR, relRRdif, and relRRrange. Using these results, we examined the performance of different ML classifiers for different numbers of the best features determined by the MRMR algorithm.

To conclude, the relevance of particular HRV parameters in distinguishing between AF and SR (based on the results from MRMR) is not strictly related to their AUC. The distributions of features in the training set in AF and SR are presented as histograms in Figure 3. In general, histograms of the features for AF and SR have a smaller overlap in features with higher AUC (see Figure 1).

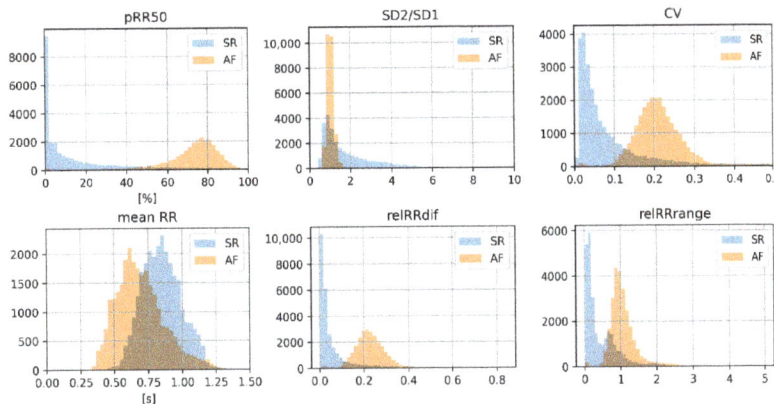

Figure 3. Histograms of six heart rate variability parameters with the highest score from minimum redundancy maximum relevance algorithm (blue—sinus rhythm, SR; orange—atrial fibrillation, AF).

pRR50—percentage of successive differences between RR intervals greater or equal to 50 ms; SD1 and SD2—standard deviation of points in the Poincare plot across and along the identity line, respectively; CV—coefficient of variance; mean RR—mean of RR intervals; relRRdif—mean of absolute differences between successive RR divided by mean RR; relRRrange = (max(RR) − min(RR))/(mean RR) (relative RRrange).

2.7. Classification Algorithms

The following standard classification algorithms were employed and compared in this study for AF detection:

- Decision Tree (DT),
- K Nearest Neighbors (KNN),
- Support Vector Machine with the linear kernel (SVM linear),
- Support Vector Machine with radial basis function kernel (SVM RBF),
- Ada Boost (ADA),
- Random Forest (RF),
- Artificial Neural Network (ANN).

In DT, a set of conditional statements (nodes) forming a tree are used for classification. Values of particular features are compared with threshold values in the nodes. During DT's training (building), new nodes in the tree are added by choosing the feature that splits the tree best according to some metric. We used Gini impurity as a metric of split quality [61].

In KNN, classification is made by measuring the distances between a new sample (whose class is unknown) and all the training samples (with known classes). K samples with the smallest distances (nearest neighbors) are selected, and the most common class among them is chosen as the class of the new sample [62].

SVM is a classification algorithm in which a hyperplane is chosen as a decision boundary separating two classes. Ideally, entire classes should be on opposite sides of the hyperplane. Moreover, the minimal distance of the training examples from the hyperplane is maximized by SVM. If the classes are not linearly separable, the problem can be mapped to a higher dimension using a transform (kernel), such as Radial Basis Function (RBF) [63].

ADA is an ensemble learning method where classification is based on decisions from multiple simple classifiers. Training of the classifiers is sequential. For each classifier, the training set is modified by adjusting the weights of particular examples. The weight is increased if the example was incorrectly classified by the previous classifier and decreased otherwise. The final classification decision is a weighted majority vote of all classifiers [64].

RF is another ensemble learning method. Classifications from multiple decision trees are used as votes, and the most commonly voted class is used as the final classification decision. Each of the trees in the forest is built using a different subset of the training dataset [65].

ANN is a vast class of algorithms based on applying an artificial neural network concept that is also used in classification problems. We used the simplest feedforward ANN with one hidden layer and ReLU (rectified linear unit) activation function.

3. Results

The methodology of classifier training in the study is presented in Figure 4. First, MRMR was used for feature selection (on the training set).

Then, sets of one to six features with the highest MRMR scores were used for the metaparameter tuning of the classifiers (in case of DT—the maximum depth of the tree, in KNN—the number of neighbors K, in SVM with linear kernel—the soft margin C, in SVM with RBF kernel—both the soft margin C and inverse of kernel's width gamma, in RF—the maximum depth and number of classifiers, in ADA—the number of classifiers, in ANN—the number of hidden neurons). The 5-fold cross-validation on the training set was used to find the best metaparameters of the classifiers. The metaparameters for which the highest average accuracy in the 5-fold cross-validation was achieved were chosen as the best for each feature set. Then, the classifiers with optimal metaparameters were trained on the training set, and their performance was validated on the test set. The results were then compared with the results obtained for the 5-fold cross-validation. We calculated the accuracy, sensitivity, specificity, positive predictive value (PPV), and diagnostic odds ratio (DOR) [66] of the classification. We decided to include DOR as a useful single metric in diagnostic testing. DOR is rarely reported in the literature on AF detection, with exceptions like [40].

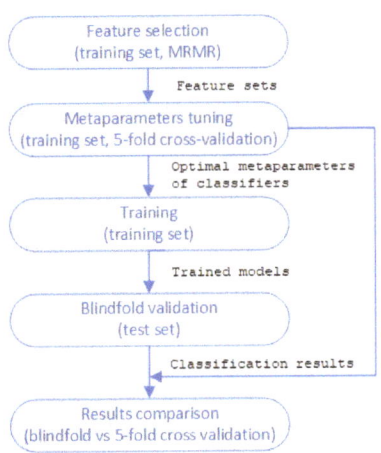

Figure 4. Diagram of training and validation methodology. MRMR—minimum redundancy maximum relevance.

3.1. Feature Sets with pRR50

The classification metrics (accuracy, sensitivity, specificity, positive predictive value, and diagnostic odds ratio—DOR [66]) obtained by the ML classifiers in the 5-fold cross-validation and blindfold validation are presented in Figures 4–8. For each classifier, one to six features with the highest MRMR scores were used for training, as summarized in Table 3.

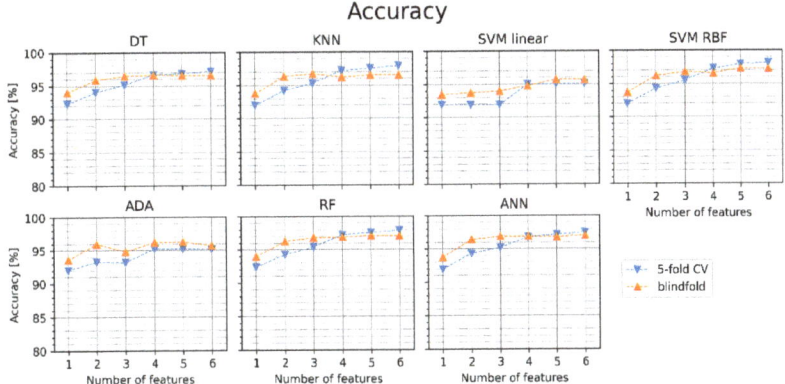

Figure 5. Accuracy of AF detection for different classifiers with sets of one to six features (orange points—blindfold validation, blue points—5-fold cross-validation). DT—decision tree, KNN—K nearest neighbors, SVM linear—support vector machine with linear kernel, SVM RBF—support vector machine with radial basis function kernel, ADA—Ada Boost, RF—random forest, ANN—artificial neural network.

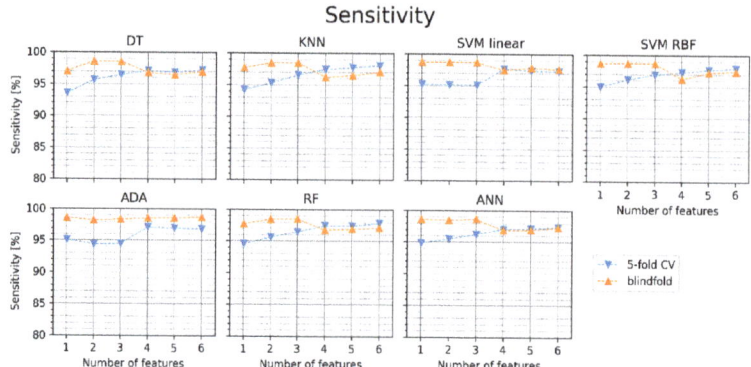

Figure 6. Sensitivity of atrial fibrillation detection for different classifiers with sets of one to six features (orange points—blindfold validation, blue points—5-fold cross-validation). DT—decision tree, KNN—K nearest neighbors, SVM linear—support vector machine with linear kernel, SVM RBF—support vector machine with radial basis function kernel, ADA—Ada Boost, RF—random forest, ANN—artificial neural network.

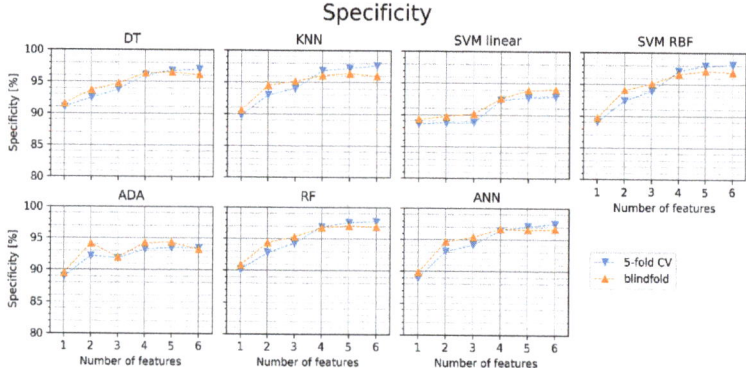

Figure 7. Specificity of AF detection for different classifiers with sets of one to six features (orange points—blindfold validation, blue points—5-fold cross-validation). DT—decision tree, KNN—K nearest neighbors, SVM linear—support vector machine with linear kernel, SVM RBF—support vector machine with radial basis function kernel, ADA—Ada Boost, RF—random forest, ANN—artificial neural network.

Table 3. Feature sets used for the classification.

No. of Features	Feature Set
1	pRR50
2	pRR50, SD2/SD1,
3	pRR50, SD2/SD1, CV
4	pRR50, SD2/SD1, CV, mean RR
5	pRR50, SD2/SD1, CV, mean RR, relRRdif
6	pRR50, SD2/SD1, CV, mean RR, relRRdif, relRRrange

pRR50—percentage of successive differences between RR intervals greater or equal to 50 ms; SD1 and SD2—standard deviation of points in the Poincare plot across and along the identity line, respectively; CV—coefficient of variance; mean RR—mean of RR intervals; relRRdif—mean of absolute differences between successive RR divided by mean RR; relRRrange = max(RR) − min(RR)/(mean RR) (relative RRrange).

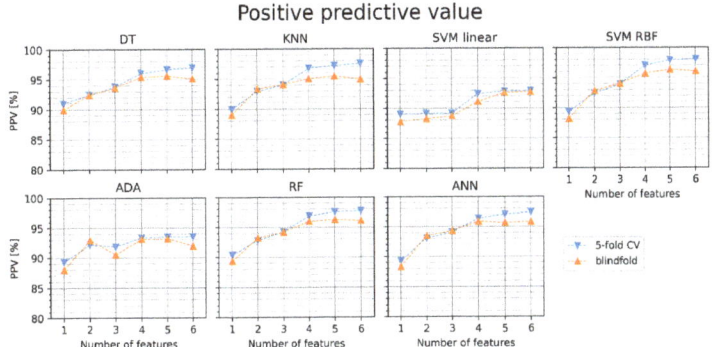

Figure 8. Positive predictive value (PPV) of AF detection for different classifiers with sets of one to six features (orange points—blindfold validation, blue points—5-fold cross-validation). DT—decision tree, KNN—K nearest neighbors, SVM linear—support vector machine with linear kernel, SVM RBF—support vector machine with radial basis function kernel, ADA—Ada Boost, RF—random forest, ANN—artificial neural network.

Figure 5 presents the accuracy obtained in our experiments. The orange points in the figure relate to the blindfold validation on the test set and the blue points to the 5-fold cross-validation. The same convention of presenting the results has been applied to other classification metrics in Figures 6–9. Average values and standard deviations of accuracy are shown in Table 4. Standard deviations are small (below 0.5 pp), which is why similar tables are not included further in this paper for other classification metrics. Figure 4 indicates that for most ML classifiers, the increase in the number of features improves the accuracy of AF detection in both cases: for the cross-validation and the blindfold validation. In all classifiers, except for SVM linear and ADA, accuracy in blindfold validation drops below the 5-fold CV level for four-six features. The obtained results are better for DT, KNN, RF, SVM RBF, and ANN than for SVM linear and ADA. SVM RBF with five features achieved the highest accuracy in the blindfold validation (97.2%). The results suggest that using the simpler classification algorithms as DT and KNN can provide comparable or slightly worse accuracy and other performance metrics (see Figures 6–9) than the relatively more complex algorithms such as SVM RBF, RF, or ANN.

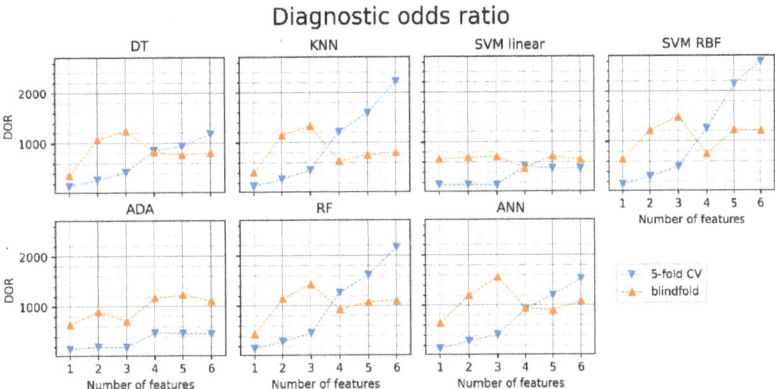

Figure 9. The diagnostic odds ratio (DOR) of AF detection for different classifiers with sets of one to six features (orange points—blindfold validation, blue points—5-fold cross-validation). DT—decision tree, KNN—K nearest neighbors, SVM linear—support vector machine with linear kernel, SVM RBF—support vector machine with radial basis function kernel, ADA—Ada Boost, RF—random forest, ANN—artificial neural network.

Table 4. Average values and standard deviations of accuracy in 5-fold cross-validation in 60 s recordings (in percentages).

Classifier \ Features	1	2	3	4	5	6
DT	92.29 (0.27)	94.06 (0.27)	95.15 (0.15)	96.65 (0.13)	96.84 (0.10)	97.16 (0.09)
KNN	92.00 (0.38)	94.20 (0.32)	95.32 (0.19)	97.18 (0.13)	97.53 (0.14)	97.90 (0.12)
SVM linear	91.91 (0.35)	91.93 (0.34)	91.92 (0.31)	95.00 (0.16)	95.04 (0.16)	95.08 (0.16)
SVM RBF	91.99 (0.34)	94.26 (0.31)	95.45 (0.11)	97.25 (0.07)	97.87 (0.13)	98.06 (0.10)
ADA	92.01 (0.35)	93.28 (0.40)	93.18 (0.37)	95.21 (0.23)	95.24 (0.26)	95.19 (0.23)
RF	92.40 (0.32)	94.26 (0.26)	95.42 (0.13)	97.24 (0.15)	97.57 (0.09)	97.88 (0.13)
ANN	91.89 (0.30)	94.32 (0.36)	95.20 (0.11)	96.79 (0.21)	97.16 (0.29)	97.48 (0.23)

DT—decision tree, KNN—K nearest neighbors, SVM linear—support vector machine with linear kernel, SVM RBF—support vector machine with radial basis function kernel, ADA—Ada Boost, RF—random forest, ANN—artificial neural network.

Figure 6 shows the sensitivity for the particular classifiers obtained in the same experiments as the accuracy in Figure 5. The achieved sensitivity values are similar for all classifiers. In the 5-fold cross-validation, the increase in the number of features improves sensitivity, but most classifiers reach the maximum for three features in the blindfold validation. Similarly, as in the case of accuracy, the obtained sensitivities are often greater for the blindfold validation than for cross-validation. SVM linear with one feature achieved the highest sensitivity in the blindfold validation (98.8%).

In Figure 7, the specificity of the particular classifiers is presented. Interestingly, in many cases, the specificity is higher in the blindfold validation than in the 5-fold cross-validation. Increasing the number of features generally improves the results. SVM RBF achieved the highest specificity in the blindfold validation with five features (97.2%).

Figure 8 shows the positive predictive value (PPV) obtained for the particular classifiers. In the 5-fold cross-validation and blindfold validation, increasing the number of features increases PPV in most classifiers. SVM RBF achieved the highest PPV in the blindfold validation with five features (96.4%).

Figure 9 shows the diagnostic odds ratio obtained for the particular classifiers. We can observe how the odds of AF detection grow with the increased number of features for different classifiers. ANN with three features achieved the highest DOR in the blindfold validation (1566). Similarly to accuracy, DOR in blindfold validation is higher than in 5-fold CV for 1–3 features and lower for 4–6 features in all classifiers, except for SVM linear and ADA.

3.2. Feature Sets without pRR50

In the next series of experiments, we repeated the feature selection process after excluding pRR50 from the analyzed features to verify how much diagnostic information was derived from pRR50, the highest scored parameter in MRMR. To provide the best comparable conditions, we repeated the MRMR analysis without pRR50, and the obtained MRMR scores are presented in Figure 10.

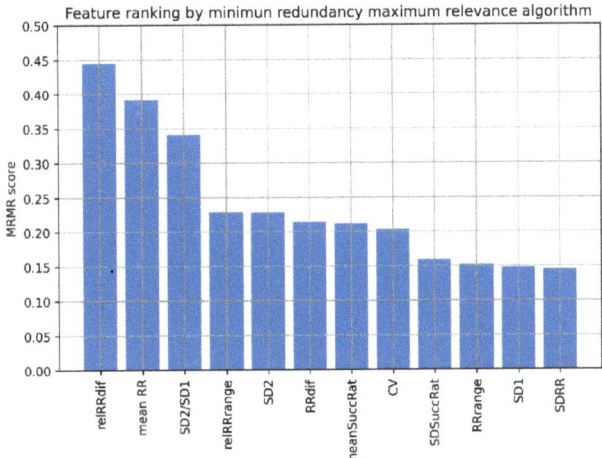

Figure 10. Ranking of heart rate variability features by minimum redundancy maximum relevance (MRMR) algorithm after excluding percentage of successive differences between RR intervals greater or equal to 50 ms (pRR50). SD1 and SD2—standard deviation of points in the Poincare plot across and along the identity line, respectively; mean RR—mean of RR intervals; SDRR—standard deviation of RR intervals; RRdif—mean of absolute differences between successive RR; CV—coefficient of variance; relRRdif = RRdif/(mean RR); meanSuccRat—mean ratio of successive RR; SDSuccRat—standard deviation of ratios of successive RR; RRrange = max(RR) − min(RR); relRRrange = RRrange/(mean RR) (relative RRrange).

The metaparameter tuning in the 5-fold cross-validation was repeated for new feature sets. The tuned classifiers were then trained and blindfold-validated. The accuracy obtained in this case is presented in Figure 11. Comparing Figure 11 with Figure 5, one can see the impact of the pRR50 parameter in AF detection procedures. SVM RBF achieved the highest accuracy in blindfold validation with five features (95.4%).

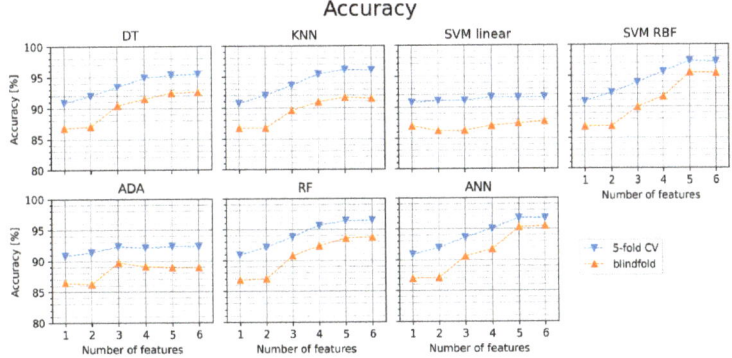

Figure 11. Accuracy of atrial fibrillation detection for different classifiers with sets of one to six features without pRR50 (orange points—blindfold validation, blue points—5-fold cross-validation). DT—decision tree, KNN—K nearest neighbors, SVM linear—support vector machine with linear kernel, SVM RBF—support vector machine with radial basis function kernel, ADA—Ada Boost, RF—random forest, ANN—artificial neural network.

The diagnostic odds ratios obtained for different classifiers and different sets of features are presented in Figure 12. The obtained DORs are notably lower than when the pRR50 was included (see Figure 9). Without pRR50, the highest DOR in the blindfold validation was achieved by ANN with six features (585).

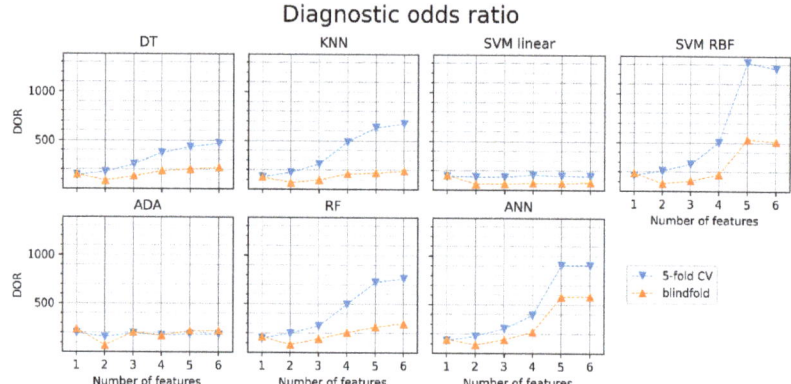

Figure 12. Diagnostic odds ratio (DOR) of atrial fibrillation detection for different classifiers with sets of one to six features (orange points—blindfold validation, blue points—5-fold cross-validation). DT—decision tree, KNN—K nearest neighbors, SVM linear—support vector machine with linear kernel, SVM RBF—support vector machine with radial basis function kernel, ADA—Ada Boost, RF—random forest, ANN—artificial neural network.

4. Discussion

Our findings demonstrate several things about discerning AF from SR using HRV parameters, selecting features for ML models, and different ML algorithms. The diagnostic properties of the applied ML algorithms are sensitive to the method used for choosing HRV parameters and the set of parameters entering the selection process. Feature selection based on AUC and MRMR gives different results. One might also see SR and AF histograms of various HRV parameters (Figure 3). Such a visual comparison shows which parameters may separate SR from AF. It is worth noting that for some features, such as mean RR and SD2/SD1, the distributions in AF and SR are not well separated, so these features are not good sole predictors of AF, but they bring additional information valuable in the presence of other features. Of the top six HRV features selected by MRMR, only four (66.7%) were in the top six with the highest AUC. In both methods, however, pRR50 was the number one HRV feature.

Furthermore, the analyzed HRV parameters describe distinguishing features of RR interval time series based on the absolute or relative differences between consecutive RR intervals, their ratios, and distributions. Interestingly, the most complex six-element MRMR-derived set mostly included the relative HRV parameters except for the mean RR.

In all six MRMR-selected feature sets, pRR50 was included. When pRR50 was excluded from the MRMR analysis, the order of selected parameters differed notably (see Figures 3 and 10). ML algorithms always performed better with pRR50 than without pRR50, regardless of the number of features between 1 and 6 (as measured by blindfold validation DOR—see Figures 9 and 12). For example, in SVM RBF with six features, the DOR was around 1200 when pRR50 was used and around 500 without pRR50.

We showed (Figure 2) which HRV parameters (features) contribute to the maximal diagnostic value, simultaneously providing minimal redundancy between subsequent features in AF detection. The 5-fold cross-validation (blue points in Figures 5–9, 11 and 12) confirmed the gradual growth of the statistical measures of AF detection with the increase in the number of the best HRV parameters chosen by the MRMR algorithm. Adding the subsequent sixth feature no longer causes a noticeable increase in the statistical measures, and in the case of some measures, even a very slight decrease. The blindfold validation results (orange points in Figures 5–9, 11 and 12) behave similarly for most algorithms. By increasing the number of features, especially from one to four, accuracy and sensitivity improved. Nevertheless, the blindfold validation results do not differ considerably from the results obtained through the 5-fold cross-validation, especially for the best algorithms.

Moreover, slightly worse results in accuracy for the blindfold validation are typical in many classification problems. The differences between the 5-fold cross-validation and blindfold validation are noticeably significant, but not in all cases; using a separate dataset for validation results in worse performance. SVM RBF achieved the highest accuracy in blindfold validation with five features (97.2%). On the other hand, ANN achieved the highest DOR in blindfold validation with three features (1566). However, it is worth noting that comparatively good results were also achieved with relatively computationally simple classifiers such as KNN or even DT, while the worst results were obtained for SVM linear and ADA.

Notably, the performance of the considered ML algorithms for AF detection is significantly higher when the feature set includes pRR50. Even if only pRR50 is used, very good diagnostic results are obtained (accuracy between 93.4 and 93.9%). In comparison, similar accuracy without pRR50 is achieved for at least four features (87.3–95.4%). Moreover, performance in blindfold validation is noticeably worse than in 5-fold cross-validation, which was not always the case when pRR50 was used.

The use of a specific length of the ECG, i.e., 60 s, limits to some extent our conclusions only to the ECG recordings or AF episodes of such a length. Our preliminary results (data not shown) with other lengths do not change the overall conclusions. Nevertheless, the impact of ECG length on the statistical measures of AF detection performance using HRV parameters selected by means of the MRMR algorithm requires further detailed investigations. It should also be noted that the goal of our research was not to study various feature selection algorithms and determine the best one which is a very general and complex task.

The MRMR algorithm proved useful and valuable in selecting HRV parameters with the potential to distinguish AF from SR in the 60 s ECGs. Three HRV parameters, i.e., pRR50, SD2/SD1, and CV, were ranked highest by MRMR for ML-based AF detection and pRR50 appears to outperform other HRV parameters for this task. It has the highest AUC, and the feature sets containing it achieve higher accuracies than those without it (see Figures 5 and 11).

The proposed methods and results presented in the paper might contribute to developing practical AF detection solutions in miniature wearable, bio-patches, implantable devices, and hand-held single- or multi-lead ECG devices [3,67–70].

It should be, however, kept in mind that the newer modes of ECG acquisition have their technical limitations, which may impact the quality of the recorded ECG signal and its noise level. If ECG quality declines, then the noise level increases, and there are a couple of reasons for it. Even if silver/silver chloride (Ag/AgCl) hydrogel electrodes are attached to a patient, there is always sweating and skin cell necrosis—this problem is particularly important in very long ECGs lasting for several consecutive days. Different materials are used to produce ECG electrodes. Metal ECG electrodes are a part of hand-held devices or smart-watches. Textile, polymer graphene, or rubber electrodes are used in the bio-patches, chest straps, or ECG vests. However, the ECG signal is usually not as good as the specialized Ag/AgCl electrodes [68,71–76]. Finally, electrical skin properties, including skin-electrode impedance, differ between patients; it changes with age, amount of subcutaneous adipose tissue or fluid accumulation, or the presence of some diseases [68,72].

For an ECG recorded with good quality, HRV parameters combined with ML methods are valuable for their potential clinical use. The number of devices dedicated to long-term ECG monitoring increases as they are vital in transient AF detection [3,68–70]. In these solutions, computational and energy efficiency are of crucial importance. Therefore, using straightforward ML classifiers and a small set of adequately selected simple HRV parameters is advisable. Having the results presented in the paper, we can consciously, i.e., based on the quantitative numerical results, choose both the ML algorithm and the extremely small sets of simple HRV features needed to achieve the assumed AF detection performance.

Recent studies have shown that advanced computational methods such as artificial intelligence may predict AF using the 12-lead and even a single-lead ECG acquired in patients with sinus rhythm [77–79]. The possibility of foreseeing the disease dramatically changes our perspective and clinical potential. Zachi et al. have proposed that with the artificial intelligence tools and modeling applied to proper data, it is possible to select previvors, i.e., individuals who are still healthy but have a substantial risk of developing a disease in the future [77]. Using artificial intelligence and structural analysis of resting ECG, it is possible to identify previvors of AF and start preventive actions before this arrhythmia and its complications occur. It might save lives, reduces morbidity, and probably the cost of AF management.

Very recently, Sagnard A. et al. [5] have shown that HRV analysis (mainly reduced LF/HF and increased pNN50 and RMSSD) predicted the new-onset in-hospital AF in over 2000 survivors of acute myocardial infarction. Their study suggests that HRV features also identify previvors of AF. However, it is unknown whether the employment of ML or artificial intelligence algorithms to an ECG in patients without AF would translate into the prediction of AF and identification of its previvors.

If HRV parameters and ML techniques can be implemented for diagnostic purposes in mobile e-health technologies, then why not use them to predict AF before it even happens? We are convinced that it is possible and that studying such a concept deserves future investigations.

The current clinical use of HRV deserves a short comment. For many years, HRV has been demonstrated to predict total or various forms of mortality, mainly in survivors of myocardial infarction and heart failure patients [12,14,80–82]. However, the constant progress in the healthcare and management of patients after myocardial infarction and heart failure has substantially reduced mortality and improved the long-term prognosis. Nowadays, more patients receive quick myocardial reperfusion and modern pharmacological treatment. These are just some of the many reasons why HRV is no longer recommended for the mortality risk stratification in cardiac patients. Nevertheless, both patients who suffer from heart attacks and those with heart failure are at risk of future developing AF. If HRV helped identify AF previvors, i.e., people at risk of the new onset of this arrhythmia, it would translate into a great return of this method to clinical practice.

5. Conclusions

HRV parameters combined with ML techniques differentiate ECGs with AF from those in SR. However, methods used for choosing HRV features may impact the outcome of the ML algorithm. Using straightforward ML classifiers and the extremely small sets of simple HRV features, regardless of the features selection methods used (AUC or MRMR), pRR50 has consistently been selected at the top HRV parameter differentiating AF from SR in ECGs of 60 s duration. The proposed methodology and the presented results of the selection of HRV parameters have the potential to develop practical solutions and devices for automatic AF detection with minimal sets of simple HRV parameters.

Author Contributions: Conceptualization, S.B., K.J. and P.G.; methodology, S.B., K.J. and P.G.; software, S.B.; validation, S.B., K.J. and P.G.; formal analysis, S.B., K.J. and P.G.; investigation, S.B., K.J. and P.G.; data curation, S.B.; writing—original draft preparation, S.B., K.J. and P.G.; writing—review and editing, S.B., K.J. and P.G.; visualization, S.B.; supervision, K.J. and P.G. All authors have read and agreed to the published version of the manuscript.

Funding: This research was funded in part by the Scientific Council for the discipline of Automatic Control, Electronics and Electrical Engineering of Warsaw University of Technology, Poland, grant "Studies on the effectiveness of atrial fibrillation detection based on the analysis of PPG signal and ECG signal using machine learning techniques, including proposals for new solutions".

Institutional Review Board Statement: Not applicable.

Informed Consent Statement: Not applicable.

Data Availability Statement: MIT-BIH Atrial Fibrillation Database (AFDB), [50,51] and Long Term AF Database (LTAFDB) [51,52] were used in the study. They are available at https://physionet.org/content/afdb/1.0.0/ (accessed on 1 June 2022) and https://physionet.org/content/ltafdb/1.0.0/ (accessed on 1 June 2022), respectively.

Conflicts of Interest: The authors declare no conflict of interest.

References

1. Kirchhoff, P.; Benussi, S.; Kotecha, D.; Ahlsson, A.; Atar, D.; Casadei, B. 2016 ESC Guidelines for the Management of Atrial Fibrillation Developed in Collaboration with EACTS. *Eur. J. Cardio-Thorac. Surg.* **2016**, *50*, e1–e88. [CrossRef] [PubMed]
2. Hindricks, G.; Potpara, T.; Dagres, N.; Arbelo, E.; Bax, J.J.; Blomström-Lundqvist, C.; Boriani, G.; Castella, M.; Dan, G.A.; Dilaveris, P.E.; et al. 2020 ESC Guidelines for the Diagnosis and Management of Atrial Fibrillation Developed in Collaboration with the European Association for Cardio-Thoracic Surgery (EACTS) The Task Force for the Diagnosis and Management of Atrial Fibrillation of the European Society of Cardiology (ESC) Developed with the Special Contribution of the European Heart Rhythm Association (EHRA) of the ESC. *Eur. Heart J.* **2021**, *42*, 373–498. [CrossRef] [PubMed]
3. Tonko, J.B.; Wright, M.J. Review of the 2020 ESC Guidelines for the Diagnosis and Management of Atrial Fibrillation—What Has Changed and How Does This Affect Daily Practice. *J. Clin. Med.* **2021**, *10*, 3922. [CrossRef] [PubMed]
4. Magnussen, C.; Niiranen, T.J.; Ojeda, F.M.; Gianfagna, F.; Blankenberg, S.; Njølstad, I.; Vartiainen, E.; Sans, S.; Pasterkamp, G.; Hughes, M. Sex Differences and Similarities in Atrial Fibrillation Epidemiology, Risk Factors, and Mortality in Community Cohorts: Results from the BiomarCaRE Consortium (Biomarker for Cardiovascular Risk Assessment in Europe). *Circulation* **2017**, *136*, 1588–1597. [CrossRef]
5. Sagnard, A.; Guenancia, C.; Mouhat, B.; Maza, M.; Fichot, M.; Moreau, D.; Garnier, F.; Lorgis, L.; Cottin, Y.; Zeller, M. Involvement of Autonomic Nervous System in New-Onset Atrial Fibrillation during Acute Myocardial Infarction. *J. Clin. Med.* **2020**, *9*, 1481. [CrossRef]
6. Ble, M.; Benito, B.; Cuadrado-Godia, E.; Pérez-Fernández, S.; Gómez, M.; Mas-Stachurska, A.; Tizón-Marcos, H.; Molina, L.; Martí-Almor, J.; Cladellas, M. Left Atrium Assessment by Speckle Tracking Echocardiography in Cryptogenic Stroke: Seeking Silent Atrial Fibrillation. *J. Clin. Med.* **2021**, *10*, 3501. [CrossRef]
7. Sörnmo, L.; Stridh, M.; Husser, D.; Bollmann, A.; Olsson, S.B. Analysis of Atrial Fibrillation: From Electrocardiogram Signal Processing to Clinical Management. *Philos. Trans. R. Soc. A Math. Phys. Eng. Sci.* **2009**, *367*, 235–253. [CrossRef]
8. Langley, P.; Bourke, J.P.; Murray, A. Frequency Analysis of Atrial Fibrillation. In Proceedings of the Computers in Cardiology 2000 (Cat. 00CH37163), Cambridge, MA, USA, 24–27 September 2000; Volume 27, pp. 65–68. [CrossRef]
9. Rieta, J.J.; Castells, F.; Sánchez, C.; Zarzoso, V.; Millet, J. Atrial Activity Extraction for Atrial Fibrillation Analysis Using Blind Source Separation. *IEEE Trans. Biomed. Eng.* **2004**, *51*, 1176–1186. [CrossRef]
10. Alcaraz, R.; Rieta, J.J. Adaptive Singular Value Cancelation of Ventricular Activity in Single-Lead Atrial Fibrillation Electrocardiograms. *Physiol. Meas.* **2008**, *29*, 1351–1369. [CrossRef]
11. Buś, S.; Jędrzejewski, K. Two Stage SVD-Based Method for QRST Waves Cancellation in Atrial Fibrillation Detection. In Proceedings of the 2019 Signal Processing Symposium (SPSympo), Krakow, Poland, 17–19 September 2019; pp. 24–28. [CrossRef]
12. Heart Rate Variability: Standards of Measurement, Physiological Interpretation and Clinical Use. Task Force of the European Society of Cardiology and the North American Society of Pacing and Electrophysiology. *Circulation* **1996**, *93*, 1043–1065. [CrossRef]
13. Bauer, A.; Camm, A.J.; Cerutti, S.; Guzik, P.; Huikuri, H.; Lombardi, F.; Malik, M.; Peng, C.-K.; Porta, A.; Sassi, R. Reference Values of Heart Rate Variability. *Heart Rhythm* **2017**, *14*, 302–303. [CrossRef]
14. Guzik, P.; Piskorski, J.; Barthel, P.; Bauer, A.; Müller, A.; Junk, N.; Ulm, K.; Malik, M.; Schmidt, G. Heart Rate Deceleration Runs for Postinfarction Risk Prediction. *J. Electrocardiol.* **2012**, *45*, 70–76. [CrossRef]
15. Guzik, P.; Piekos, C.; Pierog, O.; Fenech, N.; Krauze, T.; Piskorski, J.; Wykretowicz, A. Classic Electrocardiogram-Based and Mobile Technology Derived Approaches to Heart Rate Variability Are Not Equivalent. *Int. J. Cardiol.* **2018**, *258*, 154–156. [CrossRef]
16. Michel, P.; Ngo, N.; Pons, J.-F.; Delliaux, S.; Giorgi, R. A Filter Approach for Feature Selection in Classification: Application to Automatic Atrial Fibrillation Detection in Electrocardiogram Recordings. *BMC Med. Inform. Decis. Mak.* **2021**, *21*, 130. [CrossRef]
17. Buś, S.; Jędrzejewski, K.; Guzik, P. A Study on Selection of HRV-based Features for Different Classifiers in Atrial Fibrillation Detection. In Proceedings of the 2021 Signal Processing Symposium (SPSympo), Lodz, Poland, 20–23 September 2021; pp. 31–34. [CrossRef]
18. Boon, K.H.; Khalil-Hani, M.; Malarvili, M.B.; Sia, C.W. Paroxysmal Atrial Fibrillation Prediction Method with Shorter HRV Sequences. *Comput. Methods Programs Biomed.* **2016**, *134*, 187–196. [CrossRef]
19. Mustaqeem, A.; Anwar, S.M.; Majid, M.; Khan, A.R. Wrapper Method for Feature Selection to Classify Cardiac Arrhythmia. In Proceedings of the 2017 39th Annual International Conference of the IEEE Engineering in Medicine and Biology Society (EMBC), Jeju, Korea, 11–15 July 2017; pp. 3656–3659. [CrossRef]
20. de Chazal, P.; Heneghan, C. Automated Assessment of Atrial Fibrillation. In Proceedings of the Computers in Cardiology 2001 (Cat. No.01CH37287), Rotterdam, The Netherlands, 23–26 September 2001; Volume 28, pp. 117–120. [CrossRef]

21. Clifford, G.D.; Liu, C.; Moody, B.; Li-wei, H.L.; Silva, I.; Li, Q.; Johnson, A.E.; Mark, R.G. AF Classification from a Short Single Lead ECG Recording: The PhysioNet/Computing in Cardiology Challenge 2017. In Proceedings of the 2017 Computing in Cardiology (CinC), Rennes, France, 24–27 September 2017; pp. 1–4. [CrossRef]
22. Datta, S.; Puri, C.; Mukherjee, A.; Banerjee, R.; Dutta Choudhury, A.; Singh, R.; Ukil, A.; Bandyopadhyay, S.; Pal, A.; Khandelwal, S. Identifying Normal, AF and Other Abnormal ECG Rhythms Using a Cascaded Binary Classifier. In Proceedings of the 2017 Computing in Cardiology (CinC), Rennes, France, 24–27 September 2017.
23. Jiménez Serrano, S.; Yagüe Mayans, J.; Simarro-Mondéjar, E.; Calvo, C.; Castells Ramon, F.; Roig, J. Atrial Fibrillation Detection Using Feedforward Neural Networks and Automatically Extracted Signal Features. In Proceedings of the 2017 Computing in Cardiology (CinC), Rennes, France, 24–27 September 2017; pp. 1–4. [CrossRef]
24. Zabihi, M.; Rad, A.B.; Katsaggelos, A.K.; Kiranyaz, S.; Narkilahti, S.; Gabbouj, M. Detection of Atrial Fibrillation in ECG Hand-Held Devices Using a Random Forest Classifier. In Proceedings of the 2017 Computing in Cardiology (CinC), Rennes, France, 24–27 September 2017; pp. 1–4. [CrossRef]
25. Krasteva, V.; Christov, I.; Naydenov, S.; Stoyanov, T.; Jekova, I. Application of Dense Neural Networks for Detection of Atrial Fibrillation and Ranking of Augmented ECG Feature Set. *Sensors* **2021**, *21*, 6848. [CrossRef]
26. Christov, I.; Krasteva, V.; Simova, I.; Neycheva, T.; Schmid, R. Ranking of the Most Reliable Beat Morphology and Heart Rate Variability Features for the Detection of Atrial Fibrillation in Short Single-Lead ECG. *Physiol. Meas.* **2018**, *39*, 094005. [CrossRef]
27. Shao, M.; Zhou, Z.; Bin, G.; Bai, Y.; Wu, S. A Wearable Electrocardiogram Telemonitoring System for Atrial Fibrillation Detection. *Sensors* **2020**, *20*, 606. [CrossRef]
28. Parsi, A.; Glavin, M.; Jones, E.; Byrne, D. Prediction of Paroxysmal Atrial Fibrillation Using New Heart Rate Variability Features. *Comput. Biol. Med.* **2021**, *133*, 104367. [CrossRef]
29. Biton, S.; Gendelman, S.; Ribeiro, A.H.; Miana, G.; Moreira, C.; Ribeiro, A.L.P.; Behar, J.A. Atrial Fibrillation Risk Prediction from the 12-Lead Electrocardiogram Using Digital Biomarkers and Deep Representation Learning. *Eur. Heart J.-Digit. Health* **2021**, *2*, 576–585. [CrossRef]
30. Zhu, J.; Pu, Y.; Huang, H.; Wang, Y.; Li, X.; Yan, T. A Feature Selection-Based Algorithm for Detection of Atrial Fibrillation Using Short-Term ECG. *J. Mech. Med. Biol.* **2021**, *21*, 2140013. [CrossRef]
31. Kotynia, M.M. Application for Atrial Fibrillation Classification Based on ECG Recordings. Bachelor's Thesis, Warsaw University of Technology, Warsaw, Poland, 2021.
32. Jiang, F.; Xu, B.; Zhu, Z.; Zhang, B. Topological Data Analysis Approach to Extract the Persistent Homology Features of Ballistocardiogram Signal in Unobstructive Atrial Fibrillation Detection. *IEEE Sens. J.* **2022**, *22*, 6920–6930. [CrossRef]
33. Parsi, A.; Byrne, D.; Glavin, M.; Jones, E. Heart Rate Variability Feature Selection Method for Automated Prediction of Sudden Cardiac Death. *Biomed. Signal Process. Control* **2021**, *65*, 102310. [CrossRef]
34. Oster, J.; Behar, J.; Colloca, R.; Li, Q.; Li, Q.; Clifford, G.D. Open Source Java-Based ECG Analysis Software and Android App for Atrial Fibrillation Screening. In Proceedings of the Computing in Cardiology 2013, Zaragoza, Spain, 22–25 September 2013; pp. 731–734.
35. Mohebbi, M.; Ghassemian, H. Detection of Atrial Fibrillation Episodes Using SVM. *IEEE Eng. Med. Biol. Soc.* **2008**, *2008*, 177–180. [CrossRef]
36. Sepulveda-Suescun, J.P.; Murillo-Escobar, J.; Urda-Benitez, R.D.; Orrego-Metaute, D.A.; Orozco-Duque, A. Atrial Fibrillation Detection through Heart Rate Variability Using a Machine Learning Approach and Poincare Plot Features. In Proceedings of the VII Latin American Congress on Biomedical Engineering CLAIB 2016, Bucaramanga, Colombia, 26–28 October 2016; pp. 565–568. [CrossRef]
37. Nguyen, A.; Ansari, S.; Hooshmand, M.; Lin, K.; Ghanbari, H.; Gryak, J.; Najarian, K. Comparative Study on Heart Rate Variability Analysis for Atrial Fibrillation Detection in Short Single-Lead ECG Recordings. In Proceedings of the 2018 40th Annual International Conference of the IEEE Engineering in Medicine and Biology Society (EMBC), Honolulu, HI, USA, 18–21 July 2018; pp. 526–529. [CrossRef]
38. Mei, Z.; Gu, X.; Chen, H.; Chen, W. Automatic Atrial Fibrillation Detection Based on Heart Rate Variability and Spectral Features. *IEEE Access* **2018**, *6*, 53566–53575. [CrossRef]
39. Kara, S.; Okandan, M. Atrial Fibrillation Classification with Artificial Neural Networks. *Pattern Recognit.* **2007**, *40*, 2967–2973. [CrossRef]
40. Pourbabaee, B.; Roshtkhari, M.J.; Khorasani, K. Deep Convolutional Neural Networks and Learning ECG Features for Screening Paroxysmal Atrial Fibrillation Patients. *IEEE Trans. Syst. Man Cybern. Syst.* **2018**, *48*, 2095–2104. [CrossRef]
41. Faust, O.; Shenfield, A.; Kareem, M.; San, T.R.; Fujita, H.; Acharya, U.R. Automated Detection of Atrial Fibrillation Using Long Short-Term Memory Network with RR Interval Signals. *Comput. Biol. Med.* **2018**, *102*, 327–335. [CrossRef]
42. Malakhov, A.I.; Schookin, S.I.; Ivancov, V.I.; Tikhomirov, A.N. A Combined Algorithm for Identification and Differentiation of Atrial Flutter and Atrial Fibrillation Based on ECG Analysis. *Biomed. Eng.* **2013**, *47*, 14–17. [CrossRef]
43. Ma, F.; Zhang, J.; Liang, W.; Xue, J. Automated Classification of Atrial Fibrillation Using Artificial Neural Network for Wearable Devices. *Math. Probl. Eng.* **2020**, *2020*, 9159158. [CrossRef]
44. Marsili, I.A.; Mase, M.; Pisetta, V.; Ricciardi, E.; Andrighetti, A.O.; Ravelli, F.; Nollo, G. Optimized Algorithms for Atrial Fibrillation Detection by Wearable Tele-Holter Devices. In Proceedings of the 2016 IEEE International Smart Cities Conference (ISC2), Trento, Italy, 12–15 September 2016; pp. 1–4. [CrossRef]

45. Erdenebayar, U.; Kim, H.; Park, J.-U.; Kang, D.; Lee, K.-J. Automatic Prediction of Atrial Fibrillation Based on Convolutional Neural Network Using a Short-Term Normal Electrocardiogram Signal. *J. Korean Med. Sci.* **2019**, *34*, e64. [CrossRef] [PubMed]
46. Mousavi, S.; Afghah, F.; Acharya, U.R. HAN-ECG: An Interpretable Atrial Fibrillation Detection Model Using Hierarchical Attention Networks. *Comput. Biol. Med.* **2020**, *127*, 104057. [CrossRef] [PubMed]
47. Faust, O.; Kareem, M.; Shenfield, A.; Ali, A.; Acharya, U.R.; Sheffield, B. Validating the Robustness of an Internet of Things Based Atrial Fibrillation Detection System. *Pattern Recognit. Lett.* **2020**, *133*, 55–61. [CrossRef]
48. Peng, H.C.; Long, F.; Ding, C. Feature selection based on mutual information: Criteria of max-dependency, max-relevance, and min-redundancy. *IEEE Trans. Pattern Anal. Mach. Intell.* **2005**, *27*, 1226–1238. [CrossRef] [PubMed]
49. Ding, C.; Peng, H. Minimum redundancy feature selection from microarray gene expression data. *J. Bioinform. Comput. Biol.* **2005**, *3*, 185–205. [CrossRef]
50. Moody, G. A New Method for Detecting Atrial Fibrillation Using RR Intervals. *Comput. Cardiol.* **1983**, *10*, 227–230.
51. Goldberger, A.L.; Amaral, L.A.; Glass, L.; Hausdorff, J.M.; Ivanov, P.C.; Mark, R.G.; Mietus, J.E.; Moody, G.B.; Peng, C.-K.; Stanley, H.E. PhysioBank, PhysioToolkit, and PhysioNet: Components of a New Research Resource for Complex Physiologic Signals. *Circulation* **2000**, *101*, e215–e220. [CrossRef]
52. Petrutiu, S.; Sahakian, A.V.; Swiryn, S. Abrupt Changes in Fibrillatory Wave Characteristics at the Termination of Paroxysmal Atrial Fibrillation in Humans. *Europace* **2007**, *9*, 466–470. [CrossRef]
53. Hastie, T.; Tibshirani, R.; Friedman, J. *The Elements of Statistical Learning: Data Mining, Inference, and Prediction*, 2nd ed.; Springer: New York, NY, USA, 2017; ISBN 978-0-387-84858-7.
54. Vabalas, A.; Gowen, E.; Poliakoff, E.; Casson, A.J. Machine Learning Algorithm Validation with a Limited Sample Size. *PLoS ONE* **2019**, *14*, e0224365. [CrossRef]
55. Walsh, I.; Pollastri, G.; Tosatto, S. Correct Machine Learning on Protein Sequences: A Peer-Reviewing Perspective. *Brief. Bioinform.* **2015**, *17*, 831–840. [CrossRef]
56. Shaffer, F.; Ginsberg, J.P. An Overview of Heart Rate Variability Metrics and Norms. *Front. Public Health* **2017**, *5*, 258. [CrossRef]
57. Guzik, P.; Piskorski, J.; Krauze, T.; Schneider, R.; Wesseling, K.H.; Wykretowicz, A.; Wysocki, H. Correlations between the Poincaré plot and conventional heart rate variability parameters assessed during paced breathing. *J. Physiol. Sci.* **2007**, *57*, 63–71. [CrossRef]
58. Kleiger, R.E.; Stein, P.K.; Bigger, J.T., Jr. Heart Rate Variability: Measurement and Clinical Utility. *Ann. Noninvasive Electrocardiol.* **2005**, *10*, 88–101. [CrossRef]
59. Rizwan, A.; Zoha, A.; Mabrouk, I.B.; Sabbour, H.M.; Al-Sumaiti, A.S.; Alomainy, A.; Imran, M.A.; Abbasi, Q.H. A Review on the State of the Art in Atrial Fibrillation Detection Enabled by Machine Learning. *IEEE Rev. Biomed. Eng.* **2020**, *14*, 219–239. [CrossRef]
60. Bolon-Candedo, V.; Alonso-Betanzos, A. *Recent Advances in Ensembles for Feature Selection*; Springer: Heidelberg, Germany, 2018.
61. Quinlan, J.R. Simplifying Decision Trees. *Int. J. Man-Mach. Stud.* **1987**, *27*, 221–234. [CrossRef]
62. Altman, N.S. An Introduction to Kernel and Nearest-Neighbor Nonparametric Regression. *Am. Stat.* **1992**, *46*, 175–185. [CrossRef]
63. Cortes, C.; Vapnik, V. Support-Vector Networks. *Mach. Learn.* **1995**, *20*, 273–297. [CrossRef]
64. Freund, Y.; Schapire, R.E. A Decision-Theoretic Generalization of on-Line Learning and an Application to Boosting. *J. Comput. Syst. Sci.* **1997**, *55*, 119–139. [CrossRef]
65. Ho, T.K. Random Decision Forests. In Proceedings of the 3rd International Conference on Document Analysis and Recognition, Montreal, QC, Canada, 14–16 August 1995; Volume 1, pp. 278–282. [CrossRef]
66. Glas, A.S.; Lijmer, J.G.; Prins, M.H.; Bonsel, G.J.; Bossuyt, P.M.M. The Diagnostic Odds Ratio: A Single Indicator of Test Performance. *J. Clin. Epidemiol.* **2003**, *56*, 1129–1135. [CrossRef]
67. Mitrega, K.; Lip, G.Y.; Sredniawa, B.; Sokal, A.; Streb, W.; Przyludzki, K.; Zdrojewski, T.; Wierucki, L.; Rutkowski, M.; Bandosz, P. Predicting Silent Atrial Fibrillation in the Elderly: A Report from the NOMED-AF Cross-Sectional Study. *J. Clin. Med.* **2021**, *10*, 2321. [CrossRef]
68. Boriani, G.; Palmisano, P.; Malavasi, V.L.; Fantecchi, E.; Vitolo, M.; Bonini, N.; Imberti, J.F.; Valenti, A.C.; Schnabel, R.B.; Freedman, B. Clinical Factors Associated with Atrial Fibrillation Detection on Single-Time Point Screening Using a Hand-Held Single-Lead ECG Device. *J. Clin. Med.* **2021**, *10*, 729. [CrossRef]
69. Guzik, P.; Malik, M. ECG by Mobile Technologies. *J. Electrocardiol.* **2016**, *49*, 894–901. [CrossRef] [PubMed]
70. Roten, L.; Goulouti, E.; Lam, A.; Elchinova, E.; Nozica, N.; Spirito, A.; Wittmer, S.; Branca, M.; Servatius, H.; Noti, F. Age and Sex Specific Prevalence of Clinical and Screen-Detected Atrial Fibrillation in Hospitalized Patients. *J. Clin. Med.* **2021**, *10*, 4871. [CrossRef]
71. Jin, H.; Abu-Raya, Y.S.; Haick, H. Advanced Materials for Health Monitoring with Skin-Based Wearable Devices. *Adv. Healthc. Mater.* **2017**, *6*, 1700024. [CrossRef] [PubMed]
72. Kaminski, M.; Prymas, P.; Konobrodzka, A.; Filberek, P.; Sibrecht, G.; Sierocki, W.; Osinska, Z.; Wykretowicz, A.; Lobodzinski, S.; Guzik, P. Clinical Stage of Acquired Immunodeficiency Syndrome in HIV-Positive Patients Impacts the Quality of the Touch ECG Recordings. *J. Electrocardiol.* **2019**, *55*, 87–90. [CrossRef]
73. Tsukada, S.; Nakashima, H.; Torimitsu, K. Conductive Polymer Combined Silk Fiber Bundle for Bioelectrical Signal Recording. *PLoS ONE* **2012**, *7*, e33689. [CrossRef]

74. Yapici, M.K.; Alkhidir, T.E. Intelligent Medical Garments with Graphene-Functionalized Smart-Cloth ECG Sensors. *Sensors* **2017**, *17*, 875. [CrossRef]
75. Cvach, M.M.; Biggs, M.; Rothwell, K.J.; Charles-Hudson, C. Daily Electrode Change and Effect on Cardiac Monitor Alarms: An Evidence-Based Practice Approach. *J. Nurs. Care Qual.* **2013**, *28*, 265–271. [CrossRef] [PubMed]
76. Xiao, Y.; Wang, M.; Li, Y.; Sun, Z.; Liu, Z.; He, L.; Liu, R. High-Adhesive Flexible Electrodes and Their Manufacture: A Review. *Micromachines* **2021**, *12*, 1505. [CrossRef] [PubMed]
77. Attia, Z.I.; Noseworthy, P.A.; Lopez-Jimenez, F.; Asirvatham, S.J.; Deshmukh, A.J.; Gersh, B.J.; Carter, R.E.; Yao, X.; Rabinstein, A.A.; Erickson, B.J. An Artificial Intelligence-Enabled ECG Algorithm for the Identification of Patients with Atrial Fibrillation during Sinus Rhythm: A Retrospective Analysis of Outcome Prediction. *Lancet* **2019**, *394*, 861–867. [PubMed]
78. Khurshid, S.; Friedman, S.; Reeder, C.; Di Achille, P.; Diamant, N.; Singh, P.; Harrington, L.X.; Wang, X.; Al-Alusi, M.A.; Sarma, G. ECG-Based Deep Learning and Clinical Risk Factors to Predict Atrial Fibrillation. *Circulation* **2022**, *145*, 122–133. [CrossRef]
79. Attia, Z.I.; Harmon, D.M.; Behr, E.R.; Friedman, P.A. Application of Artificial Intelligence to the Electrocardiogram. *Eur. Heart J.* **2021**, *42*, 4717–4730. [CrossRef]
80. Bauer, A.; Malik, M.; Schmidt, G.; Barthel, P.; Bonnemeier, H.; Cygankiewicz, I.; Guzik, P.; Lombardi, F.; Müller, A.; Oto, A. Heart Rate Turbulence: Standards of Measurement, Physiological Interpretation, and Clinical Use: International Society for Holter and Noninvasive Electrophysiology Consensus. *J. Am. Coll. Cardiol.* **2008**, *52*, 1353–1365. [CrossRef]
81. Sassi, R.; Cerutti, S.; Lombardi, F.; Malik, M.; Huikuri, H.V.; Peng, C.-K.; Schmidt, G.; Yamamoto, Y.; Reviewers, D.; Gorenek, B. Advances in Heart Rate Variability Signal Analysis: Joint Position Statement by the e-Cardiology ESC Working Group and the European Heart Rhythm Association Co-Endorsed by the Asia Pacific Heart Rhythm Society. *Europace* **2015**, *17*, 1341–1353. [CrossRef]
82. Cygankiewicz, I.; Zareba, W.; Vazquez, R.; Bayes-Genis, A.; Pascual, D.; Macaya, C.; Almendral, J.; Fiol, M.; Bardaji, A.; Gonzalez-Juanatey, J.R. Risk Stratification of Mortality in Patients with Heart Failure and Left Ventricular Ejection Fraction > 35%. *Am. J. Cardiol.* **2009**, *103*, 1003–1010. [CrossRef]

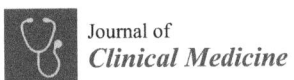

Systematic Review

Structural Heart Alterations in Brugada Syndrome: Is it Really a Channelopathy? A Systematic Review

Antonio Oliva [1,†], Simone Grassi [2,†], Vilma Pinchi [2], Francesca Cazzato [1], Mónica Coll [3,4], Mireia Alcalde [3], Marta Vallverdú-Prats [3], Alexandra Perez-Serra [3], Estefanía Martínez-Barrios [5,6,7], Sergi Cesar [5,6,7], Anna Iglesias [3], José Cruzalegui [5,6,7], Clara Hernández [5], Victoria Fiol [5,6,7], Elena Arbelo [4,6,7], Nuria Díez-Escuté [8], Vincenzo Arena [9], Josep Brugada [4,5,6,7,8], Georgia Sarquella-Brugada [5,6,7,10], Ramon Brugada [3,4,9,11,*,‡] and Oscar Campuzano [3,4,10,*,‡]

[1] Department of Health Surveillance and Bioethics, Section of Legal Medicine, Fondazione Policlinico A. Gemelli IRCCS, Università Cattolica del Sacro Cuore, 00168 Rome, Italy; antonio.oliva@unicatt.it (A.O.); francescacazzato993@gmail.com (F.C.)

[2] Department of Health Sciences, Section of Forensic Medical Sciences, University of Florence, Largo Brambilla 3, 50134 Florence, Italy; simone.grassi@unicatt.it (S.G.); vilma.pinchi@unifi.it (V.P.)

[3] Cardiovascular Genetics Center, University of Girona-IDIBGI, 17190 Girona, Spain; mcoll@gencardio.com (M.C.); malcalde@gencardio.com (M.A.); mvallverdu@gencardio.com (M.V.-P.); aperez@idibgi.org (A.P.-S.); annai@brugada.org (A.I.)

[4] Centro de Investigación Biomédica en Red. Enfermedades Cardiovasculares (CIBERCV), 28029 Madrid, Spain; earbelo@clinic.cat (E.A.); jbrugada@clinic.cat (J.B.)

[5] Pediatric Arrhythmias, Inherited Cardiac Diseases and Sudden Death Unit, Cardiology Department, Sant Joan de Déu Hospital de Barcelona, 08950 Barcelona, Spain; estefania.martinez@sjd.es (E.M.-B.); sergi.cesar@gmail.com (S.C.); josecarlos.cruzalegui@sjd.es (J.C.); clara.hernandez@sjd.es (C.H.); jvfiolramis@gmail.com (V.F.); georgia@brugada.org (G.S.-B.)

[6] European Reference Network for Rare, Low Prevalence and Complex Diseases of the Heart (ERN GUARD-Heart), 1105 AZ Amsterdam, The Netherlands

[7] Arrítmies Pediàtriques, Cardiologia Genètica i Mort Sobtada, Malalties Cardiovasculars en el Desenvolupament, Institut de Recerca Sant Joan de Déu, Esplugues de Llobregat, 08950 Barcelona, Spain

[8] Arrhythmias Unit, Hospital Clinic, University of Barcelona-IDIBAPS, 08036 Barcelona, Spain; nuria.andrews@gmail.com

[9] Institute of Pathological Anatomy, School of Medicine, Catholic University, 00168 Rome, Italy; vincenzo.arena@policlinicogemelli.it

[10] Medical Science Department, School of Medicine, University of Girona, 17003 Girona, Spain

[11] Cardiology Service, Hospital Josep Trueta, University of Girona, 17007 Girona, Spain

* Correspondence: ramon@brugada.org (R.B.); oscar@brugada.org (O.C.)

† These authors contributed equally to this work.

‡ These authors contributed equally to this work.

Abstract: Brugada syndrome (BrS) is classified as an inherited cardiac channelopathy attributed to dysfunctional ion channels and/or associated proteins in cardiomyocytes rather than to structural heart alterations. However, hearts of some BrS patients exhibit slight histologic abnormalities, suggesting that BrS could be a phenotypic variant of arrhythmogenic cardiomyopathy. We performed a systematic review of the literature following Preferred Reporting Items for Systematic Reviews and Meta-Analyses Statement (PRISMA) criteria. Our comprehensive analysis of structural findings did not reveal enough definitive evidence for reclassification of BrS as a cardiomyopathy. The collection and comprehensive analysis of new cases with a definitive BrS diagnosis are needed to clarify whether some of these structural features may have key roles in the pathophysiological pathways associated with malignant arrhythmogenic episodes.

Keywords: sudden cardiac death; Brugada syndrome; histopathology; forensic pathology; endomyocardial biopsy

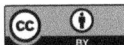

1. Introduction

Brugada syndrome (BrS) is an inherited cardiac syndrome associated with the increased risk of ventricular tachycardia, ventricular fibrillation (VF), and sudden cardiac death (SCD) in a structurally normal heart. On an electrocardiogram (ECG), the diagnosis of BrS is based on *"ST-segment elevation with type 1 morphology ≥2 mm in one or more leads among the right precordial leads V1 and/or V2 positioned in the second, third, or fourth intercostal space, occurring either spontaneously or after provocative drug test with intravenous administration of sodium channel blockers"* [1]. The type 1 ECG pattern described above is the only one diagnostic of BrS, whereas other repolarization patterns (type 2 and type 3) found in more than one right precordial lead should be considered suggestive of the disease and require further confirmatory investigations. Other known causes of ST-segment elevation in the right precordial leads (phenocopies) must be excluded. BrS is traditionally classified as an inherited cardiac channelopathy because it is associated with ion channel dysfunction or the altered expression/function of proteins associated with ion channels in ventricular cardiomyocytes. It is characterized by incomplete penetrance and variable expressivity. A comprehensive genetic test can identify ~35% of diagnosed BrS patients and covers more than 20 potential genes encoding mainly ion channel components and associated proteins but also structural proteins. The sodium channel protein type 5 subunit alpha (*SCN5A*) gene, in particular, shows deleterious alterations in 30% of diagnosed patients. As the pathophysiological mechanism and functional effects of variants in other genes is still to be clarified, current guidelines recommend genetic analysis of *SCN5A* alone in patients with a BrS ECG [2–4].

BrS was first reported in 1992 and was classified as purely of electrical origin; since then, structural cardiac abnormalities have been identified in hearts of some patients with BrS [5–8]. For instance, right ventricular (RV) enlargement, reduced RV function, larger RV end-diastolic and end-systolic volumes, and left ventricular (LV) midfall late gadolinium enhancement (LGE) are apparent by cardiovascular magnetic resonance (CMR) imaging. LGE may be an early marker of an underlying cardiomyopathy in patients who do not fulfill all the current BrS diagnostic criteria [9,10]. BrS and arrhythmogenic cardiomyopathy (ACM) frequently show overlapping clinical and histopathological features and represent a highly challenging differential diagnosis, thus, leading to a high risk of misdiagnosis when ill-defined features are found [11–13]. Commonalities in clinical/histopathologic features and pathophysiological pathways (disorders of the connexome) between BrS and ACM prompted a hypothesis that BrS could be a phenotypic variant of ACM [14–18]; however, this hypothesis remains to be thoroughly tested.

In this review, given these findings and the commonalities between BrS and heart diseases of structural origin, such as ACM, we sought to evaluate if the pathological classification of BrS as a pure channelopathy remains appropriate. To achieve this, we performed a comprehensive review of the topic focusing on the reported macroscopic and microscopic structural alterations in BrS, observed in explanted hearts, autopsies, and endomyocardial biopsies.

2. Material and Methods

We performed a systematic literature search according to the current Preferred Reporting Items for Systematic Reviews and Meta-Analyses Statement (PRISMA) criteria (Figure 1). We searched PubMed and Scopus databases for papers published between 1 January 1997 (note that the first paper on the genetic basis of BrS was published at the end of 1996) and 25 December 2021. We used a search string (restricted to the terms in the paper titles and abstracts) in which, using the Boolean operator "AND", we combined the term "Brugada Syndrome" with the terms "fibrosis or scar or myocardial inflammation or structural heart disease or structural anomalies or structural abnormalities or histological anomalies or histological abnormalities or histological substrate or biopsies or fatty infiltration or ACM or ARVD or ARVC". We developed and applied one search strategy for each database. Two authors independently performed a preliminary search and retrieved and selected articles that fulfilled the inclusion criteria: research studies written in English that evaluated a possible correlation between BrS and certain structural cardiac alterations (macroscopic/microscopic) and/or cardiomyopathies.

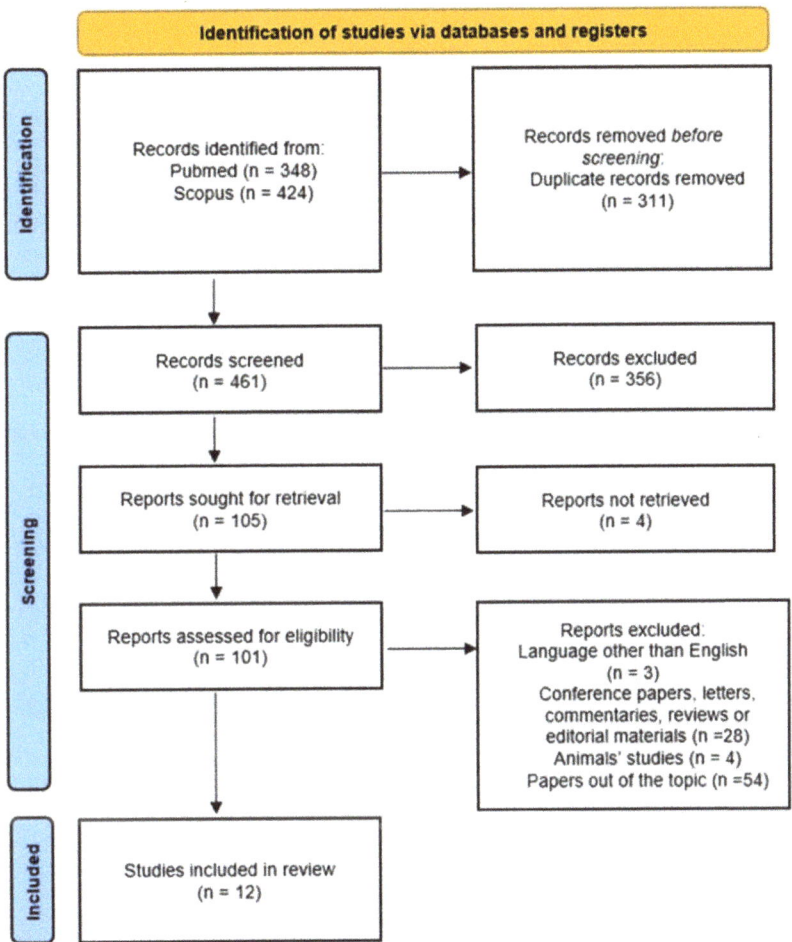

Figure 1. PRISMA flow diagram followed in this review.

Our preliminary research identified 772 papers, 348 through PubMed and 424 through Scopus. After the removal of 311 duplicates, 356 papers were excluded as they did not meet the inclusion criteria based on the title and abstract analyses. Of the 105 articles remaining, 4 were excluded due to the unavailability of the full text. Hence, a total of 101 papers were assessed for eligibility. Full texts of reviews, case reports, experimental studies in animal models, conference articles, articles that did not focus on structural cardiac abnormalities in BrS, and articles that were not published in English were removed from the pool of eligible papers. Following the exclusion of all articles that did not meet our inclusion criteria, 12 eligible publications were included in our analysis and were critically reviewed by three investigators who extracted data relevant to the purpose of the present study. Selected studies are presented in two different paragraphs depending on the kinds of samples that were processed for histological analysis (samples collected from explanted heart or during autopsies versus endomyocardial biopsy samples). All authors agreed on the final data included in our study. Eligible papers were synthetized in a table, considering these variables: number of the reference, number of the cases and of the controls, kind of samples (endomyocardial biopsy vs explanted heart/autopsy samples), technique used for microscopic analysis, main microscopic findings, and whether genetic testing was performed.

3. Results

3.1: Explanted Heart/Autopsy Samples

Two relevant case reports and two relevant case-series studies were identified. Assessment of formalin-fixed paraffin-embedded explanted heart tissue from a young individual with BrS and a clinical history of recurring VF [19], revealed moderate hypertrophy of the right ventricular wall (12 mm) and focal endocardial fibroelastosis. Moreover, in the RV (in the lateral wall and, especially, in the right ventricular outflow tract [RVOT]), significant fatty infiltration that reached the subendocardium was evident and was associated with interstitial fibrosis. The report excluded ACM because there was no evidence of transmural fatty infiltration, myocyte alterations, or inflammatory infiltrates (Table 1).

Table 1. Summary of the literature review regarding explanted hearts/autopsy samples.

Reference	Cases	Controls	Samples	Technique for Microscopy	Main Findings	Genetic Testing
Coronel [19]	1	0	Explanted heart	Hematoxylin-eosin and picrosirius red	Hypertrophy of the right ventricular wall, focal endocardial fibroelastosis, fatty infiltration, interstitial fibrosis	Yes
Moritomo [20]	1	0	Autopsy samples	Hematoxylin-eosin, Masson's trichrome and Azan Mallory	Reduction number of node cells and increased fatty tissue and fibrosis in the sinus node	No
Nademanee [21]	6	6	Autopsy samples	Hematoxylin-eosin and elastic Van Gieson and connexin-43 immunofluorescent	An increased collagen and fibrosis, (RVOT), reduction in connexin-43 signal	Yes
Miles [22]	28	29	Autopsy samples	Hematoxylin-eosin and picrosirius red	Increased collagen content in both ventricles, especially in RVOT epicardium	Yes

An autopsy of a 30-year-old victim of BrS [20] revealed biventricular contraction band necrosis and significant fatty tissue deposition in the RVOT. There were fewer cells of the sinus node, which was surrounded by fatty tissue and prominent fibrosis. Additionally, in two autopsy populations, including six autopsy-negative sudden deaths cases with (at least) a first-degree blood relative affected by BrS and six cases of non-cardiac deaths (as controls), individuals with BrS showed an increased amount of collagen [21]. The RVOT and epicardium demonstrated the greatest amount of fibrosis, and reduced expression of connexin-43 was observed in the RVOT. All hearts exhibited fibrosis, independent of the presence of *SCN5A* pathogenic variants. Together, these data suggested that in BrS, at the epicardial surface, interstitial fibrosis and reduced gap junction expression in the RVOT could lead to electrical anomalies. In further support of this finding, in 28 hearts from SCD cases with a non-confirmed diagnosis of BrS, the ventricular myocardium exhibited a higher proportion of collagen, irrespective of sampling location or myocardial layer (the highest proportion was found in the RVOT epicardium in individuals with suspected BrS) (Table 1) [22]. There was no statistically significant association reported between *SCN5A* genotype and histotype.

3.2. Endomyocardial Biopsies

Two relevant case reports and six relevant case-series studies were identified. Explanted heart and autopsy samples showed the presence of fibrosis and collagen deposition and reduced expression of connexin-43, together potentially leading to electrical anomalies associated with BrS; however, endomyocardial biopsies exhibited inflammation and fatty infiltration (hallmarks of ACM). For example, a relationship between BrS and ACM was suggested, due to the observation of the fatty replacement of myocardium in a biopsy sample of an RV septum from a 73-old-year man with a history of syncopal episodes and precordial oppression, who was then diagnosed with BrS (Table 2) [23]. After identification of this possible association, biopsies in the septal-apical region of the LV and RV of 18 patients with BrS were performed [24]. From these samples, lymphocytic myocarditis (mainly activated T lymphocytes) associated with focal areas of myocyte necrosis in 14 cases was identified (myocarditis was biventricular in 6 cases, while in 8 cases inflammatory infiltrates were exclusively in the RV). Additionally, 4 cases showed evidence of viral genomes. The remaining 4 cases carried rare *SCN5A* variants, which are potentially associated with BrS (but not with a conclusive role) and presented abnormal levels of myocyte apoptosis. These data suggest a potential link between inflammation and BrS. Among biopsies collected from the RVOT areas of abnormal voltage identified under 3-dimensional electroanatomic mapping (3D-EAM) guidance from 30 BrS cases [25], 12 cases demonstrated myocardial inflammation with lymphomononuclear infiltrates, while 3 demonstrated an association between inflammatory infiltrates and myocyte necrosis (indicating an active myocarditis). All cases with abnormal structural findings also had interstitial and replacement fibrosis, as well as a statistically significant association between inflammation and inducibility with programmed ventricular stimulation (PVS)/extent of bipolar low voltage areas [25]. No statistically significant association between genotype and clinical/microscopic phenotype was reported. In stained myocardial samples obtained from one young case of SCD and from nine BrS patients, the expression of three proteins (α-cardiac actin, keratin-24, and connexin-43) and a sodium channel was assessed [26]. All cases exhibited abnormal aggregates of the three proteins and sodium channel within the sarcoplasm of the myocardium compared to healthy controls, suggesting that trafficking defects may be implicated in the pathogenesis of BrS. These findings were associated with the presence of antibodies against α-cardiac actin, α-skeletal actin, keratin, and connexin-43 in the sera of BrS patients, suggesting an autoimmune response. The authors stressed the relevance of connexin-43 anomalies, highlighting that in animal models, this protein is less abundant in the RVOT epicardium (Table 2).

Table 2. Summary of the literature review regarding biopsies.

Reference	Cases	Controls	Samples	Technique for Microscopy	Main Findings	Genetic Testing
Izumi [23]	1	0	Biopsy	Hematoxylin-eosin	Fatty replacement of myocardium	No
Frustaci [24]	18	0	Biopsies	Hematoxylin-eosin, Miller's elastic Van Gieson, and Masson's trichrome	Lymphocytic myocarditis with focal areas of myocytes necrosis, hypertrophy, and diffuse vacuolization of cardiomyocytes with cytoplasm degeneration	Yes
Zumhagen [27]	21	12	Biopsies	Hematoxylin-eosin and Miller's elastic Van Gieson	Moderate hypertrophy and fatty replacement of the myocardium, moderate fibrosis	Yes
Marras [28]	1	0	Biopsy	Masson's trichrome	Fibro-fatty replacement and mild endocardial fibrous thickening	No

Table 2. Cont.

Reference	Cases	Controls	Samples	Technique for Microscopy	Main Findings	Genetic Testing
Ohkubo [29]	25	0	Biopsies	Hematoxylin-eosin	Moderate-to-severe fatty infiltration/myocyte degeneration, arrangement disorder, interstitial fibrosis, and lymphocyte infiltration	No
Tanaka [30]	68	0	Biopsies	Hematoxylin-eosin, Masson's trichrome, and immunohistochemical CD45, CD68, 4-hydroxy-2-nonenal-modified protein	Large 4-hydroxy-2-nonenal-modified protein areas in those without SCN5A mutation and with history of ventricular fibrillation	Yes
Pieroni [25]	30	0	Biopsies	Hematoxylin-eosin, Masson's trichrome, and immunohistochemistry anti-CD45RO	Myocardial inflammation with lymphomononuclear infiltrates	Yes
Chatterejee [26]	9	1	Biopsies	Immunohistochemistry	Abnormal myocardial expression of alfa-cardiac actin, alfa-skeletal actin, keratin-24, connexin-43, Nav1.5	Yes

Fat deposition and oxidative stress may also trigger fibrosis and structural abnormalities that could potentially be associated with BrS. Endomyocardial biopsies from the septum (86%) and/or the RV/RVOT (76%) and/or the RV apex (57%) of 21 patients with a clinical BrS diagnosis showed no signs of acute inflammation [27]. However, approximately 50% of cases exhibited moderate cellular hypertrophy and fatty replacement of the myocardium, and less than one-fourth of cases had moderate fibrosis. In 4 patients in which there was predominant fatty replacement, criteria for ACM were not definitively met. Histotype and genotype were not correlated. The authors considered it unlikely that the reported findings could represent an arrhythmogenic origin. Biopsies at the junction between the septum and anterior RV free wall of a 65-year-old man with BrS demonstrated areas of fibro-fatty replacement covering 66% of the biopsy area [28]. The histomorphometric criteria for diagnosis of ACM were not definitively met. Additionally, biopsies on the upper septal region of the RV of 25 patients with a clinical diagnosis of BrS and inducible VF [29] showed moderate-to-severe fatty infiltration in 5 patients and showed myocyte degeneration (apoptotic zone), fibrosis, and lymphocyte infiltration in 4 patients. There was no detected correlation between clinical/electrophysiological phenotype and histotype, but a relationship between histological anomalies and slow conduction at the RVOT is possible. In patients with a documented history of VF, the 4-hydroxy-2-nonenal (HNE)-modified protein-positive area (a marker of lipid peroxidation and indicator of oxidative stress levels) was larger in endomyocardial biopsies from the RV side of the septum of 68 patients with a clinical diagnosis of BrS [30]. This finding was especially true if only patients without SCN5A variants were considered. Therefore, in individuals who do not carry SCN5A variants, oxidative stress could be involved in arrhythmogenesis, likely inactivating cardiac Na$^+$ channels (Table 2).

3.3. Genetics

All manuscripts focused on structural alterations in BrS included a total of 209 cases. Genetic testing was performed in 161, and 36 cases carried a rare variant in the SCN5A gene (22.36%). This percentage is according to the widely accepted genetic yield in BrS [31], with SCN5A being the main gene currently associated with this arrhythmogenic syndrome [32]. Other minor genes encoding sodium subunits or associated proteins have been proposed as potential causes of BrS, but further studies should be conducted to conclude their definite role [3]. Due to some of the manuscripts being published more than five years ago, we performed an update following the American College of Medical Genetics and Genomics (ACMG) recommendations [33], according to our recent approach in the clinical translation of genetic diagnosis [31,34]. We identified only 16 cases (9.93%) who had a Likely Pathogenic (LP) or Pathogenic (P) variant explaining the genetic origin of BrS (Table 3). Most rare variants currently remain as VUS (Variant of Unknown Significance) due to the lack of enough conclusive data. Other cases diagnosed with BrS but without a positive *SCN5A* genetic diagnosis could be due to other genetic alterations in this gene [35] or in other genes [36]. However, it is also important to remark that only in 57 cases reported in the three most recent studies [22,25,26], a comprehensive genetic analysis including gene encoding cardiomyopathies were performed.

Table 3. Genetic data of variants in the *SCN5A* gene.

Publication	Zone	Region	Nucleotide	Protein	dbSNP/ClinVar	GnomAD (MAF)	ACMG 2022	Genes Analysed
Coronel et al. 2005 [19]	C-Terminal	Intracellular	c.5803G>A	p.Gly1935Ser	rs199473637/VUS	7/248912 (0.0028%)	VUS	PKP2, DSP, RyR2
Zumhagen et al. 2008 [27]	S5 (DII)	Pore	c.2582_2583del	p.Phe861TrpfsTer90	rs794728914/P	NA	P	No
Zumhagen et al. 2008 [27]	Loop DII-DIII	Intracellular	NA	p.Pro1002HisfsTer25	NA	NA	VUS	No
Zumhagen et al. 2008 [27]	Loop DIII-DIV	Intracellular	c.4477_4479del	p.Lys1493del	rs869025522/LP	1/151978 (0.0006%)	LP	No
Zumhagen et al. 2008 [27]	S2 (DIV)	Voltage Sensor	c.4720G>A	p.Glu1574Lys	rs199473620/VUS	NA	VUS	No
Zumhagen et al. 2008 [27]	S6 (DIV)	Pore	c.5290G>T	p.Val1764Phe	rs199473309/NA	NA	VUS	No
Zumhagen et al. 2008 [27]	C-Terminal	Intracellular	c.5435C>A	p.Ser1812Ter	rs371891414/LP	NA	LP	No
Frustaci et al. 2009 [24]	Loop S5-S6 (DI)	Extracellular	c.1127G>A	p.Arg376His	rs199473101/LP	2/247596 (0.0008%)	LP	PKP2, RyR2
Frustaci et al. 2009 [24]	Loop DII-DIII	Intracellular	c.3068G>A	p.Arg1023His	rs199473592/VUS	70/247778 (0.0283%)	LB	PKP2, RyR2
Frustaci et al. 2009 [24]	S4 (DIV)	Voltage Sensor	c.4930C>T	p.Arg1644Cys	rs199473287/P	1/251472 (0.0003%)	P	PKP2, RyR2
Frustaci et al. 2009 [24]	C-Terminal	Intracellular	c.5903T>G	p.Ile1968Ser	rs199473639/VUS	4/244136 (0.0016%)	VUS	PKP2, RyR2
Nademanee et al. 2015 [21]	Loop DI-DII	Intracellular	c.1582A>T	p.Ser528Cys	NA	NA	VUS	No
Nademanee et al. 2015 [21]	S5 (DII)	Pore	c.2537T>G	p.Leu846Arg	NA	NA	VUS	No
Nademanee et al. 2015 [21]	S6 (DIII)	Pore	c.4385T>A	p.Leu1462Gln	NA	NA	VUS	No
Pieroni et al. 2018 [25]	S6 (DII)	Pore	c.2798T>C	p.Leu933Pro	NA	NA	VUS	147 genes (panel)
Pieroni et al. 2018 [25]	Loop (S5-S6) DIV	Extracellular	c.5102T>G	p.Met1701Arg	NA	NA	VUS	147 genes (panel)
Pieroni et al. 2018 [25]	Loop S5-S6 (DIII)	Extracellular	c.4300_4311del	p.Tyr1434_Gln1437del	NA	NA	LP	147 genes (panel)
Pieroni et al. 2018 [25]	S2 (DIV)	Voltage Sensor	c.4720G>A	p.Glu1574Lys	rs199473620/VUS	NA	VUS	147 genes (panel)
Pieroni et al. 2018 [25]	S4 (DIV)	Voltage Sensor	c.4930C>T	p.Arg1644Cys	rs199473287/P	1/251472 (0.0003%)	P	147 genes (panel)
Pieroni et al. 2018 [25]	Loop DII-DIII	Intracellular	c.3352C>T	p.Gln1118Ter	rs869025520/P	NA	P	147 genes (panel)
Chatterjee et al. 2020 [26]	Loop S5-S6 (DI)	Extracellular	c.1007C>T	p. Pro336Leu	rs199473093/VUS	NA	LP	Gene panel
Chatterjee et al. 2020 [26]	Loop DII-DIII	Intracellular	c.3352C>T	p.Gln1118Ter	rs869025520/P	NA	P	Gene panel

Table 3. Cont.

Publication	Zone	Region	Nucleotide	Protein	dbSNP/ClinVar	GnomAD (MAF)	ACMG 2022	Genes Analysed
Chatterjee et al. 2020 [26]	Loop S5-S6 (DI)	Extracellular	c.844C>G	p.Arg282Gly	rs199473082/VUS	NA	VUS	Gene panel
Chatterjee et al. 2020 [26]	NA	NA	c.3508+1G>A	NA	NA	NA	VUS	Gene panel
Chatterjee et al. 2020 [26]	Loop DIII-DIV	Intracellular	c.4501C>G	p.Leu1501Val	rs199473266/VUS	5/251446 (0.0019%)	VUS	Gene panel
Chatterjee et al. 2020 [26]	S6 (DIII)	Pore	c.4387A>T	p.Asn1463Tyr	rs199473614/VUS	NA	VUS	Gene panel
Chatterjee et al. 2020 [26]	Loop DIII-DIV	Intracellular	c.4477_4479del	p.Lys1493del	rs869025522/LP	1/151978 (0.0006%)	LP	Gene panel
Chatterjee et al. 2020 [26]	Loop S5-S6 (DI)	Extracellular	c.1127G>A	p.Arg376His	rs199473101/LP	2/247596 (0.0008%)	LP	Gene panel
Chatterjee et al. 2020 [26]	Loop S5-S6 (DIV)	Extracellular	c.5027T>C	p.Met1676Thr	rs750013499/LP	1/251494 (0.0003%)	LP	Gene panel
Chatterjee et al. 2020 [26]	Loop S1-S2 (DIII)	Extracellular	c.3695G>A	p.Arg1232Trp	rs199473206/VUS	6/250110 (0.0023%)	VUS	Gene panel
Miles et al. 2021 [22]	Loop S3-S4 (DIII)	Intracellular	c.3944C>G	p.Ser1315Ter	rs1261656894/NA	NA	LP	174 genes (panel)
Miles et al. 2021 [22]	N-Terminal	Intracellular	c.50C>T	p.Thr17Ile	NA	NA	VUS	174 genes (panel)
Miles et al. 2021 [22]	Loop S5-S6 (DIV)	Extracellular	c.5038G>A	p.Ala1680Thr	rs199473294/VUS	10/251494 (0.0039%)	VUS	174 genes (panel)
Miles et al. 2021 [22]	S5 (DI)	Pore	c.673C>T	p.Arg225Trp	rs199473072/LP	3/242066 (0.0012%)	LP	174 genes (panel)
Miles et al. 2021 [22]	S1 (DIII)	Voltage Sensor	c.3665T>G	p.Leu1222Arg	NA	NA	VUS	174 genes (panel)
Miles et al. 2021 [22]	S3 (DIV)	Voltage Sensor	c.4850_4852delTCT	p.Phe1617del	rs749697698/LP	5/250930 (0.0019%)	LP	174 genes (panel)

dbSNP, database single nucleotide polymorphism; MAF, Minor Allele Frequency; ACMG, American College of Molecular Genetics; VUS, Variant of Unknown Significance; P, Pathogenic.

4. Discussion

BrS is currently classified as a purely electrical cardiac disease, but structural alterations identified in some cases suggest a potential reclassification of BrS as a cardiomyopathy. It is possible that dysfunctional ion channels lead to abnormal apoptosis and to a significant inflammatory/immune reaction and subsequent fibrosis in RV. An alternative hypothesis is that certain ion channel mutations result in altered excitation–contraction coupling causing cardiac remodeling [37]. Despite current arguments about this point, during the 30 years since first publication, none of the published cases with a definitive diagnosis of BrS have progressed to the definitive diagnosis of any cardiomyopathy during follow-up. Of all the analyzed manuscripts concerning structural alterations, few were performed by expert cardiopathologists, and this fact may represent a limitation due to the particular technical difficulty of microscopic diagnosis. Some centers included cardiac magnetic resonance (CMR) as part of BrS assessment despite not being included in current guidelines [32]. Therefore, further studies focused on analyzing potential correlations between BrS and structural abnormalities are needed to clarify whether BrS can definitively be reclassified as a cardiomyopathy.

Our comprehensive analysis identified recurring microscopic features of acute and chronic inflammation in the RVOT of BrS cases. Despite signs of acute inflammation, it is not a definitive hallmark of BrS but may trigger arrhythmias, especially in genetically predisposed hearts [25,26]. However, no conclusive studies have been published to date specifically examining this association, and the cause of myocardial inflammation remains undetermined. Increased collagen inside the myocardium represents a frequent feature of BrS and is predominant in the RV in both autopsy and endocardial biopsy samples [22]. However, this evidence is limited, as many of the patients studied did not have a confirmed clinical diagnosis of BrS. Another issue concerning fibrosis localization is the significance given to the collagen localized in the extraventricular parts of the conduction system [20]. The presence of collagen in this area is considered physiological; however, a significant amount of fibrosis can be abnormal, especially in young individuals [38]. For instance, an autopsy-negative case of sudden death in the young showed abnormal fibrosis of the sino-atrial node and the presence of a rare variant in the *SLMAP* gene (a minor gene potentially associated with BrS) [38]. In general, the presence of fibrosis in both the subendocardium and subepicardium has also been observed in other conditions (e.g., early repolarization syndrome) that are referred as "J-waves syndromes" and share the same arrhythmogenesis and the ECG changes of BrS [21,38].

As with inflammation, there is no clear evidence to date about fibrosis as a hallmark in BrS despite the presence of fibrosis in heart walls being widely accepted as proarrhythmogenic. Currently, data published identifies histological alterations in RV and in the RVOT of BrS patients. Transduction of electrical signals through myocytes is mainly due to connexin-43, and a reduction in this protein in the RVOT in BrS cases has been reported [21]; however, it is unclear if this phenomenon occurs before or after fibrosis. Therefore, further studies should seek to clarify if fibrosis identified in BrS samples could be a cause or consequence of arrhythmogenesis. In addition, electron beam computed tomography detected structural abnormalities on the RVOT and on the inferior wall of the RV that seem to be related to the onset of premature ventricular contractions and the initiation of VF [7]. RVOT is a critical part of the conduction system; thus, BrS may involve the abnormal expression of cardiac neural crest cells during embryonic myocardial development of the RVOT (whose characteristics differ from those of the surrounding myocardium) [39].

Recurrent histological features identified in BrS cases (myocardial fibrosis and the presence of inflammatory infiltrates) suggest a potential overlap between BrS and ACM histotypes. Debate persists surrounding whether BrS could be a cardiomyopathy or a phenotypic variant of ACM. Having the ability to make a differential diagnosis between BrS and ACM is crucial because in BrS cases that present ACM features, arrhythmic risk can be higher, and, in general, deciding the therapeutic strategy can be challenging [40,41]. This differential diagnosis is not always easier if clinical information is considered. For instance, patients with a definite diagnosis of ACM may exhibit an ECG pattern of BrS with a longer PQ interval and longer QRS duration, even if transient [42]. Therefore, in these cases, imaging data should also be considered. For instance, echocardiography can help in this differential diagnosis because BrS patients tend to have a mild alteration of RVOT morphology and motion but in the absence of overall dilation and dysfunction of the RV, typical of ACM [43,44]. Moreover, CMR can help to evaluate the fatty infiltration of the myocardium and the RV wall kinetics, helping in the differential diagnosis [45–48]. Data published to date state that early stages of ACM show alterations in ECG readings that are also observed in BrS cases, and discerning both entities is a challenge. Therefore, it cannot be ruled out that BrS and ACM share pathophysiological mechanisms and represent phenotypic and dynamic expressions of the same disease spectrum. Long-term follow-up is, therefore, required. Identification of the phenotype is important because of the clinical implications for both risk stratification and patient management. High-risk patients with a purely symptomatic electrical disorder may be more suitable for implantable cardioverter defibrillator (ICD). Whereas depending on the extent of the structural changes, selective ablation or drug therapy might be preferred. Future studies should focus on developing better standardized methods to differentiate BrS from ACM, to be evaluated by a multidisciplinary team of experts to ensure maximum diagnostic yield.

Improvement in genetic screening may help to clarify the diagnosis; however, it is not currently a viable solution, as the role of some potentially pathogenic variants has yet to be clarified, and a contribution of several genes in the development of the phenotype cannot be excluded. A comprehensive genetic analysis including all genes currently associated with BrS and ACM should be used in clinical or forensic settings [49]. However, even with genetic testing, differential diagnosis can be difficult because, for instance, rare variants located in the *PKP2* gene may be a potential cause of both ACM and BrS [12]. Yet, recent work identified one of these rare variants that was previously associated with BrS as a definitive cause in an ACM family [50]. Our group performed a comprehensive genetic interpretation of all rare variants in *PKP2* potentially associated with BrS, and none allowed a definite genotype–phenotype association [11]. In addition, less than 2% of ACM patients harbor rare *SCN5A* variants [51], but no conclusive role of these rare variants in ACM has been reported to date. These findings reinforce the necessity of further studies that include patients with a clear BrS diagnosis and ACM and a comprehensive genetic diagnosis, which would clarify the deleterious role of the identified rare variants. We recommend including a complete genotype–phenotype segregation in relatives to conclude a definitive genetic component, which could be translated into clinical practice.

Limitations

We cannot definitively state that all manuscripts detailing structural alterations in BrS patients are included in our search using the PRISMA system at the time of our search. To assure a comprehensive search, we performed additional searches in Index Copernicus (www.en.indexcopernicus.com), Google Scholar (www.scholar.google.es), Springer Link (www.link.springer.com), Science Direct (www.sciencedirect.com), the Excerpta Medica Database (www.elsevier.com/solutions/embase-biomedical-research), and the IEEE Xplore Digital Library (www.ieeexplore.ieee.org/Xplore/home.jsp (all accessed on 25 December 2021)). After performing these additional searches, no other data was included. BrS patients who suddenly died or had a clinical indication for an ablation are high-risk patients and do not cover the entire spectrum of BrS patients.

5. Conclusions

BrS is currently considered a channelopathy; however, the identification of structural findings in some cases highlights the potential complex interplay between these structural alterations and ion channel dysfunction. The recurrence of some structural features in BrS should be carefully considered because in some of these cases there was an ECG pattern mimicking BrS (BrS phenocopies), but no definite diagnosis of BrS was reported. To overcome these issues, we recommend always performing a comprehensive investigation including all possible sources of information to select cases with a certain diagnosis of BrS. In addition, a close follow-up is strongly recommended, as throughout the 30 years since the first BrS publication, none of the published cases with a definitive diagnosis of BrS have progressed to the definitive diagnosis of any cardiomyopathy. Taking all data into account, we conclude that there is currently not enough evidence supporting a reclassification of BrS as a cardiomyopathy or an autoimmune disease. However, it should be noted that in autopsies, the observation of microscopic heart anomalies does not justify the exclusion of BrS as a possible diagnosis, so far. Therefore, new data may help to clarify the widely accepted classification of a "classic" channelopathy without structural heart alterations.

Author Contributions: A.O., S.G., G.S.-B., J.B., R.B. and O.C., conceptualization; A.O., S.G., V.P., F.C. and O.C., protocol development; M.C., M.A., M.V.-P., A.P.-S., E.M.-B., S.C., A.I., J.C., C.H., V.F., E.A., N.D.-E. and V.A., data analysis; A.O., S.G., and O.C., manuscript writing; A.O., S.G., G.S.-B., J.B., R.B. and O.C., data interpretation. All authors have read and agreed to the published version of the manuscript.

Funding: Grant n. R4124501052 Fondi di Ateneo D3.1 to Antonio Oliva. Universita' Cattolica del Sacro Cuore contributed to the funding of this research project and its publication. Funders had no role in study design, data collection, data analysis, interpretation, or writing of the report.

Institutional Review Board Statement: Not applicable.

Informed Consent Statement: Not applicable.

Data Availability Statement: Not applicable.

Conflicts of Interest: The authors declare no conflict of interest.

References

1. Priori, S.G.; Blomstrom-Lundqvist, C. 2015 European Society of Cardiology Guidelines for the management of patients with ventricular arrhythmias and the prevention of sudden cardiac death summarized by co-chairs. *Eur. Heart J.* **2015**, *36*, 2757–2759. [CrossRef] [PubMed]
2. Brugada, J.; Campuzano, O.; Arbelo, E.; Sarquella-Brugada, G.; Brugada, R. Present Status of Brugada Syndrome: JACC State-of-the-Art Review. *J. Am. Coll. Cardiol.* **2018**, *72*, 1046–1059. [CrossRef] [PubMed]
3. Campuzano, O.; Sarquella-Brugada, G.; Fernandez-Falgueras, A.; Cesar, S.; Coll, M.; Mates, J.; Arbelo, E.; Perez-Serra, A.; Del Olmo, B.; Jorda, P.; et al. Genetic interpretation and clinical translation of minor genes related to Brugada syndrome. *Hum. Mutat.* **2019**, *40*, 749–764. [CrossRef] [PubMed]
4. Mates, J.; Mademont-Soler, I.; Fernandez-Falgueras, A.; Sarquella-Brugada, G.; Cesar, S.; Arbelo, E.; Garcia-Alvarez, A.; Jorda, P.; Toro, R.; Coll, M.; et al. Sudden Cardiac Death and Copy Number Variants: What Do We Know after 10 Years of Genetic Analysis? *Forensic Sci. Int. Genet.* **2020**, *47*, 102281. [CrossRef]
5. Brugada, P.; Brugada, J. Right bundle branch block, persistent ST segment elevation and sudden cardiac death: A distinct clinical and electrocardiographic syndrome. A multicenter report. *J. Am. Coll. Cardiol.* **1992**, *20*, 1391–1396. [CrossRef]
6. Lippi, G.; Montagnana, M.; Meschi, T.; Comelli, I.; Cervellin, G. Genetic and clinical aspects of Brugada syndrome: An update. *Adv. Clin. Chem.* **2012**, *56*, 197–208.
7. Takagi, M.; Aihara, N.; Kuribayashi, S.; Taguchi, A.; Shimizu, W.; Kurita, T.; Suyama, K.; Kamakura, S.; Hamada, S.; Takamiya, M. Localized right ventricular morphological abnormalities detected by electron-beam computed tomography represent arrhythmogenic substrates in patients with the Brugada syndrome. *Eur. Heart J.* **2001**, *22*, 1032–1041. [CrossRef]
8. Takagi, M.; Aihara, N.; Kuribayashi, S.; Taguchi, A.; Kurita, T.; Suyama, K.; Kamakura, S.; Takamiya, M. Abnormal response to sodium channel blockers in patients with Brugada syndrome: Augmented localised wall motion abnormalities in the right ventricular outflow tract region detected by electron beam computed tomography. *Heart* **2003**, *89*, 169–174. [CrossRef]
9. Bastiaenen, R.; Cox, A.T.; Castelletti, S.; Wijeyeratne, Y.D.; Colbeck, N.; Pakroo, N.; Ahmed, H.; Bunce, N.; Anderson, L.; Moon, J.C.; et al. Late gadolinium enhancement in Brugada syndrome: A marker for subtle underlying cardiomyopathy? *Heart Rhythm* **2017**, *14*, 583–589. [CrossRef]
10. Papavassiliu, T.; Wolpert, C.; Fluchter, S.; Schimpf, R.; Neff, W.; Haase, K.K.; Duber, C.; Borggrefe, M. Magnetic resonance imaging findings in patients with Brugada syndrome. *J. Cardiovasc. Electrophysiol.* **2004**, *15*, 1133–1138. [CrossRef]
11. Campuzano, O.; Fernandez-Falgueras, A.; Iglesias, A.; Brugada, R. Brugada Syndrome and PKP2: Evidences and uncertainties. *Int. J. Cardiol.* **2016**, *214*, 403–405. [CrossRef]
12. Cerrone, M.; Delmar, M. Desmosomes and the sodium channel complex: Implications for arrhythmogenic cardiomyopathy and Brugada syndrome. *Trends Cardiovasc. Med.* **2014**, *24*, 184–190. [CrossRef]
13. Kataoka, S.; Serizawa, N.; Kitamura, K.; Suzuki, A.; Suzuki, T.; Shiga, T.; Shoda, M.; Hagiwara, N. An overlap of Brugada syndrome and arrhythmogenic right ventricular cardiomyopathy/dysplasia. *J. Arrhythmia* **2016**, *32*, 70–73. [CrossRef]
14. Peters, S. Brugada phenocopy or Brugada ECG pattern in patients characterized by early repolarization pattern and additional arrhythmogenic right ventricular cardiomyopathy. *Int. J. Cardiol.* **2014**, *172*, 278. [CrossRef]
15. Peters, S. Association between arrhythmogenic cardiomyopathy and Brugada syndrome—The influence of novel electrocardiographic features of Brugada syndrome. *Int. J. Cardiol.* **2015**, *191*, 301–302. [CrossRef]
16. Peters, S. Is Brugada syndrome a variant of arrhythmogenic cardiomyopathy? *Int. J. Cardiol.* **2015**, *189*, 88–90. [CrossRef]
17. Peters, S. Is early sudden death in the course of arrhythmogenic cardiomyopathy due to initial Brugada syndrome? *Int. J. Cardiol.* **2015**, *182*, 107–108. [CrossRef]
18. Ben-Haim, Y.; Asimaki, A.; Behr, E.R. Brugada syndrome and arrhythmogenic cardiomyopathy: Overlapping disorders of the connexome? *Europace* **2021**, *23*, 653–664. [CrossRef]
19. Coronel, R.; Casini, S.; Koopmann, T.T.; Wilms-Schopman, F.J.; Verkerk, A.O.; de Groot, J.R.; Bhuiyan, Z.; Bezzina, C.R.; Veldkamp, M.W.; Linnenbank, A.C.; et al. Right ventricular fibrosis and conduction delay in a patient with clinical signs of Brugada syndrome: A combined electrophysiological, genetic, histopathologic, and computational study. *Circulation* **2005**, *112*, 2769–2777. [CrossRef]
20. Morimoto, S.; Uemura, A.; Hishida, H. An autopsy case of Brugada syndrome with significant lesions in the sinus node. *J. Cardiovasc. Electrophysiol.* **2005**, *16*, 345–347. [CrossRef]
21. Nademanee, K.; Raju, H.; de Noronha, S.V.; Papadakis, M.; Robinson, L.; Rothery, S.; Makita, N.; Kowase, S.; Boonmee, N.; Vitayakritsirikul, V.; et al. Fibrosis, Connexin-43, and Conduction Abnormalities in the Brugada Syndrome. *J. Am. Coll. Cardiol.* **2015**, *66*, 1976–1986. [CrossRef] [PubMed]
22. Miles, C.; Asimaki, A.; Ster, I.C.; Papadakis, M.; Gray, B.; Westaby, J.; Finocchiaro, G.; Bueno-Beti, C.; Ensam, B.; Basu, J.; et al. Biventricular Myocardial Fibrosis and Sudden Death in Patients with Brugada Syndrome. *J. Am. Coll. Cardiol.* **2021**, *78*, 1511–1521. [CrossRef] [PubMed]
23. Izumi, T.; Ajiki, K.; Nozaki, A.; Takahashi, S.; Tabei, F.; Hayakawa, H.; Sugimoto, T. Right ventricular cardiomyopathy showing right bundle branch block and right precordial ST segment elevation. *Intern. Med.* **2000**, *39*, 28–33. [CrossRef] [PubMed]
24. Frustaci, A.; Priori, S.G.; Pieroni, M.; Chimenti, C.; Napolitano, C.; Rivolta, I.; Sanna, T.; Bellocci, F.; Russo, M.A. Cardiac histological substrate in patients with clinical phenotype of Brugada syndrome. *Circulation* **2005**, *112*, 3680–3687. [CrossRef]

25. Pieroni, M.; Notarstefano, P.; Oliva, A.; Campuzano, O.; Santangeli, P.; Coll, M.; Nesti, M.; Carnevali, A.; Fraticelli, A.; Iglesias, A.; et al. Electroanatomic and Pathologic Right Ventricular Outflow Tract Abnormalities in Patients with Brugada Syndrome. *J. Am. Coll. Cardiol.* **2018**, *72*, 2747–2757. [CrossRef]
26. Chatterjee, D.; Pieroni, M.; Fatah, M.; Charpentier, F.; Cunningham, K.S.; Spears, D.A.; Chatterjee, D.; Suna, G.; Bos, J.M.; Ackerman, M.J.; et al. An autoantibody profile detects Brugada syndrome and identifies abnormally expressed myocardial proteins. *Eur. Heart J.* **2020**, *41*, 2878–2890. [CrossRef]
27. Zumhagen, S.; Spieker, T.; Rolinck, J.; Baba, H.A.; Breithardt, G.; Bocker, W.; Eckardt, L.; Paul, M.; Wichter, T.; Schulze-Bahr, E. Absence of pathognomonic or inflammatory patterns in cardiac biopsies from patients with Brugada syndrome. *Circ. Arrhythmia Electrophysiol.* **2009**, *2*, 16–23. [CrossRef]
28. Marras, E.; Basso, C.; Sciarra, L.; Delise, P. Unexplained syncope, Brugada-like ECG and minimal structural right ventricular abnormalities: Which is the right diagnosis? *J. Cardiovasc. Med.* **2009**, *10*, 273–275. [CrossRef]
29. Ohkubo, K.; Watanabe, I.; Okumura, Y.; Takagi, Y.; Ashino, S.; Kofune, M.; Sugimura, H.; Nakai, T.; Kasamaki, Y.; Hirayama, A.; et al. Right ventricular histological substrate and conduction delay in patients with Brugada syndrome. *Int. Heart J.* **2010**, *51*, 17–23. [CrossRef]
30. Tanaka, M.; Nakamura, K.; Kusano, K.F.; Morita, H.; Ohta-Ogo, K.; Miura, D.; Miura, A.; Nakagawa, K.; Tada, T.; Murakami, M.; et al. Elevated oxidative stress is associated with ventricular fibrillation episodes in patients with Brugada-type electrocardiogram without SCN5A mutation. *Cardiovasc. Pathol.* **2011**, *20*, e37–e42. [CrossRef]
31. Milman, A.; Behr, E.R.; Gray, B.; Johnson, D.C.; Andorin, A.; Hochstadt, A.; Gourraud, J.B.; Maeda, S.; Takahashi, Y.; Jm Juang, J.; et al. Genotype-Phenotype Correlation of SCN5A Genotype in Patients with Brugada Syndrome and Arrhythmic Events: Insights from the SABRUS in 392 Probands. *Circ. Genom. Precis. Med.* **2021**, *14*, e003222. [CrossRef]
32. Wilde, A.A.M.; Semsarian, C.; Marquez, M.F.; Sepehri Shamloo, A.; Ackerman, M.J.; Ashley, E.A.; Sternick, E.B.; Barajas-Martinez, H.; Behr, E.R.; Bezzina, C.R.; et al. European Heart Rhythm Association (EHRA)/Heart Rhythm Society (HRS)/Asia Pacific Heart Rhythm Society (APHRS)/Latin American Heart Rhythm Society (LAHRS) Expert Consensus Statement on the State of Genetic Testing for Cardiac Diseases. *Heart Rhythm* **2022**, *19*, e1–e60. [CrossRef]
33. Richards, S.; Aziz, N.; Bale, S.; Bick, D.; Das, S.; Gastier-Foster, J.; Grody, W.W.; Hegde, M.; Lyon, E.; Spector, E.; et al. Standards and guidelines for the interpretation of sequence variants: A joint consensus recommendation of the American College of Medical Genetics and Genomics and the Association for Molecular Pathology. *Genet. Med.* **2015**, *17*, 405–424. [CrossRef]
34. Campuzano, O.; Sarquella-Brugada, G.; Fernandez-Falgueras, A.; Coll, M.; Iglesias, A.; Ferrer-Costa, C.; Cesar, S.; Arbelo, E.; Garcia-Alvarez, A.; Jorda, P.; et al. Reanalysis and reclassification of rare genetic variants associated with inherited arrhythmogenic syndromes. *EBioMedicine* **2020**, *54*, 102732. [CrossRef]
35. Perez-Agustin, A.; Pinsach-Abuin, M.L.; Pagans, S. Role of Non-Coding Variants in Brugada Syndrome. *Int. J. Mol. Sci.* **2020**, *21*, 8556. [CrossRef] [PubMed]
36. Campuzano, O.; Sarquella-Brugada, G.; Cesar, S.; Arbelo, E.; Brugada, J.; Brugada, R. Update on Genetic Basis of Brugada Syndrome: Monogenic, Polygenic or Oligogenic? *Int. J. Mol. Sci.* **2020**, *21*, 7155. [CrossRef]
37. Antzelevitch, C.; Yan, G.X.; Ackerman, M.J.; Borggrefe, M.; Corrado, D.; Guo, J.; Gussak, I.; Hasdemir, C.; Horie, M.; Huikuri, H.; et al. J-Wave syndromes expert consensus conference report: Emerging concepts and gaps in knowledge. *Europace* **2017**, *19*, 665–694.
38. Grassi, S.; Vidal, M.C.; Campuzano, O.; Arena, V.; Alfonsetti, A.; Rossi, S.S.; Scarnicci, F.; Iglesias, A.; Brugada, R.; Oliva, A. Sudden Death without a Clear Cause after Comprehensive Investigation: An Example of Forensic Approach to Atypical/Uncertain Findings. *Diagnostics* **2021**, *11*, 886. [CrossRef]
39. Elizari, M.V.; Levi, R.; Acunzo, R.S.; Chiale, P.A.; Civetta, M.M.; Ferreiro, M.; Sicouri, S. Abnormal expression of cardiac neural crest cells in heart development: A different hypothesis for the etiopathogenesis of Brugada syndrome. *Heart Rhythm* **2007**, *4*, 359–365. [CrossRef]
40. Scheirlynck, E.; Chivulescu, M.; Lie, O.H.; Motoc, A.; Koulalis, J.; de Asmundis, C.; Sieira, J.; Chierchia, G.B.; Brugada, P.; Cosyns, B.; et al. Worse Prognosis in Brugada Syndrome Patients with Arrhythmogenic Cardiomyopathy Features. *JACC Clin. Electrophysiol.* **2020**, *6*, 1353–1363. [CrossRef]
41. Moncayo-Arlandi, J.; Brugada, R. Unmasking the molecular link between arrhythmogenic cardiomyopathy and Brugada syndrome. *Nat. Rev. Cardiol.* **2017**, *14*, 744–756. [CrossRef] [PubMed]
42. Ueda, N.; Nagase, S.; Kataoka, N.; Nakajima, K.; Kamakura, T.; Wada, M.; Yamagata, K.; Ishibashi, K.; Inoue, Y.; Miyamoto, K.; et al. Prevalence and characteristics of the Brugada electrocardiogram pattern in patients with arrhythmogenic right ventricular cardiomyopathy. *J. Arrhythmia* **2021**, *37*, 1173–1183. [CrossRef] [PubMed]
43. Gray, B.; Gnanappa, G.K.; Bagnall, R.D.; Femia, G.; Yeates, L.; Ingles, J.; Burns, C.; Puranik, R.; Grieve, S.M.; Semsarian, C.; et al. Relations between right ventricular morphology and clinical, electrical and genetic parameters in Brugada Syndrome. *PLoS ONE* **2018**, *13*, e0195594. [CrossRef] [PubMed]
44. Jeevaratnam, K.; Rewbury, R.; Zhang, Y.; Guzadhur, L.; Grace, A.A.; Lei, M.; Huang, C.L. Frequency distribution analysis of activation times and regional fibrosis in murine $Scn5a^{+/-}$ hearts: The effects of ageing and sex. *Mech. Ageing Dev.* **2012**, *133*, 591–599. [CrossRef]

45. Corrado, D.; Zorzi, A.; Cerrone, M.; Rigato, I.; Mongillo, M.; Bauce, B.; Delmar, M. Relationship between Arrhythmogenic Right Ventricular Cardiomyopathy and Brugada Syndrome: New Insights from Molecular Biology and Clinical Implications. *Circ. Arrhythmia Electrophysiol.* **2016**, *9*, e003631. [CrossRef]
46. Sato, Y.; Kato, K.; Hashimoto, M.; Akiyama, H.; Matsumoto, N.; Takase, H.; Ogawa, K.; Sakamaki, T.; Yagi, H.; Kanmatsuse, K. Localized right ventricular structural abnormalities in patients with idiopathic ventricular fibrillation: Magnetic resonance imaging study. *Heart Vessel.* **1996**, *11*, 100–103. [CrossRef]
47. Heermann, P.; Hedderich, D.M.; Paul, M.; Schulke, C.; Kroeger, J.R.; Baessler, B.; Wichter, T.; Maintz, D.; Waltenberger, J.; Heindel, W.; et al. Biventricular myocardial strain analysis in patients with arrhythmogenic right ventricular cardiomyopathy (ARVC) using cardiovascular magnetic resonance feature tracking. *J. Cardiovasc. Magn. Reson.* **2014**, *16*, 75. [CrossRef]
48. Heermann, P.; Fritsch, H.; Koopmann, M.; Sporns, P.; Paul, M.; Heindel, W.; Schulze-Bahr, E.; Schulke, C. Biventricular myocardial strain analysis using cardiac magnetic resonance feature tracking (CMR-FT) in patients with distinct types of right ventricular diseases comparing arrhythmogenic right ventricular cardiomyopathy (ARVC), right ventricular outflow-tract tachycardia (RVOT-VT), and Brugada syndrome (BrS). *Clin. Res. Cardiol.* **2019**, *108*, 1147–1162.
49. Gerull, B.; Brodehl, A. Insights into Genetics and Pathophysiology of Arrhythmogenic Cardiomyopathy. *Curr. Heart Fail. Rep.* **2021**, *18*, 378–390. [CrossRef]
50. Persampieri, S.; Pilato, C.A.; Sommariva, E.; Maione, A.S.; Stadiotti, I.; Ranalletta, A.; Torchio, M.; Dello Russo, A.; Basso, C.; Pompilio, G.; et al. Clinical and Molecular Data Define a Diagnosis of Arrhythmogenic Cardiomyopathy in a Carrier of a Brugada-Syndrome-Associated PKP2 Mutation. *Genes* **2020**, *11*, 571. [CrossRef]
51. Te Riele, A.S.; Agullo-Pascual, E.; James, C.A.; Leo-Macias, A.; Cerrone, M.; Zhang, M.; Lin, X.; Lin, B.; Sobreira, N.L.; Amat-Alarcon, N.; et al. Multilevel analyses of SCN5A mutations in arrhythmogenic right ventricular dysplasia/cardiomyopathy suggest non-canonical mechanisms for disease pathogenesis. *Cardiovasc. Res.* **2017**, *113*, 102–111. [CrossRef]

Article

Statistical and Diagnostic Properties of pRRx Parameters in Atrial Fibrillation Detection

Szymon Buś [1,*], Konrad Jędrzejewski [1] and Przemysław Guzik [2]

[1] Institute of Electronic Systems, Faculty of Electronics and Information Technology, Warsaw University of Technology, Nowowiejska 15/19, 00-665 Warsaw, Poland
[2] Department of Cardiology-Intensive Therapy and Internal Disease, Poznan University of Medical Sciences, 60-355 Poznan, Poland
* Correspondence: szymon.bus.dokt@pw.edu.pl; Tel.: +48-22-2345883

Abstract: Background: We studied the diagnostic properties of the percentage of successive RR intervals differing by at least x ms (pRRx) as functions of the threshold value x in a range of 7 to 195 ms for the differentiation of atrial fibrillation (AF) from sinus rhythm (SR). Methods: RR intervals were measured in 60-s electrocardiogram (ECG) segments with either AF (32,141 segments) or SR (32,769 segments) from the publicly available Physionet Long-Term Atrial Fibrillation Database (LTAFDB). For validation, we have used ECGs from the Massachusetts Institute of Technology–Beth Israel Hospital (MIT–BIH) Atrial Fibrillation Database. The pRRx distributions in AF and SR in relation to x were studied by histograms, along with the mutual association by the nonparametric Spearman correlations for all pairs of pRRx, and separately for AF or SR. The optimal cutoff values for all pRRx were determined using the receiver operator curve characteristic. A nonparametric bootstrap with 5000 samples was used to calculate a 95% confidence interval for several classification metrics. Results: The distributions of pRRx for x in the 7–195 ms range are significantly different in AF than in SR. The sensitivity, specificity, accuracy, and diagnostic odds ratios differ for pRRx, with the highest values for x = 31 ms (pRR31) rather than x = 50 (pRR50), which is most commonly applied in studies on heart rate variability. For the optimal cutoff of pRR31 (68.79%), the sensitivity is 90.42%, specificity 95.37%, and the diagnostic odds ratio is 194.11. Validation with the ECGs from the MIT–BIH Atrial Fibrillation Database confirmed our findings. Conclusions: We demonstrate that the diagnostic properties of pRRx depend on x, and pRR31 outperforms pRR50, at least for ECGs of 60-s duration.

Keywords: atrial fibrillation detection; cardiac arrhythmia; electrocardiography; heart rate variability

1. Introduction

Atrial fibrillation (AF) is a tachyarrhythmia with uncoordinated atrial electrical activation and ineffective atrial contraction [1–3]. Diagnosis of AF is based on an electrocardiogram (ECG) with irregular RR intervals (the distances between the peaks of R waves of the QRS complexes reflecting the electrical depolarization of ventricles and measuring the duration of each cardiac cycle), the absence of distinct repeating P waves, and irregular atrial activation. AF must be documented in an entire 12-lead ECG of a duration of at least 8–10-s. If a single ECG strip is used, an arrhythmic episode is considered AF if it lasts at least 30 s [1,2].

AF is the most common sustained cardiac arrhythmia, and it is the only available cardiac rhythm for many people. Heart palpitations, symptoms of irregular pulse, worsened exercise tolerance, dyspnea, and sometimes angina can accompany AF. However, many individuals are asymptomatic or experience mild or unspecific symptoms easily related to advancing age, emotions or effort, or other diseases such as hyperthyroidism [4]. Consequently, AF may be undetected or is found accidentally during a routine check-up or a medical visit for another reason [1,2].

AF increases the risk of excessive morbidity with debilitating clinical consequences and premature death. This arrhythmia always increases the risk of severe arterial thromboembolism, resulting, for example, in an ischaemic stroke of the brain. Therefore, AF must be appropriately diagnosed and actively screened for, particularly in high-risk populations such as older age and patients with hypertension, diabetes, heart failure, or valvular disease [5,6].

Many systems used for AF screening can record ECGs of various lengths, ranging from a couple-of-second 12-lead ECG to recordings of several weeks with the long-term Holter ECGs or ECG bio-patches attached to the skin. Implantable loop recorders are an invasive option for even more prolonged ECG monitoring lasting up to two years.

Visual inspection and ECG analysis are the gold standards for AF diagnosis. With technological advancement, the amount of data with long-term ECGs gradually increases, so a quick analysis of such recordings becomes challenging. New approaches to automatic or semiautomatic analysis are proposed, many of them based on heart rate variability (HRV) analysis [7]. HRV uses mathematical analysis of RR interval time series. RR interval is the cardiac cycle duration measured between two consecutive QRS complexes in a continuous ECG. HRV was developed many years ago. Its primary use was limited only to RR intervals of sinus rhythm (SR) origin for either physiological analysis or prediction of mortality in different diseases.

Due to different distributions of HRV-derived parameters in AF and SR [8], HRV has gained new interest in AF detection in ECG [9–11], as well as from wearable devices [12,13]. Several authors used feature selection methods to find the most relevant HRV parameters for AF detection [14,15]. Others incorporated HRV to predict future occurrence of AF [16,17].

The percentage of successive RR intervals differing by at least 50 ms (pRR50) is a particular form of pRRx parameter. Ewing et al. [18] proposed the total number of successive RR intervals that differ by at least x ms (RRx count) for monitoring cardiac parasympathetic activity. They analyzed two threshold values: x = 50 ms and x = 6.25% of the previous RR interval. The computationally simpler 50 ms threshold was later widely adopted, and Bigger et al. [19] proposed a relative statistic pNN50 (percentage of normal-to-normal RR interval differences over 50 ms). The "NN" in the name emphasizes that the analyzed R-waves are of sinus origin [1,19]. However, the same mathematical analysis can be conducted for different cardiac rhythms, including AF. RR intervals are not normal (i.e., of sinus origin) in AF and thus should always be labeled as RR and not as NN.

So far, the threshold values x other than 50 ms have rarely been analyzed. Mietus et al. [20] used pRRx with x ranging from 4 ms to 100 ms to compare various groups such as healthy people versus patients with heart failure, sleeping vs. awake states, or young vs. elderly subjects. In all cases, thresholds <50 ms allowed for better discrimination between the studied groups. Torres et al. [21] applied pRRx with x from 10 ms to 50 ms to distinguish healthy subjects from survivors of acute myocardial infarction, and thresholds <50 ms performed better. Saiz-Vivo et al. [22,23] used HRV indices, including pRR20 and pRR50, to analyze 500 beats preceding onsets of AF and distinguish between healthy and AF subjects. In several studies [24–27], various pRRx indices with x from 5 ms to 500 ms were used to distinguish between four cardiac rhythms (AF/SR/noisy/other) [28]. Jovic et al. [29] combined various HRV parameters with pRR5, pRR10, pRR20, and pRR50 to differentiate between nine cardiac rhythms, including AF [30].

We have recently analyzed the diagnostic properties of several HRV parameters, including the mean of RR intervals (mean RR); the standard deviation of RR intervals (SDRR); the standard deviation of points perpendicular to the line of identity (SD1) and along the line of identity (SD2) from the Poincare plot analysis; the power of low-frequency (LF: 0.04–0.15 Hz) and high-frequency (HF: 0.15–0.4 Hz); and pRR10, pRR30, pRR50, pRR70, and pRR90 [31]. Among these parameters, pRR30 had the highest area under the curve (AUC) [32]. Different combinations of the HRV parameters, used as input features for ML classifiers, showed that the sets with pRR30 outperformed other HRV feature sets, including those with pRR50. Conroy et al. [33] used parameters analogous to pRRx to detect AF in the photoplethysmographic signal (PPG). Instead of RR intervals, interbeat intervals (IBI) from PPG were used, and the highest AUC was yielded for x = 35 ms. Ramesh et al. [34] used HRV features, including pRR20, RR20, pRR50, and RR50 (and analogous parameters from PPG), for AF detection in ECG and PPG.

Altogether, these data strongly suggest that various x threshold values for the difference between two successive RR intervals might be more helpful in detecting AF. However, the 50 ms threshold (pRR50) has been used for many years as a commonly accepted practice in HRV analysis.

The primary aim of this study was to systematically explore the diagnostic properties of the pRRx as a function of the different x thresholds for differentiating AF from SR in 60-s ECG segments. The secondary aim was to compare the diagnostic properties of the pRR50 with the pRRx found to have the optimal diagnostic properties for AF detection in the same 60-s ECG segments. This part of the study is presented separately in Appendix A.

2. Materials and Methods

2.1. Data

For this study, we used anonymized data from the Long-Term Atrial Fibrillation Database (LTAFDB) [35,36]. It contains 84 long 24-h Holter electrocardiographic (ECG) recordings sampled at a rate of 128 Hz, the information about locations of R-waves, and the type of corresponding cardiac beats (normal, supraventricular, ventricular, atrial fibrillation, and technical artifact). The LTAFDB database contains ECG recordings from patients with paroxysmal AF and other arrhythmias. We selected only uninterrupted ECG fragments with either AF or SR of at least 60-s duration for further analysis. We discarded the segments labelled as different rhythms.

The data-preprocessing scheme is presented in Figure 1. The RR interval time series were cut into 60-s separate, neighboring segments. For a segment to be labeled SR, each RR interval had to be of SR origin. If it was not, for example, it was a atrial or ventricular beat, the segment was removed from further analysis. For AF segments, each cardiac beat needed to be AF, and if a ventricular beat was found, such a segment was also excluded.

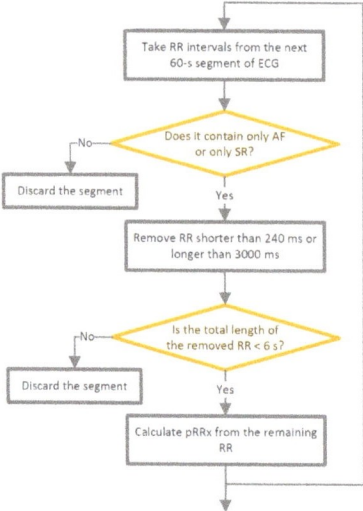

Figure 1. Data preprocessing scheme. RR—interval between peaks of consecutive R-waves; ECG—electrocardiogram; AF—atrial fibrillation; SR—sinus rhythm; and pRRx—percentage of successive RR intervals differing by at least x ms.

For SR and AF, to limit the number of potentially unidentified technical artifacts, RR intervals shorter than 240 ms or longer than 3000 ms were removed. Additionally, RR intervals corresponding to ventricular premature beats were also removed from both SR and AF ECGs. For SR only, premature supraventricular beats were removed too. Segments with a total length of excluded RR intervals exceeding 6 s were also discarded from the analysis. The total number of 60-s RR series after preprocessing was 64,910 (32,141 AF, 32,769 SR).

As the sampling rate of 128 Hz corresponds to the precision of 7.8125 ms, we quantized pRRx thresholds x into 7.8125 ms bins. The absolute values of the differences between consecutive RR intervals were measured and used to calculate pRRx for the x ranging from 7.8125 to 195.3125 ms in 7.8125 ms steps for both SR and AF 60-s segments. To improve the paper's readability, we use only the integer part of x in ms in the names of parameters, e.g., pRR7 instead of pRR7.8125.

2.2. Software Tools

We used Python programming language (version 3.9, Python Software Foundation, Wilmington, DE, USA) for all the analyses.

2.3. Statistical Analysis

First, we analyzed the distributions of pRRx obtained for different x values separately for SR and AF using histograms. Based on the histograms and Shapiro–Wilk test results, we concluded that pRRx do not have normal distributions either in AF or in SR. Consequently, we used a percentile scale to describe the distributions and mostly applied nonparametric statistical techniques for data analysis.

Next, using the Wilcoxon test [37], we made paired comparisons for pRRx with different x (separately for SR and AF). We conducted the unpaired analysis comparing pRRx for the same x between SR and AF using the Mann–Whitney test [38]. The associations between pRRx values for different x were analyzed with the Spearman correlation [39] and presented as heatmaps with rho correlation coefficients. To analyze the differences between two pRRx with different x, we calculated the mean difference for quantifying bias, and the standard deviation (SD) of the differences for each pair of pRRx. As the data distribution was not normal, we defined the limits of agreement (LoA) as the range between the 2.5th and 97.5th percentile of the distribution of the differences. To analyze the diagnostic properties of pRRx with different x, the area under the curve (AUC) from the receiver operator curve (ROC) characteristics was calculated [32]. We identified the optimal cutoff values for each x using Youden's Index [40], which maximizes the sum of sensitivity and specificity of AF/SR differentiation.

For each threshold x with the optimal cutoff value for differentiating between AF and SR, we calculated several classification metrics [41], namely, accuracy, specificity, sensitivity, F1-score [42], positive predictive value (PPV), negative predictive value (NPV), and diagnostic odds ratio (DOR) [43]. For the estimation of classification metrics' 95% confidence interval (CI), we used a nonparametric bootstrap with 5000 samples [44]. We analyzed all measures as functions of the threshold value x of pRRx in the range of 7 to 195 ms.

As the use of the pRR50 parameter is a de facto standard, we decided to compare its diagnostic properties against the optimal pRRx for AF detection. The optimal cutoff values for both parameters were estimated with the Youden criterion [40], and we used a nonparametric bootstrap to compare the distributions of the classification metrics with optimal cutoffs to verify whether the diagnostic properties of different thresholds are not random. For the sampling frequency of 128 Hz in the LTAFDB, the threshold x = 54 ms is equivalent to x = 50 ms, so pRR54 was used as an equivalent of pRR50.

3. Results

3.1. Data Distribution Analysis

Figure 2 shows pRRx histograms for SR and AF for different x threshold values between 7 and 195 ms. The histograms for SR and AF partially overlap—for the same x, the left part of the SR distribution covers the right part of the AF distribution. The overlap is notable for very low (pRR7, pRR15) and very high values of the threshold x (pRR101–pRR195), but the distributions are better separated between these extremes.

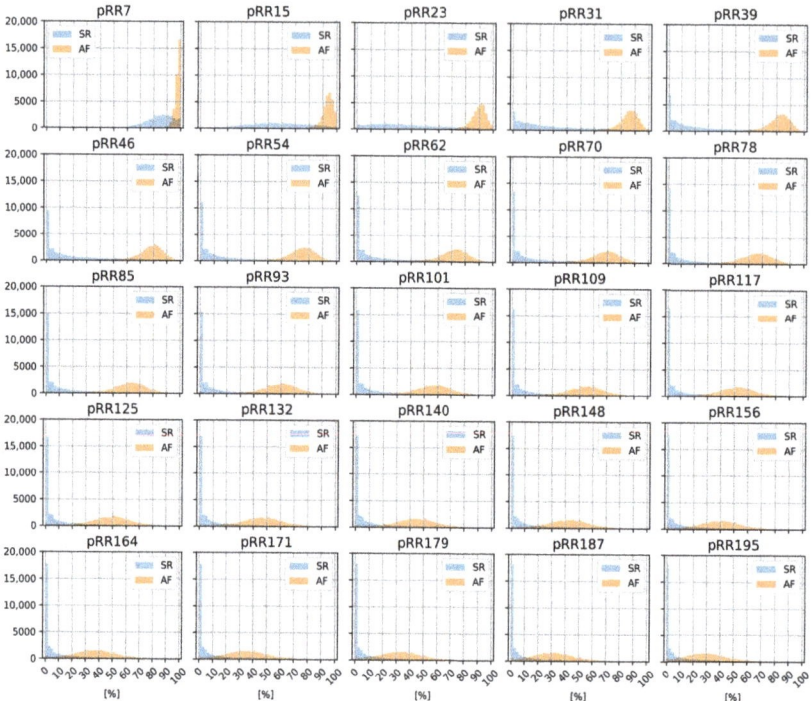

Figure 2. Histograms of percentages of successive RR intervals differing by at least x ms (pRRx) for sinus rhythm (SR) and atrial fibrillation (AF) for different x thresholds.

Figure 3 presents medians (bolder line), the 25th to 75th percentile range (darker band), and the 10th to 90th percentile range (lighter band) for AF (orange) and SR (blue). Median values of SR and AF never cross or overlap in the whole range of studied x. Interestingly, there is also no overlap between the 75th percentiles of pRRx for SR and the 25th percentiles of pRRx for AF. Additionally, the 90th percentile of pRRx for SR does not cross with the 10th percentile for AF in the range of x from 15 to 85 ms. It suggests that the optimal value of threshold x for differentiating between AF and SR lies within this range.

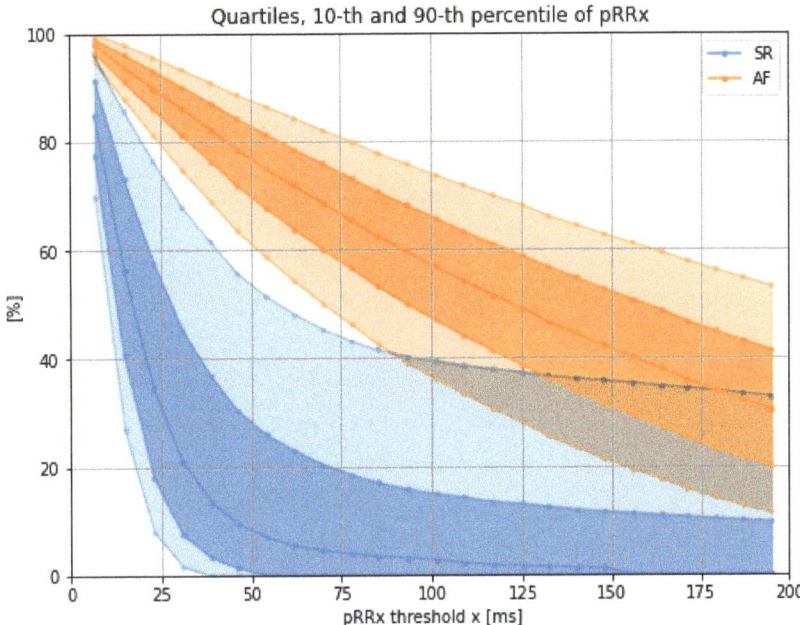

Figure 3. Medians (bolder line), interquartile ranges (darker band), and 10th to 90th percentile ranges (lighter band) of the percentages of successive RR intervals differing by at least x ms (pRRx) for sinus rhythm (SR) and atrial fibrillation (AF) for different x thresholds.

3.2. Correlation

Figure 4 shows two heatmaps with rho coefficients of Spearman correlations between pRRx for the different x thresholds in SR (the upper panel) and AF (the lower panel). For most x thresholds, particularly for lower values, the correlation coefficients are higher for SR than for AF. For the highest values of x, these correlations are above 0.95, both for SR and AF.

The rho coefficients decrease for SR and AF as the distance between two pRRx increases. Interestingly, this effect is more pronounced for lower x. For instance, in AF recordings, the rho coefficient drops from 0.7 for the pair (pRR7, pRR15) to 0.63 for (pRR7, pRR23). In contrast, rho is 1 for two pairs (pRR195, pRR187) and (pRR195, pRR179).

In AF, the pRRx with the lowest x (pRR7) has the strongest correlation with pRR15 (0.7), which is lower than in SR (0.92). However, the weakest correlation (between pRR7 and pRR195) is higher in AF (0.42) than in SR (0.38). It shows that for the lower values of x, the range of correlations is much wider for SR than for AF. Additionally, it suggests that the strength of correlations between various pRRx changes non-linearly for SR and AF.

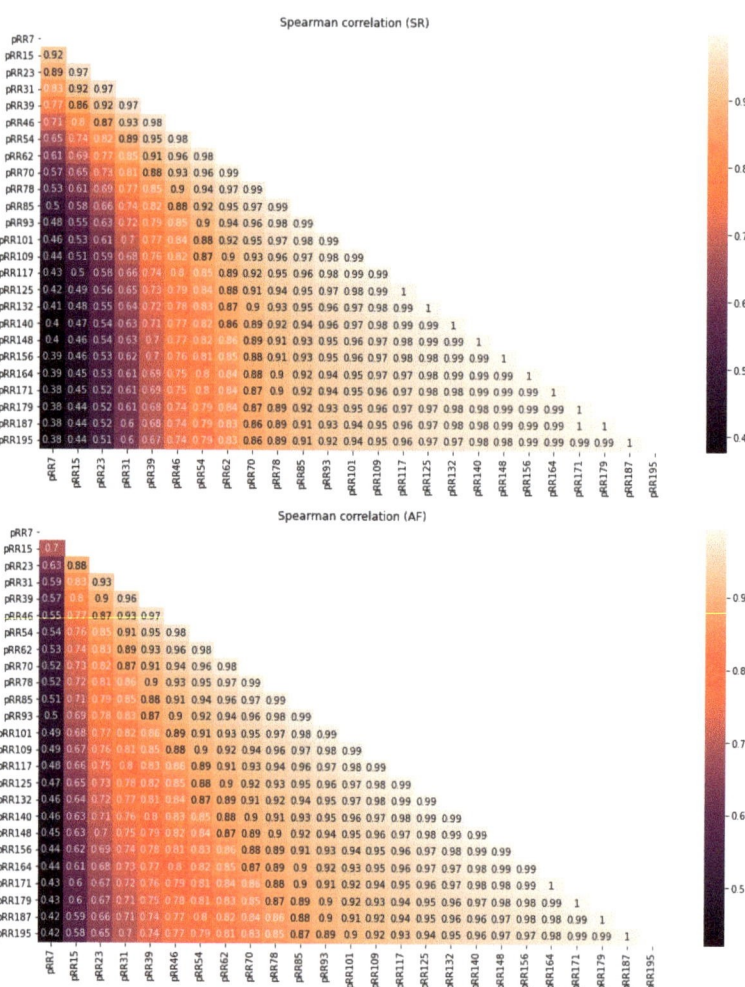

Figure 4. Heatmaps of Spearman correlation with rho coefficients between the percentages of successive RR intervals differing by at least x ms (pRRx parameters) for different x thresholds for sinus rhythm (SR, **top panel**) and atrial fibrillation (AF, **bottom panel**) segments of 60-s electrocardiograms.

3.3. Difference Analysis

Figure 5 separately summarizes the differences between all pairs of pRRx parameters for AF and SR. For each pair of pRRx parameters, e.g., pRR7 and pRR46, the mean difference (bias) and LoA (the range between 2.5th and 97.5th percentile of the differences' distribution) were computed.

There are visible differences in the relations of biases or LoAs of the differences for all possible pairs of pRRx with various x values. The bias distributions for different x resemble one of the reciprocal functions and are non-linear for SR and nearly linear with a negative slope for AF. In SR, for the x thresholds starting from 78 ms onward, the LoA values of the differences between different pairs of pRRx initially increase to their peak and then decline reciprocally. No similar early increase in such LoA is present for AF, in which these lines nearly linearly decrease from the maximal values for the closest to minimal values for the most distant pRRx pairs.

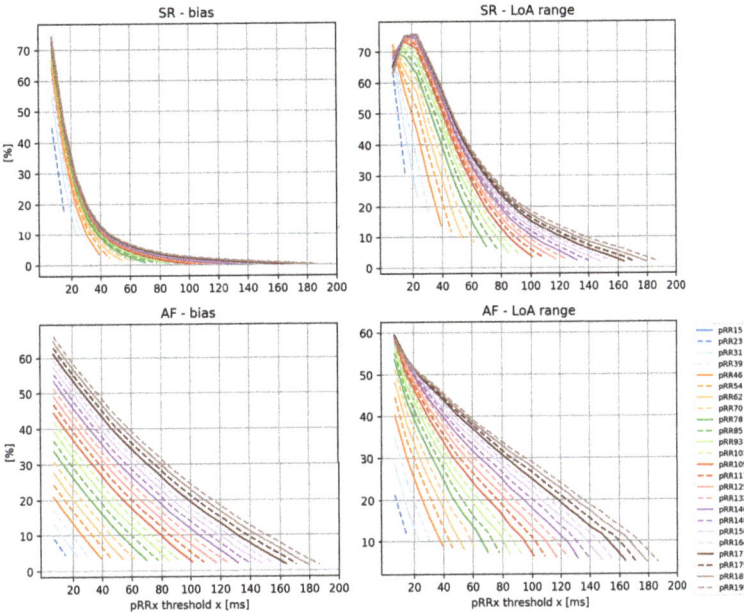

Figure 5. Summary of the analysis of the differences between the pairs of the percentages of successive RR intervals differing by at least x ms (pRRx parameters). Mean difference (bias) and 95% limits of agreement (LoA) range in sinus rhythm (SR, **top**) and atrial fibrillation (AF, **bottom**).

3.4. Area under ROC Curve (AUC)

The AUCs for the differentiation of AF from SR, shown in Figure 6, have their peak values exceeding 0.94 for the range of x from 15 ms to 85 ms (identical with the no overlapping zone between the 90th percentile of the pRRx distribution of SR and 10th percentile for AF as visible in Figure 3). AUCs gradually decrease to 0.87 for the highest x thresholds. In other words, pRRx for lower x values has a much better AUC for distinguishing the SR from AF recordings. The maximal AUC value can be one of the criteria for selecting the optimal x threshold for differentiating SR from AF with pRRx. In our study, the maximal AUC value (0.958) was for x = 31 ms, i.e., pRR31.

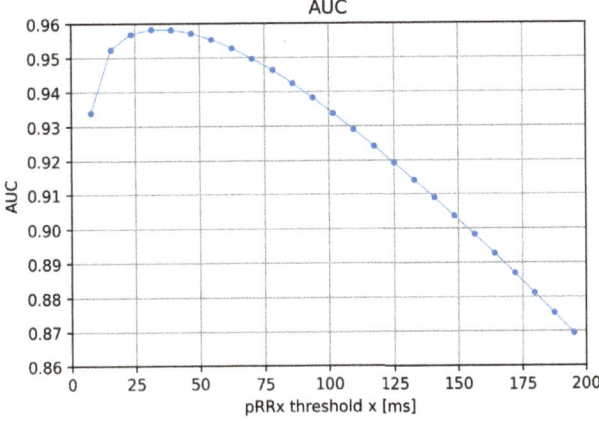

Figure 6. Area under curve (AUC) of the percentages of successive RR intervals differing by at least x ms (pRRx parameters) for the differentiation of AF from SR as a function of the x threshold.

3.5. Determining Optimal Cutoff Values for Different pRRx

Using Youden's index, we selected optimal cutoff values for all pRRx (Figure 7). Notably, the cutoff values for pRRx strongly and negatively depended on their x threshold.

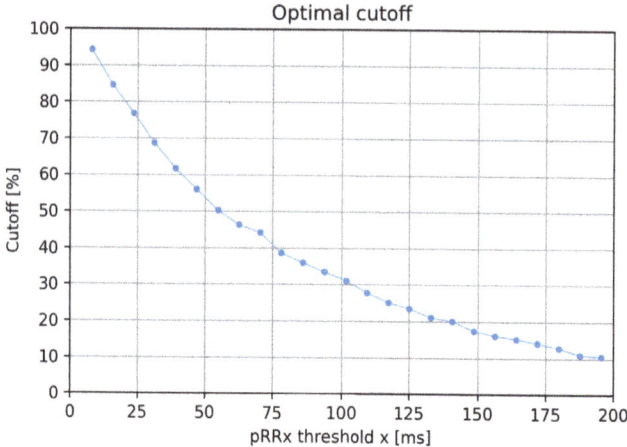

Figure 7. Optimal cutoff values based on Youden Index the percentages of successive RR intervals differing by at least x ms (pRRx parameters) as a function of the x threshold.

Next, the nonparametric bootstrap estimated the statistical metrics of AF detection using pRRx parameters with the optimal cutoffs. Figure 8 shows the median values and 95% CI of the classification metrics for optimal cutoffs of pRRx in relation to the x threshold. Although there is a gradual slow decline in the sensitivity of pRRx, its median exceeds 0.9 in the whole studied range of x. For the NPV, this relation is similar, with the lowest values above 0.89 for the largest x = 195 ms. Gradual decline with the increasing x values is also visible for both PPV and specificity. However, the decline is more rapid and deeper, from 0.89 to 0.77 (PPV), and from 0.88 to 0.72 (specificity) for x thresholds above 50 ms.

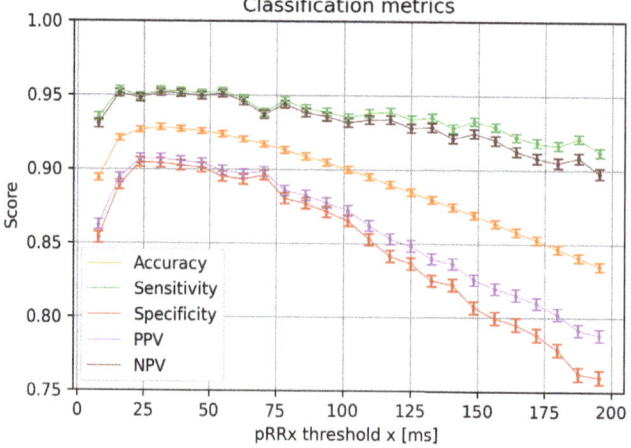

Figure 8. Medians and 95% confidence intervals of diagnostic classification metrics for optimum cutoff values for the percentages of successive RR intervals differing by at least x ms (pRRx parameters) as a function of the x threshold. PPV—positive predictive value, NPV—negative predictive value.

3.6. The Diagnostic Odds Ratios for Optimal Cutoffs for Different pRRx

Figure 9 presents median values of DOR with 95% CI for optimal cutoffs for different pRRx in relation to the x value. The highest DOR of 194.01 is observed for pRR31. In other words, the odds of pRR31 being greater or equal to the cutoff = 68.79% (Figure 7) is nearly 200 higher for the AF presence than in its absence. The next highest DORs are for pRR39, pRR46, and pRR25, all exceeding 175. DORs for pRRx for x up to 81 ms are at least 125, then gradually decline with increasing x values, reaching a minimum of 32.68 for x = 195 ms.

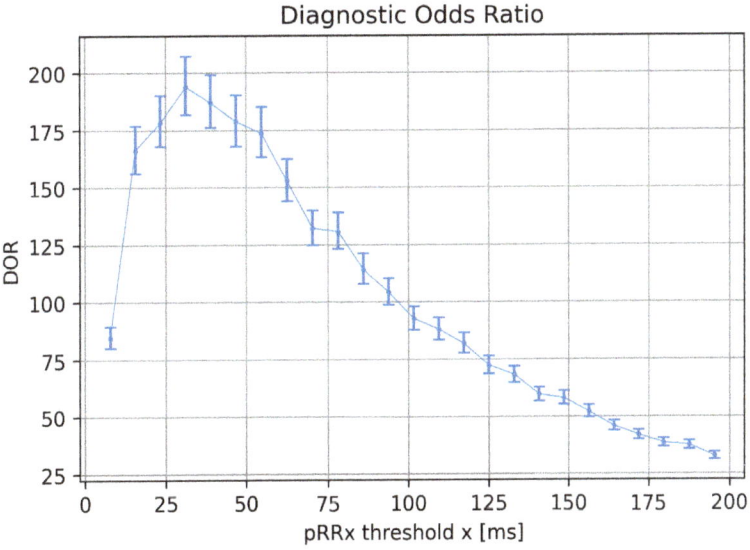

Figure 9. Medians and 95% confidence intervals of diagnostic odds ratio (DOR) for optimum cutoff values for the percentages of successive RR intervals differing by at least x ms (pRRx parameters) as a function of the x threshold.

3.7. Comparison of pRR50 and pRR31

The threshold x = 50 ms of pRRx is most broadly used and analyzed in HRV literature, including HRV-based AF detection methods. On the other hand, in our study, pRR31 achieved the highest accuracy (Figure 8) and DOR (Figure 9). We used a nonparametric bootstrap to compare the distributions of classification metrics obtained by pRR31 and pRR50 with optimal cutoffs to verify whether better diagnostic properties of different thresholds are not random. For the sampling frequency of 128 Hz in the LTAFDB, the threshold x = 54 ms is equivalent to x = 50 ms, so pRR54 was used as an equivalent of pRR50. Figure 10 shows the histograms of accuracy, sensitivity, specificity, and DOR for pRR50 and pRR31. All the metrics are visibly higher for pRR31 than for pRR50, except for sensitivity, which is only slightly higher for pRR31. The Shapiro–Wilk test verified that accuracy, sensitivity, and specificity have normal distributions and DOR does not. The histograms and the results of paired t-test (accuracy, sensitivity, and specificity) and Wilcoxon test (DOR) demonstrate that better performance of pRR31 is not random.

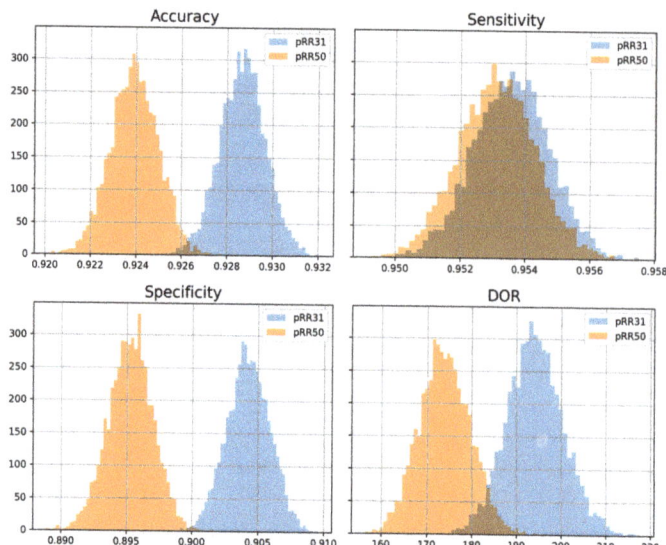

Figure 10. Histograms of classification metrics for optimum cutoff values for pRR31 and pRR50 (the percentages of successive RR intervals differing by at least 31 ms and 50 ms, respectively). DOR—diagnostic odds ratio.

4. Discussion

In this study, we summarize various statistical properties of pRRx as functions of the x threshold both for AF and SR. All possible pairs of pRRx, regardless of the x distance separating them, are well correlated (Figure 4). Good correlations with rho at least 0.7 were present for all pRRx starting from x = 46 ms and most for x = 39 ms in SR recordings. In AF, all pairs of pRRx are well correlated, starting from x = 31 ms and then for most x = 23 ms. For higher x, pairs of pRRx are perfectly correlated. Lower pRRx values provide more information than higher pRRx. For instance, compared to pRR100, the pRR31 informs about the percentage of neighboring RR intervals, which differ not only from 100 ms but also in the lower range between 31 and 100 ms. In other words, using pRRx with higher x thresholds is more aggressive as it filters out much important information in the lower x ranges. Another issue is that good correlation does not mean that all pRRx parameters are the same and thus replaceable. Besides, caution should be exercised for the lowest x = 7 ms, for which the rho values drop to 0.38 and 0.42 for SR and AF, respectively. This analysis shows that various pRRx provide different information, particularly those with lower x.

The analysis of differences between different pRRx (Figure 5) reveals that their mean difference (bias) and the 95% limits of agreement range have distinct properties in AF and in SR. It shows that the decline of pRRx differences is more dynamic for SR than AF, even for the neighboring x. This analysis also demonstrates that pRRx with different x, even for the closest pairs of pRRx, do not provide identical information.

The optimal cutoffs for pRRx depended differently on the threshold x in a wide range from 7 ms to 195 ms. The best diagnostic features for AF detection are for the x range between 15 and 85 ms. It was repeatedly indicated by comparing pRRx 90th percentile for SR and 10th percentile for AF (Figure 3), then AUC over 0.94 (Figure 6), and finally with odds ratios exceeding 110 for specific cutoffs (Figure 9). Out of several possible x values within this range, x = 31 ms appears to be the best.

pRR50 is the most broadly studied pRRx parameter in physiological and clinical studies with ECG with sinus rhythm and for the differentiation of AF from SR [45–48]. Only a few studies explored pRRx with threshold values x different than 50 ms in AF detection [22,23,25–27,29,31,33]. Among them, only one study contained an analysis of the distribution of pRRx in AF and SR [26], and two had AUCs of the parameters [31,33]. However, neither analysis was in-depth.

Our study is more detailed, systematic, and focused on the whole pRRx family in a broad range of x thresholds. It is probably the first analysis investigating various statistical properties of pRRx exclusively as a function of x for the differentiation of AF from SR.

This study provides practical consequences for distinguishing AF from SR in 60-s ECG segments. First, although pRR50 is within the range of x values with very good diagnostic properties, it is not the best. Second, for the 60-s ECG segments, the x = 31 ms outperforms other pRRx (including pRR50), particularly when comparing DORs. The odds of pRR31 exceeding 68.79% (Figure 9) is nearly 200 times higher in the presence of AF than in the absence of AF. Third, we demonstrate how distinct the statistical properties of pRRx are in SR and AF. Fourth, if HRV parameters are used to differentiate AF from SR, for example, in the machine learning algorithms, pRRx with x shorter than 50 should be applied.

In SR, the differences between the duration of successive RR intervals are much more limited than in AF. The RR interval for SR usually falls within 80 to 120% of the previous RR interval. For AF, no such limit exists. It results from a couple of physiological regulatory mechanisms controlling SR, which have weaker or no effect on the heart rate during AF.

SR originates in the sinus node, where pacemaker depolarization activity is regulated by several controlling mechanisms. The electrical depolarization from the sinus nodes travels across the right atrium and reaches the atrioventricular node. The atrioventricular conduction undergoes additional controlling regulations. During AF, thousands of cells from the border of pulmonary veins and the left atrium or both atria depolarize spontaneously in a relatively uncontrolled way. Atrial depolarizations reach the atrioventricular node in a more or less random order, which may or may not conduct them through the His system to both ventricles. The refractory period is probably the most important physiological mechanism that is still functioning; it may control the ventricle rate in AF. All cells of the atrioventricular node, His system, and ventricles have various refractory periods. During this period, cardiac cells below the atria cannot respond to electrical depolarization. The refractory period, particularly in the atrioventricular node, is under the strong control of the autonomic nervous system during SR. This control is less effective but is still present during AF. In other words, less controlling mechanisms over the ventricular rate in AF introduce some randomness to RR intervals and thus higher values of pRRx than in SR.

The limitations of the study must be recognized. It is an observational and retrospective study using ECG recordings from a single (Long-Term AF Database) database. To verify whether the results are not database-specific, we used optimal cutoffs of pRRx from LTAFDB and employed them to classify 60-s segments from MIT–BIH Atrial Fibrillation Database (250 Hz sampling frequency) [35,49]. The highest DOR (median 276) and accuracy (median 0.944) were obtained for pRR31 (in LTAFDB 194 and 0.928, respectively—the detailed results are shown in Appendix A). Moreover, these public databases have been used in several studies, and others can easily replicate our results. Other limitations are the arbitrary use of 60-ss ECG segments and the application of additional filters removing too short (<240 ms) or too long (>3000 ms) RR intervals to select ECG segments that might result in "too perfect" results. Thus, the interpretation of our findings must be limited only to the specific settings of the filters and ECG recording of 60-s duration.

Comparison of different methods and parameters is always complex and should never be based on a single approach or descriptor. As demonstrated, visual inspection is always essential—such a simple approach as the distribution analysis clearly shows how pRRx changes for various x, both for SR and AF. Unfortunately, presenting the actual data distribution is not a common approach. Next, correlation analysis is the most popular in many studies to present how well some parameters are correlated. Presented correlation heatmaps also show strong correlations for pRRx in a wide range of x values. Many studies stop at this point, without further and more detailed exploration. However, additional analyses with classic statistical methods, starting with differences analysis, followed by more advanced analyses such as ROC, the identification of cutoff points, and various classification measures, reveal huge differences between parameters that appear so well related. Summarizing this part, a set of several classical statistical methods for comparing various methods or parameters should be constantly employed in clinical medicine. Referring to one method, usually correlation analysis, can produce misleading conclusions and false diagnoses.

5. Conclusions

In conclusion, pRRx values for various x thresholds are not the same or interchangeable. Although most pRRx help detect AF, the parameters around pRR31 outperform others. If in a 60-s ECG the pRR31 is at least 68.79%, it is far more likely to be AF than SR. Using optimal pRRx instead of pRR50 should improve machine learning models for AF detection. Our results potentially apply to different biomedical systems used for screening for AF, e.g., long-term ECG Holter or bio-patch systems. However, we are aware that this potential should be validated using real-life ECG recordings acquired in clinical conditions, and it requires further prospective studies. It is worth noticing that the proposed approach for searching for the most valuable, from the point of view of AF detection, pRRx parameters can be repeated in other conditions and applied, for example, to specific ECG devices. Finally, pRR50 has been used in several studies as one of the HRV features incorporated in various machine learning models detecting AF. Replacing pRR50 with pRRx with a smaller x might improve the diagnostic properties of such models.

Author Contributions: Conceptualization, S.B., K.J. and P.G.; methodology, S.B., K.J. and P.G.; software, S.B.; validation, S.B., K.J. and P.G.; formal analysis, S.B., K.J. and P.G.; investigation, S.B., K.J. and P.G.; data curation, S.B.; writing—original draft preparation, S.B., K.J. and P.G.; writing—review and editing, S.B., K.J. and P.G.; visualization, S.B.; and supervision, K.J. and P.G. All authors have read and agreed to the published version of the manuscript.

Funding: This research was funded in part by the Scientific Council for the discipline of Automatic Control, Electronics, and Electrical Engineering of Warsaw University of Technology, Poland, grant "Studies on the effectiveness of atrial fibrillation detection based on the analysis of PPG signal and ECG signal using machine learning techniques, including proposals for new solutions".

Institutional Review Board Statement: Not applicable.

Informed Consent Statement: Not applicable.

Data Availability Statement: MIT–BIH Atrial Fibrillation Database (AFDB) [35,49], and Long-Term AF Database (LTAFDB) [35,36] were used in the study. They are available at https://physionet.org/content/afdb/1.0.0/ (accessed on 1 June 2022) and https://physionet.org/content/ltafdb/1.0.0/ (accessed on 1 June 2022), respectively.

Conflicts of Interest: The authors declare no conflict of interest.

Appendix A. Results of Validation on MIT–BIH AF Database

We used the optimal cutoff values of pRRx parameters from the training set long-term Atrial Fibrillation Database (LTAFDB) to detect AF in the test set from the Massachusetts Institute of Technology–Beth Israel Hospital (MIT–BIH) Atrial Fibrillation Database (AFDB) [35,49]. Data preparation was the same as in the training set (Figure 1), and a nonparametric bootstrap with 5000 samples was used to estimate classification results' distribution.

Appendix A.1. Comparison between Training Set and Test Set Results

A comparison of the results of AF detection in the training set and the test set is presented in Figure A1. The classification metrics include the diagnostic odds ratio (DOR), accuracy, sensitivity, specificity, positive predictive value (PPV), and negative predictive value (NPV). In the test set, the highest DOR (median 276) and accuracy (median 0.944) are achieved for pRR31 (in training set 194 and 0.928, respectively). Peak values of DOR, accuracy, PPV, NPV, and specificity are higher in the test set AFDB, while sensitivity is higher in the training set LTAFDB in the whole range of threshold values x.

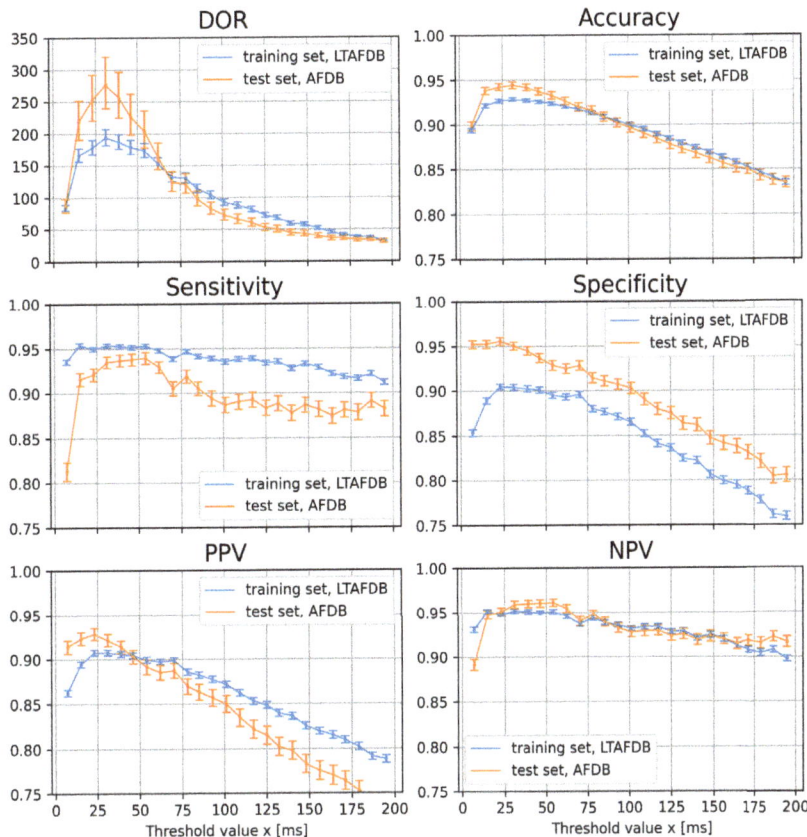

Figure A1. Medians and 95% confidence intervals of AF detection results in the training set Long-Term Atrial Fibrillation Database (LTAFDB) and the test set MIT–BIH Atrial Fibrillation Database (AFDB): diagnostic odds ratio (DOR, **top left**), accuracy (**top right**), sensitivity (**middle left**), specificity (**middle right**), positive predictive value (PPV, **bottom left**), and negative predictive value (NPV, **bottom right**).

The difference between performance in the training set and the test set can be a result of one or more factors, including:

- Distinct patient populations in two databases:
  - LTAFDB: 84 subjects;
  - AFDB: 25 subjects.
- Various sampling frequencies:
  - LTAFDB: 128 Hz;
  - AFDB: 250 Hz.
- The different lengths of the ECG recording:
  - LTAFDB: 24 h (night and day);
  - AFDB: 10 h (unspecified time of day).
- Unequal proportions of 60-s segments with AF and SR:
  - LTAFDB: 32,769 SR, 32,141 AF (49.5% AF);
  - AFDB: 8836 SR, 5490 AF (38.3% AF).

Appendix A.2. Comparison between pRR31 and pRR50

The histograms in Figure A2 show the distribution of four classification metrics (accuracy, sensitivity, specificity, and DOR) in AF detection in the test set using pRR31 and pRR50. For accuracy, specificity, and DOR, the results are higher for pRR31 than for pRR50. For sensitivity, there is an overlap between the distributions for pRR31 and pRR50, but the average is higher for pRR50.

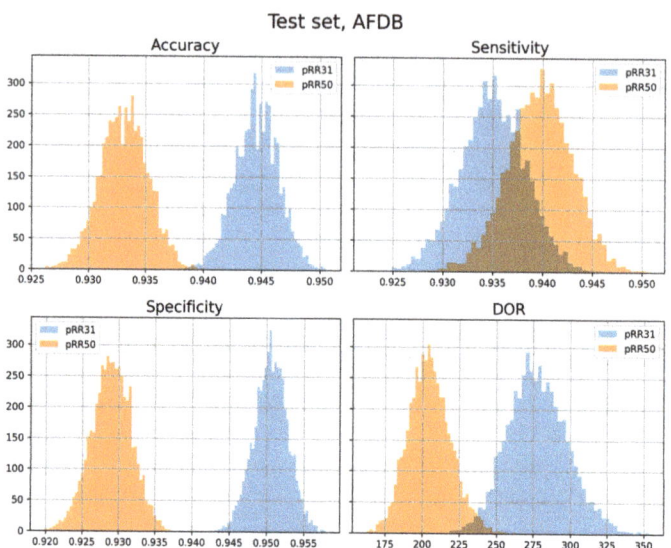

Figure A2. Histograms of atrial fibrillation detection results in the test set MIT–BIH Atrial Fibrillation Database (AFDB) for pRR31 and pRR50 (the percentages of successive RR intervals differing by at least 31 ms and 50 ms, respectively). DOR - diagnostic odds ratio.

Since not all the metrics had normal distribution (Shapiro–Wilk test) both for pRR31 and pRR50, we used the Wilcoxon test to compare the performance of pRR31 and pRR50. In all cases, the differences between the classification results cannot be explained by randomness.

Appendix A.3. Conclusions from the Validation

The results presented in the Appendix A confirm the study's findings. For AF detection in 60-s ECG, the most effective threshold value x in pRRx is not 50 ms (pRR50). Both in the training set LTAFDB and in the test set AFDB, pRR31 achieves the best performance, measured by accuracy and DOR. This phenomenon is not limited to a single ECG database; thus, pRR50 should not necessarily be a default pRRx parameter used in AF detection.

References

1. Hindricks, G.; Potpara, T.; Dagres, N.; Arbelo, E.; Bax, J.J.; Blomström-Lundqvist, C.; Boriani, G.; Castella, M.; Dan, G.A.; Dilaveris, P.E. 2020 ESC Guidelines for the diagnosis and management of atrial fibrillation developed in collaboration with the European Association for Cardio-Thoracic Surgery (EACTS) The Task Force for the diagnosis and management of atrial fibrillation of the European Society of Cardiology (ESC) Developed with the special contribution of the European Heart Rhythm Association (EHRA) of the ESC. *Eur. Heart J.* **2021**, *42*, 373–498. [CrossRef] [PubMed]
2. Tonko, J.B.; Wright, M.J. Review of the 2020 ESC Guidelines for the Diagnosis and Management of Atrial Fibrillation—What Has Changed and How Does This Affect Daily Practice. *J. Clin. Med.* **2021**, *10*, 3922. [CrossRef] [PubMed]
3. Roten, L.; Goulouti, E.; Lam, A.; Elchinova, E.; Nozica, N.; Spirito, A.; Wittmer, S.; Branca, M.; Servatius, H.; Noti, F. Age and Sex Specific Prevalence of Clinical and Screen-Detected Atrial Fibrillation in Hospitalized Patients. *J. Clin. Med.* **2021**, *10*, 4871. [CrossRef]

4. Ble, M.; Benito, B.; Cuadrado-Godia, E.; Pérez-Fernández, S.; Gómez, M.; Mas-Stachurska, A.; Tizón-Marcos, H.; Molina, L.; Martí-Almor, J.; Cladellas, M. Left Atrium Assessment by Speckle Tracking Echocardiography in Cryptogenic Stroke: Seeking Silent Atrial Fibrillation. *J. Clin. Med.* **2021**, *10*, 3501. [CrossRef]
5. Krisai, P.; Roten, L.; Zeljkovic, I.; Pavlovic, N.; Ammann, P.; Reichlin, T.; Auf der Maur, E.; Streicher, O.; Knecht, S.; Kühne, M.; et al. Prospective Evaluation of a Standardized Screening for Atrial Fibrillation after Ablation of Cavotricuspid Isthmus Dependent Atrial Flutter. *J. Clin. Med.* **2021**, *10*, 4453. [CrossRef]
6. Boriani, G.; Palmisano, P.; Malavasi, V.L.; Fantecchi, E.; Vitolo, M.; Bonini, N.; Imberti, J.F.; Valenti, A.C.; Schnabel, R.B.; Freedman, B. Clinical Factors Associated with Atrial Fibrillation Detection on Single-Time Point Screening Using a Hand-Held Single-Lead ECG Device. *J. Clin. Med.* **2021**, *10*, 729. [CrossRef]
7. Electrophysiology Task Force of the European Society of Cardiology the North American Society of Pacing. Heart Rate Variability. Standards of measurement, physiological interpretation, and clinical use. *Circulation* **1996**, *93*, 1043–1065. [CrossRef]
8. Sagnard, A.; Guenancia, C.; Mouhat, B.; Maza, M.; Fichot, M.; Moreau, D.; Garnier, F.; Lorgis, L.; Cottin, Y.; Zeller, M. Involvement of Autonomic Nervous System in New-Onset Atrial Fibrillation during Acute Myocardial Infarction. *J. Clin. Med.* **2020**, *9*, 1481. [CrossRef] [PubMed]
9. Rizwan, A.; Zoha, A.; Mabrouk, I.B.; Sabbour, H.M.; Al-Sumaiti, A.S.; Alomainy, A.; Imran, M.A.; Abbasi, Q.H. A Review on the State of the Art in Atrial Fibrillation Detection Enabled by Machine Learning. *IEEE Rev. Biomed. Eng.* **2020**, *14*, 219–239. [CrossRef] [PubMed]
10. Khan, A.A.; Lip, G.Y.H.; Shantsila, A. Heart rate variability in atrial fibrillation: The balance between sympathetic and parasympathetic nervous system. *Eur. J. Clin. Investig.* **2019**, *49*, e13174. [CrossRef] [PubMed]
11. Krasteva, V.; Christov, I.; Naydenov, S.; Stoyanov, T.; Jekova, I. Application of Dense Neural Networks for Detection of Atrial Fibrillation and Ranking of Augmented ECG Feature Set. *Sensors* **2021**, *21*, 6848. [CrossRef] [PubMed]
12. Kareem, M.; Lei, N.; Ali, A.; Ciaccio, E.J.; Acharya, U.R.; Faust, O. A review of patient-led data acquisition for atrial fibrillation detection to prevent stroke. *Biomed. Signal Process. Control* **2021**, *69*, 102818. [CrossRef]
13. Marinucci, D.; Sbrollini, A.; Marcantoni, I.; Morettini, M.; Swenne, C.A.; Burattini, L. Artificial Neural Network for Atrial Fibrillation Identification in Portable Devices. *Sensors* **2020**, *20*, 3570. [CrossRef] [PubMed]
14. Michel, P.; Ngo, N.; Pons, J.F.; Delliaux, S.; Giorgi, R. A filter approach for feature selection in classification: Application to automatic atrial fibrillation detection in electrocardiogram recordings. *BMC Med. Inform. Decis. Mak.* **2021**, *21*, 130. [CrossRef] [PubMed]
15. Buś, S.; Jędrzejewski, K.; Guzik, P. Using Minimum Redundancy Maximum Relevance Algorithm to Select Minimal Sets of Heart Rate Variability Parameters for Atrial Fibrillation Detection. *J. Clin. Med.* **2022**, *11*, 4004. [CrossRef]
16. Parsi, A.; Glavin, M.; Jones, E.; Byrne, D. Prediction of paroxysmal atrial fibrillation using new heart rate variability features. *Comput. Biol. Med.* **2021**, *133*, 104367. [CrossRef]
17. Biton, S.; Gendelman, S.; Ribeiro, A.H.; Miana, G.; Moreira, C.; Ribeiro, A.L.P.; Behar, J.A. Atrial fibrillation risk prediction from the 12-lead electrocardiogram using digital biomarkers and deep representation learning. *Eur. Heart J.-Digit. Health* **2021**, *2*, 576–585. [CrossRef]
18. Ewing, D.J.; Neilson, J.M.; Travis, P. New method for assessing cardiac parasympathetic activity using 24 hour electrocardiograms. *Heart* **1984**, *52*, 396–402. [CrossRef]
19. Bigger Jr, J.T.; Kleiger, R.E.; Fleiss, J.L.; Rolnitzky, L.M.; Steinman, R.C.; Miller, J.P. Components of heart rate variability measured during healing of acute myocardial infarction. *Am. J. Cardiol.* **1988**, *61*, 208–215. [CrossRef]
20. Mietus, J.E.; Peng, C.K.; Henry, I.; Goldsmith, R.L.; Goldberger, A.L. The pNNx files: Re-examining a widely used heart rate variability measure. *Heart* **2002**, *88*, 378–380. [CrossRef]
21. Torres, B.; Naranjo Orellana, J. Use of pNNx statistics in the evaluation of heart rate variability at rest and during exercise. *Arch. Med. Deporte* **2010**, *27*, 255–259.
22. Saiz-Vivo, J.; Corino, V.D.; de Melis, M.; Mainardi, L.T. Unsupervised Classification of Atrial Fibrillation Triggers Using Heart Rate Variability Features Extracted from Implantable Cardiac Monitor Data. In Proceedings of the 2020 42nd Annual International Conference of the IEEE Engineering in Medicine & Biology Society (EMBC), Montreal, QC, Canada, 20–24 July 2020; pp. 426–429. [CrossRef]
23. Saiz-Vivo, J.; Corino, V.D.A.; Hatala, R.; de Melis, M.; Mainardi, L.T. Heart Rate Variability and Clinical Features as Predictors of Atrial Fibrillation Recurrence After Catheter Ablation: A Pilot Study. *Front. Physiol.* **2021**, *12*, 672896. [CrossRef] [PubMed]
24. Liu, Y.; Chen, J.; Bao, N.; Gupta, B.B.; Lv, Z. Survey on atrial fibrillation detection from a single-lead ECG wave for Internet of Medical Things. *Comput. Commun.* **2021**, *178*, 245–258. [CrossRef]
25. Datta, S.; Puri, C.; Mukherjee, A.; Banerjee, R.; Dutta Choudhury, A.; Singh, R.; Ukil, A.; Bandyopadhyay, S.; Pal, A.; Khandelwal, S. Identifying Normal, AF and other Abnormal ECG Rhythms using a Cascaded Binary Classifier. In Proceedings of the 2017 Computing in Cardiology (CinC), Rennes, France, 24–27 September 2017. [CrossRef]
26. Jiménez Serrano, S.; Yagüe Mayans, J.; Simarro-Mondéjar, E.; Calvo, C.; Castells Ramon, F.; Roig, J. Atrial Fibrillation Detection Using Feedforward Neural Networks and Automatically Extracted Signal Features. In Proceedings of the 2017 Computing in Cardiology (CinC), Rennes, France, 24–27 September 2017. [CrossRef]
27. Teijeiro, T.; Garcia, C.A.; Castro, D.; Félix, P. Arrhythmia Classification from the Abductive Interpretation of Short Single-Lead ECG Records. In Proceedings of the 2017 Computing in Cardiology (CinC), Rennes, France, 24–27 September 2017. [CrossRef]

28. Clifford, G.D.; Liu, C.; Moody, B.; Li-wei, H.L.; Silva, I.; Li, Q.; Johnson, A.E.; Mark, R.G. AF Classification from a Short Single Lead ECG Recording: The PhysioNet/Computing in Cardiology Challenge 2017. In Proceedings of the 2017 Computing in Cardiology (CinC), Rennes, France, 24–27 September 2017; pp. 1–4.
29. Jovic, A.; Bogunovic, N. Evaluating and comparing performance of feature combinations of heart rate variability measures for cardiac rhythm classification. *Biomed. Signal Process. Control* **2012**, *7*, 245–255. [CrossRef]
30. Moody, G.; Mark, R. The impact of the MIT-BIH Arrhythmia Database. *IEEE Eng. Med. Biol. Mag.* **2001**, *20*, 45–50. [CrossRef] [PubMed]
31. Buś, S.; Jędrzejewski, K.; Guzik, P. A Study on Selection of HRV-based Features for Different Classifiers in Atrial Fibrillation Detection. In Proceedings of the 2021 Signal Processing Symposium (SPSympo), Lodz, Poland, 20–23 September 2021; pp. 31–34. [CrossRef]
32. Fawcett, T. An introduction to ROC analysis. *Pattern Recognit. Lett.* **2006**, *27*, 861–874. [CrossRef]
33. Conroy, T.; Guzman, J.H.; Hall, B.; Tsouri, G.; Couderc, J.P. Detection of atrial fibrillation using an earlobe photoplethysmographic sensor. *Physiol. Meas.* **2017**, *38*, 1906–1918. [CrossRef]
34. Ramesh, J.; Solatidehkordi, Z.; Aburukba, R.; Sagahyroon, A. Atrial Fibrillation Classification with Smart Wearables Using Short-Term Heart Rate Variability and Deep Convolutional Neural Networks. *Sensors* **2021**, *21*, 7233. [CrossRef]
35. Goldberger, A.L.; Amaral, L.A.; Glass, L.; Hausdorff, J.M.; Ivanov, P.C.; Mark, R.G.; Mietus, J.E.; Moody, G.B.; Peng, C.K.; Stanley, H.E. PhysioBank, PhysioToolkit, and PhysioNet: Components of a new research resource for complex physiologic signals. *Circulation* **2000**, *101*, e215–e220. [CrossRef]
36. Petrutiu, S.; Sahakian, A.V.; Swiryn, S. Abrupt changes in fibrillatory wave characteristics at the termination of paroxysmal atrial fibrillation in humans. *EP Eur.* **2007**, *9*, 466–470. [CrossRef] [PubMed]
37. Wilcoxon, F. Individual Comparisons by Ranking Methods. *Biom. Bull.* **1945**, *1*, 80–83. [CrossRef]
38. Mann, H.B.; Whitney, D.R. On a Test of Whether one of Two Random Variables is Stochastically Larger than the Other. *Ann. Math. Stat.* **1947**, *18*, 50–60. [CrossRef]
39. Spearman, C. The Proof and Measurement of Association between Two Things. *Am. J. Psychol.* **1904**, *15*, 72–101. [CrossRef]
40. Youden, W.J. Index for rating diagnostic tests. *Cancer* **1950**, *3*, 32–35. [CrossRef]
41. Butkuvienė, M.; Petrėnas, A.; Sološenko, A.; Martín-Yebra, A.; Marozas, V.; Sörnmo, L. Considerations on performance evaluation of atrial fibrillation detectors. *IEEE Trans. Biomed. Eng.* **2021**, *68*, 3250–3260. [CrossRef]
42. Chinchor, N.; Sundheim, B.M. MUC-5 evaluation metrics. In Proceedings of the Fifth Message Understanding Conference (MUC-5), Baltimore, MD, USA, 25–27 August 1993.
43. Glas, A.S.; Lijmer, J.G.; Prins, M.H.; Bonsel, G.J.; Bossuyt, P.M.M. The diagnostic odds ratio: A single indicator of test performance. *J. Clin. Epidemiol.* **2003**, *56*, 1129–1135. [CrossRef]
44. Efron, B. Bootstrap Methods: Another Look at the Jackknife. *Ann. Stat.* **1979**, *7*, 1–26. [CrossRef]
45. Nguyen, A.; Ansari, S.; Hooshmand, M.; Lin, K.; Ghanbari, H.; Gryak, J.; Najarian, K. Comparative Study on Heart Rate Variability Analysis for Atrial Fibrillation Detection in Short Single-Lead ECG Recordings. In Proceedings of the 2018 40th Annual International Conference of the IEEE Engineering in Medicine and Biology Society (EMBC), Honolulu, HI, USA, 18–21 July 2018; pp. 526–529. [CrossRef]
46. Christov, I.; Krasteva, V.; Simova, I.; Neycheva, T.; Schmid, R. Ranking of the most reliable beat morphology and heart rate variability features for the detection of atrial fibrillation in short single-lead ECG. *Physiol. Meas.* **2018**, *39*, 094005. [CrossRef]
47. Kim, D.; Seo, Y.; Jung, W.R.; Youn, C.H. Detection of Long Term Variations of Heart Rate Variability in Normal Sinus Rhythm and Atrial Fibrillation ECG Data. In Proceedings of the 2008 International Conference on BioMedical Engineering and Informatics, Sanya, China, 27–30 May 2008; pp. 404–408. [CrossRef]
48. Rubin, J.; Parvaneh, S.; Asif, R.; Conroy, B.; Babaeizadeh, S. Densely Connected Convolutional Networks and Signal Quality Analysis to Detect Atrial Fibrillation Using Short Single-Lead ECG Recordings. In Proceedings of the 2017 Computing in Cardiology (CinC), Rennes, France, 24–27 September 2017. [CrossRef]
49. Moody, G. A new method for detecting atrial fibrillation using RR intervals. *Comput. Cardiol.* **1983**, *10*, 227–230.

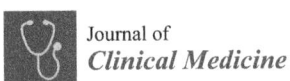

Article

Heart Rate Variability Impairment Is Associated with Right Ventricular Overload and Early Mortality Risk in Patients with Acute Pulmonary Embolism

Monika Lisicka [1], Marta Skowrońska [1], Bartosz Karolak [1], Jan Wójcik [2], Piotr Pruszczyk [1] and Piotr Bienias [1,*]

[1] Department of Internal Medicine and Cardiology, Medical University of Warsaw, 02-005 Warsaw, Poland
[2] Students' Scientific Association Zator, Department of Internal Medicine and Cardiology, Medical University of Warsaw, 02-005 Warsaw, Poland
* Correspondence: pbienias@mp.pl; Tel.: +48-22-502-1144; Fax: +48-22-502-2142

Abstract: The association between heart rate variability (HRV) and mortality risk of acute pulmonary embolism (APE), as well as its association with right ventricular (RV) overload is not well established. We performed an observational study on consecutive patients with confirmed APE. In the first 48 h after admission, 24 h Holter monitoring with assessment of time-domain HRV, echocardiography and NT-proBNP (N-terminal pro-B-type natriuretic peptide) measurement were performed in all participants. We pre-examined 166 patients: 32 (20%) with low risk of early mortality, 65 (40%) with intermediate–low, 65 (40%) with intermediate–high, and 4 (0.02%) in the high risk category. The last group was excluded from further analysis due to sample size, and finally, 162 patients aged 56.3 ± 18.5 years were examined. We observed significant correlations between HRV parameters and echocardiographic signs of RV overload. SDNN (standard deviation of intervals of all normal beats) correlated with echocardiography-derived RVSP (right ventricular systolic pressure; r = −0.31, p = 0.001), TAPSE (tricuspid annulus plane systolic excursion; r = 0.21, p = 0.033), IVC (inferior vena cava diameter; r = −0.27, p = 0.002) and also with NT-proBNP concentration (r = −0.30, p = 0.004). HRV indices were also associated with APE risk stratification, especially in the low-risk category (r = 0.30, p = 0.004 for SDNN). Univariate and multivariate analyses confirmed that SDNN values were associated with signs of RV overload. In conclusion, we observed a significant association between time-domain HRV parameters and echocardiographic and biochemical signs of RV overload. Impaired HRV parameters were also associated with worse a clinical risk status of APE.

Keywords: acute pulmonary embolism; electrocardiography; Holter monitoring; heart rate variability; right ventricle overload

1. Introduction

Venous thromboembolism, clinically presenting as deep vein thrombosis or acute pulmonary embolism (APE), is globally the third most frequent acute cardiovascular syndrome. Even though the annual fatality rates of the disease across Europe and Northern America have decreased over a 15 year period, APE is still associated with adverse clinical outcomes, including deterioration and death [1]. Numerous electrocardiographic abnormalities are observed during APE, especially in the 12-lead ECG. However, the evidence on the role of 24 h Holter or other long-term electrocardiography monitoring in controlling the clinical status or evaluating the prognosis of APE is scarce. This also applies to the heart rate variability (HRV) obtained during Holter monitoring, which is a reflection of cardiac autonomic nervous system (cANS) activity, both sympathetic and parasympathetic. Several studies revealed that cANS imbalances are associated with a worse clinical prognosis in patients with impaired left ventricular function, especially as a consequence of myocardial infarction or heart failure [2]. It is postulated that the sympathetic–parasympathetic imbalance might be associated with various adverse events, including severe and life-threatening ventricular arrhythmias [2,3]. The right side of the heart, especially the right atrium, is an area with even more autonomous innervation than the left side. Thus, HRV analysis is presumed to be especially effective in monitoring autonomic function in patients with conditions affecting mainly the right side of the heart, such as APE [3]. A potential model, linking HRV parameters with echocardiographic features of right ventricular (RV) overload may lead to improved prognosis assessment, and consequently, improvement of clinical practice in these patients. However, the clinical utility of HRV has not yet been established in large cohorts of APE patients.

We make the assumption that time-domain HRV analysis, which can be easily performed by standard Holter monitoring [4], might be a promising tool for risk stratification of patients with APE. Therefore, the aim of our study was to evaluate the relationship between Holter-derived HRV indices and specific echocardiographic and laboratory parameters, well established in the assessment of the prognosis of APE, along with their analysis in the context of APE risk stratification according to the European Society of Cardiology (ESC) [1].

2. Materials and Methods

We performed a prospective, single-center, cross-sectional, observational study, running for 10 years between 2009 and 2019. At baseline, consecutive adult patients with APE confirmed by imaging (mostly computed tomography pulmonary angiogram) were included. Detailed evaluation of clinical status, past medical history and laboratory tests were performed at admission, while echocardiography and 24 h Holter monitoring were conducted within 48 h of admission at the latest (most often <24 h). Then, the prognosis of APE was assessed according to the ESC guidelines. All participants were assessed according to current ESC guidelines but, in terms of the present data analysis, retrospectively assigned to risk categories stated in the 2019 guidelines, i.e., low, intermediate–low, intermediate–high and high risk. This classification provides information about the APE severity and the risk of early (in-hospital or 30-day) mortality. Patients with clinical signs of hemodynamic instability were classified in the high risk category. Patients without hemodynamic instability, but with presence of both RV dysfunction (on echocardiography or computed tomography angiography) and elevation of laboratory biomarkers (mainly cardiac troponin, but N-terminal pro-B-type natriuretic peptide (NT-proBNP) also provides prognostic information) were referred to the intermediate–high risk category. The presence of only one of the aforementioned signs of RV disfunction (in cardiac imaging or biochemical) enabled the identification of the intermediate–low risk category, while the absence of both of them to the low risk category, provided that the simplified pulmonary embolism severity index score was 0 points [1].

Transthoracic echocardiography was performed using a Philips iE33 ultrasound system (Philips Medical System, Andover, MA, USA) with a 2.5–3.5 MHz transducer. Patients were examined in the left lateral position. According to current American and European recommendations, all standard dimensions, valve morphology and function, left ventricular ejection fraction and right heart parameters were evaluated [5]. The emphasis was put on the RV assessment, including following parameters: TRPG (tricuspid regurgitation peak gradient), RVSP (right ventricular systolic pressure), AcT (right ventricular outflow Doppler acceleration time), IVC (inferior vena cava diameter) and TAPSE (tricuspid annulus plane systolic excursion) measurement. Considering the extensive experience of our experts in the field of diagnostic imaging, verified by the certificate of the Section of Echocardiography of the Polish Cardiac Society, which is a part of the ESC, as well as the high repeatability (inter/intra-observer), which was confirmed in one of the studies on patients with APE carried out in our center, echocardiographic examination was performed at a time by one experienced physician [6].

Ambulatory Holter monitoring was conducted using three-channel digitized recordings (Lifecard CF, Spacelabs Healthcare, Snoqualmie, WA, USA). Routine evaluations of heart rates and arrhythmias were performed (Sentinel Impresario, Spacelabs Healthcare, USA). Careful manual review and filtering algorithms were used to eliminate inappropriate electrocardiographic strips, aimed to eliminate fragments illegible for further analysis. Time-domain HRV parameters were obtained from 24 h Holter monitoring, including SDNN (standard deviation of intervals of all normal beats), SDNN-I (the average of the standard deviations of N-N intervals for each 5-min), SDANN (standard deviation of five-minute mean N-N interval), RMSSD (root mean square standard deviation), pNN50 (percentage of intervals that are more than 50 ms different from previous interval) and triangular index (integral of the density of the NN interval histogram divided by its height) [4]. These parameters were chosen as sufficient for time-domain HRV analysis, considering that many parameters closely correlate with others. SDNN and HRV-Index estimate overall HRV, SDANN and SDNN-I estimate long-term components of HRV, RMSSD and pNN50 estimate short-term components of HRV [4]. For each HRV parameter, the results of the entire 24 h evaluation were taken for further analysis, without the division into day and night periods. Each Holter recording was analyzed by a qualified and certified cardiologist without blinding.

Echocardiographic and Holter examinations were performed by different members of the research staff who knew the full protocol but did not know the detailed results obtained, which were later transferred to the database. Taking in the relatively modest data on long-term electrocardiographic monitoring and Holter-derived cANS assessment in APE patients, we decided to conduct an exploratory study to provide new information on this topic without a pre-existing hypothesis.

3. Statistical Analysis and Data Presentation

The data collection was not blinded. Continuous variables were compared with Student's t test or the Wilcoxon test, according to data distribution. Categorical variables were compared using Fisher's exact test. All tests were double-sided. Variables with a normal distribution are presented as mean followed by standard deviation. Deletions of outliers' data were not performed. Variables not showing normal distribution, as well as those with skewed distribution, were presented as median with range and also with interquartile range values. Pearson's correlation coefficient was used to assess the significance of the connections between parameters considered to show normal distribution. Abridged logistic regression analysis was performed to explore the influence of confounding factors on the values of SDNN, the most important HRV parameter. Both univariate and multivariate analyses were carried out with the examination of multiple models. Statistical significance was determined at $p < 0.05$. Results of univariate and multivariate analyses are presented as odds ratios (OR) with 95% confidence intervals (95% CI). All statistical analyses were performed using Statistica 14.0 (StatSoft Inc., Tulsa, OK, USA).

4. Results

The study cohort consisted of 166 consecutive patients with confirmed APE admitted to our specialist center, almost all of them to our cardiac care unit. As described above, all participants were assigned to the APE risk classification groups according to ESC guidelines. The majority of the patients was allocated to the intermediate risk category (130 persons, 80%), of which exactly half belonged to the intermediate–low risk APE category (65 persons) and the other half to the intermediate–high risk APE. Low risk APE consisted of 32 (20%) patients, while only four (0.02%) participants had the high risk disease. Patients with the high clinical risk category were excluded from further statistical analysis due to small sample size, which cannot give conclusive results in the context of the whole study population. Then, to reach the needs of statistical equations and provide results, more plausible and representative for our study population, we merged the intermediate–low and intermediate–high risk groups into one group of patients with the intermediate risk APE. All patients received standard anticoagulation therapy and other medications needed for their specific comorbidities.

The general characteristics at baseline are shown in Table 1 and did not differ significantly between groups of patients with low and intermediate risk. Results were not different for males and females either—detailed results are not shown. As expected, due to right RV overload, the NT-proBNP level was significantly higher in intermediate risk APE. For the same reason, echocardiographic parameters related to impaired RV function were worse in this group of patients in comparison with the low risk APE population. During a follow-up of 48 h, none of the patients finally enrolled in the study died, required thrombolysis, or were transferred to an intensive/critical care unit.

Table 1. The general characteristics, laboratory data, echocardiographic parameters and 24 h Holter and time-domain heart rate variability data in all enrolled patients with acute pulmonary embolism (APE), as well as in subgroups with low and intermediate early mortality risk.

	All APE Patients (n = 162) [a]	Low Risk APE (n = 32)	Intermediate Risk APE (n = 130)	p Value Low vs. Intermediate Risk APE
General characteristics and laboratory data at admission				
Age (years) [b]	56.3 ± 18.5 (18–86)	54.6 ± 17.2 (20–82)	53.4 ± 18.0 (18–86)	0.39
Females (n, %)	89 (54%)	18 (56%)	68 (52%)	0.8
BMI (kg/m^2)	29.1 ± 5.6	27.2 ± 5.5	31.1 ± 5.7	**0.04**
HR at admission (bpm)	88 ± 18	87 ± 22	91 ± 16	0.21
SBP at admission (mmHg)	128.1 ± 18.8	128.0 ± 16.5	130.8 ± 18.7	0.48
NT-proBNP (pg/mL) *	627 (52.5–2795.5, 160.0–2321.0)	95 (18.0–272.0, 52.5–201.0)	1443 (59.0–29,071.0, 486.0–2795.5)	**0.02**
Echocardiography parameters				
LVEF (%)	59.7 ± 6.9	62.3 ± 2.6	59.5 ± 7.6	0.09
LVDD (mm)	41.4 ± 6.6	43.6 ± 6.3	41.2 ± 7.6	0.28
RVD (mm)	38.2 ± 9.0	32.8 ± 6.8	38.6 ± 8.0	**0.02**
TRPG (mmHg)	34.4 ± 16.3	21.6 ± 6.7	37.6 ± 15.5	**0.005**
RVSP (mmHg)	41.5 ± 17.3	27.0 ± 6.7	46.6 ± 16.0	**0.005**
IVC (mm)	15.5 ± 4.6	13.6 ± 2.9	16.2 ± 4.7	**0.02**
AcT (ms)	83.5 ± 27.5	105.3 ± 22.2	75.8 ± 26.5	**0.005**
TAPSE (mm)	21.1 ± 4.9	23.9 ± 3.7	20.5 ± 4.9	0.06
24 h Holter and time-domain heart rate variability data				
Mean heart rate (bpm)	77 ± 14	75 ± 11	79 ± 13	0.26
Non-sustained SVT (n, %)	47 –29.00%	5 –15.70%	41 –31.50%	0.3
Non-sustained VT (n, %)	9 –5.40%	2 –6.30%	7 –5.40%	0.4
Paroxysmal atrial fibrillation (n., %)	2 –0.01%	0 -	2 –0.01%	-
SDNN (ms) *	92 (39.6–222.9, 68.8–121.4)	113.6 (65.5–222.9, 93–154.2)	87.9 (39.6–193.1, 65–116)	0.05
SDNN-I (ms) *	30.2 (10.1–90.4, 21.2–39.3)	35.7 (15.9–90.4, 32.9–52.4)	28 (10.1–85.9, 20.7–37.3)	0.06
SDANN (ms) *	85.1 (29.0–190.4, 61.0–110.8)	100.1 (35.2–190.4, 82.6–126.9)	80.6 (29.0–182.9, 58–107.9)	0.1
RMSSD (ms) *	26.8 (12.4–96.2, 20.2–38.2)	32.8 (12.6–96.2, 22.9–54)	26.8 (12.4–94.2, 19.9–36.9)	**0.02**
pNN50 (%) *	2.8 (0.1–74.8, 1.0–16.0)	6.8 (0.1–74.8, 2.1–16.0)	2.45 (0.1–37.7, 1.0–7.1)	**0.03**
Triangular Index *	12.3 (4.1–33.3, 9.6–17.3)	15.7 (6.7–33.3, 10.8–20.1)	11.7 (4.1–28.4, 9.5–16.2)	0.21

* value expressed as median with range and also interquartile range. [a] Four high risk patients were excluded from the pre-screened consecutive 166 individuals. [b] For age, the range is additionally shown. APE—acute pulmonary embolism; BMI—body mass index; HR—heart rate; SBP—systolic blood pressure; LVDD—left ventricle diastolic diameter; LVEF—left ventricle ejection fraction; RVD—right ventricle diameter; NT-proBNP—N-terminal pro-B-type natriuretic peptide; TRPG—tricuspid regurgitation peak gradient; RVSP—right ventricular systolic pressure; IVC—inferior vena cava diameter; AcT—right ventricular outflow Doppler acceleration time; TAPSE—tricuspid annulus plane systolic excursion; SDNN—standard deviation of intervals of all normal beats; SDNN-I—the average of the standard deviations of N-N intervals for each 5 min; SDANN—standard deviation of five-minute mean N-N interval; pNN50—percentage of intervals that are more than 50 ms different from previous interval; RMSSD—root mean square standard deviation; triangular index—integral of the density of the NN interval histogram divided by its height; Bold values show significant results.

The results of 24 h Holter monitoring in APE patients are also displayed in Table 1. For all APE patients, the median Holter recording time was 23 h and 22 min and was similar in the low and intermediate risk category groups (23:16 vs. 23:37, $p = 0.82$), while the shortest recording was 21 h and 12 min. However, the results of our HRV analysis are not obvious and easy to explain. While the values of SDNN, pNN50 and RMSSD were significantly lower in the intermediate than in the low risk APE group, no remarkable difference was found in the values of other parameters.

The next step was analysis of the potential relations between HRV and parameters obtained in echocardiography and biochemical tests. It was made collectively for the entire study population. Interestingly, while the mean HR was not associated with any of the echocardiographic measurements, its correlation with NT-proBNP levels reached statistical significance. We also found a lot of significant correlations between HRV and echocardiographic parameters describing RV function (Figure 1). Notably, most HRV parameters showed an inverse correlation with NT-proBNP concentration—detailed results are presented in Table 2.

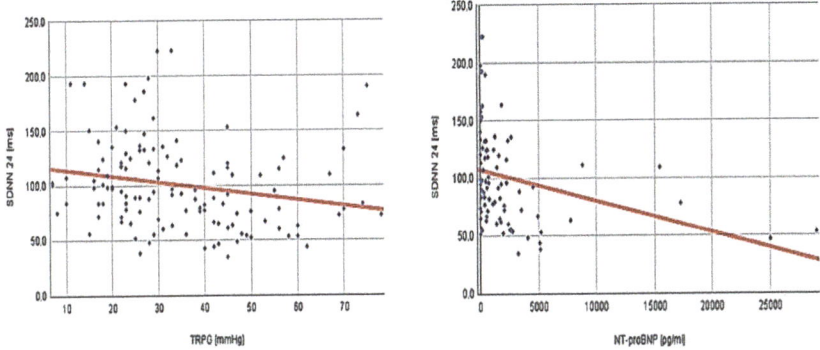

SDNN 24—standard deviation of intervals of all normal beats in 24-h Holter monitoring
TRPG—tricuspid regurgitation peak gradient
NT-proBNP—N-terminal pro B type natriuretic peptide concentration

Figure 1. Correlations in all low and intermediate risk patients with acute pulmonary embolism (n = 162) between standard deviation of intervals of all normal beats in 24 h Holter monitoring and tricuspid regurgitation peak gradient ($r = 0.22$, $p = 0.016$)—left side of the figure—and N-terminal pro-B type natriuretic peptide concentration ($r = -0.30$, $p = 0.004$)—right side of the figure.

Table 2. Correlations between time-domain heart rate variability indices, right ventricle overload echocardiographic parameters and also N-terminal pro B type natriuretic peptide concentration in all low and intermediate risk patients with acute pulmonary embolism ($n = 162$) [a].

	Mean HR	SDNN (ms)	SDNN-I (ms)	SDANN (ms)	RMSSD (ms)	pNN50 (%)	Triangular Index
TRPG (mmHg)	r = 0.08, p = 0.36	r = −0.22, p = 0.02	r = −0.14, p = 0.11	r = −0.16, p = 0.07	r = −0.30, p = 0.003	r = −0.80, p = 0.41	r = −0.19, p = 0.04
RVSP (mmHg)	r = 0.09, p = 0.33	r = −0.31, p = 0.001	r = −0.21, p = 0.03	r = −0.31, p = 0.001	r = −0.80, p = 0.45	r = −1.10, p = 0.29	r = −0.28, p = 0.003
TAPSE (mm)	r = −0.11, p = 0.11	r = 0.21, p = 0.03	r = 0.09, p = 0.39	r = 0.27, p = 0.006	r = 0.50, p = 0.61	r = 0.70, p = 0.49	r = 0.22, p = 0.49
IVC (mm)	r = 0.06, p = 0.11	r = −0.27, p = 0.002	r = −0.18, p = 0.01	r = −0.18, p = 0.04	r = −1.00, p = 0.31	r = −0.80, p = 0.44	r = −0.29, p = 0.44
AcT (ms)	r = −0.10, p = 0.24	r = 0.31, p = 0.001	r = 0.29, p = 0.01	r = 0.38, p = 0.001	r = 1.60, p = 0.12	r = 2.10, p = 0.36	r = 0.30, p = 0.04
NT-proBNP (pg/mL)	r = 0.22, p = 0.03	r = −0.30, p = 0.004	r = −0.24, p = 0.02	r = −0.35, p = 0.001	r = −0.60, p = 0.52	r = −1.10, p = 0.28	r = −0.26, p = 0.01

[a] four high risk patients were excluded from the pre-screened consecutive 166 individuals. Abbreviations—see Table 1.

Moreover, we performed abridged univariate and multivariate logistic regression analysis to assess the association of the echocardiographic parameters and NT-proBNP concentration on the values of SDNN, the principal parameter in the HRV analysis. The results are presented in Table 3. In univariate analysis TRPG, RVSP, TAPSE, IVC, AcT and NT-proBNP were examined and all of them showed a significant association with SDNN values. However, in the multivariate analysis only IVC diameter and NT-proBNP level remained statistically relevant.

Table 3. Logistic regression analysis assessing the influence of right ventricle overload echocardiographic parameters and N-terminal pro B type natriuretic peptide concentration on the standard deviation of intervals of all normal beats (SDNN) corrected for its increase of 10 ms.

	Univariate Analysis		Multivariate Analysis *	
	Odds Ratio (95% CI)	p-Value	Odds Ratio (95% CI)	p-Value
TRPG (mmHg) [a]	0.52 (0.11–0.92)	0.013	-	-
RVSP (mmHg) [a]	0.39 (0.26–0.93)	0.001	-	-
TAPSE (mm) [b]	2.50 (1.18–3.10)	0.027	-	-
IVC (mm) [b]	0.69 (0.39–0.83)	0.002	0.91 (0.21–0.92)	0.014
AcT (ms) [c]	1.38 (1.33–5.98)	0.002	-	-
NT-proBNP (pg/mL) [d]	0.23 (0.18–0.31)	0.002	0.83 (0.04–0.91)	0.041

Abbreviations—see Table 1. * results of multivariate analysis shown only for statistically significant parameters. [a] Odds ratio and 95% CI corrected for an increase of 10 mmHg. [b] Odds ratio and 95% CI corrected for an increase of 1 mm. [c] Odds ratio and 95% CI corrected for an increase of 10 ms. [d] Odds ratio and 95% CI corrected for an increase of 100 pg/mL.

5. Discussion

In our study we put impact on analyzing the connection between time-domain HRV and APE in the context of its severity and prognosis. We revealed novel associations between 24 h Holter monitoring HRV parameters and clinical status, as well as the echocardiographic and biochemical signs of RV overload. Extensive analysis of HRV parameters and their correlation with indices of RV overload have given us promising results with potential clinical value. The strength of our research is also a large cohort of patients observed in the severe phase of APE.

Over the last decades, HRV parameters were increasingly considered as indicators of the cANS activity [4,7,8]. However, there is limited research depicting HRV as an important indicator of cANS dysfunction in patients with RV disorders. Among others, Bienias et al. and Witte et al. demonstrated that Holter-derived parameters depict significant cANS impairment in patients with pulmonary hypertension of various etiologies [9–12]. Several studies have demonstrated that patients with arterial or chronic thromboembolic pulmonary hypertension are characterized by significant impairment of heart rate turbulence, which was related to the disease severity [9,13]. Patients with impaired RV due to pulmonary arterial hypertension were also found to have decreased post-exercise HRV parameters in comparison with healthy individuals, which reflects the prolonged recovery of cANS control in this population [14]. HRV parameters were also shown to be impaired in other chronic RV overload conditions, e.g., in arrhythmogenic right ventricular cardiomyopathy and tetralogy of Fallot [3,15]. In some studies the main and the simplest cANS parameter, i.e., mean HR, reflecting an increased sympathetic and decreased parasympathetic tone, was also found to be a prognostic factor in venous thromboembolism occurrence [16,17].

Lower values of HRV parameters can be considered to be predictors of various cardiac arrhythmia occurrences, including life-threatening ventricular arrhythmias and atrial fibrillation [2,18]. According to the literature, the most common serious arrhythmia appearing in the first days of APE is atrial fibrillation, followed by other supraventricular tachycardias [19–21]. Surprisingly, in our study population, atrial fibrillation was extremely uncommon, while short supraventricular tachycardias were recorded in 29% of patients but without clinical deterioration. It remains unclear whether this is an effect of the sample size or the reason for the relatively high proportion of patients in relatively good clinical status after admission.

Clinical observations indicate that the occurrence of serious ventricular arrhythmias immediately after APE is very rare with unclear recommendations for long-term management and prognosis [22]. Cardiac arrest being a result of APE is usually related to pulseless electrical activity [3]. In our study no significant ventricular arrhythmias were found either. Syncope (usually as one of the first sign of the diseases) may occur in about 10% of patients with APE, it is mainly related to cANS dysfunction, and may worsen the prognosis [23,24]. As such, they are another potential coefficient, the risk of which could be identified using HRV parameters. Yet, in our study population we did not identify any cases of syncope during hospitalization.

It is important to remark that most of the clinical characteristics of our participants did not differ significantly between groups with low and intermediate risk of APE. It is especially compelling that one half of the intermediate risk group consisted of patients with intermediate–high risk of APE. It is clear that RV overload in our cohort observed in diagnostic imaging did not cause major changes in the parameters describing the general status at admission and did not remarkably increase the risk of shock in the study population.

Even though, echocardiographic parameters describing the RV function remarkably differed between groups, indicating that patients with the intermediate risk APE had significantly higher overload of RV, in spite of similar general status parameters at admission. Importantly, echocardiographic parameters describing the left ventricular function did not differ between low and intermediate risk APE groups, which provides a conclusion that cANS dysfunction observed in our patients was triggered mainly by RV overload. Supporting this suspicion is the fact that we revealed significant correlations between HRV parameters and echocardiographic-derived TRPG, RVSP, IVC, TAPSE and AcT (Table 2). Additional correlations between HRV indices and NT-proBNP level are also consistent. Logistic regression analysis confirmed that the increase in SDNN values was associated with better echocardiography-derived indices of RV function and lower values of NT-proBNP (in contrast, worse echocardiographic parameters and increased NT-proBNP concentration were associated with lower SDNN values). It is a novel finding, and to our knowledge, has not yet been described in the literature regarding APE.

Most of the HRV parameters, including SDNN and SDANN, are assumed to express mainly sympathetic nervous system activity, whereas RMSSD and pNN50 were found to reflect rather the parasympathetic composition of the cANS [2,4]. Considering that in our study the relationship between the tested HRV parameters and APE risk status reached statistical significance, there is a need for further research in this area. Our results might indicate the prominent role of relative parasympathetic dysfunction in the course of APE.

6. Limitations

Our study also has several limitations. First, our study cohort consisted of only few individuals with high risk APE (we excluded them from the statistical analysis). Second, we observed a relatively good clinical status of patients with intermediate–high risk APE. It might have been a reason for the inconclusive incidence of arrhythmia and undetected syncope in the severe phase of APE during our observation, as well as the unclear results of comparison between different HRV parameters in both analyzed risk groups. Third, the relationship between HRV and echocardiographic markers of RV overload reached statistical significance, but there is no proven causality between them, which makes their results hypothesis-generating. Moreover, it remains unclear whether more and stronger associations between HRV parameters and APE prognosis could be found in larger study cohorts, with more representative proportions of individual APE risk categories, especially with more patients at high risk. Fourth, the observation time was short, up to 24–48 h after admission, with no follow-up in our protocol. Therefore, it is not possible to predict adverse events in the long-term. Fifth, in our analysis, we skipped the assessment of cardiac troponins because during the study the methods of laboratory assessment in our center, and thus, normal values changed (standard high-sensitive troponins). Sixth, another possible limitation is the lack of frequency-domain (power spectral) HRV analysis. However, we are convinced that well-performed time-domain HRV is sufficient for the first line cANS function evaluation. In addition, frequency-domain analysis should be performed under controlled registration conditions, preferably in a laboratory, similar for all patients, which was not possible and planned in our study protocol. It is important to take into account that all the conditions, such as concomitant clinical diseases, medications taken or the time of admission of the patient to the ward, will have a significant impact on the results of such an analysis and will make the interpretation of the results difficult and error-prone.

7. Conclusions

We revealed a significant association between time-domain HRV parameters and echocardiographic, as well as biochemical signs of RV overload. Moreover, some HRV parameters were associated with the clinical risk classification of APE, differing significantly between groups with intermediate and low risk of early mortality. As Holter monitoring with HRV analysis is an easy-to-obtain and cost-effective diagnostic method, our observations indicate the need for further evaluation to determine the clinical significance and standardization of HRV analysis in patients with acute pulmonary embolism.

Author Contributions: Conceptualization, P.B.; data curation, P.B., M.L., M.S., B.K. and J.W.; formal analysis, M.L.; investigation, P.B., M.S., B.K. and J.W.; methodology, P.B., M.L. and P.P.; project administration, P.B. and P.P.; supervision, P.B. and P.P.; writing—original draft, P.B. and M.L.; writing—review and editing, P.B. All authors have read and agreed to the published version of the manuscript.

Funding: This research received no external funding.

Institutional Review Board Statement: This study was conducted in accordance with the amended Declaration of Helsinki and approved by the local independent ethics board.

Informed Consent Statement: Informed consent was obtained from all subjects involved in the study.

Data Availability Statement: No publicly archived datasets were analyzed or generated during the study.

Conflicts of Interest: The authors have no conflict of interest to declare.

References

1. Konstantinides, S.V.; Meyer, G.; Becattini, C.; Bueno, H.; Geersing, G.J.; Harjola, V.-P.; Huisman, M.V.; Humbert, M.; Jennings, C.S.; Jiménez, D.; et al. 2019 ESC Guidelines for the diagnosis and management of acute pulmonary embolism developed in collaboration with the European Respiratory Society (ERS). *Eur. Heart J.* **2020**, *41*, 543–603. [CrossRef] [PubMed]
2. Huikuri, H.V.; Stein, P.K. Heart rate variability in risk stratification of cardiac patients. *Prog. Cardiovasc. Dis.* **2013**, *56*, 153–159. [CrossRef]
3. Lisicka, M.; Radochońska, J.; Bienias, P. Arrhythmias and autonomic nervous system dysfunction in acute and chronic diseases with right ventricle involvement. *Folia Cardiologica* **2019**, *14*, 445–455. [CrossRef]
4. Heart Rate Variability: Standards of Measurement, Physiological Interpretation, and Clinical Use. Task Force of the European Society of Cardiology the North American Society of Pacing Electrophysiology. *Circulation* **1996**, *93*, 1043–1065.
5. Lang, R.M.; Badano, L.P.; Mor-Avi, V.; Afilalo, J.; Armstrong, A.; Ernande, L.; Flachskampf, F.A.; Foster, E.; Goldstein, S.A.; Kuznetsova, T.; et al. Recommendations for cardiac chamber quantification by echocardiography in adults: An update from the American Society of Echocardiography and the European Association of Cardiovascular Imaging. *Eur. Heart J. Cardiovasc. Imaging* **2015**, *16*, 233–270. [CrossRef]
6. Kurnicka, K.; Lichodziejewska, B.; Goliszek, S.; Dzikowska-Diduch, O.; Zdończyk, O.; Kozłowska, M.; Kostrubiec, M.; Ciurzyński, M.; Palczewski, P.; Grudzka, K.; et al. Echocardiographic Pattern of Acute Pulmonary Embolism: Analysis of 511 Consecutive Patients. *J. Am. Soc. Echocardiogr.* **2016**, *29*, 907–913. [CrossRef]
7. Hayano, J.; Yuda, E. Pitfalls of assessment of autonomic function by heart rate variability. *J. Physiol. Anthropol.* **2019**, *38*, 3. [CrossRef]
8. Shaffer, F.; Ginsberg, J.P. An Overview of Heart Rate Variability Metrics and Norms. *Front. Public Health* **2017**, *5*, 258. [CrossRef]

9. Bienias, P.; Kostrubiec, M.; Rymarczyk, Z.; Korczak, D.; Ciurzyński, M.; Kurzyna, M.; Torbicki, A.; Fijałkowska, A.; Pruszczyk, P. Severity of arterial and chronic thromboembolic pulmonary hypertension is associated with impairment of heart rate turbulence. *Ann. Noninvasive Electrocardiol.* **2015**, *20*, 69–78. [CrossRef]
10. Bienias, P.; Ciurzynski, M.; Kostrubiec, M.; Rymarczyk, Z.; Kurzyna, M.; Korczak, D.; Roik, M.; Torbicki, A.; Fijalkowska, A.; Pruszczyk, P. Functional class and type of pulmonary hypertension determinate severity of cardiac autonomic dysfunction assessed by heart rate variability and turbulence. *Acta Cardiol.* **2015**, *70*, 286–296. [CrossRef] [PubMed]
11. Witte, C.; Meyer Zur Heide Genannt Meyer-Arend, J.U.; Andrié, R.; Schrickel, J.W.; Hammerstingl, C.; Schwab, J.O.; Nickenig, G.; Skowasch, D.; Pizarro, C. Heart Rate Variability and Arrhythmic Burden in Pulmonary Hypertension. *Adv. Exp. Med. Biol.* **2016**, *934*, 9–22. [CrossRef] [PubMed]
12. Peters, E.L.; Bogaard, H.J.; Vonk Noordegraaf, A.; de Man, F.S. Neurohormonal modulation in pulmonary arterial hypertension. *Eur. Respir. J.* **2021**, *58*, 2004633. [CrossRef]
13. Stratmann, G.; Gregory, G.A. Neurogenic and humoral vasoconstriction in acute pulmonary thromboembolism. *Anesth. Analg.* **2003**, *97*, 341–354. [CrossRef] [PubMed]
14. Paula-Ribeiro, M.; Ribeiro, I.C.; Aranda, L.C.; Silva, T.M.; Costa, C.M.; Ramos, R.P.; Ota-Arakaki, J.S.; Cravo, S.L.; Nery, L.E.; Stickland, M.K.; et al. Carotid chemoreflex activity restrains post-exercise cardiac autonomic control in healthy humans and in patients with pulmonary arterial hypertension. *J. Physiol.* **2019**, *597*, 1347–1360. [CrossRef] [PubMed]
15. Okólska, M.; Łach, J.; Matusik, P.T.; Pająk, J.; Mroczek, T.; Podolec, P.; Tomkiewicz-Pająk, L. Heart Rate Variability and Its Associations with Organ Complications in Adults after Fontan Operation. *J. Clin. Med.* **2021**, *10*, 4492. [CrossRef]
16. Folsom, A.R.; Lutsey, P.L.; Pope, Z.C.; Fashanu, O.E.; Misialek, J.R.; Cushman, M.; Michos, E.D. Atherosclerosis Risk in Communities (ARIC) Study Investigators. Resting heart rate and incidence of venous thromboembolism. *Res. Pract. Thromb. Haemost.* **2019**, *4*, 238–246. [CrossRef]
17. Awotoye, J.; Fashanu, O.E.; Lutsey, P.L.; Zhao, D.; O'Neal, W.T.; Michos, E.D. Resting heart rate and incident venous thromboembolism: The Multi-Ethnic Study of Atherosclerosis. *Open Heart* **2020**, *7*, e001080. [CrossRef]
18. Khan, A.A.; Lip, G.Y.H.; Shantsila, A. Heart rate variability in atrial fibrillation: The balance between sympathetic and parasympathetic nervous system. *Eur. J. Clin. Invest.* **2019**, *49*, e13174. [CrossRef]
19. Ng, A.C.; Adikari, D.; Yuan, D.; Lau, J.K.; Yong, A.S.; Chow, V.; Kritharides, L. The Prevalence and Incidence of Atrial Fibrillation in Patients with Acute Pulmonary Embolism. *PLoS ONE* **2016**, *11*, e0150448. [CrossRef]
20. Krajewska, A.; Ptaszynska-Kopczynska, K.; Kiluk, I.; Kosacka, U.; Milewski, R.; Krajewski, J.; Musial, W.J.; Sobkowicz, B. Paroxysmal Atrial Fibrillation in the Course of Acute Pulmonary Embolism: Clinical Significance and Impact on Prognosis. *Biomed. Res. Int.* **2017**, *2017*, 5049802. [CrossRef]
21. Majos, E.; Dąbrowski, R.; Szwed, H. The right ventricle in patients with chronic heart failure and atrial fibrillation. *Cardiol. J.* **2013**, *20*, 220–226. [CrossRef]
22. Radochońska, J.; Lisicka, M.; Bienias, P. The purpose of electrocardiography in acute and chronic diseases with right ventricular involvement. *Folia Cardiol.* **2019**, *14*, 572–582. [CrossRef]
23. Keller, K.; Beule, J.; Balzer, J.O.; Dippold, W. Syncope and collapse in acute pulmonary embolism. *Am. J. Emerg. Med.* **2016**, *34*, 1251–1257. [CrossRef] [PubMed]
24. Liesching, T.; O'Brien, A. Significance of a syncopal event. Pulmonary embolism. *Postgrad. Med.* **2002**, *111*, 19–20. [CrossRef] [PubMed]

Disclaimer/Publisher's Note: The statements, opinions and data contained in all publications are solely those of the individual author(s) and contributor(s) and not of MDPI and/or the editor(s). MDPI and/or the editor(s) disclaim responsibility for any injury to people or property resulting from any ideas, methods, instructions or products referred to in the content.

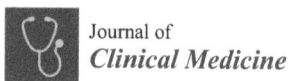

Article

Prevalence and Clinical Characteristics of Patients with Torsades de Pointes Complicating Acquired Atrioventricular Block

Sok-Sithikun Bun *, Nathan Heme, Florian Asarisi, Fabien Squara, Didier Scarlatti, Pamela Moceri and Emile Ferrari

Faculty of Medicine, Pasteur University Hospital, 06000 Nice, France
* Correspondence: sithi.bun@gmail.com

Abstract: Background: Female gender, degree of QT prolongation, and genetic susceptibility are known risk factors for developing torsades de pointes (TdP) during high-grade atrioventricular block (HG-AVB). Our objective was to analyze the prevalence and clinical characteristics of patients presenting with TdP and AVB (TdP [+]) in comparison with non-TdP patients with AVB (TdP [−]). Methods: All the ECGs from patients prospectively admitted for AVB (2 to 1, HG, and complete) at the University Hospital of Nice were analyzed. Automated corrected QT (QTc), manual measurements of QT and JT intervals, and Tpeak-to-end were performed at the time of the most severe bradycardia. Results: From September 2020 to November 2021, 100 patients were admitted for HG-AVB. Among them, 17 patients with TdP were identified (8 men; 81 ± 10 years). No differences could be identified concerning automated QTc, manual QTc (Bazett correction), baseline QRS width, or mean left ventricular ejection fraction between the two groups. Potassium serum level on admission and mean number of QT-prolonging drugs per patient were not significantly different between the two groups, respectively: 4.34 ± 0.5 mmol/L in TdP [+] versus 4.52 ± 0.6 mmol/L ($p = 0.33$); and 0.6 ± 0.7 in TdP [+] versus 0.3 ± 0.5 ($p = 0.15$). In contrast, manual QTc$_{FR}$ (Fridericia correction), JT (Fridericia correction), Tpeak-to-end, and Tpe/QT ratio were significantly increased in the TdP [+] group, respectively: 486 ± 70 ms versus 456 ± 53 ms ($p = 0.04$); 433 ± 98 ms versus 381 ± 80 ms ($p = 0.02$); 153 ± 57 ms versus 110 ± 40 ms ($p < 0.001$); and 0.27 ± 0.08 versus 0.22 ± 0.06 ($p < 0.001$). Conclusions: The incidence of TdP complicating acquired AVB was 17%. Longer QTc$_{FR}$, JT, and Tpeak-to-end were significantly increased in the case of TdP but also in the presence of permanent AVB during the hospitalization.

Keywords: atrioventricular block; torsades de pointes; QT interval

1. Introduction

Torsades de pointes (TdP) are a specific form of polymorphic ventricular tachycardia that is preceded by QT interval prolongation and occurs in a variety of conditions [1]. TdP is a known but uncommon complication of atrioventricular block (AVB) and may recur in some patients, even after permanent cardiac pacing [2]. Female gender [3], degree of QT prolongation [4], and genetic susceptibility [5] are all known risk factors for developing TdP during acquired AVB. While electrocardiographic (ECG) parameters predicting the occurrence of TdP have been well described, little is known about the clinical characteristics of the patients presenting with this life-threatening complication. Identifying predisposing factors for developing TdP may help in better discriminating a higher-risk group and avoiding any recurrence of TdP.

Our objective was to analyze the prevalence, clinical, and ECG characteristics of patients prospectively admitted for AVB and TdP (TdP [+] group) in comparison with non-TdP patients (TdP [−] group).

2. Materials and Methods

All the patients admitted at the University Hospital of Nice for acquired AVB were prospectively included in this study, and their electrocardiograms (ECGs) were systematically collected. The cohort included patients presenting with 2 to 1, high grade (HG), and complete AVB leading to bradycardia that was severe enough to justify hospital admission. The patients with the following forms of AVB were excluded from this study: AVB in the setting of acute myocardial infarction, drug toxicity, or vagally mediated episodes. All the patients underwent continuous cardiac monitoring during their hospitalization stay, until pacemaker implantation (if needed). The ECG tracings (12 lead surface and telemonitoring during hospitalization) were reviewed by one experienced electrophysiologist (S.-S.B.). AVB was classified as permanent in this study if complete AVB was observed throughout the hospitalization stay during cardiac monitoring, or intermittent if complete AVB was observed in alternation with 1:1 conduction (eventually facilitated by isoproterenol infusion).

TdP was defined as polymorphic ventricular tachycardia (faster than 120 beats per minute and at least three consecutive QRS complexes originating from the ventricles), with axis rotation and variable QRS complex amplitudes. Patients were assigned to the TdP [+] group if more than 10 TdP beats were recorded during telemetry. The clinical and electrocardiographic characteristics of the patients were analyzed, as well as the number of QT prolonging agents and potassium serum level on admission. ECGs were recorded at a gain of 10 mm/mV and a paper speed of 25 mm/s. Automated corrected QT intervals (QTc_{AUTO}) were collected, and manual measurements of the following intervals were performed at the time of the most severe bradycardia: RR, QT, JT, and Tpeak-to-end intervals (Figure 1). For manual measurements, QT intervals were measured from the onset of the QRS complex to the end of the T wave, which was defined as the point of its merger with the isoelectric line. QTc is the QT for the heart rate using the Bazett formula (QTc = QT/square root of RR) [6], whereas QTc_{FR} uses the Fridericia heart rate correction formula [7]. T peak-to-end was measured from the summit of the T wave to the end of the QT interval. These intervals were determined as a mean value derived from three consecutive cardiac cycles. Both QT, JT, and Tpeak-to-end intervals were measured in the ECG leads with the longest value. Corrected (JTc) is the JT interval for the heart rate with the Fridericia formula correction.

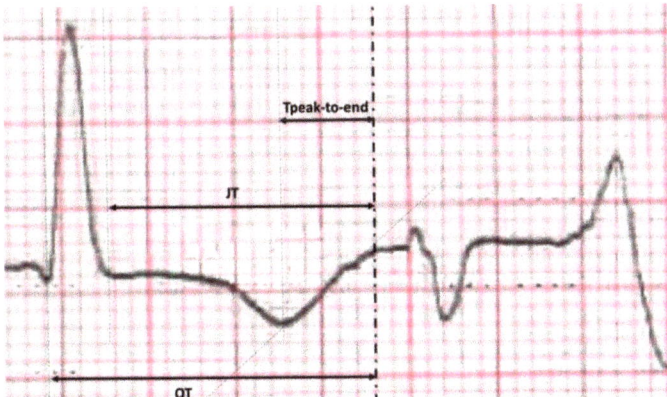

Figure 1. Method of manual measurement for QT, JT, and Tpeak-to-end intervals at the moment of most severe bradycardia.

This study was approved by the Institutional Review Board. According to our institutional guidelines, all patients gave written informed consent for the pacemaker implant (if needed).

Statistical Analysis

The statistical analysis was performed using Excel (San Diego, CA, USA). Categorical variables are described as numbers and percentages. Continuous variables are described as mean ± SD for normal distributions or median for a range for non-normal distributed. Between-group differences in categorical variables were compared using a chi-squared test. Differences between continuous variables were compared using a Student's t test. To test whether different variables were influencing the occurrence of TdP, a binary logistic regression was performed with TdP as the dependent variable and other variables as covariates.

3. Results

From September 2020 to November 2021, 100 patients were admitted for HG or complete AVB in our institution. Among them, 17 patients (17%) with TdP were identified (8 men; 81 ± 9 years). A total of 13 out of 17 patients presented with several episodes of TdP (76%). An example is shown in Figure 2. Arterial hypertension was present in 10/17 (59%), with a mean left ventricular ejection fraction = 57 ± 6%. A comparison with the other patients admitted with complete AVB but without TdP is shown in Table 1. No clinical characteristics could distinguish patients presenting with TdP complicating AVB, in comparison with other patients admitted without TdP [−], except concerning the intermittent nature of AVB. Permanent AVB during the hospitalization stay was statistically more prevalent in TdP [+] patients (14 out of 17, 83%) versus 43/83 (52%) in TdP [−], $p = 0.02$. Two patients (12%) in TdP [+] elicited a pause-dependent (phase 4) AVB mechanism versus 12 (14%) in TdP [−], $p = 0.77$ [8].

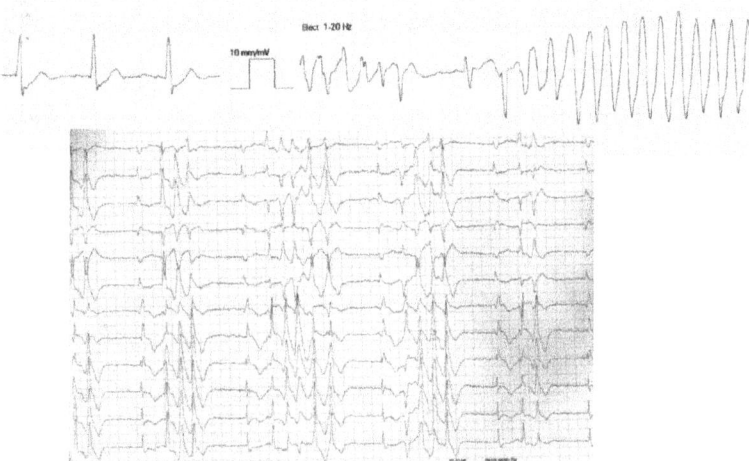

Figure 2. Twelve-lead ECG from an 82-year-old female patient admitted to the emergency department for syncope with brain trauma. The initial ECG shows atrial fibrillation with complete atrioventricular block and ventricular escape rhythm (with right bundle branch block morphology) and salvos of torsades de pointes. The initial episode required urgent electrical cardioversion.

Table 1. Characteristics of patients with TdP.

	TdP [+] (n = 17)	TdP [−] (n = 83)	p-Value
Age (years)	81 ± 10 (57–94)	83 ± 12 (14–102)	0.62
Men, n (%)	8 (47)	46 (55)	0.72
Arterial hypertension, n (%)	10 (59)	56 (67)	0.13
Syncope, n (%)	13 (76)	46 (55)	0.11
Permanent AVB, n (%)	14 (82)	43 (51)	0.02
LVEF (%)	57 ± 6	55 ± 8	0.73
eGFR (mL/min/1.73 m^2)	54 ± 29	56 ± 25	0.77
Mean QRS duration (ms)	119 ± 24	118 ± 33	0.86
QT$_{cAUTO}$ (ms)	479 ± 55	465 ± 51	0.31
R-R interval (ms)	1414 ± 429	1360 ± 408	0.62
Heart rate (beats per min)	46 ± 14	49 ± 17	0.58
QT$_c$ interval (ms)	462 ± 64	438 ± 55	0.11
QT$_{cFR}$ interval (ms)	486 ± 70	456 ± 53	0.045
JT$_c$ interval (ms)	433 ± 98	381 ± 80	0.023
Tpeak-to-end interval (ms)	153 ± 57	110 ± 40	0.0003
Tpe/QT ratio	0.27 ± 0.08	0.22 ± 0.06	0.0005

No differences could be identified between the two groups concerning QT$_{cAUTO}$, baseline QRS width, or mean left ventricular ejection fraction. Potassium serum level on admission and mean number of QT-prolonging drugs (Supplementary Materials) per patient were not significantly different between the two groups, respectively: 4.34 ± 0.5 mmol/L in group TdP [+] versus 4.53 ± 0.6 mmol/L (p = 0.13) and 0.57 ± 0.7 in group TdP [+] versus 0.34 ± 0.5 (p = 0.13). QTc, QT$_{cFR}$, the JTc interval, and Tpeak-to-end were significantly prolonged in the TdP group in comparison with the TdP [-] group (Figure 3). Univariable analysis with logistic regression was statistically significant for the presence of permanent AVB during hospitalization, QT$_{cFR}$, Tpeak-to-end, and Tpeak-to-end/QT (Table 2). QTc was an independent predictor of TdP in a logistic regression model using age, gender, the presence of permanent AVB, the R-R interval, and Tpeak-to-end as covariates (p = 0.04).

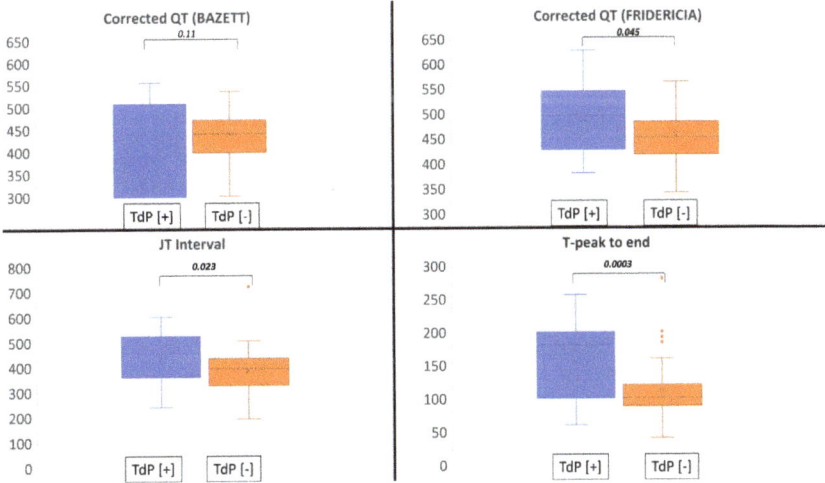

Figure 3. Box plots of corrected QT with Bazett's formula (**upper left**), Fridericia's formula (**upper right**), the JTc interval (**lower left**), and Tpeak-to-end (**lower right**) between the two groups. Bold, significant on statistical analysis.

Table 2. Summary of univariable and multivariable analysis (logistic regression) with TdP.

	Odds Ratio 95% Confidence Intervals	p-Value
Univariable analysis		
Age (for a 10 year increase)	1.11 (0.70–1.66)	0.62
Female gender	1.44 (0.50–4.19)	0.5
Permanent AVB †	4.44 (1.33–20.3)	0.02
Potassium serum level on admission (+0.1 mmol/L)	1.06 (0.96–1.19)	0.26
Number of QT prolonging drugs (+ 0.1)	0.93 (0.85–1.03)	0.17
Mean QRS duration (+10 ms)	1.02 (0.86–1.21)	0.82
R-R interval (+100 ms)	0.96 (0.85–1.08)	0.48
Heart rate (+10 bpm)	1.01 (0.98–1.05)	0.47
Corrected QT (Bazett) (+10 ms)	1.08 (0.99–1.18)	0.09
Corrected QT (Fridericia) (+10 ms)	1.09 (1.00–1.19)	0.05
Corrected JT (Fridericia) (+10 ms)	1.06 (0.99–1.15)	0.09
Tpeak-to-end (+10 ms)	1.20 (1.07–1.35)	<0.01
Tpeak-Tend/QT (+0.01)	1.14 (1.04–1.26)	<0.01
Multivariable analysis		
Age (for a 10 year increase)	0.99 (0.95–1.04)	0.92
Female gender	1.79 (0.64–5.22)	0.27
Permanent AVB †	2.51 (0.8–7.69)	0.71
R-R interval (+100 ms)	1.00 (0.99–1.00)	0.46
Corrected QT (Bazett) (+10 ms)	0.99 (0.98–0.99)	0.04
Tpeak-to-end (+10 ms)	0.98 (0.97–0.99)	<0.01

All electrocardiographic parameters refer to values during an atrioventricular block. † in comparison to intermittent AVB.

4. Discussion

4.1. Prevalence of TdP in Patients with Atrioventricular Block

Available data are sparse concerning the prevalence of TdP in AVB patients, reaching 11% in older reports [2]. In this initial report describing ventricular tachycardia-ventricular fibrillation (and not TdP), the proportion could rise to 30% in the case of permanent AVB, as compared to partial AVB (4%). Later, Cho et al. reported a prevalence of TdP of around 2.2% in a recent retrospective study including 898 AVB patients from three tertiary hospitals over a 20 year period [9]. In this retrospective study, the authors excluded at least one third of the initial cohort of patients with TdP for various reasons: drug-induced QT prolongation, electrolyte disturbance, TdP during pacing rhythm, or absence of baseline ECG. Our study reports a prevalence of TdP (17%) complicating AVB in a tertiary medium- to high-volume center. This is in line with the most recent study, which reported an incidence rate of 25% of TdP in their retrospective cohort (100 patients), 12.6% of TdP in a cohort of 87 patients admitted with AVB in the prospective group, and a final prevalence of 18.8% among a pooled number of 250 patients from three distinct cohorts [4]. These variations may also be attributed to the classification of the patients: QT-prolonging agents were excluded in previous reports, whereas patients taking QT-prolonging drugs were included in our analysis.

4.2. Clinical Characteristics of Patients with TdP and Atrioventricular Block

As reported in early observations, TdP may be associated with Adams–Stokes seizures in addition to syncopal episodes related to the asystole itself [2]. This may produce another aggravating situation for trauma to occur at initial presentation. The observation of TdP during AVB may suggest the possibility of prompt management of AVB using a temporary pacing lead or externalized reusable permanent pacemaker (in the case of drug toxicity inducing QT prolongation, for example, allowing time for drug wash-out) [10,11]. There are no current recommendations for pacing programming after implantation in patients with TdP during AVB at presentation. It has been reported that TdP may recur in these patients even after permanent cardiac pacing, with the necessity for increasing the lower pacing rate from 60 to 80 or 90 beats/min, and eventually, adding a β-blocking agent. Identifying predisposing factors for developing TdP may help in better discriminating a higher-risk group and avoiding any recurrence of TdP, for instance, by anticipating pacemaker programming.

Another concern should be the development of pacing-induced cardiomyopathy and the likelihood of ventricular arrhythmia recurrence in patients with initial TdP on admission [12]. It is also not known whether conduction system pacing could represent a better strategy in this subgroup of patients with TdP complicating AVB by avoiding any recurrence during long-term pacing [13].

The majority of studies published in the literature focused on ECG features that could predict the occurrence of TdP during acquired AVB, but few studies exist on the clinical characteristics associated with TdP. In our study, no significant differences concerning the clinical features could be found between the two groups. Other parameters such as serum potassium level, renal function, or the number of QT-prolonging agents at the time of TdP were also not different between the two groups. Cho et al. did not find any difference in clinical data (hypertension or diabetes mellitus) in the TdP patients when compared to the control group [9]. In our study, there were more syncopal episodes in the TdP [+] group, but without reaching statistical significance ($p = 0.11$). Finally, the most discriminant factor was the presence of permanent AVB at presentation, which was significantly increased in the TdP [+] group as compared to the TdP [−] group ($p = 0.02$). In previous studies, female gender was found to be an independent risk factor for TdP occurrence; this was not the case in our study [4].

4.3. ECG Predictors of TdP in Atrioventricular Block Patients

Different QTc cut-off values (that predicted the occurrence of TdP) have been reported in the literature (Table 3), ranging from 440 to 565 ms. This wide range of values may be explained by several factors. The method of QT measurement may vary from one study to another. For instance, the correction of the QT interval using the Bazett formula was the most frequently used correction in the majority of the studies concerning TdP complicating AVB. Noteworthily, limitations of QTc with the Bazett formula at slow rates have also been demonstrated, with higher performance of the Fridericia formula during bradycardia [14,15]. The measurements were usually performed by a single operator, except in the study by Cho et al., with very low inter-observer variability. In our study, one electrophysiologist performed the QT measurements to limit inter-observer variability, but QT automatic measurements were also performed [9]. Automatic QT measurements have been shown to be accurate with high agreement when compared to manual measurements [16,17]. In contrast with previous reports, QTc and QTc_{AUTO} values were not statistically different between the two groups in our study, but only QTc_{FR}. Concerning the other ECG parameters, our findings were in total agreement with previously published studies, with JT interval and Tpeak-to-end values being significantly increased in the TdP [+] group [18]. The JT interval and the $J\text{-}T_{peak}$ have been reported to be a more reliable marker of the torsadogenic risk in patients with long QT syndrome, ventricular conduction defect, or in receiving a QT prolonging agent [19–21].

Table 3. Summary of published studies of ECG parameters in TdP patients during AVB.

Author	Design Number of TdP [+]/TdP [−]	Parameter	TdP [+]	TdP [−]
Strasberg B, 1986 [22]	Retrospective 9 vs. 12	QTc (ms)	510 ± 60 *	400 ± 40
Moroe K, 1988 [23]	Retrospective 6 vs. 9	QTc (ms)	580 ± 112 *	459 ± 37
Kurita T, 1992 [24]	Retrospective 6 vs. 8	QTc (ms)	585 ± 45 *	476 ± 58
Subbiah, 2010 [5]	Retrospective 11 vs. 33	QTc (ms) Tpeak-to-end (ms)	440 ± 93 * 147 ± 25 *	376 ± 40 94 ± 25
Cho MS, 2015 [9]	Retrospective 20 vs. 80	QT (ms) Tpeak-to-end (ms) Tpe/QT	716.4 ± 98.9 * 334.2 ± 59.1 * 0.49 ± 0.09 *	523.2 ± 91.3 144 ± 73.7 0.27 ± 0.11
Chorin, 2017 [4]	Retrospective and prospective 47 vs. 203	QTc (ms)	564 ± 81 *	422 ± 62
Our series, 2023	Prospective 17 vs. 83	QTc$_{FR}$ (ms) Tpeak-to-end (ms) Tpe/QT JTc (ms)	486 ± 70 * 160 ± 57 * 0.29 ± 0.08 * 437 ± 89 *	456 ± 53 106 ± 35 0.21 ± 0.06 375 ± 71

* Variables are statistically significant in comparison with TdP [−] group.

4.4. Limitations

This is a monocentric study with a limited number of patients, but its prospective nature provided some new information about the expected prevalence of TdP complicating acquired AVB. Genetic testing was not systematically performed in our elderly TdP [+] group. Recent studies [5,25] found that the presence of a genetic disposition ranged from 17 to 36%. Chevalier et al. found 17% of HERG mutations only in patients with a QT interval above 600 ms and AVB. Of note, our TdP [+] patients were discharged with a list of medications that were contraindicated in the long QT syndrome.

5. Conclusions

The prevalence of TdP complicating acquired AVB was 17%. Longer QTc$_{FR}$, increased JT interval, and Tpeak-to-end were electrocardiographic predictors of TdP. The presence of permanent AVB was more likely associated with TdP in comparison with intermittent AVB at initial presentation.

Supplementary Materials: The following supporting information can be downloaded at: https://www.mdpi.com/article/10.3390/jcm12031067/s1, Table S1: Usual treatments favoring QT prolongation in the TdP [+] group.

Author Contributions: Conceptualization, S.-S.B.; methodology, S.-S.B.; validation, S.-S.B.; formal analysis, S.-S.B.; investigation, F.A. and N.H.; writing—original draft preparation, S.-S.B.; writing—review and editing, S.-S.B.; visualization, F.S. and D.S.; supervision, P.M. and E.F. All authors have read and agreed to the published version of the manuscript.

Funding: This research received no external funding.

Institutional Review Board Statement: The study was conducted according to the guidelines of the Declaration of Helsinki and approved by the Institutional Review Board of Nice University Hospital (protocol code SB-CHU22).

Informed Consent Statement: Informed consent was obtained from all subjects involved in the study. Written informed consent has been obtained from the patient(s) to publish this paper.

Data Availability Statement: The datasets used and analyzed during the current study are available from the corresponding author on reasonable request.

Conflicts of Interest: The authors declare no conflict of interest.

References

1. Dessertenne, F. La tachycardie ventriculaire à deux foyers opposés variables [Ventricular tachycardia with 2 variable opposing foci]. *Arch. Mal. Coeur Vaiss.* **1966**, *59*, 263–272. [PubMed]
2. Jensen, G.; Sigurd, B.; Sandoe, E. Adams-Stokes seizures due to ventricular tachydysrhythmias in patients with heart block: Prevalence and problems of management. *Chest* **1975**, *67*, 43–48. [CrossRef] [PubMed]
3. Kawasaki, R.; Machado, C.; Reinoehl, J.; Fromm, B.; Baga, J.J.; Steinman, R.T.; Lehmann, M.H. Increased propensity of women to develop torsades de pointes during complete heart block. *J. Cardiovasc. Electrophysiol.* **1995**, *6*, 1032–1038. [CrossRef] [PubMed]
4. Chorin, E.; Hochstadt, A.; Viskin, S.; Rozovski, U.; Havakuk, O.; Baranchuk, A.; Enriquez, A.; Strasberg, B.; Guevara-Valdivia, M.E.; Márquez, M.F.; et al. Female gender as independent risk factor of torsades de pointes during acquired atrioventricular block. *Heart Rhythm* **2017**, *14*, 90–95. [CrossRef]
5. Subbiah, R.N.; Gollob, M.H.; Gula, L.J.; Davies, R.W.; Leong-Sit, P.; Skanes, A.C.; Yee, R.; Klein, G.J.; Krahn, A.D. Torsades de pointes during complete atrioventricular block: Genetic factors and electrocardiogram correlates. *Can. J. Cardiol.* **2010**, *26*, 208–212. [CrossRef]
6. Bazett, H.C. An analysis of the time-relations of electrocardiograms. *Heart* **1920**, *7*, 353–370. [CrossRef]
7. Fridericia, L.S. Dir Systolendaeur in Elektrokardiogram bei normalen Menchen und bei Herzkranken. *Acta Med. Scand.* **1920**, *53*, 469–486. [CrossRef]
8. Bun, S.S.; Asarisi, F.; Heme, N.; Squara, F.; Scarlatti, D.; Taghji, P.; Deharo, J.C.; Moceri, P.; Ferrari, E. Prevalence and Clinical Characteristics of Patients with Pause-Dependent Atrioventricular Block. *J. Clin. Med.* **2022**, *11*, 449. [CrossRef]
9. Cho, M.S.; Nam, G.B.; Kim, Y.G.; Hwang, K.W.; Kim, Y.R.; Choi, H.; Kim, S.H.; Rhee, K.S.; Kim, N.J.; Kim, J.S.; et al. Electrocardiographic predictors of bradycardia-induced torsades de pointes in patients with acquired atrioventricular block. *Heart Rhythm* **2015**, *12*, 498–505. [CrossRef]
10. Bun, S.S.; Taïeb, J.; Scarlatti, D.; Squara, F.; Taghji, P.; Errahmouni, A.; Hasni, K.; Enache, B.; Amara, W.; Deharo, J.C.; et al. Organisation et gestion aiguë du bloc atrioventriculaire complet: Résultats d'une enquête multicentrique nationale [Organization and management of acute complete atrioventricular block: Results from a Multicenter National Survey]. *Ann. Cardiol. Angeiol.* **2021**, *70*, 68–74. [CrossRef]
11. Beneyto, M.; Seguret, M.; Taranzano, M.; Mondoly, P.; Biendel, C.; Rollin, A.; Bounes, F.; Elbaz, M.; Maury, P.; Delmas, C. Externalized Reusable Permanent Pacemaker for Prolonged Temporary Cardiac Pacing in Critical Cardiac Care Units: An Observational Monocentric Retrospective Study. *J. Clin. Med.* **2022**, *11*, 7206. [CrossRef] [PubMed]
12. Fruelund, P.Z.; Sommer, A.; Frøkjær, J.B.; Lundbye-Christensen, S.; Zaremba, T.; Søgaard, P.; Graff, C.; Vraa, S.; Mahalingasivam, A.A.; Thøgersen, A.M.; et al. Risk of Pacing-Induced Cardiomyopathy in Patients with High-Degree Atrioventricular Block-Impact of Right Ventricular Lead Position Confirmed by Computed Tomography. *J. Clin. Med.* **2022**, *11*, 7228. [CrossRef] [PubMed]
13. Haeberlin, A.; Canello, S.; Kummer, A.; Seiler, J.; Baldinger, S.H.; Madaffari, A.; Thalmann, G.; Ryser, A.; Gräni, C.; Tanner, H.; et al. Conduction System Pacing Today and Tomorrow. *J. Clin. Med.* **2022**, *11*, 7258. [CrossRef] [PubMed]
14. Rautaharju, P.M.; Zhou, S.H.; Wong, S.; Prineas, R.; Berenson, G.S. Functional characteristics of QT prediction formulas. The concepts of QTmax and QT rate sensitivity. *Comput. Biomed. Res.* **1993**, *26*, 188–204. [CrossRef]
15. Vandenberk, B.; Vandael, E.; Robyns, T.; Vandenberghe, J.; Garweg, C.; Foulon, V.; Ector, J.; Willems, R. QT correction across the heart rate spectrum, in atrial fibrillation and ventricular conduction defects. *Pacing. Clin. Electrophysiol.* **2018**, *41*, 1101–1108. [CrossRef]
16. Fosser, C.; Duczynski, G.; Agin, M.; Wicker, P.; Darpo, B. Comparison of manual and automated measurements of the QT interval in healthy volunteers: An analysis of five thorough QT studies. *Clin. Pharm.* **2009**, *86*, 503–506. [CrossRef]
17. Bun, S.S.; Taghji, P.; Courjon, J.; Squara, F.; Scarlatti, D.; Theodore, G.; Baudouy, D.; Sartre, B.; Labbaoui, M.; Dellamonica, J.; et al. QT Interval Prolongation Under Hydroxychloroquine/Azithromycin Association for Inpatients With SARS-CoV-2 Lower Respiratory Tract Infection. *Clin. Pharm.* **2020**, *108*, 1090–1097. [CrossRef]
18. Can, L.H.; Kültürsay, H.; Hasdemir, C. Repolarization characteristics and incidence of Torsades de Pointes in patients with acquired complete atrioventricular block. *Anadolu Kardiyol. Derg.* **2007**, *7*, 98–100.
19. Shah, M.J.; Wieand, T.S.; Rhodes, L.A.; Berul, C.I.; Vetter, V.L. QT and JT dispersion in children with long QT syndrome. *J. Cardiovasc. Electrophysiol.* **1997**, *8*, 642–648. [CrossRef]
20. Zhou, S.H.; Wong, S.; Rautaharju, P.M.; Karnik, N.; Calhoun, H.P. Should the JT rather than the QT interval be used to detect prolongation of ventricular repolarization? An assessment in normal conduction and in ventricular conduction defects. *J. Electrocardiol.* **1992**, *25*, 131–136. [CrossRef]
21. Vicente, J.; Zusterzeel, R.; Johannesen, L.; Ochoa-Jimenez, R.; Mason, J.W.; Sanabria, C.; Kemp, S.; Sager, P.T.; Patel, V.; Matta, M.K.; et al. Assessment of Multi-Ion Channel Block in a Phase I Randomized Study Design: Results of the CiPA Phase I ECG Biomarker Validation Study. *Clin. Pharm.* **2019**, *105*, 943–953. [CrossRef] [PubMed]
22. Strasberg, B.; Kusniec, J.; Erdman, S.; Lewin, R.F.; Arditti, A.; Sclarovsky, S. Polymorphous ventricular tachycardia and atrioventricular block. *Pacing Clin. Electrophysiol.* **1986**, *9*, 522–526. [CrossRef]
23. Moroe, K.; Saku, K.; Tashiro, N.; Hiroki, T.; Arakawa, K. "Torsades de pointes" and atrioventricular block. *Clin. Cardiol.* **1988**, *11*, 9–13. [CrossRef] [PubMed]

24. Kurita, T.; Ohe, T.; Marui, N.; Aihara, N.; Takaki, H.; Kamakura, S.; Matsuhisa, M.; Shimomura, K. Bradycardia-induced abnormal QT prolongation in patients with complete atrioventricular block with torsades de pointes. *Am. J. Cardiol.* **1992**, *69*, 628–633. [CrossRef] [PubMed]
25. Chevalier, P.; Bellocq, C.; Millat, G.; Piqueras, E.; Potet, F.; Schott, J.J.; Baró, I.; Lemarec, H.; Barhanin, L.; Rousson, R.; et al. Torsades de pointes complicating atrioventricular block: Evidence for a genetic predisposition. *Heart Rhythm* **2007**, *4*, 170–174. [CrossRef]

Disclaimer/Publisher's Note: The statements, opinions and data contained in all publications are solely those of the individual author(s) and contributor(s) and not of MDPI and/or the editor(s). MDPI and/or the editor(s) disclaim responsibility for any injury to people or property resulting from any ideas, methods, instructions or products referred to in the content.

Systematic Review

Rhythm vs. Rate Control in Patients with Postoperative Atrial Fibrillation after Cardiac Surgery: A Systematic Review and Meta-Analysis

Muneeb Ahmed [1], Emilie P. Belley-Coté [1], Yuan Qiu [2], Peter Belesiotis [1], Brendan Tao [3], Alex Wolf [4], Hargun Kaur [1], Alex Ibrahim [4], Jorge A. Wong [1], Michael K. Wang [1], Jeff S. Healey [1], David Conen [1], Philip James Devereaux [1], Richard P. Whitlock [1] and William F. Mcintyre [1,*]

[1] Faculty of Health Sciences, McMaster University, Hamilton, ON L8L 2X2, Canada
[2] Ottawa Heart Institute, University of Ottawa, Ottawa, ON K1Y 4W7, Canada
[3] Department of Medicine, University of British Columbia, Vancouver, BC V6T 1Z1, Canada
[4] Department of Medicine, Western University, Hamilton, ON N6A 5C1, Canada
* Correspondence: william.mcintyre@phri.ca

Abstract: Background: Postoperative atrial fibrillation (POAF) is the most common complication after cardiac surgery; it is associated with morbidity and mortality. We undertook this review to compare the effects of rhythm vs. rate control in this population. Methods: We searched MEDLINE, Embase and CENTRAL to March 2023. We included randomized trials and observational studies comparing rhythm to rate control in cardiac surgery patients with POAF. We used a random-effects model to meta-analyze data and rated the quality of evidence using GRADE. Results: From 8,110 citations, we identified 8 randomized trials (990 patients). Drug regimens used for rhythm control included amiodarone in four trials, other class III anti-arrhythmics in one trial, class I anti-arrhythmics in four trials and either a class I or III anti-arrhythmic in one trial. Rhythm control compared to rate control did not result in a significant difference in length of stay (mean difference −0.8 days; 95% CI −3.0 to +1.4, I^2 = 97%), AF recurrence within 1 week (130 events; risk ratio [RR] 1.1; 95%CI 0.6–1.9, I^2 = 54%), AF recurrence up to 1 month (37 events; RR 0.9; 95%CI 0.5–1.8, I^2 = 0%), AF recurrence up to 3 months (10 events; RR 1.0; 95%CI 0.3–3.4, I^2 = 0%) or mortality (25 events; RR 1.6; 95%CI 0.7–3.5, I^2 = 0%). Effect measures from seven observational studies (1428 patients) did not differ appreciably from those in randomized trials. Conclusions: Although atrial fibrillation is common after cardiac surgery, limited low-quality data guide its management. Limited available evidence suggests no clear advantage to either rhythm or rate control. A large-scale randomized trial is needed to inform this important clinical question.

Keywords: rhythm control; rate control; atrial fibrillation; cardiac surgery; length of stay

1. Introduction

Annually, over half a million adults undergo cardiac surgery in North America [1]. These numbers are expected to increase as the global burden of cardiovascular disease grows [2,3]. Atrial fibrillation (AF) is the most common complication after cardiac surgery; postoperative AF (POAF) occurs in up to 40% of patients [4]. Patients who experience POAF are more likely to have adverse events, including up to a fourfold increase in the odds of stroke and a doubling in the odds of death [4–6]. Patients with POAF spend, on average, an additional 48 h in the intensive care unit, 3 more days in the hospital, and have a 30% greater chance of hospital readmission in the 30 days after surgery [5–8].

Two strategies are used to manage POAF: rhythm and rate control. Rhythm control focuses on restoring sinus rhythm with anti-arrhythmic drugs (most commonly amiodarone) or electrical cardioversion. Rate control uses one or more negative chronotropic drugs to control ventricular rate. The optimal strategy remains unclear [9–11]. Guidelines issued by the Canadian Cardiovascular Society (CCS), the European Society of Cardiology (ESC), the Cardiac Society of Australia and New Zealand, and the European Association for Cardio-Thoracic Surgery (EACTS) have all addressed the issue of rhythm vs. rate control after cardiac surgery, with differing conclusions [9–12].

This systematic review and meta-analysis aimed to synthesize all of the evidence (randomized trials and observational studies) on the safety and efficacy of a rhythm control strategy as compared to a rate control strategy in adult patients without a history of AF who developed POAF after cardiac surgery.

2. Materials and Methods

We registered the protocol with PROSPERO (2021 CRD42021259249). Supplementary File S1 lists the differences between the registered protocol and the final manuscript. This systematic review adheres to Preferred Reporting Items for Systematic Reviews and Meta-Analyses (PRISMA) guidelines [13].

2.1. Eligibility Criteria

We searched for published randomized trials and observational studies comparing a rhythm control to a rate control strategy in cardiac surgery patients who developed POAF after cardiac surgery. We included studies if they reported at least one of the predetermined outcomes of interest. Rhythm control was defined by the use of an anti-arrhythmic drug (i.e., a class I or III agent, including amiodarone) or electrical cardioversion, irrespective of the use of rate-controlling agents. Rate control was defined as a strategy based on any of beta blockers, non-dihydropyridine calcium channel blockers or digoxin. We did not place restrictions on language and considered both full texts and studies published only as abstracts.

2.2. Search Methods

We searched MEDLINE, Embase and CENTRAL from inception to March 2023. We also screened trial registries and contacted experts to identify additional studies. We designed a search strategy and reviewed it with a librarian to capture pharmacologic rhythm control with a class I or III anti-arrhythmic agent, electrical cardioversion, and pharmacologic rate control with beta blockers, non-dihydropyridine calcium channel blockers or digoxin. We present the search strategy in Supplementary File S2.

2.3. Selection of Studies

We selected studies using Covidence Systematic review software (Veritas Health Innovation, Melbourne, VIC, Australia). Two reviewers screened titles and abstracts independently and in duplicate and retrieved full-text reports for all items deemed potentially relevant by either reviewer. Subsequently, two authors independently compared full-text reports against eligibility criteria. We resolved any disagreements through discussion with the senior author.

2.4. Data Extraction

We abstracted descriptive data (e.g., patient population, intervention, comparator) from selected studies. Outcomes of interest were length of the index hospital stay, hospital readmission, new or worsening heart failure, days out of hospital, quality of life, freedom from AF (within 1 week, up to 1 month, and up to 3 months), bleeding, myocardial infarction, mortality, and stroke. We used studies' definitions for clinical outcomes. Two reviewers independently and in duplicate extracted data using pre-designed data collection forms. We resolved disagreements through discussion with the senior author.

2.5. Risk of Bias

We assessed risk of bias in randomized trials using the Cochrane Risk of **Bias** 2 (RoB 2) tool [14]. We independently assessed the following domains in duplicate: (i) random sequence generation; (ii) allocation concealment; (iii) blinding of study participants, personnel, and outcome assessors; (iv) incomplete outcome data (we considered $\geq 20\%$ missing data at high risk of bias); and (v) performance bias. We compared the assessments and discussed them to resolve disagreements. For analysis and presentation purposes, we dichotomized risk of bias as high (or likely high) or low (or likely low). We categorized a trial as high risk of bias if it was at risk of selection, performance, detection, or reporting bias for that outcome.

We assessed risk of bias in observational studies using the Cochrane-endorsed CLARITY tool [15]. We rated the risk of bias in studies as low, moderate, serious, or critical across seven domains: (i) bias due to confounding; (ii) selection of patients into the study; (iii) classification of the intervention; (iv) bias due to deviations from the intended intervention; (v) missing data; (vi) measurement of outcomes; and (vii) selection of reported results [15].

2.6. Statistical Analysis

We analyzed randomized trials and observational studies separately. We used mean difference (MD) as the standard measure of association for length of the index hospital stay and risk ratios (RRs) for all other clinical outcomes. We present 95% confidence intervals (CI) around estimates of effect. We assessed clinical and methodological heterogeneity based on study characteristics. We transformed the median and a measure of dispersion to mean and standard deviation for our meta-analyses, assuming a normal distribution [16]. We measured statistical heterogeneity using the I^2 statistic. We considered an I^2 greater than 50% as showing substantial heterogeneity [17]. We used RevMan 5.3 (The Cochrane Collaboration, Denmark) to combine data quantitatively. We decided a priori to use a random-effects model with Mantel–Haenszel weighting because it is conservative, and we expected clinical and methodological heterogeneity. We analyzed according to the participant's first assigned group (intention-to-treat principle) in randomized trials where participants crossed over to the other treatment. We considered two-sided p-values < 0.05 to be statistically significant.

We performed pre-specified subgroup analyses comparing studies in which participants received amiodarone-based rhythm control to those in which they received other regimens (Supplementary File S3). We evaluated for interaction between subgroups and treatment effect and reported p-values.

2.7. Quality Assessment

We assessed the quality of evidence using the GRADE (Grading of Recommendations Assessment, Development and Evaluation) approach [18]. We appraised our confidence in the estimates of effects by considering risk of bias in individual studies, directness of the evidence, precision of effect estimates for individual clinical outcomes, heterogeneity of the data and potential for publication bias.

3. Results
3.1. Selection of Included Studies

From 8110 citations, we identified eight randomized trials that evaluated 10 different rhythm control regimens and included a total of 990 patients [19–26]. Table 1 outlines the characteristics of the included trials. Supplementary File S4 outlines the study selection process. Drug regimens used for rhythm control included amiodarone in four trials, other class III anti-arrhythmics in one trial, class I anti-arrhythmics in four trials and either a class I or III anti-arrhythmic in one trial. For rate control, four trials permitted choice between beta blockers, calcium channel blockers or digoxin, one trial allowed choice between calcium channel blockers or digoxin, one trial used beta blockers alone, one trial used calcium channel blockers alone and one trial used digoxin alone. Supplementary file S5 describes the rhythm monitoring methods that were used in each trial.

Table 1. Characteristics of included randomized trials.

Study ID	N	Surgery Type	Rhythm Control	Rate Control	Follow-Up Duration	Outcomes Reported
Demirkilic 1996 [24]	120	Isolated CABG: 120/120 (100%)	Choice between: -Quinidine PO 550 mg/day -Amiodarone PO 600 mg/day for 7 days then 200 mg/day	Verapamil PO 240 mg/day	1 week	AF recurrence (within 1 week, up to 1 month & up to 3 months)
Gillinov 2016 [25]	523	Isolated CABG: 212/523 (40.5%) CABG + valve repair: 17/523 (3.3%) CABG + valve replacement: 86/523 (16.4%) Non-CABG: 208/523 (39.8%)	Amiodarone 3 g PO load then 200 mg per day Both arms received rate control for HR < 100 and got DCCV if AF was persistent beyond 24–48 h	Beta blocker and/or calcium channel blocker and/or Digoxin Both arms received rate control for HR < 100 and got DCCV if AF was persistent beyond 24–48 h	60 days	Length of stay AF recurrence (within 1 week, up to 1 month & up to 3 months) Mortality Stroke
Hjelms 1992 [19]	30	Isolated CABG: 25/30 (83.3%) Non-CABG: 5/30 (16.7%)	IV Procainamide, then PO Procainamide for 1 week	Choice between: -IV Digoxin -PO Digoxin maintenance dose 0.1–0.3 mg	1 week	Length of stay AF recurrence (within 1 week) Mortality
Kamali 2017 [20]	146	Isolated CABG: 146/146 (100%)	Amiodarone PO or IV 300 mg followed by 1–3 mg/kg every 6 h and 0.5 mg/kg 18 h later	Beta blocker IV 1–3 mg/kg/h for 24 h	24 h	Length of stay AF Recurrence (within 1 week) Mortality
Karacaglar 2019 [26]	50	Isolated CABG: 43/50 (86%) CABG + valve surgery: 7/50 (14%)	IV amiodarone DCCV if in AF at 24 h then PO amiodarone for 28 days	Beta blocker, calcium channel blocker or Digoxin DCCV if in AF at 24 h	30 days	Length of stay AF Recurrence (within 1 week, up to 1 month) Bleeding Mortality Stroke
Lee 2000 [21]	50	Isolated CABG: 34/50 (68%) CABG + valve surgery: 7/50 (14%) Non-CABG: 9/50 (18%)	Choice between: -Sotalol PO 120–360 mg/day -Propafenone PO 300–900 mg/day -Procainamide IV 500–1000 mg followed by a continuous infusion of 1 to 4 mg/h or 2 to 3 g/day in divided oral doses. -Amiodarone IV 200 mg/day after a loading dose of 1200 to 1600 mg for 4 to 5 days DCCV if in AF at 48 h	Beta blocker, calcium channel blocker or Digoxin	Rhythm: 48 h Rate: Until HR ≤ 110 BPM or 110–120 BPM with no heart failure	Length of stay AF recurrence (within 1 week, up to 1 month & up to 3 months) Mortality
Soucier 2003 [22]	42	Isolated CABG: 34/42 (81%) CABG + valve surgery: 6/42 (14.3%) Non-CABG: 2/42 (4.8%)	Choice between: -IV Ibutilide -Propafenone	Physician choice beta blocker encouraged	1 week	AF recurrence (within 1 week) Stroke
Wafa 1989 [23]	29	Isolated CABG: 29/29 (100%)	Flecainide IV for up to 24 h	IV Digoxin +/− Verapamil	24 h	Length of stay AF recurrence (within 1 week)

PO: taken orally; IV: given intravenously; AF: atrial fibrillation; N: number of randomized patients; DCCV: direct current cardioversion; CABG: coronary artery bypass graft.

We identified seven observational studies that included a total of 1428 patients (Supplementary File S6) [27–33]. For rhythm control, five studies used amiodarone while two studies permitted choice between a class I or III anti-arrhythmic. For rate control, two studies allowed choice between beta blockers, calcium channel blockers or digoxin, one study permitted choice between beta blockers or digoxin, one study allowed choice between beta blockers or calcium channel blockers, two studies used digoxin alone and one study used beta blockers alone.

3.2. Risk of Bias Assessment

We outline judgments about risk of bias in included studies in Supplementary Files S7–S9. Only one out of eight randomized trials reported blinding of participants and personnel and blinding of outcome assessment [20,23]. We judged risks of bias related to randomization, allocation, incomplete outcome data, and selective reporting as either low or likely low in all studies. All observational studies had serious or moderate risk of bias.

4. Outcomes

4.1. Data from Randomized Trials

Compared to rate control, rhythm control did not result in a significant reduction in length of stay (Table 2, Figure 1, Supplementary file S3). There was no statistical evidence of a subgroup effect on length of stay between studies that used amiodarone-based and non-amiodarone-based rhythm control. We rated the quality of evidence for this outcome as very low due to its skewed distribution, imprecision, inconsistency and risk of bias (Supplementary Files S7, S9, and S10).

Table 2. Summary of length of stay and subgroup analyses for the comparison of rhythm vs. rate control.

Group	N Studies (References)	Total Patients	Mean Length of Stay in Days+/− Standard Deviation		Mean Difference (95%CI)	p-Value	I^{2n}	Quality of Evidence Reason for Judgement (Supplementary Files S7, S9a–h and S10)
			Rhythm Control	Rate Control				
All trials	5 [20–22,25,26]	815	6.6 ± 0.7	6.3 ± 0.7	−0.8 days (−3.0 to +1.4)	0.47	97%	Very low Skewed distribution, risk of bias, imprecision
Amiodarone-based rhythm control	3 [20,24,25]	723	6.1 ± 0.6	5.7 ± 0.6	0.5 days (−1.5 to +2.5)	0.63	95%	
Nonamiodarone-based rhythm control	2 [21,22]	92	9.8 ± 1.3	12.6 ± 1.3	−3.1 days (−6.2 to +0.1)	0.06	64%	

No significant subgroup differences for length of stay (p = 0.06).

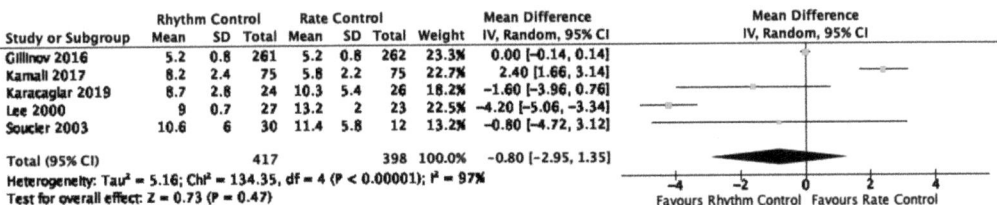

Figure 1. Length of stay in randomized trials. Forest plot displaying an inverse-variance weighted random-effects meta-analysis comparing rhythm and rate control on length of the index hospital stay in days (mean difference). Columns of data are displayed in the plot for all figures. The drugs and dosages in each trial are documented in Table 1 for all figures. We used studies' definitions for clinical outcomes for all figures. The size of data markers indicates the weight of the study in all figures. Error bars indicate 95% CIs for all figures. We used RevMan 5.3 (The Cochrane Collaboration, Odense, Denmark) to combine data quantitatively for all figures [20–22,25,26].

Compared to rate control, rhythm control did not result in a significant reduction in AF recurrence within 1 week, up to 1 month or up to 3 months, mortality or stroke (Table 3,

Figures 2–4, Supplementary File S3). There was no statistical evidence of a subgroup effect on mortality between studies that used amiodarone-based and non-amiodarone-based rhythm control. We rated the quality of evidence for most outcomes as low due to imprecision and risk of bias (Supplementary Files S7, S9 and S10). We rated the quality of evidence for stroke as very low due to very serious imprecision and risk of bias (Supplementary Files S7, S9 and S10).

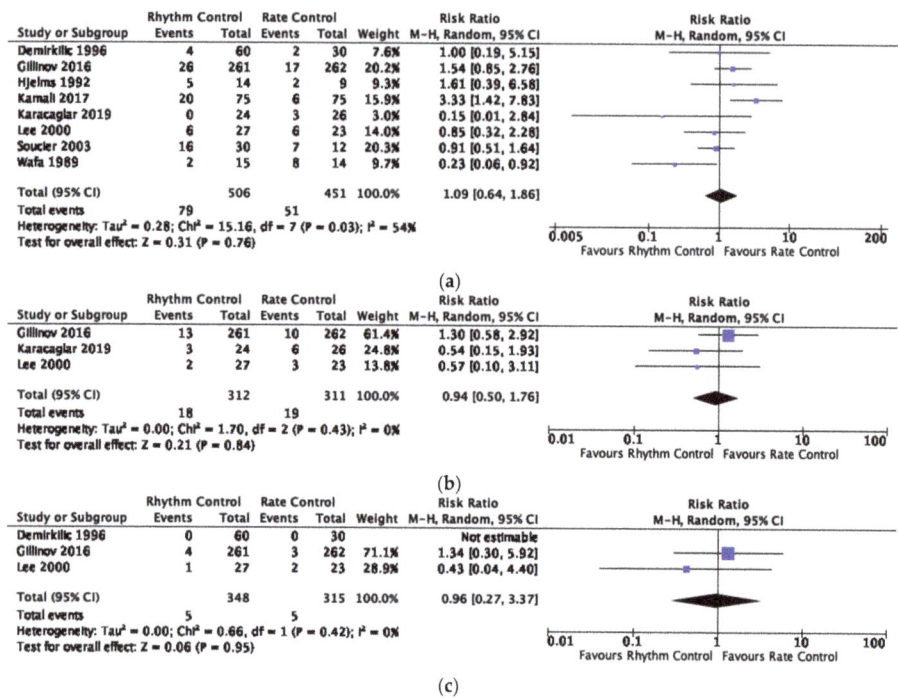

Figure 2. (**a**) AF recurrence within 1 week in randomized trials. Forest plot displaying relative risks calculated using a random-effects model with Mantel-Haenszel weighting comparing rhythm and rate control on atrial fibrillation recurrence within 1 week. The relative risks were calculated using a random-effects model with Mantel-Haenszel weighting for all figures [19–26]; (**b**) AF recurrence up to 1 month in randomized trials. Forest plot displaying relative risks calculated using a random-effects model with Mantel-Haenszel weighting comparing rhythm and rate control on atrial fibrillation recurrence up to 1 month [21,25,26]; (**c**) AF recurrence up to 3 months in randomized trials; Forest plot displaying relative risks calculated using a random-effects model with Mantel-Haenszel weighting comparing rhythm and rate control on atrial fibrillation recurrence up to 3 months [21,24,25].

Table 3. Summary of AF recurrence, mortality and stroke and sensitivity analyses for the comparison of rhythm vs. rate control.

Group	N Studies (References)	Number of Patients with Events/Number of Patients at Risk		Relative Risk			Quality of Evidence Reason for Judgement (Supplementary Files S7, S9 and S10)
		Rhythm Control	Rate Control	Risk Ratio (95% CI)	p-Value	I^2	
AF recurrence							
AF recurrence within one week	8 [19–26]	79/605	51/451	1.1 (0.6–1.9)	0.76	54%	Low Imprecision, risk of bias
AF recurrence up to one month	3 [21,25,26]	18/312	19/311	0.9 (0.5–1.8)	0.84	0%	

Table 3. Cont.

Group	N Studies (References)	Number of Patients with Events/Number of Patients at Risk		Relative Risk			Quality of Evidence Reason for Judgement (Supplementary Files S7, S9 and S10)
		Rhythm Control	Rate Control	Risk Ratio (95% CI)	p-Value	I²	
AF recurrence up to three months	3 [21,24,25]	5/348	5/315	1.0 (0.3–3.4)	0.95	0%	
Mortality							
All studies	5 [20–22,25,26]	16/419	9/396	1.6 (0.7–3.5)	0.24	0%	
Amiodarone-based rhythm control	3 [20,25,26]	14/360	9/363	1.5 (0.7–3.4)	0.33	0%	Low Imprecision, risk of bias
NonAmiodarone-based rhythm control	2 [21,22]	2/57	0/35	4.3 (0.2–85.0)	0.34	N/A	
No significant subgroup differences for mortality (p = 0.51)							
Stroke							
All studies	3 [22,25,26]	4/297	6/318	0.7 (0.1–4.6)	0.73	44%	Very low Very serious imprecision, risk of bias

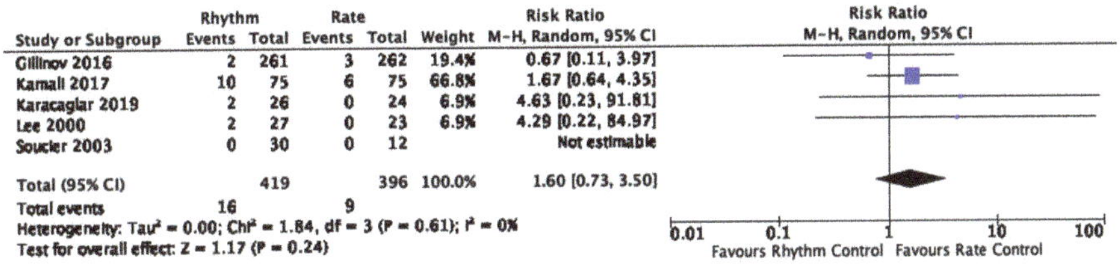

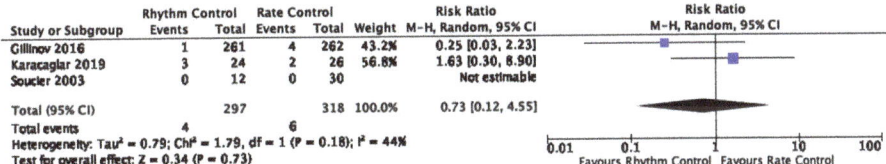

Figure 3. Mortality in randomized trials. Forest plot displaying relative risks calculated using a random-effects model with Mantel-Haenszel weighting comparing rhythm and rate control on mortality as defined by the respective study [20–22,25,26].

Figure 4. Stroke in randomized trials. Forest plot displaying relative risks calculated using a random-effects model with Mantel-Haenszel weighting comparing rhythm and rate control on stroke as defined by the respective study [22,25,26].

4.2. Data from Observational Studies

Among observational studies, four studies reported data on length of stay, three studies reported on AF recurrence within 1 week, two studies reported on AF recurrence up to 1 month, three studies reported on AF recurrence up to 3 months and two studies reported on mortality. Effect measures from observational studies did not differ appreciably from those in randomized trials (Supplementary File S5). We rated the quality of evidence for all outcomes as very low. All outcomes were downgraded due to risk of bias. Length of stay was downgraded for non-normal distribution. All other outcomes were downgraded for serious imprecision (Supplementary File S11).

5. Discussion

The current literature, when synthesized, fails to demonstrate significant differences in length of stay, AF recurrence, mortality or stroke between rhythm and rate control strategies for patients with POAF after cardiac surgery. This lack of significant difference is consistent between studies that used both amiodarone-based and non-amiodarone-based rhythm control. However, this body of evidence has important limitations. The number of patients enrolled in trials evaluating rhythm and rate control strategies in postoperative atrial fibrillation is small, with fewer than 1000 participants in total. Most of these studies were open-label. Moreover, substantial variability in interventions and follow-up durations reduced confidence in estimates of effect.

To our knowledge, this systematic review and meta-analysis is the first to compare rhythm vs. rate control specifically in patients with POAF after cardiac surgery. A 2018 systematic review of RCTs comparing rhythm to rate control for patients with AF in general only included one study with POAF [34]. This meta-analysis of 12 studies showed no significant difference between rhythm and rate control groups for mortality, bleeding, and thromboembolic events but demonstrated a higher rehospitalization rate with rhythm control [34].

The largest trial in this review was conducted by the Cardiothoracic Surgical Trials Network from 2014 to 2015; it accounts for 523 of the 990 participants (52.8% of patients, 23.3% of the weight for length of stay) in the meta-analysis [25]. This trial has important limitations that deserve mention, some of which are highlighted in the 2017 EACTS Guidelines [12]. The treatment regimen of this trial included amiodarone for the rhythm control group and beta blocker/calcium channel blocker or digoxin for the rate control group. However, both groups received rate control for patients with a heart rate less than 100 and were cardioverted electrically if AF was persistent beyond 24–48 h, which may have minimized differences in treatment effect. The cross-over rate was very high (25%), and rhythm status was assessed using intermittent rather than continuous ECG. In addition, the trial included patients with short episodes of POAF—these low-risk patients may have obscured benefits seen in higher-risk patients.

As neither rhythm nor rate control is superior for the treatment of POAF in cardiac surgery patients, both strategies can be considered for the treatment of individual patients. Both the ESC and CCS guidelines suggest tailoring treatment. The 2020 ESC guidelines state that "*...rate or rhythm control treatment decisions should be based on symptoms* (Class I Recommendation, Level A Evidence)". The 2016 CCS Guidelines state that "*choice of strategy should therefore be individualized on the basis of the degree of symptoms* (Strong Recommendation, Moderate-Quality Evidence)" [9,10]. In contrast, the 2017 EACTS guidelines state that "*In patients with postoperative haemodynamically stable POAF, rhythm control is recommended* (Class I Recommendation, Level B Evidence)" [12].

Our study suggests that large, randomized trials are required to compare rhythm and rate control for POAF in cardiac surgery patients. Future studies should assess adverse events and seek to understand clinician, economic and patient values in decision-making. This review also highlights the lack of data on other important outcomes, such as bleeding, hospital readmission, new or worsening heart failure, days out of hospital, quality of life, bleeding and thrombotic events. The International Consortium for Health Outcomes Measurement has identified these outcomes to be meaningful to both patients and clinicians and recommends them as standard outcomes for trials in AF [35,36].

6. Strengths and Weaknesses

Our search was comprehensive, using three large trial databases (MEDLINE, Embase, and CENTRAL) for published data, and we screened trial registries and enquired with specialists about additional studies. The review was pre-registered and used the GRADE framework to evaluate the quality of the evidence.

The principal limitations of this review are inherent to the studies that met the eligibility criteria. Variability in intervention types, follow-up periods, drug types, doses and durations, as well as a high proportion of patients lost to follow-up in the included studies, may have obscured a signal. It is worth noting that some drugs primarily intended for rhythm control, such as amiodarone, dronedarone and sotalol, can also have an impact on reducing ventricular rate during atrial fibrillation. Amiodarone, in particular, has shown effectiveness in slowing the ventricular rate in patients with atrial fibrillation and heart failure who are intolerant to high-dose β-blockade in combination with digoxin or in whom calcium channel blockers are contraindicated. However, in our review, we focused exclusively on assessing amiodarone as a rhythm control agent, and its potential role in acute heart rate control in the context of cardiac surgery was not specifically examined. Studies reported overall adverse events rather than comparative counts between rhythm and rate control, which obviated meta-analysis. Included studies ascertained AF recurrence using 12 lead-ECG and/or short-duration Holter monitoring. Implantable loop recorders (ILRs) are the most sensitive tool for detecting AF recurrence and have become increasingly used in post-ablation studies. ILRs may have led to detectable differences in AF recurrence outcomes [37]. Furthermore, since many cardiac surgery patients receive oral anticoagulation, the risk of thromboembolic events in the perioperative period overall was low, which may have affected the signal between rhythm and rate control for reducing thromboembolic events.

7. Conclusions

Currently, limited, low-quality data inform on the efficacy of a rhythm control vs. a rate control approach for patients with new-onset AF following cardiac surgery. A large-scale randomized trial is needed to inform this important clinical question.

Supplementary Materials: The following supporting information can be downloaded at: https://www.mdpi.com/article/10.3390/jcm12134534/s1.

Author Contributions: Conceptualization, M.A., J.S.H. and W.F.M.; Methodology, M.A., Y.Q., P.B. and W.F.M.; Formal analysis, M.A.; Data curation, B.T., A.W., H.K. and A.I.; Writing—original draft, M.A.; Writing—review & editing, E.P.B.-C., Y.Q., J.A.W., M.K.W., J.S.H., D.C., P.J.D., R.P.W. and W.F.M.; Supervision, W.F.M. All authors have read and agreed to the published version of the manuscript.

Funding: This research received no external funding.

Institutional Review Board Statement: Not applicable.

Informed Consent Statement: Not applicable.

Data Availability Statement: All relevant data are within the manuscript and Supplementary Materials.

Acknowledgments: We thank Toru Inami for his assistance in assessing articles written in Japanese; the members of the McMaster Interdisciplinary Investigative Outcomes Node—Cardiac Sciences, Intensive Care and Anesthesia (McMaster University), for their methodological support; Jack Young, MLIS (McMaster Health Sciences Library), for reviewing our search strategy; Stephanie Sanger (McMaster Health Sciences Library), for assistance with full-text retrieval. They did not receive compensation for their contributions.

Conflicts of Interest: All authors have completed and submitted the ICMJE Form for Disclosure of Potential Conflicts of Interest.

Abbreviations and Acronyms

Atrial fibrillation	(AF)
Canadian Cardiovascular Society	(CCS)
Coronary artery bypass graft	(CABG)
Direct current cardioversion	(DCCV)
European Society of Cardiology	(ESC)
European Association for Cardio-Thoracic Surgery	(EACTS)
Given intravenously	(IV)
GRADE	(Grading of Recommendations Assessment, Development and Evaluation)
Postoperative atrial fibrillation	(POAF)
Preferred Reporting Items for Systematic Reviews and Meta-Analyses	(PRISMA)
Taken orally	(PO)

References

1. Writing Group Members; Roger, V.L.; Go, A.S.; Lloyd-Jones, D.M.; Benjamin, E.J.; Berry, J.D.; Borden, W.B.; Bravata, D.M.; Dai, S.; Ford, E.S.; et al. Heart Disease and Stroke Statistics—2012 Update. *Circulation* **2012**, *125*, e2–e220.
2. Yusuf, S.; Reddy, S.; Ounpuu, S.; Anand, S. Global burden of cardiovascular diseases: Part II: Variations in cardiovascular disease by specific ethnic groups and geographic regions and prevention strategies. *Circulation* **2001**, *104*, 2855–2864. [CrossRef]
3. Baghai, M.; Wendler, O.; Grant, S.W.; Goodwin, A.T.; Trivedi, U.; Kendall, S.; Jenkins, D.P. Aortic valve surgery in the UK, trends in activity and outcomes from a 15-year complete national series. *Eur. J. Cardio-Thorac. Surg.* **2021**, *60*, 1353–1357. [CrossRef] [PubMed]
4. Bessissow, A.; Khan, J.; Devereaux, P.J.; Alvarez-Garcia, J.; Alonso-Coello, P. Postoperative atrial fibrillation in non-cardiac and cardiac surgery: An overview. *J. Thromb. Haemost.* **2015**, *13* (Suppl. S1), S304–S312. [CrossRef] [PubMed]
5. Eikelboom, R.; Sanjanwala, R.; Le, M.-L.; Yamashita, M.H.; Arora, R.C. Postoperative Atrial Fibrillation after Cardiac Surgery: A Systematic Review and Meta-Analysis. *Ann. Thorac. Surg.* **2021**, *111*, 544–554. [CrossRef] [PubMed]
6. Wang, M.K.; Meyre, P.B.; Heo, R.; Devereaux, P.J.; Birchenough, L.; Whitlock, R.; McIntyre, W.F.; Chen, Y.C.P.; Ali, M.Z.; Biancari, F.; et al. Short-term and Long-term Risk of Stroke in Patients with Perioperative Atrial Fibrillation after Cardiac Surgery: Systematic Review and Meta-analysis. *CJC Open* **2022**, *4*, 85–96. [CrossRef]
7. Goyal, P.; Kim, M.; Krishnan, U.; Mccullough, S.A.; Cheung, J.W.; Kim, L.K.; Pandey, A.; A Borlaug, B.; Horn, E.M.; Safford, M.M.; et al. Post-operative atrial fibrillation and risk of heart failure hospitalization. *Eur. Heart J.* **2022**, *43*, 2971–2980. [CrossRef]
8. LaPar, D.J.; Speir, A.M.; Crosby, I.K.; Fonner, E., Jr.; Brown, M.; Rich, J.B.; Quader, M.; Kern, J.A.; Kron, I.L.; Ailawadi, G. Postoperative Atrial Fibrillation Significantly Increases Mortality, Hospital Readmission, and Hospital Costs. *Ann. Thorac. Surg.* **2014**, *98*, 527–533. [CrossRef]
9. Macle, L.; Cairns, J.; Leblanc, K.; Tsang, T.; Skanes, A.; Cox, J.L.; Healey, J.S.; Bell, A.; Pilote, L.; Andrade, J.G.; et al. 2016 Focused Update of the Canadian Cardiovascular Society Guidelines for the Management of Atrial Fibrillation. *Can. J. Cardiol.* **2016**, *32*, 1170–1185. [CrossRef]
10. Hindricks, G.; Potpara, T.; Dagres, N.; Arbelo, E.; Bax, J.J.; Blomström-Lundqvist, C.; Boriani, G.; Castella, M.; Dan, G.A.; Dilaveris, P.E.; et al. 2020 ESC Guidelines for the diagnosis and management of atrial fibrillation developed in collaboration with the European Association for Cardio-Thoracic Surgery (EACTS): The Task Force for the diagnosis and management of atrial fibrillation of the European Society of Cardiology (ESC) Developed with the special contribution of the European Heart Rhythm Association (EHRA) of the ESC. *Eur. Heart J.* **2021**, *42*, 373–498.
11. Brieger, D.; Amerena, J.; Attia, J.; Bajorek, B.; Chan, K.H.; Connell, C.; Freedman, B.; Ferguson, C.; Hall, T.; Haqqani, H.; et al. National Heart Foundation of Australia and the Cardiac Society of Australia and New Zealand: Australian Clinical Guidelines for the Diagnosis and Management of Atrial Fibrillation 2018. *Heart Lung Circ.* **2018**, *27*, 1209–1266. [CrossRef] [PubMed]
12. Sousa-Uva, M.; Head, S.J.; Milojevic, M.; Collet, J.-P.; Landoni, G.; Castella, M.; Dunning, J.; Gudbjartsson, T.; Linker, N.J.; Sandoval, E.; et al. 2017 EACTS Guidelines on perioperative medication in adult cardiac surgery. *Eur. J. Cardiothorac. Surg.* **2018**, *53*, 5–33. [CrossRef] [PubMed]
13. Page, M.J.; McKenzie, J.E.; Bossuyt, P.M.; Boutron, I.; Hoffmann, T.C.; Mulrow, C.D.; Shamseer, L.; Tetzlaff, J.M.; Akl, E.A.; Brennan, S.E.; et al. The PRISMA 2020 statement: An updated guideline for reporting systematic reviews. *PLoS Med.* **2021**, *18*, e1003583. [CrossRef] [PubMed]
14. Sterne, J.A.C.; Savović, J.; Page, M.J.; Elbers, R.G.; Blencowe, N.S.; Boutron, I.; Cates, C.J.; Cheng, H.Y.; Corbett, M.S.; Eldridge, S.M.; et al. RoB 2: A revised tool for assessing risk of bias in randomised trials. *BMJ* **2019**, *366*, l4898. [CrossRef] [PubMed]
15. The Clarity Review Group, McMaster University. Tool to Assess Risk of Bias in Cohort Studies. Available online: http://help.magicapp.org/knowledgebase/articles/327941-tool-to-assess-risk-of-bias-in-cohort-studies (accessed on 10 May 2023).
16. Wan, X.; Wang, W.; Liu, J.; Tong, T. Estimating the sample mean and standard deviation from the sample size, median, range and/or interquartile range. *BMC Med. Res. Methodol.* **2014**, *14*, 135. [CrossRef]
17. Cumpston, M.; Li, T.; Page, M.J.; Chandler, J.; Welch, V.A.; Higgins, J.P.; Thomas, J. Updated guidance for trusted systematic reviews: A new edition of the Cochrane Handbook for Systematic Reviews of Interventions. *Cochrane Database Syst. Rev.* **2019**, *10*, ED000142. [CrossRef]
18. Guyatt, G.H.; Oxman, A.D.; Schünemann, H.J.; Tugwell, P.; Knottnerus, A. GRADE guidelines: A new series of articles in the Journal of Clinical Epidemiology. *J. Clin. Epidemiol.* **2011**, *64*, 380–382. [CrossRef]
19. Hjelms, E. Procainamide conversion of acute atrial fibrillation after open-heart surgery compared with digoxin treatment. *Scand. J. Thorac. Cardiovasc. Surg.* **1992**, *26*, 193–196. [CrossRef]
20. Kamali, A.; Sanatkar, A.; Sharifi, M.; Moshir, E. Evaluation of amiodarone versus metoprolol in treating atrial fibrillation after coronary artery bypass grafting. *Interv. Med. Appl. Sci.* **2017**, *9*, 51–55. [CrossRef]
21. Lee, J.K.; Klein, G.J.; Krahn, A.D.; Yee, R.; Zarnke, K.; Simpson, C.; Skanes, A.; Spindler, B. Rate-control versus conversion strategy in postoperative atrial fibrillation: A prospective, randomized pilot study. *Am. Heart J.* **2000**, *140*, 871–877. [CrossRef]
22. Soucier, R.; Silverman, D.; Abordo, M.; Jaagosild, P.; Abiose, A.; Madhusoodanan, K.P.; Therrien, M.; Lippman, N.; Dalamagas, H.; Berns, E. Propafenone versus ibutilide for post operative atrial fibrillation following cardiac surgery: Neither strategy improves outcomes compared to rate control alone (the PIPAF study). *Med. Sci. Monit. Int. Med. J. Exp. Clin. Res.* **2003**, *9*, PI19–PI23.

23. Wafa, S.S.; Ward, D.E.; Parker, D.J.; Camm, A.J. Efficacy of flecainide acetate for atrial arrhythmias following coronary artery bypass grafting. *Am. J. Cardiol.* **1989**, *63*, 1058–1064. [CrossRef]
24. Yilmaz, A.T.; Demírkiliç, U.; Arslan, M.; Kurulay, E.; Ozal, E.; Tatar, H.; Öztürk, Y. Long-term prevention of atrial fibrillation after coronary artery bypass surgery: Comparison of quinidine, verapamil, and amiodarone in maintaining sinus rhythm. *J. Card. Surg.* **1996**, *11*, 61–64. [CrossRef]
25. Gillinov, A.M.; Bagiella, E.; Moskowitz, A.J.; Raiten, J.M.; Groh, M.A.; Bowdish, M.E.; Ailawadi, G.; Kirkwood, K.A.; Perrault, L.P.; Parides, M.K.; et al. Rate Control versus Rhythm Control for Atrial Fibrillation after Cardiac Surgery. *N. Engl. J. Med.* **2016**, *374*, 1911–1921. [CrossRef] [PubMed]
26. Karaçağlar, E.; Atar, İ.; Özbiçer, S.; Sezgin, A.; Özçobanoğlu, S.; Yazici, A.C.; Özin, B.; Müderrisoğlu, H. Amiodarone Versus Direct Current Cardioversion in Treatment of Atrial Fibrillation after Cardiac Surgery. *Turk. J. Clin. Lab.* **2019**, *10*, 26–32. Available online: https://dergipark.org.tr/en/pub/tjcl/issue/44073/519537#article_cite (accessed on 8 December 2021). [CrossRef]
27. Kowey, P.R.; Stebbins, D.; Igidbashian, L.; Goldman, S.M.; Sutter, F.P.; Rials, S.J.; Marinchak, R.A. Clinical outcome of patients who develop PAF after CABG surgery. *Pacing Clin. Electrophysiol.* **2001**, *24*, 191–193. [CrossRef]
28. Abbas, S.; Gul, S.; Dhahri, A.; Iqbal, M.; Khan, T.; Khan, S. Amiodarone vs digoxin in the treatment of atrial fibrillation in postoperative rheumatic cardiac valvular patients. *J. Pak. Med. Assoc.* **2016**, *66*, 1098–1101.
29. Bruggmann, C.; Astaneh, M.; Lu, H.; Tozzi, P.; Ltaief, Z.; Voirol, P.; Sadeghipour, F. Management of Atrial Fibrillation Following Cardiac Surgery: Observational Study and Development of a Standardized Protocol. *Ann. Pharmacother.* **2021**, *55*, 830–838. [CrossRef] [PubMed]
30. Cioffi, G.; Cemin, C.; Russo, T.E.; Pellegrini, A.; Terrasi, F.; Ferrario, G. Post-discharge recurrences of new-onset atrial fibrillation following cardiac surgery: Impact of low-dose amiodarone and beta-blocker prophylaxis. *Ital. Heart J.* **2000**, *1*, 691–697. [PubMed]
31. List of Abstracts: Suppl. 1 to Vol. 12 (May 20, 2011). *Interact. Cardiovasc. Thorac. Surg.* **2011**, *12* (Suppl. S1), iv–xxiii. [CrossRef]
32. Guaragna, J.C.; Martins, V.; Brunini, T.M.; Linhatti, J.L.; Brauner, F.B.; Pires, R.C.; Bodanese, L.C. Use of high-dose oral amiodarone for the reversion of atrial fibrillation during the postoperative period of cardiac surgery. *Arq. Bras. Cardiol.* **1997**, *69*, 401–405. [CrossRef]
33. Shah, P.; Shpigel, A.; Wasser, T.; Sabo, M.; Feldman, B. Morbidity of Post-Coronary Artery Bypass Surgery Patients with Atrial Fibrillation Treated with Rate Control versus Sinus-Restoring Therapy. *Heart Drug* **2001**, *1*, 192–196. [CrossRef]
34. Abushouk, A.I.; Ashraf Ali, A.; Mohamed, A.; el Sherif, L.; Abdelsamed, M.; Kamal, M.; Sayed, M.K.; Mohamed, N.A.; Osman, A.A.; Shaheen, S.M.; et al. Rhythm Versus Rate Control for Atrial Fibrillation: A Meta-analysis of Randomized Controlled Trials. *Biomed. Pharmacol. J.* **2018**, *11*, 609–620. [CrossRef]
35. ICHOM Our Mission. Available online: https://www.ichom.org/mission/ (accessed on 8 March 2022).
36. Seligman, W.H.; Das-Gupta, Z.; Jobi-Odeneye, A.O.; Arbelo, E.; Banerjee, A.; Bollmann, A.; Caffrey-Armstrong, B.; A Cehic, D.; Corbalan, R.; Collins, M.; et al. Development of an international standard set of outcome measures for patients with atrial fibrillation: A report of the International Consortium for Health Outcomes Measurement (ICHOM) atrial fibrillation working group. *Eur. Heart J.* **2020**, *41*, 1132–1140. [CrossRef] [PubMed]
37. Rovaris, G.; Ciconte, G.; Schiavone, M.; Mitacchione, G.; Gasperetti, A.; Piazzi, E.; Negro, G.; Montemerlo, E.; Rondine, R.; Pozzi, M.; et al. Second-generation laser balloon ablation for the treatment of atrial fibrillation assessed by continuous rhythm monitoring: The LIGHT-AF study. *Europace* **2021**, *23*, 1380–1390. [CrossRef] [PubMed]

Disclaimer/Publisher's Note: The statements, opinions and data contained in all publications are solely those of the individual author(s) and contributor(s) and not of MDPI and/or the editor(s). MDPI and/or the editor(s) disclaim responsibility for any injury to people or property resulting from any ideas, methods, instructions or products referred to in the content.

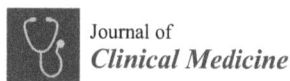 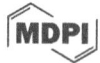

Review

Echocardiographic Evaluation of Atrial Remodelling for the Prognosis of Maintaining Sinus Rhythm after Electrical Cardioversion in Patients with Atrial Fibrillation

Paweł Wałek [1,2,*], Joanna Roskal-Wałek [1,3], Patryk Dłubis [1] and Beata Wożakowska-Kapłon [1,2]

1. Collegium Medicum, Jan Kochanowski University, 25-317 Kielce, Poland; joanna.roskal.walek@wp.pl (J.R.-W.); patryk.dlubis@gmail.com (P.D.); bw.kaplon@poczta.onet.pl (B.W.-K.)
2. 1st Clinic of Cardiology and Electrotherapy, Swietokrzyskie Cardiology Centre, 25-736 Kielce, Poland
3. Ophthalmology Clinic, Voivodeship Regional Hospital, 25-736 Kielce, Poland
* Correspondence: pawel.walek@o2.pl

Abstract: Atrial fibrillation (AF) is the most common atrial tachyarrhythmia. One of the methods of AF treatment is direct current cardioversion (DCCV), but in the long-term follow-up we observe quite a high percentage of AF recurrences after this procedure. In order to assess the prognosis of DCCV effectiveness, we use clinical, biochemical and echocardiographic parameters. The objective of this review is to systematise the current knowledge on echocardiographic measurements in patients with persistent AF used to assess the progress of remodelling of the atrial wall, which affects the likelihood of maintaining sinus rhythm after DCCV. In this article, echocardiographic parameters for the evaluation of remodelling of the atrial wall are divided into groups referring to structural, mechanical, and electrical remodelling, as well as parameters for the evaluation of left ventricular filling pressure. The article aims to draw attention to the clinical value of echocardiographic measurements, which is the selection of patients who will maintain sinus rhythm after DCCV in the long-term follow-up, which will allow to avoid unnecessary risks associated with the procedure and enable the selection of the appropriate treatment strategy.

Keywords: atrial fibrillation; tissue Doppler; strain; strain rate; remodelling; echocardiography; cardioversion

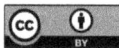

1. Introduction

Atrial fibrillation (AF) is the most common atrial tachyarrhythmia. It is estimated that up to 33.5 million patients may be affected worldwide, which does not include those with an asymptomatic form of the disease. The prevalence expected in 2030 is more than 15 million Europeans and 12.1 million Americans. It is estimated that 886,000 European citizens are first diagnosed with AF each year and that one in four adults over the age of 40 will experience AF in their lifetime [1–5].

The most serious complication of atrial fibrillation is arterial embolism of cardiac origin, including stroke and TIA (transient ischemic attack), with AF one of the main causes. AF is also associated with the progression of systolic and diastolic heart failure, decreased quality of life, and increased all-cause mortality [6–8]. Because AF does not always have obvious symptoms, diagnosis is often a challenge.

The mechanisms leading to the development of atrial fibrillation are not fully understood. The probable cause of AF is considered to be damage to the atrial muscle and the development of remodelling. Widely described modifiable and non-modifiable risk factors contribute significantly to this phenomenon. Persistent AF also leads to further damage and, in consequence, to progressive remodelling [9]. There are currently three main types of atrial remodelling: electrical, mechanical and structural. Electrical remodelling consists in shortening the action potential and refractory period of atrial cells, as well as changes in sarcolemmal sodium ion channels and gap junctions. Mechanical remodelling consists in the impairment and dyssynchrony of atrial wall muscle contraction caused mainly by the replacement of myocardial cells by fibroblasts and fibrous tissue. Structural remodelling is the enlargement of the atrial cavities. Changes in the structure and function of atrial wall cells may lead to the induction of atrial fibrillation. Each of these types of remodelling can be evaluated indirectly by means of echocardiography.

The main goal of AF treatment is to eliminate or reduce the symptoms associated with arrhythmia and to prevent thromboembolic complications [10]. Reduction of AF symptoms is achieved by restoring and maintaining sinus rhythm (SR) or by controlling the heart rate. For this purpose, pharmacotherapy, ablation, or pharmacological or electrical cardioversion (DCCV–direct current cardioversion) are used [10]. One of the most commonly applied methods of restoring SR is DCCV, which is characterised by easy performance and low cost, so it is frequently offered to patients with AF. The effectiveness of cardioversion in restoring SR in patients with persistent and paroxysmal AF is estimated at 75–88%, while SR can be maintained for 12 months in 70% of patients [11].

The objective of this review is to systematise the current knowledge on echocardiographic measurements in patients with persistent AF used to assess the progress of remodelling, which affects the likelihood of maintaining sinus rhythm after DCCV. In this article, echocardiographic parameters for the evaluation of remodelling are divided into groups referring to structural, mechanical, and electrical remodelling, as well as parameters for the evaluation of left ventricular filling pressure (Table 1). The article aims to draw attention to the clinical value of echocardiographic measurements, which is the selection of patients who will maintain sinus rhythm after DCCV in the long-term follow-up. Appropriate selection of patients with persistent AF for an appropriate treatment strategy will avoid unnecessary risks associated with the procedure.

Table 1. Echocardiographic parameters evaluating atrial remodelling.

Structural Remodelling	Mechanical Remodelling	Electrical Remodelling
1. Left atrial anteroposterior diameter (LAAP)	1. Mitral inflow A-wave velocity	1. Total atrial conduction time (TACT) *
2. Left atrial volume (LAV) in the late systolic phase and left atrial volume in the late systolic phase indexed with body surface–left atrial volume index (LAVI).	2. Left and right atrial emptying fraction (LAEF and RAEF)	
3. Right atrial volume (RAV) in the late systolic phase and right atrial volume in the late systolic phase indexed with body surface–right atrial volume index (RAVI).	3. Measurement of mitral inflow velocity in the LV (Afc)	
4. Total atrial conduction time (TACT) *	4. Inflow and outflow velocity in the appendage of the LA–left atrial appendage flow velocity (LAAFV)	
	5. Left and right atrial wall motion velocity (LAWMV and RAWMV)	
	6. Left atrial appendage wall motion velocity (LAAWMV)	
	7. Left atrial strain and strain rate	

* Depends on the size (structural remodelling) and the conduction velocity of the electrical excitation (electrical remodelling).

2. Material and Methods

In March 2023, an extensive manual search was performed through the major electronic databases (PubMed, Google Scholar) in order to identify relevant studies published on atrial remodelling. The following search terms were used: "atrial fibrillation echocardiography", "atrial fibrillation remodeling", "atrial fibrillation cardioversion", "atrial fibrillation atrial strain", "atrial fibrillation emptying fraction", "predictors for maintenance of sinus rhythm after cardioversion, echocardiography", and "atrial fibrillation recurrence after successful cardioversion", in different combinations. With regard to echocardiographic parameters with prognostic values in the prognosis of sinus rhythm failure after DCCV, original studies were selected and the latest review articles were included in the analysed reports. A total of 65 compatible research publications were identified and used to compile this review.

3. Structural Remodelling

Structural remodelling is the final stage of atrial remodelling resulting from preceding and accompanying electrical and mechanical remodelling. It is not confirmed whether AF is due to remodelling or remodelling is due to AF, although both mechanisms seem likely.

Parameters for structural remodelling evaluation are rather well described, and their correlation with the persistence of SR after DCCV has been thoroughly studied. The most commonly performed measurement is of the left atrium anteroposterior diameter (LAAP) during TTE (transthoracic echocardiogram). This is the least accurate parameter for evaluating the size of the left atrium (LA), since the enlargement of the LA is visible in the top–bottom measurement, so the real size of the LA is often underestimated. Despite numerous studies, the predictive value of this parameter remains unclear [12–18]. A more precise measurement of the LA size is the measurement of the left atrial volume (LAV) in the late systolic phase, indexed with the body surface as the left atrial volume index (LAVI). It has been shown that patients with recurrent AF have significantly increased LA sizes compared to those with SR, and that LA enlargement significantly increases the risk of AF recurrence [16,19–21]. LAVI measurements provide a reliable estimation of LA size. The introduction of LAVI improved the accuracy of prognosing AF recurrence after effective DCCV, both during AF and SR [15,22–24]. Compared to LAAP, LAVI has a significantly higher predictive value in terms of AF recurrence after DCCV [15].

In addition to evaluating the structure of the left atrium, assessment of the right atrium (RA) is also important. There are data indicating the superiority of the right atrial volume index (RAVI) over LAVI in evaluating the risk of AF recurrence after DCCV [25]. Atrial volume can also be measured with contrast computed tomography. The diagnostic value of such measurements, together with RAVI and LAVI for the evaluation of AF recurrence after PVI (pulmonary vein isolation), was studied [26]. The results of the study indicate that determining the ratio of RAVI to LAVI can be a useful and valuable indicator of the recurrence of arrhythmia [26].

4. Mechanical Remodelling

It is estimated that mechanical and structural remodelling of the LA is caused by excessive tension of the LA wall, which leads to the replacement of muscle fibres with connective tissue. Increased tension of the LA wall and a reduced number of muscle fibres lead to impaired contractility of the LA wall and the wall of its appendage, which in turn causes a dilation of the LA cavity and a decrease in myocardial velocity. The degree of mechanical remodelling is correlated with the duration of AF, as well as with the presence of mitral insufficiency [27]. An increasing number of researchers emphasise the superiority of parameters for measuring mechanical remodelling over parameters for measuring structural remodelling in evaluating the chances of maintaining SR in patients with AF [28–31]. These parameters can be evaluated after DCCV, but parameters during AF are also available for testing. The ability to assess the likelihood of maintaining SR prior to performing DCCV is extremely valuable, as it can provide a better assessment of the patient before qualifying for DCCV or an alternative treatment. In addition to the prognostic value in terms of AF recurrence after DCCV, some parameters measured during transoesophageal echocardiography (TEE), such as left atrial appendage wall motion velocity (LAAWMV) and peak atrial contraction strain (PACS), are also useful for evaluating the risk of thromboembolic complications in AF patients [32–36].

Assessment of mechanical remodelling of the LA can be performed using standard echocardiography, as well as new techniques, such as assessment of deformation of the LA wall during TEE or TTE. Standard echocardiographic measurements during TTE help in assessing mechanical remodelling by means of such parameters as LAEF (left atrial emptying fraction) and RAEF (right atrial emptying fraction), or AFc (left atrial fibrillatory contraction flow). During a TEE, it is possible to assess LAAFV (left atrial appendage flow velocity) using pulse Doppler imaging or LAAWMV (left atrial appendage wall motion velocity) using tissue Doppler imaging. New imaging techniques such as strain and strain rate allow us to more accurately assess the systolic function of the LA muscle. Strain and strain rate measurements can be performed by means of tissue Doppler imaging (TDI), but measurements taken with this technique are prone to error due to its angle dependence. Strain and strain rate measurements can also be performed by means of STE (speckle tracking echocardiography), which is free from angle dependence error but requires better visualisation than TDI. Using strain and strain rate techniques, we can assess the extensibility and contractility of the left atrial wall, as well as the dispersion of deformation of the LA walls and local motility disorders of the LA walls.

4.1. Mitral Inflow A-Wave Velocity

With the damage to the atria and the progression of remodelling, the mechanical function becomes impaired, which leads to a decrease in mitral inflow velocity. Cardioversion can restore the sinus rhythm, but not necessarily the mechanical function of the atria. The time to regain correct atrial mechanical function has been linked to several factors, one of which is the duration of AF [37]. Among the Doppler examination parameters evaluating the flow through the mitral valve, the A-wave velocity proved to be an independent risk factor for AF recurrence after DCCV in studies by Spiecker et al. and Grundvold et al. [38,39]. Using the functions of tissue Doppler imaging, the velocity of the A wave of mitral inflow can be assessed during TTE after successful cardioversion of atrial fibrillation. In a study by Spiecker et al., sinus rhythm was restored pharmacologically in 14% of patients and with DCCV in 77% of patients. Echocardiography was performed up to 4 h after cardioversion and then on the first, second and third day after restoring SR. In a multivariate regression analysis, the A-wave velocity of the mitral inflow measured one day after DCCV proved to be an independent predictor of AF recurrence. In subsequent studies, there was a gradual increase in the A-wave velocity from the day of cardioversion (mean 44 cm/s) until four weeks after it (72 cm/s). Patients whose AF duration was less than six weeks demonstrated a higher A-wave velocity after successful cardioversion. The E-wave mitral inflow velocity was comparable between patients with maintained SR and with recurrent AF [38]. Grundvold et al. also described the effect of low A-wave velocities of mitral flow on an increased risk of AF recurrence after cardioversion. Significantly lower mitral A-wave velocity (≤ 0.1 m/s) was reported in the 6-month follow-up in the group of patients with AF recurrence compared to the group where SR was maintained (≥ 0.45 m/s). There were no differences in atrial size or left ventricular function between the groups with recurrent AF and maintained SR [39].

4.2. Left and Right Atrial Emptying Fraction

One of the parameters for evaluation of the mechanical function of the left and right atria is their emptying fraction. This is the ratio of the volume of blood ejected into the ventricle during atrial contraction to the volume of blood in the atrium before its contraction. It is calculated as follows: (LA maximum volume − LA minimum volume)/LA maximum volume × 100%. It allows for indirect assessment of the atrial contractility and the degree of progression of mechanical remodelling. Higher values of emptying fraction mean a larger volume of blood transported to the ventricles during ventricular diastole so that less blood remains in the atria. It is connected with a lower degree of stretching of the atria and, over a longer period, slower development of structural remodelling, which results mainly from mechanical remodelling. Mechanical remodelling has a negative effect on atrial contractility, and studies show that patients with maintained SR after DCCV had higher LAEF and RAEF than patients with recurrent AF, and that RAEF and LAEF had greater prognostic value in evaluating recurrent AF after DCCV than LAVI and RAVI [28]. Until recently, it was believed that atrial contractility during an episode of AF was disturbed to such an extent that it did not generate an LA emptying volume. Studies show that the emptying volume is still generated, despite contractility impairment during an episode of AF. In addition, measurement of the LA emptying fraction during AF has prognostic value in terms of the maintenance of SR after DCCV [40,41]. Kim et al. presented a method for evaluating the contractility of LA during an episode of AF, which consists in measuring the wave of mitral inflow to the LV that occurs between successive E waves of mitral inflow. This parameter was called Afc (atrial fibrillatory contraction flow), and it is assumed that the larger the Afc wave, the better the contractility of LA is preserved (Figure 1) [41]. Based on these analyses, the authors concluded that the velocity time integral of the Afc wave and its velocity predict AF recurrence after DCCV more accurately than LAVI. In our study, we found that patients who have a higher LAEF during AF also have a better prognosis in terms of maintaining sinus rhythm after DCCV than patients with a lower LAEF. In addition, the parameter that evaluates mechanical remodelling had greater prognostic value than parameters that evaluate structural remodelling [40].

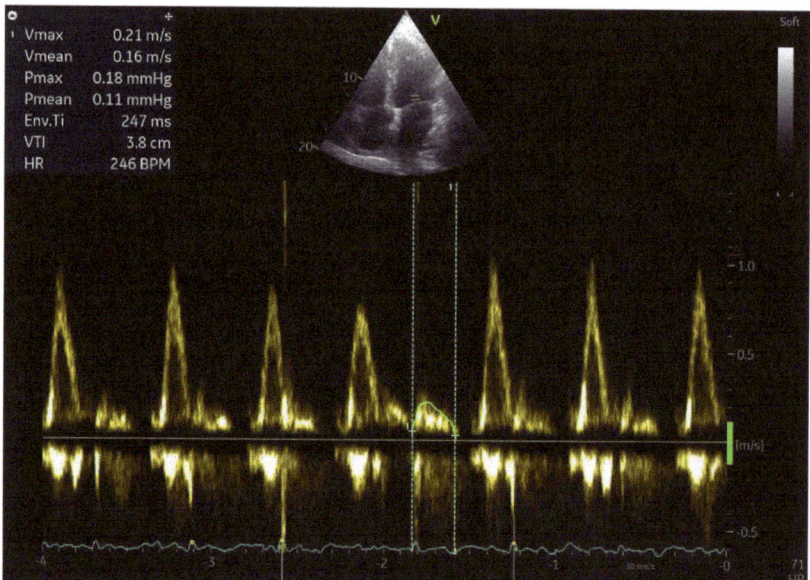

Figure 1. Left atrial fibrillatory contraction flow (Afc). Pulsed-wave Doppler of mitral filling in the apical four-chamber projection during atrial fibrillation. Velocity time integral (VTI) and AFc velocity measurement. AFc VTI 3.8 cm. AFc V 21 cm/s.

4.3. Left Atrial Appendage Flow Velocity

Another echocardiographic parameter that allows us to assess the systolic function, and thus mechanical remodelling of the left atrium, is the left atrial appendage flow velocity (LAAFV), measured both during sinus rhythm and atrial fibrillation. The limitation of this parameter is that it must be measured during a TEE examination. In a healthy person, during the sinus rhythm, when the contractility of the left atrium appendage (LAA) is preserved, the top of the appendage during contraction almost completely closes. As a result of wall hardening, which occurs in remodelling, the contractility of the LAA decreases, which results in a decrease in the velocity of blood inflow and outflow. Measurement of LAAFV during TEE provides an indirect assessment of the systolic function of the LAA. The left atrium appendage has a characteristic emptying pattern during SR [42]. The highest emptying velocity occurs in the proximal part of the LAA: 50 to 83 cm/s in healthy individuals [43]. A velocity below 40 cm/s increases the risk of stroke and AF recurrence after successful DCCV. The higher the value, the higher the probability of maintaining SR after DCCV. In a study by Melduni et al., LAAFV was shown to have prognostic value in terms of assessment of sinus rhythm maintenance after DCCV, risk of stroke, and death in patients with atrial fibrillation. In the study, it was demonstrated that the risk of the above events increases with a decrease in LAAFV values [44]. Similarly, Antonelli et al. presented LAAFV as a predictor of the maintenance of SR after DCCV. In their study, LAAFV had greater predictive value in terms of the maintenance of SR after DCCV than the structural remodelling parameter LAAP [21].

4.4. Left and Right Atrial Wall Motion Velocity

Another parameter with high prognostic value for evaluation of the maintenance of SR after DCCV measured in TTE is the left and right atrial wall motion velocity—LAWMV and RAWMV. De Vos et al. evaluated the prognostic value of measurements of atrial wall motion velocity and duration of an AF cycle for evaluating the immediate success of DCCV and the maintenance of SR over one year after DCCV in patients with persistent AF. LAWMV and RAWMV were measured using TDI, and the measurements were performed retrospectively using the Q-analysis software on colour Doppler images. Measurements were performed during late diastole in the left lateral atrial wall just below the mitral valve ring and in the right lateral atrial wall just below the tricuspid valve ring. LAWMV did not have prognostic value for the immediate success of DCCV, but it was shown that patients with higher LAWMV values were more likely to maintain sinus rhythm after DCCV over a 12-month follow-up. In the case of RAWMV, it was shown that the higher the result of this measurement, the higher the chances of immediate success of DCCV and maintenance of sinus rhythm over a 12-month follow-up. In this study, the group of patients with maintained SR after DCCV did not differ in terms of structural remodelling parameters (LAAP, RAV, LAV) from the group of patients who had recurrent AF [45]. In addition, it was demonstrated that the longer the duration of AF, the lower the LAWMV values during atrial fibrillation, which suggests that the LAA wall motion velocity reflected mechanical remodelling [27]. A limitation of RAWMV and LAWMV measurements is that they are much more difficult in patients with high ventricular rhythm.

Recently, left and right atrial wall motion velocity was proven to possess prognostic value in terms of predicting the maintenance of the sinus rhythm after electrical cardioversion performed due to persistent AF, in which velocity measurements were performed directly using tissue Doppler imaging (TDI) (Figure 2) [46]. In this study, in a multivariate regression analysis including clinical and echocardiographic factors, only LAWMV was a significant predictor of SR maintenance over 12 months. Direct measurement, compared to the Q-analysis from colour Doppler imaging used by De Vos et al., has some advantages. Direct measurement is much less time-consuming and does not require additional software. Additionally, in Q-analysis, the sampling rate of the velocity measurement is affected by the size of the colour Doppler image that is recorded. Direct measurement of the left atrial wall motion velocity by means of tissue Doppler imaging is performed in the same way as a' and e' measurements of the velocity of diastolic motion of the mitral valve ring, but the Doppler gate should be located approximately 10 mm below the ring. A clear advantage of using colour Doppler imaging and the Q-analysis software is the ability to perform retrospective measurements from recordings made earlier.

Assessment of the myocardial velocity in the atria appears to be a promising method for evaluating the likelihood of SR maintenance after DCCV in persistent atrial fibrillation, and hence it is important to further evaluate these parameters in a larger patient population.

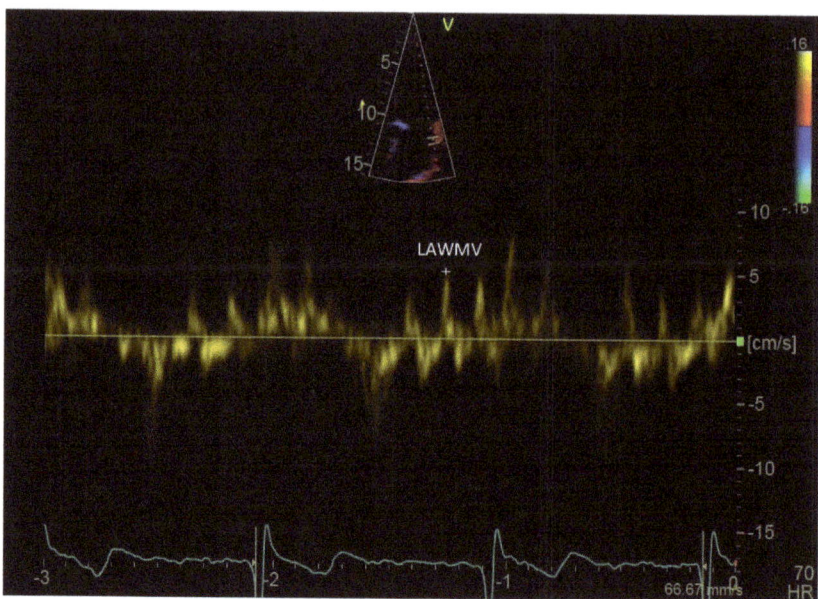

Figure 2. Left atrial wall motion velocity (LAWMV). LAWMV 5 cm/s. Pulsed-wave tissue Doppler in the apical four-chamber projection during atrial fibrillation.

4.5. Left Atrial Appendage Wall Motion Velocity

Another parameter in the direct evaluation of the mechanical function of the left atrial appendage is left atrial appendage wall motion velocity (LAAWMV) (Figure 3). Left atrial appendage wall motion velocity correlates with the degree of mechanical remodelling, which leads to a decrease in myocardial velocity. Patients whose LAAWMV is measured during AF have lower LAAWMV values than patients with sinus rhythm [47]. One of the advantages of LAAWMV over other markers of mechanical remodelling is that it can be measured before cardioversion during AF. There are two techniques available for evaluating LAA wall motion velocity: TDI (tissue Doppler imaging) and STE (speckle tracking echocardiography). Currently, STE is considered to be the preferred technique for evaluating myocardial velocity and deformity because it is free from angle dependence, which is the main limitation of TDI. The weakness of the STE technique is the need to obtain very good imaging quality, which is difficult in the case of thin walls of the LAA, whereas TDI does not have this limitation. Unfortunately, measurements of LAA wall motion velocity and deformation with STE can only be performed during TEE, while LAA wall motion velocity measurements with TDI can be performed using both TTE and TEE. The measurement of LAAWMV requires a break in the systolic function of the ventricle in order to visualise the systolic wave of the LAA wall motion. Rapid motion of the ventricles makes measurement difficult, but the stimulation of the vagus nerve that occurs during TEE slows down the heart rate, making reliable measurement of LAAWMV possible. In our study, LAAWMV had prognostic value both in terms of SR restoration after DCCV and SR maintenance over a 12-month follow-up after DCCV. Among the analysed echocardiographic parameters evaluated before DCCV during AF, only LAAWMV and E/e' had prognostic value in terms of maintenance of SR after DCCV, both in multivariate models containing only echocardiographic parameters, including parameters for structural remodelling evaluation, and in the model with clinical parameters [31].

A recently discovered phenomenon is LAAWMV reduction in the lateral LAA wall compared to the LAA medial wall in patients with AF, while in patients without diagnosed AF, there is an opposite relation. The chances of identifying a patient with paroxysmal AF using this phenomenon was 22.14 (95% CI, 12.06–40.64; $p < 0.001$) [47].

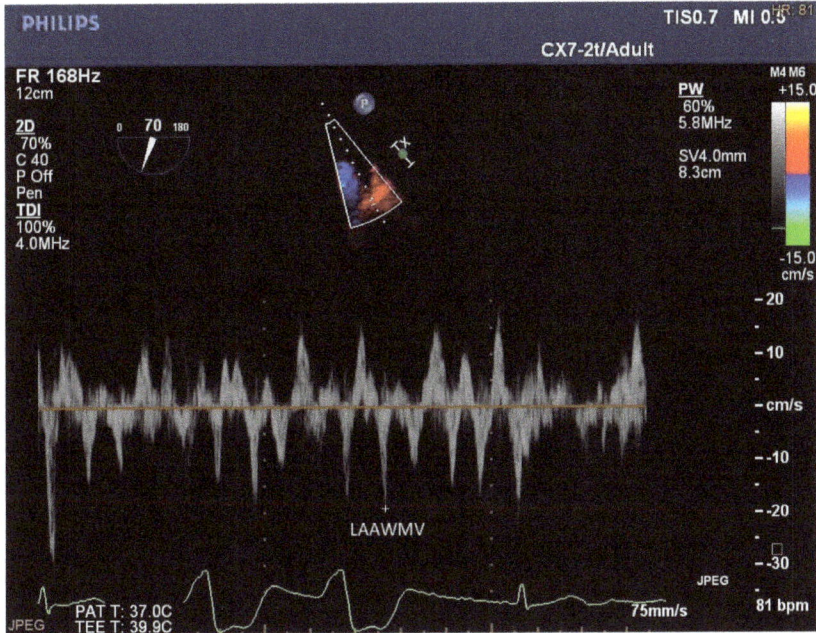

Figure 3. Left atrial appendage wall motion velocity (LAAWMV). LAAWMV 18 cm/s. Pulsed-wave tissue Doppler in two-chamber 60–90° projection in transoesophageal echocardiography during atrial fibrillation.

4.6. Left Atrial Strain and Strain Rate

A parameter called left atrial strain (LAS) is used to assess the degree of mechanical deformation of the myocardium. Progressive remodelling leading to atrial wall rigidity leads to a decrease in strain and strain rate during AF. Using the above-mentioned STE and TDI techniques, it is possible to assess the strain and strain rate during echocardiography [48]. An examination can be performed both during AF and after sinus rhythm restoration. In patients with sinus rhythm, the reservoir, conduit and contraction phases of LA can be evaluated (Figures 4 and 5). In the reservoir phase, the susceptibility of the atrial wall to stretching is assessed. During the contraction phase—the ability of the atrial muscle to contract—and the conduit phase is the difference in measurement in the reservoir and contraction phases. During AF, only the conduit phase is evaluated, while the reservoir phase is a negative value of the conduit phase. Initially, strain and strain rate assessment were performed using TDI. One of the first studies of strain and strain rate using TDI to assess the prognosis of patients after DCCV in terms of maintenance of SR demonstrated the usefulness of these parameters in patients with persistent AF [29,49].

Decreased strain and strain rate were shown to be predictive of AF occurrence, especially in patients who have suffered a cryptogenic stroke [50,51]. Strain and strain rate are not only predictors of the occurrence of the first diagnosed AF, but can also be used to assess the probability of maintaining SR after a DCCV performed to treat AF. It was demonstrated that strain and strain rate measured the day after a successful DCCV are predictive of SR maintenance [52]. Moreover, the study revealed that strain and strain rate measured in the contraction phase have greater predictive value in terms of maintaining sinus rhythm than strain and strain rate assessed in the reservoir and conduit phases [52].

Strain measurements before cardioversion can predict the maintenance of sinus rhythm after DCCV. Morenzo-Ruiz et al. showed that the reservoir phase strain measured during AF before DCCV was predictive of SR maintenance over a 6-month follow-up, both in patients with persistent AF and long-standing persistent AF [53]. Shaikh et al. found that an increase in strain measured before DCCV and then after effective DCCV has prognostic value in terms of SR maintenance. The greater the increase in PALS after cardioversion relative to the measurement during AF, the greater the probability of maintaining SR over 6 months [54]. The left atrial conduit function can also be determined using the formula [(LV maximum − LV minimum) − (LA maximum − LA minimum) volume], expressed as % LV stroke volume. In studies evaluating LA conduit function, it was demonstrated that the parameter for LA conduit function evaluation is an independent risk factor of AF recurrence after DCCV [55,56].

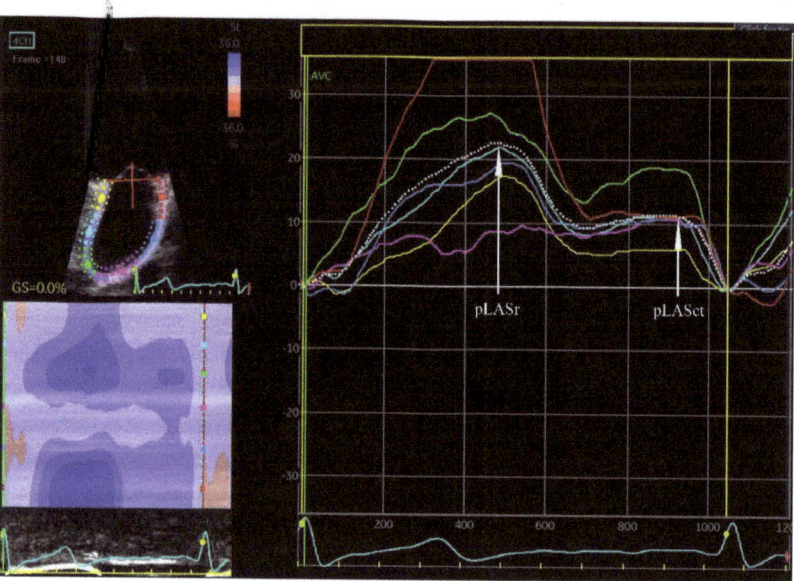

Figure 4. Left atrial strain. pLASr 22%, peak left atrial stain measured during the reservoir phase; pLASct 11%, peak left atrial stain measured during the contractile phase. The measurements are the average of the 6 assessed left atrial wall segments. The measurement was made in the apical four-chamber projection during sinus rhythm.

Loss of coordinated atrial myocardial contraction is the result of mechanical remodelling and is described as dispersion. Strain evaluation also allows for the evaluation of LA wall contractility disorders such as dispersion and dyskinesia. Dispersion is defined as the standard deviation of the time to achieve maximum deformation in different atrial segments and indicates asynchronous contraction of individual LA walls [57–59]. Under normal conditions, all segments of the LA wall should reach maximum deformation at the same time of the heart cycle. Dell'era et al. demonstrated that asynchrony of the left atrial contraction has prognostic value for the maintenance of SR after DCCV [58]. Similarly, Doruchowska et al. proved that the dispersion of time to maximum strain is an important predictor of SR maintenance after DCCV [30]. In a study by Rondano et al., the standard deviation of the time to maximum deformation was inversely dependent on the value of the maximum deformation. This study also showed that asynchronous LA contraction is a predictor of AF recurrence in patients after an effective DCCV performed to treat AF [57].

Left atrial wall dyskinesia is a new indicator that can be used to assess the likelihood of maintaining SR after DCCV in persistent AF. Left atrial wall dyskinesia means that certain segments of the atrial wall expand rather than contract during the contraction phase. In measurements of the LA strain rate in the contraction phase, dyskinetic segments demonstrate positive strain rate values, which indicates that they are stretching relative to adjacent segments that have negative strain rate values, which indicates that they are contracting (Figure 6). This phenomenon is analogous to dyskinesia of segments of the left ventricle walls. A study evaluating strain rate the day after effective DCCV showed that the appearance of dyskinetic LA wall segments increases the risk of AF recurrence after effective DCCV over a 12-month follow-up [60].

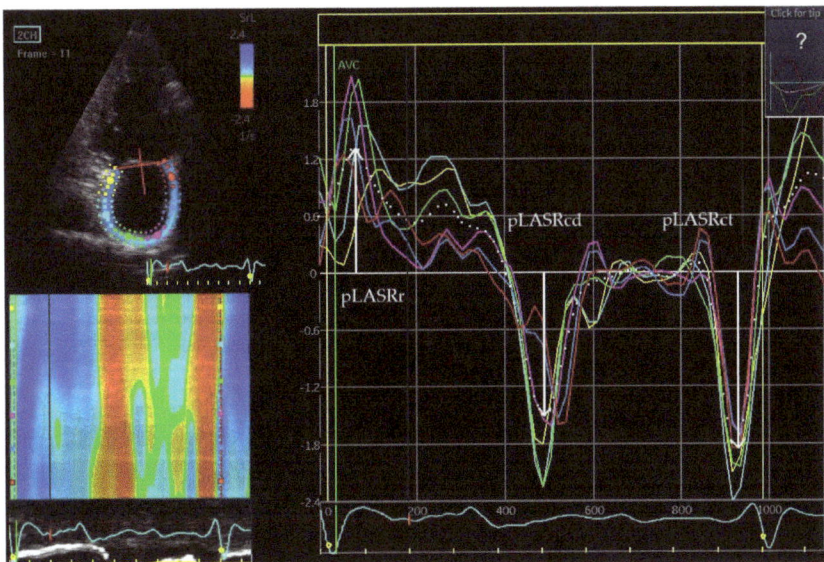

Figure 5. Left atrial strain rate. pLASRr 1.3 s^{-1} peak left atrial strain rate measured during the reservoir phase. pLASRcd −1.5 s^{-1}, peak left atrial strain rate measured during the conduit phase. pLASRct −1.9 s^{-1}, peak left atrial strain rate measured during the contractile phase. The measurements are the average of the 6 assessed left atrial wall segments. The measurement was made in the apical two-chamber projection during sinus rhythm.

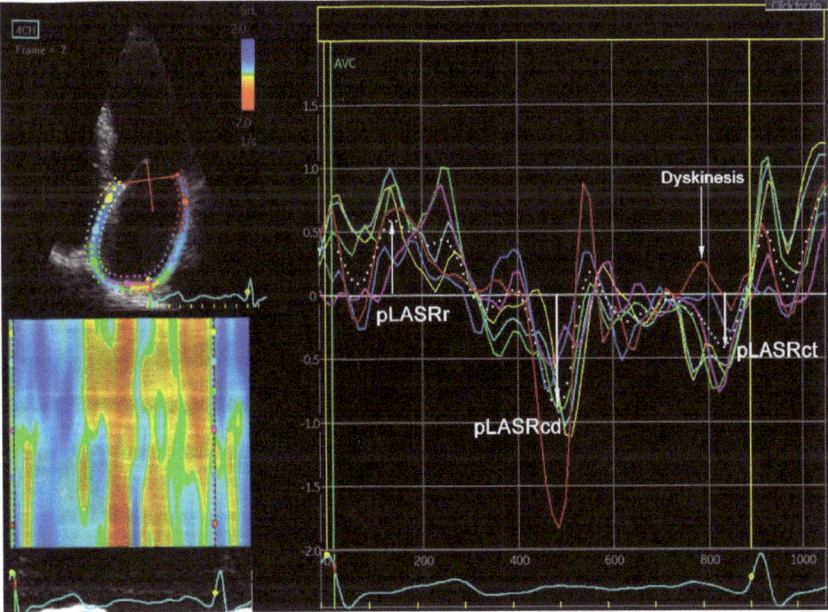

Figure 6. Left atrial wall dyskinesis. Stretching of one of the left atrial wall segments during the contractile phase. The phenomenon of left atrial wall dyskinesia is assessed during pLASRct; in the contractile phase, all segments of the left atrial wall should contract, while when dyskinesia occurs, one or several segments expand. The measurement was made in the apical four-chamber projection during sinus rhythm.

5. Electrical Remodelling

The type of remodelling that occurs first, and is also the least visible and difficult to visualise with echocardiography, is electrical remodelling. Electrical remodelling of the atrial walls is an expression of disorders in intercellular connections, change in ion channels, progressive LA wall fibrosis, and abnormalities in the conduction of electrical stimuli between the cells of the atrial wall, which results in slowing down of electrical stimuli conduction and the development of micro-re-entry substrate [61,62]. A lack of balance between collagen synthesis and degradation leads to myolysis and the development of atrial fibrosis, which in turn affects the electromechanical function of the LA, manifested by a longer atrial conduction time [63,64]. Currently, the only echocardiographic parameter that depends on electrical remodelling but also on structural remodelling is total atrial conduction time (TACT) (Figure 7). TACT is affected by both slowing down of the electrical stimuli conduction in the atrial wall, i.e., electrical remodelling, and by the length of the path that electrical stimuli must travel, i.e., enlargement of the right and left atrial cavity, which is an expression of structural remodelling. The delay between the P wave in the electrocardiogram from lead I or II and mechanical LA activation measured by tissue Doppler echocardiography, called PA-TDI, provides a reliable estimate of total atrial activation time, reflecting the degree of atrial fibrosis in biopsy samples [65]. In a study by Leung et al., PA-TDI was shown to be significantly higher in patients with AF compared to those without AF [66]. TACT prolongation reflects the slowing down of conduction and dilation of the atria and identifies individuals prone to developing atrial fibrillation [67,68].

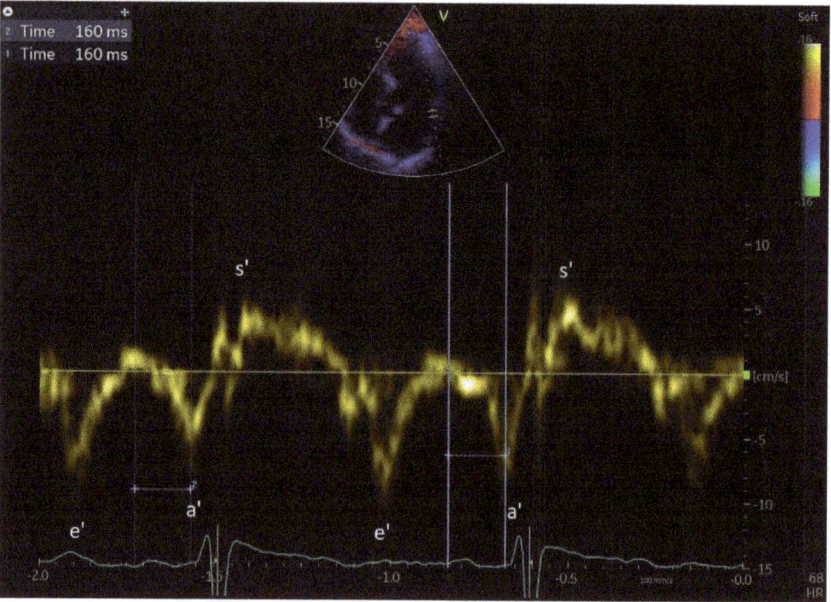

Figure 7. Total atrial conduction time (TACT). PA-TDI 160 ms. PA-TDI is the time interval between the onset of the P wave in electrocardiogram in lead I or II and the peak of the a' wave on the atrial tissue Doppler velocity curve from the lateral left atrial wall. Pulsed-wave tissue Doppler of mitral annulus velocity in the apical four-chamber projection during sinus rhythm. a', late lateral mitral annulus velocity; e', early lateral mitral annulus velocity; s', systolic mitral annulus velocity.

TACT was demonstrated to be predictive of AF recurrence after DCCV. Müller et al. showed that patients with prolonged TACT have a higher risk of early AF recurrence after DCCV. Using a multivariate regression model, they demonstrated the superiority of this parameter over a parameter for evaluation of structural remodelling, but they did not assess echocardiographic parameters representing the progression of mechanical remodelling [69]. The prognostic value of TACT for the maintenance of SR after DCCV in AF was also investigated in long-term studies. Using the same method to evaluate PA-TDI as Muller et al., Maffe et al. evaluated the prognostic value of TACT in patients with persistent AF undergoing DCCV at the annual SR maintenance assessment. Maffe et al. also confirmed the prognostic value of TACT, which was the best predictor of the chances of maintaining SR after DCCV in the studied population. The analysed parameters also included parameters for evaluating structural remodelling (LAVI, RAVI) and mechanical remodelling (a' wave, LAEF). The analysed echocardiographic parameters did not include strain or strain rate [70]. Karantoumanis et al. also showed the predictive value of TACT in terms of maintenance of SR after DCCV. In a multivariate regression model and ROC curve analysis, they proved the superiority of TACT over the parameters for evaluating structural remodelling (LAVI, RAVI) and mechanical remodelling (LAEF). The authors also evaluated left and right atrial strain defined as "left and right atrial peak longitudinal strain during ventricular systole" and the left atrial strain rate as "left atrial peak longitudinal strain rate during ventricular systole." These parameters did not differ between the group of patients with maintained sinus rhythm and the group of patients with recurrent AF. The study also analysed left atrial longitudinal strain, but it was not precisely described how this was measured, and despite obtaining statistical significance in the studied group, it was not further analysed in multivariate regression models [71].

Evaluation of electrical remodelling seems to be a very promising method for evaluating the prognosis of AF recurrence after DCCV in patients with persistent AF, but echocardiography does not currently seem to be a good tool for evaluating these types of changes in the left or right atrial wall.

6. Left Ventricular Filling Pressure

A separate parameter that does not concern the assessment of atrial remodelling but is an important predictor of AF recurrence after electrical cardioversion in persistent atrial fibrillation is left ventricular filling pressure (LVFP), which assesses left ventricular diastolic dysfunction. Left ventricular filling pressure is estimated during sinus rhythm by measuring mitral valve inflow waves E and A, the e' wave of the diastolic motion of the mitral valve ring, and the mitral inflow E wave deceleration time (DT).

Assessment of the filling pressure is also possible during AF, but estimation of the LV filling pressure is difficult because the lack of the A wave in the mitral inflow and the high variability of E and e' waves in successive heart cycles negatively affects the accuracy of the estimate and the variability of subsequent measurements.

In studies evaluating left ventricular filling pressure based on the E/e' ratio, it was demonstrated that the LV filling pressure assessed during persistent AF and after successful DCCV is a predictor of SR maintenance after DCCV [72–74]. In a study by Chung et al., an increased E/e' ratio significantly correlated with AF recurrence after cardioversion [71]. In a study by Fornengo et al., DT <150 ms (E-wave deceleration time), septal e'-wave <8 cm/s and septal E/e' ratio ≥11 were considered as the cut-off point for increased LV filling pressure [73]. Similarly, in our study, we showed that elevated values of E/a and E/e' are predictors of AF recurrence after DCCV in patients with normal systolic function of the LV muscle. In this study, in a multivariate regression model, parameters evaluating the left ventricular filling pressure had greater predictive value for SR maintenance after DCCV than parameters evaluating structural remodelling (LAVI) or mechanical remodelling LA (LAEF). The study did not measure mechanical remodelling parameters using the strain or strain rate methods [75].

7. Summary

Although ablation is becoming an increasingly common and effective method of treating patients with both paroxysmal and persistent AF, cardioversion remains one of the most frequently performed procedures in cardiology departments [76,77]. As there are no fully effective and safe antiarrhythmic drugs, the risk of recurrence of atrial fibrillation after DCCV remains high. The use of echocardiographic parameters to assess the prognosis for AF recurrence after DCCV has clear advantages in terms of availability, repeatability and better prognostic value for the maintenance of sinus rhythm after DCCV than clinical or biochemical parameters. Echocardiography remains the method of choice for evaluating the structure and function of the atria and ventricles compared to MRI and computed tomography, due to its greater availability and safety. Therefore, it is important to search for new, improved echocardiographic parameters that correlate with the progression of remodelling and allow for a more accurate assessment of the risk of AF recurrence after DCCV. Table 2 shows the optimal cut-off, area under the curve, sensitivity and specificity of the presented echocardiographic parameters for estimating the risk of recurrence of AF after DCCV. Based on this review of the available literature, it can be concluded that echocardiographic parameters evaluating mechanical remodelling of the left atrium have greater prognostic value than parameters evaluating structural remodelling in terms of prognosis of maintenance of sinus rhythm after DCCV in persistent and paroxysmal AF, and electrical remodelling can only be indirectly assessed by echocardiographic examination. Most of the echocardiographic parameters presented in this article have not yet been introduced into the daily clinical practice of qualifying patients with AF for treatment. This is because advanced software is required, some of the parameters have low repeatability, and their measurement can be time-consuming. However, some of the presented echocardiographic parameters can be performed without the involvement of additional time or advanced software, such as AFc or LAWMV. From a practical point of view, time invested in the assessment of a patient with AF allows us to more accurately qualify them for individual forms of therapy, such as pharmacotherapy, cardioversion or ablation. As ablation is a rapidly developing form of AF therapy, the above echocardiographic parameters should be studied further in terms of their prognostic value for maintaining sinus rhythm after ablation, pulmonary vein isolation or possible qualification of patients for expanded forms of standard ablation [78,79].

Table 2. Prognostic value of echocardiographic parameters in terms of maintenance of sinus rhythm/atrial fibrillation recurrence * after electrical cardioversion.

Parameter	Number of Patients	Paroxysmal/Persistent AF	Optimal Cut-Off	AUC	Sensitivity (%)	Specificity (%)	Follow-Up (months)
LAVI * [15]	76	No distinction	31 mL/m^2	0.78	71.2	78.3	>12 months
LAVI [28]	95	Persistent	48 mL/m^2	0.63	52	79	6
RAVI [28]	95	Persistent	43 mL/m^2	0.76	72	82	6
Mitral inflow A-wave velocity * [38]	112	No distinction	52 cm/s	0.710	91	43	1
LAEF in AF [28]	95	Persistent	42%	0.89	73	100	6
RAEF in AF [28]	95	Persistent	52%	0.92	88	89	6
LAEF in AF [40]	146	Persistent	23.9%	0.680	83.6	51.2	12
AFc * VTI [41]	137	Persistent	3.1 cm	0.962	97	75.7	5
AFc * velocity [41]	137	Persistent	32 cm/s	0.857	96.8	94.1	5
LAAFV in AF [21]	186	>48 h <1 year of AF	40 cm/s	0.700	56	80	12
RAWMV in AF [45]	133	Persistent	No data	0.67	No data	No data	12
LAWMV in AF [45]	133	Persistent	No data	0.66	No data	No data	12
LAWMV in AF [46]	126	Persistent	3 cm/s	0.738	92.7	49.3	12
LAAWMV in AF [31]	121	Persistent	7.16 cm/s	0.738	76.5	70	12
pLASR (inferior wall) in AF [29]	65	No distinction. ≤3 months	1.8 sek^{-1}	0.878	92	78	3

Table 2. Cont.

Parameter	Number of Patients	Paroxysmal/ Persistent AF	Optimal Cut-Off	AUC	Sensitivity (%)	Specificity (%)	Follow-Up (months)
pLAS (septal) in AF [29]	65	No distinction. ≤3 months	22%	0.852	77	86	3
pLASR cd in AF (basal left) [49]	52	No distinction. <1 year	2.18 s^{-1}	0.860	83.9	64.3	1
pLAS ct 4c in SR [52]	89	Persistent	No data	0.765	No data	No data	12
pLAS r *,[1] in AF [53]	131	Persistent	10.75%	0.954	85	99	6
TP-SD Left atrial asynchrony [57]	130	Persistent	15%	No data	82.4	35	12
dTPLS in SR [30]	80 (61 restored SR)	Persistent	128 ms	0.660	57	83	6
Left atrial wall dyskinesia * in SR [60]	89	Persistent	Binary variable	0.71	59.57	82.5	12
TACT * in SR [69]	54	Persistent	152 ms	0.990	87	100	7 days
TACT * in SR [70]	104	Persistent	152 ms	0.923	91	87	12
TACT * in SR [71]	60	39 patients paroxysmal AF and 21 with persistent AF	125.8 ms	0.989	98	100	12
E/e' in AF [40]	146	Persistent	8.7	0.645	73.8	55.4	12
E/e' * in AF [72]	66	Persistent	9.15	0.780	75	73.1	>12 months
E/e' * in AF [74]	175	Persistent	11	0.660	No data	85	3
E/e' in SR [75]	117	Persistent	9.17	0.726	72.1	74.1	12
E/A in SR [75]	117	Persistent	2.2	0.726	73.12	73.21	12

* Parameters assessing the recurrence of atrial fibrillation after electrical cardioversion. [1] pLAS (GPALS)—mean of strain results obtained from apical four and two chamber views. 4c, four-chamber view; AF, atrial fibrillation; AFc, left atrial fibrillatory contraction flow; AUC, area under the curve; cd, conduit phase; ct, contraction phase; dTPLS, dispersion of time to peak longitudinal strain; LAAFV, left atrial appendage flow velocity; LAAWMV, left atrial appendage wall motion velocity; LAEF, left atrial emptying fraction; LAVI, left atrial volume index; LAWMV, left atrial wall motion velocity; pLAS, peak left atrial strain; pLASR, peak left atrial strain rate; r, reservoir phase; RAEF, right atrial emptying fraction; RAVI, right atrial volume index; RAWMV, right atrial wall motion velocity; SR, sinus rhythm; TACT, total atrial conduction time; VTI, velocity time integral.

Author Contributions: Conceptualization: P.W., J.R.-W. and B.W.-K.; data curation: P.W., J.R.-W. and P.D.; investigation: P.W., J.R.-W. and P.D.; methodology: P.W., J.R.-W. and P.D.; project administration: B.W.-K.; resources: P.W., J.R.-W. and P.D.; supervision: B.W.-K.; validation: B.W.-K.; writing—original draft: P.W., J.R.-W. and P.D.; writing—review and editing: B.W.-K. All authors have read and agreed to the published version of the manuscript.

Funding: Project financed under the program of the Minister of Education and Science called "Regional Initiative of Excellence" in the years 2019–2023, project 024/RID/2018/19; amount of financing 11,999,000.00 PLN. This work was supported by Jan Kochanowski University, Kielce, Poland (grant SUPB.RN.23.017) to P.W.

Institutional Review Board Statement: Not applicable.

Informed Consent Statement: Not applicable.

Data Availability Statement: Not applicable.

Conflicts of Interest: The authors declare no conflict of interest.

References

1. Zoni-Berisso, M.; Lercari, F.; Carazza, T.; Domenicucci, S. Epidemiology of atrial fibrillation: European perspective. *Clin. Epidemiol.* **2014**, *6*, 213–220. [CrossRef] [PubMed]
2. Chugh, S.S.; Havmoeller, R.; Narayanan, K.; Singh, D.; Rienstra, M.; Benjamin, E.J.; Gillum, R.F.; Kim, Y.-H.; McAnulty, J.H., Jr.; Zheng, Z.-J.; et al. Worldwide epidemiology of atrial fibrillation: A Global Burden of Disease 2010 Study. *Circulation* **2014**, *129*, 837–847. [CrossRef]
3. Colilla, S.; Crow, A.; Petkun, W.; Singer, D.E.; Simon, T.; Liu, X. Estimates of current and future incidence and prevalence of atrial fibrillation in the U.S. adult population. *Am. J. Cardiol.* **2013**, *112*, 1142–1147. [CrossRef] [PubMed]
4. Global Burden of Disease Collaborative Network. *Global Burden of Disease Study 2016 (GBD 2016) Results*; Institute for Health Metrics and Evaluation (IHME): Seattle, WA, USA, 2016.
5. Lloyd-Jones, D.M.; Wang, T.J.; Leip, E.P.; Larson, M.G.; Levy, D.; Vasan, R.S.; D'Agostino, R.B.; Massaro, J.M.; Beiser, A.; Wolf, P.A.; et al. Lifetime risk for development of atrial fibrillation: The Framingham Heart Study. *Circulation* **2004**, *110*, 1042–1046. [CrossRef]
6. Mackenzie, J. Observations on the process which results in auricular fibrillation. *Br. Med. J.* **1922**, *2*, 71–73. [CrossRef]
7. Marijon, E.; Le Heuzey, J.-Y.; Connolly, S.; Yang, S.; Pogue, J.; Brueckmann, M.; Eikelboom, J.; Themeles, E.; Ezekowitz, M.; Wallentin, L.; et al. RE-LY Investigators. Causes of death and influencing factors in patients with atrial fibrillation: A competing-risk analysis from the randomized evaluation of long-term anticoagulant therapy study. *Circulation* **2013**, *128*, 2192–2201. [CrossRef]
8. Thrall, G.; Lane, D.; Carroll, D.; Lip, G.Y. Quality of life in patients with atrial fibrillation: A systematic review. *Am. J. Med.* **2006**, *119*, 448.E1–448.E19. [CrossRef]
9. Wożakowska-Kapłon, B. Effect of sinus rhythm restoration on plasma brain natriuretic peptide in patients with atrial fibrillation. *Am. J. Cardiol.* **2004**, *93*, 1555–1558. [CrossRef]
10. Kirchhof, P.; Benussi, S.; Kotecha, D.; Ahlsson, A.; Atar, D.; Casadei, B.; Castella, M.; Diener, H.-C.; Heidbuchel, H.; Hendriks, J.; et al. 2016 ESC Guidelines for the Management of Atrial Fibrillation Developed in Collaboration With EACTS. *Europace* **2016**, *18*, 1609–1678. [CrossRef] [PubMed]
11. Pisters, R.; Nieuwlaat, R.; Prins, M.H.; Le Heuzey, J.-Y.; Maggioni, A.P.; Camm, A.J.; Crijns, H.J.; for the Euro Heart Survey Investigators. Clinical correlates of immediate success and outcome at 1-year follow-up of real-world cardioversion of atrial fibrillation: The Euro Heart Survey. *Europace* **2012**, *14*, 666–674. [CrossRef]
12. Ewy, G.A.; Ulfers, L.; Hager, W.D.; Rosenfeld, A.R.; Roeske, W.R.; Goldman, S. Response of atrial fibrillation to therapy: Role of etiology and left atrial diameter. *J. Electrocardiol.* **1980**, *13*, 119–123. [CrossRef]
13. Dittrich, H.C.; Erickson, J.S.; Schneiderman, T.; Blacky, A.; Savides, T.; Nicod, P.H. Echocardiographic and clinical predictors for outcome of elective cardioversion of atrial fibrillation. *Am. J. Cardiol.* **1989**, *63*, 193–197. [CrossRef]
14. Mattioli, A.V.; Castelli, A.; Andria, A.; Mattioli, G. Clinical and echocardiographic features influencing recovery of atrial function after cardioversion of atrial fibrillation. *Am. J. Cardiol.* **1998**, *82*, 1368–1371. [CrossRef]
15. Marchese, P.; Malavasi, V.; Rossi, L.; Nikolskaya, N.; Donne, G.D.; Becirovic, M.; Colantoni, A.; Luciani, A.; Modena, M.G. Indexed left atrial volume is superior to left atrial diameter in predicting nonvalvular atrial fibrillation recurrence after successful cardioversion: A prospective study. *Echocardiography* **2012**, *29*, 276–284. [CrossRef]
16. Okçün, B.; Yigit, Z.; Küçükoglu, M.S.; Mutlu, H.; Sansoy, V.; Guzelsoy, D.; Uner, S. Predictors for maintenance of sinus rhythm after cardioversion in patients with nonvalvular atrial fibrillation. *Echocardiography* **2002**, *19*, 351–357. [CrossRef]
17. Raitt, M.H.; Volgman, A.S.; Zoble, R.G.; Charbonneau, L.; Padder, F.A.; O'Hara, G.E.; Kerr, D. Prediction of the recurrence of atrial fibrillation after cardioversion in the Atrial Fibrillation Followup Investigation of Rhythm Management (AFFIRM) study. *Am. Heart J.* **2006**, *151*, 390–396. [CrossRef]
18. Olshansky, B.; Heller, E.N.; Mitchell, L.B.; Chandler, M.; Slater, W.; Green, M.; Brodsky, M.; Barrell, P.; Greene, H.L. Are transthoracic echocardiographic parameters associated with atrial fibrillation recurrence or stroke? Results from the Atrial Fibrillation Follow-Up Investigation of Rhythm Management (AFFIRM) study. *J. Am. Coll. Cardiol.* **2005**, *45*, 2026–2033. [CrossRef] [PubMed]
19. Zhuang, J.; Wang, Y.; Tang, K.; Li, X.; Peng, W.; Liang, C.; Xu, Y. Association between left atrial size and atrial fibrillation recurrence after single circumferential pulmonary vein isolation: A systematic review and meta-analysis of observational studies. *Europace* **2012**, *14*, 638–645. [CrossRef] [PubMed]
20. Parikh, S.S.; Jons, C.; McNitt, S.; Daubert, J.P.; Schwarz, K.Q.; Hall, B. Predictive capability of left atrial size measured by CT, TEE, and TTE for recurrence of atrial fibrillation following radiofrequency catheter ablation. *Pacing Clin. Electrophysiol.* **2010**, *33*, 532–534. [CrossRef] [PubMed]
21. Antonielli, E.; Pizzuti, A.; Pálinkás, A.; Tanga, M.; Gruber, N.; Michelassi, C.; Varga, A.; Bonzano, A.; Gandolfo, N.; Halmai, L.; et al. Clinical value of left atrial appendage flow for prediction of long-term sinus rhythm maintenance in patients with nonvalvular atrial fibrillation. *J. Am. Coll. Cardiol.* **2002**, *39*, 1443–1449. [CrossRef]
22. Tsang, T.S.; Abhayaratna, W.P.; Barnes, M.E.; Miyasaka, Y.; Gersh, B.J.; Bailey, K.R.; Cha, S.S.; Seward, J.B. Prediction of cardiovascular outcomes with left atrial size: Is volume superior to area or diameter? *J. Am. Coll. Cardiol.* **2006**, *47*, 1018–1023. [CrossRef] [PubMed]

23. Toufan, M.; Kazemi, B.; Molazadeh, N. The significance of the left atrial volume index in prediction of atrial fibrillation recurrence after electrical cardioversion. *J. Cardiovasc. Thorac. Res.* **2017**, *9*, 54–59. [CrossRef] [PubMed]
24. Marchese, P.; Bursi, F.; Donne, G.D.; Malavasi, V.; Casali, E.; Barbieri, A.; Melandri, F.; Modena, M.G. Indexed left atrial volume predicts the recurrence of non-valvular atrial fibrillation after successful cardioversion. *Eur. J. Echocardiogr.* **2011**, *12*, 214–221. [CrossRef] [PubMed]
25. Luong, C.; Thompson, D.J.; Bennett, M.; Gin, K.; Jue, J.; Barnes, M.E.; Colley, P.; Tsang, T.S. Right atrial volume is superior to left atrial volume for prediction of atrial fibrillation recurrence after direct current cardioversion. *Can. J. Cardiol.* **2015**, *31*, 29–35. [CrossRef] [PubMed]
26. Sasaki, T.; Nakamura, K.; Naito, S.; Minami, K.; Koyama, K.; Yamashita, E.; Kumagai, K.; Oshima, S. The Right to Left Atrial Volume Ratio Predicts Outcomes after Circumferential Pulmonary Vein Isolation of Longstanding Persistent Atrial Fibrillation. *Pacing Clin. Electrophysiol.* **2016**, *39*, 1181–1190. [CrossRef]
27. Limantoro, I.; de Vos, C.B.; Delhaas, T.; Weijs, B.; Blaauw, Y.; Schotten, U.; Kietselaer, B.; Pisters, R.; Crijns, H.J. Clinical correlates of echocardiographic tissue velocity imaging abnormalities of the left atrial wall during atrial fibrillation. *Europace* **2014**, *16*, 1546–1553. [CrossRef] [PubMed]
28. Luong, C.L.; Thompson, D.J.; Gin, K.G.; Jue, J.; Nair, P.; Lee, P.-K.; Tsang, M.Y.; Barnes, M.E.; Colley, P.; Tsang, T.S. Usefulness of the Atrial Emptying Fraction to Predict Maintenance of Sinus Rhythm After Direct Current Cardioversion for Atrial Fibrillation. *Am. J. Cardiol.* **2016**, *118*, 1345–1349. [CrossRef]
29. Di Salvo, G.; Caso, P.; Lo Piccolo, R.; Fusco, A.; Martiniello, A.R.; Russo, M.G.; D'Onofrio, A.; Severino, S.; Calabró, P.; Pacileo, G.; et al. Atrial myocardial deformation properties predict maintenance of sinus rhythm after external cardioversion of recent-onset lone atrial fibrillation: A color Doppler myocardial imaging and transthoracic and transesophageal echocardiographic study. *Circulation* **2005**, *112*, 387–389. [CrossRef]
30. Doruchowska, A.; Wita, K.; Bochenek, T.; Szydło, K.; Filipecki, A.; Staroń, A.; Wróbel, W.; Krzych, L.; Trusz-Gluza, M. Role of left atrial speckle tracking echocardiography in predicting persistent atrial fibrillation electrical cardioversion success and sinus rhythm maintenance at 6 months. *Adv. Med. Sci.* **2014**, *59*, 120. [CrossRef]
31. Wałek, P.; Sielski, J.; Gorczyca, I.; Roskal-Wałek, J.; Starzyk, K.; Jaskulska-Niedziela, E.; Bartkowiak, R.; Wożakowska-Kapłon, B. Left atrial mechanical remodelling assessed as the velocity of left atrium appendage wall motion during atrial fibrillation is associated with maintenance of sinus rhythm after electrical cardioversion in patients with persistent atrial fibrillation. *PLoS ONE* **2020**, *15*, e0228239. [CrossRef]
32. Kupczynska, K.; Michalski, B.W.; Miskowiec, D.; Kasprzak, J.D.; Wejner-Mik, P.; Wdowiak-Okrojek, K.; Lipiec, P. Association between left atrial function assessed by speckle-tracking echocardiography and the presence of left atrial appendage thrombus in patients with atrial fibrillation. *Anatol. J. Cardiol.* **2017**, *18*, 15–22. [CrossRef]
33. Uretsky, S.; Shah, A.; Bangalore, S.; Rosenberg, L.; Sarji, R.; Cantales, D.R.; Macmillan-Marotti, D.; Chaudhry, F.A.; Sherrid, M.V. Assessment of left atrial appendage function with transthoracic tissue Doppler echocardiography. *Eur. J. Echocardiogr.* **2009**, *10*, 363–371. [CrossRef] [PubMed]
34. Tamura, H.; Watanabe, T.; Hirono, O.; Nishiyama, S.; Sasaki, S.; Shishido, T.; Miyashita, T.; Miyamoto, T.; Nitobe, J.; Kayama, T.; et al. Low wall velocity of left atrial appendage measured by trans-thoracic echocardiography predicts thrombus formation caused by atrial appendage dysfunction. *J. Am. Soc. Echocardiogr.* **2010**, *23*, 545–552.E1. [CrossRef] [PubMed]
35. Tamura, H.; Watanabe, T.; Nishiyama, S.; Sasaki, S.; Wanezaki, M.; Arimoto, T.; Takahashi, H.; Shishido, T.; Miyashita, T.; Miyamoto, T.; et al. Prognostic value of low left atrial appendage wall velocity in patients with ischemic stroke and atrial fibrillation. *J. Am. Soc. Echocardiogr.* **2012**, *25*, 576–583. [CrossRef]
36. Yoshida, N.; Okamoto, M.; Hirao, H.; Nanba, K.; Kinoshita, H.; Matsumura, H.; Fukuda, Y.; Ueda, H. Role of transthoracic left atrial appendage wall motion velocity in patients with persistent atrial fibrillation and a low CHADS2 score. *J. Cardiol.* **2012**, *60*, 310–315. [CrossRef]
37. Manning, W.J.; Silverman, D.I.; Katz, S.E.; Riley, M.F.; Come, P.C.; Doherty, R.M.; Munson, J.T.; Douglas, P.S. Impaired left atrial mechanical function after cardioversion: Relation to the duration of atrial fibrillation. *J. Am. Coll. Cardiol.* **1994**, *23*, 1535–1540. [CrossRef]
38. Spiecker, M.; Böhm, S.; Börgel, J.; Grote, J.; Görlitz, S.; Huesing, A.; Mügge, A. Doppler echocardiographic prediction of recurrent atrial fibrillation following cardioversion. *Int. J. Cardiol.* **2006**, *113*, 161–166. [CrossRef]
39. Grundvold, I.; Tveit, A.; Smith, P.; Seljeflot, I.; Abdelnoor, M.; Arnesen, H. The predictive value of transthoracic echocardiographic variables for sinus rhythm maintenance after electrical cardioversion of atrial fibrillation. Results from the CAPRAF study, a prospective, randomized, placebo-controlled study. *Cardiology* **2008**, *111*, 30–35. [CrossRef]
40. Wałek, P.; Gorczyca, I.; Sielski, J.; Wożakowska-Kapłon, B. Left atrial emptying fraction determined during atrial fibrillation predicts maintenance of sinus rhythm after direct current cardioversion in patients with persistent atrial fibrillation. *PLoS ONE* **2020**, *15*, e0238002. [CrossRef]
41. Kim, H.; Lee, J.-P.; Yoon, H.-J.; Park, H.-S.; Cho, Y.-K.; Nam, C.-W.; Hur, S.-H.; Kim, Y.-N.; Kim, K.-B. Association between Doppler flow of atrial fibrillatory contraction and recurrence of atrial fibrillation after electrical cardioversion. *J. Am. Soc. Echocardiogr.* **2014**, *27*, 1107–1112. [CrossRef] [PubMed]
42. Pollick, C.; Taylor, D. Assessment of left atrial appendage function by transesophageal echocardiography. Implications for the development of thrombus. *Circulation* **1991**, *84*, 223–231. [CrossRef]

43. Mikael Kortz, R.A.; Delemarre, B.J.; van Dantzig, J.M.; Bot, H.; Kamp, O.; Visser, C.A. Left atrial appendage blood flow determined by transesophageal echocardiography in healthy subjects. *Am. J. Cardiol.* **1993**, *71*, 976–981. [CrossRef]
44. Melduni, R.M.; Lee, H.C.; Bailey, K.R.; Miller, F.A., Jr.; Hodge, D.O.; Seward, J.B.; Gersh, B.J.; Ammash, N.M. Real-time physiologic biomarker for prediction of atrial fibrillation recurrence, stroke, and mortality after electrical cardioversion: A prospective observational study. *Am. Heart J.* **2015**, *170*, 914–922. [CrossRef]
45. De Vos, C.B.; Limantoro, I.; Pisters, R.; Delhaas, T.; Schotten, U.; Cheriex, E.C.; Tieleman, R.G.; Crijns, H.J. The mechanical fibrillation pattern of the atrial myocardium is associated with acute and long-term success of electrical cardioversion in patients with persistent atrial fibrillation. *Heart Rhythm.* **2014**, *11*, 1514–1521. [CrossRef]
46. Wałek, P.; Roskal-Wałek, J.; Dłubis, P.; Tracz, J.; Wożakowska-Kapłon, B. Left Atrial Wall Motion Velocity Assessed during Atrial Fibrillation Predicts Sinus Rhythm Maintenance after Electrical Cardioversion in Patients with Persistent Atrial Fibrillation. *Int. J. Environ. Res. Public Health* **2022**, *19*, 1550. [CrossRef] [PubMed]
47. Farese, G.E.; Tayal, B.; Stöbe, S.; Laufs, U.; Hagendorff, A. Regional Disparities of Left Atrial Appendage Wall Contraction in Patients With Sinus Rhythm and Atrial Fibrillation. *J. Am. Soc. Echocardiogr.* **2019**, *32*, 755–762. [CrossRef] [PubMed]
48. Sun, B.J.; Park, J.-H. Echocardiographic Measurement of Left Atrial Strain—A Key Requirement in Clinical Practice. *Circ. J.* **2021**, *86*, 6–13. [CrossRef]
49. Wang, T.; Wang, M.; Fung, J.W.; Yip, G.W.; Zhang, Y.; Ho, P.P.; Tse, D.M.; Yu, C.M.; Sanderson, J.E. Atrial strain rate echocardiography can predict success or failure of cardioversion for atrial fibrillation: A combined transthoracic tissue Doppler and transoesophageal imaging study. *Int. J. Cardiol.* **2007**, *114*, 202–209. [CrossRef] [PubMed]
50. Deferm, S.; Bertrand, P.B.; Churchill, T.W.; Sharma, R.; Vandervoort, P.M.; Schwamm, L.H.; Sanborn, D.M.Y. Left atrial mechanics assessed early during hospitalization for cryptogenic stroke are associated with occult atrial fibrillation: A speckle-tracking strain echocardiography study. *J. Am. Soc. Echocardiogr.* **2021**, *34*, 156–165. [CrossRef]
51. Sade, L.E.; Keskin, S.; Can, U.; Çolak, A.; Yüce, D.; Çiftçi, O.; Özin, B.; Müderrisoğlu, H. Left atrial mechanics for secondary prevention from embolic stroke of undetermined source. *Eur. Heart J. Cardiovasc. Imaging* **2022**, *23*, 381–391. [CrossRef]
52. Wałek, P.; Grabowska, U.; Cieśla, E.; Gorczyca, I.; Wożakowska-Kapłon, B. Left atrial longitudinal strain in the contractile phase as a predictor of sinus rhythm maintenance after electrical cardioversion performed due to persistent atrial fibrillation. *Kardiol. Pol.* **2021**, *79*, 458–460. [CrossRef]
53. Moreno-Ruiz, L.A.; Madrid-Miller, A.; Martínez-Flores, J.E.; González-Hermosillo, J.A.; Arenas-Fonseca, J.; Zamorano-Velázquez, N.; Mendoza-Pérez, B. Left atrial longitudinal strain by speckle tracking as independent predictor of recurrence after electrical cardioversion in persistent and long standing persistent non-valvular atrial fibrillation. *Int. J. Cardiovasc. Imaging* **2019**, *35*, 1587–1596. [CrossRef]
54. Shaikh, A.Y.; Maan, A.; A Khan, U.; Aurigemma, G.P.; Hill, J.C.; Kane, J.L.; A Tighe, D.; Mick, E.; McManus, D.D. Speckle echocardiographic left atrial strain and stiffness index as predictors of maintenance of sinus rhythm after cardioversion for atrial fibrillation: A prospective study. *Cardiovasc. Ultrasound* **2012**, *10*, 48. [CrossRef]
55. Degiovanni, A.; Boggio, E.; Prenna, E.; Sartori, C.; De Vecchi, F.; Marino, P.N.; From the Novara Atrial Fibrillation (NAIF) Study Group. Association between left atrial phasic conduit function and early atrial fibrillation recurrence in patients undergoing electrical cardioversion. *Clin. Res. Cardiol.* **2018**, *107*, 329–337. [CrossRef]
56. Giubertoni, A.; Boggio, E.; Ubertini, E.; Zanaboni, J.; Calcaterra, E.; Degiovanni, A.; Bellacosa, I.; Marino, P.N. Atrial conduit function quantitation precardioversion predicts early arrhythmia recurrence in persistent atrial fibrillation patients. *J. Cardiovasc. Med.* **2019**, *20*, 169–179. [CrossRef] [PubMed]
57. Rondano, E.; Dell'Era, G.; De Luca, G.; Piccinino, C.; Bellomo, G.; Marino, P.N. Left atrial asynchrony is a major predictor of 1-year recurrence of atrial fibrillation after electrical cardioversion. *J. Cardiovasc. Med.* **2010**, *11*, 499–506. [CrossRef] [PubMed]
58. Dell'Era, G.; Rondano, E.; Franchi, E.; Marino, P.; On behalf of the Novara Atrial Fibrillation (NAIF) Study Group. Atrial asynchrony and function before and after electrical cardioversion for persistent atrial fibrillation. *Eur. J. Echocardiogr.* **2010**, *11*, 577–583. [CrossRef] [PubMed]
59. Marino, P.N.; Degiovanni, A.; Baduena, L.; Occhetta, E.; Dell'era, G.; Erdei, T.; Fraser, A.G. Non-invasively estimated left atrial stiffness is associated with short-term recurrence of atrial fibrillation after electrical cardioversion. *J. Cardiol.* **2017**, *69*, 731. [CrossRef]
60. Wałek, P.; Ciesla, E.; Gorczyca, I.; Wozakowska-Kapłon, B. Left atrial wall dyskinesia assessed during contractile phase as a predictor of atrial fibrillation recurrence after electrical cardioversion performed due to persistent atrial fibrillation. *Medicine* **2020**, *99*, e23333. [CrossRef]
61. Hindricks, G.; Potpara, T.; Dagres, N.; Arbelo, E.; Bax, J.J.; Blomström-Lundqvist, C.; Boriani, G.; Castella, M.; Dan, G.A.; Dilaveris, P.E.; et al. 2020 ESC Guidelines for the diagnosis and management of atrial fibrillation developed in collaboration with the European Association for Cardio-Thoracic Surgery (EACTS): The Task Force for the diagnosis and management of atrial fibrillation of the European Society of Cardiology (ESC) Developed with the special contribution of the European Heart Rhythm Association (EHRA) of the ESC. *Eur. Heart J.* **2021**, *42*, 373–498. [CrossRef]
62. Goette, A.; Kalman, J.M.; Aguinaga, L.; Akar, J.; Cabrera, J.A.; Chen, S.A.; Chugh, S.S.; Corradi, D.; D'Avila, A.; Dobrev, D.; et al. EHRA/HRS/APHRS/SOLAECE expert consensus on Atrial cardiomyopathies: Definition, characterization, and clinical implication. *Europace* **2016**, *18*, 1455–1459. [CrossRef]

63. Nattel, S.; Burstein, B.; Dobrev, D. Atrial remodeling and atrial fibrillation: Mechanisms and implications. *Circ. Arrhythm. Electrophysiol.* **2008**, *1*, 62–73. [CrossRef] [PubMed]
64. Mary-Rabine, L.; Albert, A.; Pham, T.D.; Hordof, A.; Fenoglio, J.J., Jr.; Malm, J.R.; Rosen, M.R. The relationship of human atrial cellular electrophysiology to clinical function and ultrastructure. *Circ. Res.* **1983**, *52*, 188–199. [CrossRef]
65. Mueller, P.; Hars, C.; Schiedat, F.; Boesche, L.I.; Gotzmann, M.; Strauch, J.; Dietrich, J.; Vogt, M.; Tannapfel, A.; Deneke, T. Correlation between total atrial conduction time estimated via tissue Doppler imaging (PATDI interval), structural atrial remodeling and newonset of atrial fibrillation after cardiac surgery. *J. Cardiovasc. Electrophysiol.* **2013**, *24*, 626–631. [CrossRef]
66. Leung, M.; Abou, R.; van Rosendael, P.J.; van der Bijl, P.; van Wijngaarden, S.E.; Regeer, M.V.; Podlesnikar, T.; Marsan, N.A.; Leung, D.Y.; Delgado, V.; et al. Relation of echocardiographic markers of left atrial fibrosis to atrial fibrillation burden. *Am. J. Cardiol.* **2018**, *122*, 584–589. [CrossRef] [PubMed]
67. Weijs, B.; de Vos, C.B.; Tieleman, R.G.; Pisters, R.; Cheriex, E.C.; Prins, M.H.; Crijns, H.J. Clinical and echocardiographic correlates of intra-atrial conduction delay. *Europace* **2011**, *13*, 1681. [CrossRef] [PubMed]
68. Merckx, K.L.; De Vos, C.B.; Palmans, A.; Habets, J.; Cheriex, E.C.; Crijns, H.J.; Tieleman, R.G. Atrial activation time determined by transthoracic doppler tissue imaging can be used as an estimate of the total duration of atrial electrical activation. *J. Am. Soc. Echocardiogr.* **2005**, *18*, 940. [CrossRef] [PubMed]
69. Müller, P.; Schiedat, F.; Bialek, A.; Bösche, L.; Ewers, A.; Kara, K.; Dietrich, J.W.; Mügge, A.; Deneke, T. Total atrial conduction time assessed by tissue doppler imaging (PA-TDI Interval) to predict early recurrence of persistent atrial fibrillation after successful electrical cardioversion. *J. Cardiovasc. Electrophysiol.* **2014**, *25*, 161. [CrossRef]
70. Maffè, S.; Paffoni, P.; Dellavesa, P.; Cucchi, L.; Zenone, F.; Bergamasco, L.; Paino, A.M.; Franchetti Pardo, N.; Signorotti, F.; Baduena, L.; et al. Prognostic value of total atrial conduction time measured with tissue Doppler imaging to predict the maintenance of sinus rhythm after external electrical cardioversion of persistent atrial fibrillation. *Echocardiography* **2015**, *32*, 420. [CrossRef]
71. Karantoumanis, I.; Doundoulakis, I.; Zafeiropoulos, S.; Oikonomou, K.; Makridis, P.; Pliakos, C.; Karvounis, H.; Giannakoulas, G. Atrial conduction time associated predictors of recurrent atrial fibrillation. *Int. J. Cardiovasc. Imaging* **2021**, *37*, 1267–1277. [CrossRef]
72. Chung, H.; Lee, B.K.; Min, P.-K.; Choi, E.-Y.; Yoon, Y.W.; Hong, B.-K.; Rim, S.-J.; Kwon, H.M.; Kim, J.-Y. Left Ventricular Filling Pressure as Assessed by the E/e' Ratio Is a Determinant of Atrial Fibrillation Recurrence after Cardioversion. *Yonsei Med. J.* **2016**, *57*, 64–71. [CrossRef]
73. Caputo, M.; Urselli, R.; Capati, E.; Navarri, R.; Sinesi, L.; Furiozzi, F.; Ballo, P.; Palazzuoli, A.; Favilli, R.; Mondillo, S. Usefulness of left ventricular diastolic dysfunction assessed by pulsed tissue Doppler imaging as a predictor of atrial fibrillation recurrence after successful electrical cardioversion. *Am. J. Cardiol.* **2011**, *108*, 698–704. [CrossRef] [PubMed]
74. Fornengo, C.; Antolini, M.; Frea, S.; Gallo, C.; Grosso Marra, W.; Morello, M.; Gaita, F. Prediction of atrial fibrillation recurrence after cardioversion in patients with left-atrial dilation. *Eur. Heart J. Cardiovasc. Imaging* **2015**, *16*, 335–341. [CrossRef] [PubMed]
75. Wałek, P.; Sielski, J.; Starzyk, K.; Gorczyca, I.; Roskal-Wałek, J.; Wożakowska-Kapłon, B. Echocardiographic assessment of left atrial morphology and function to predict maintenance of sinus rhythm after electrical cardioversion in patients with non-valvular persistent atrial fibrillation and normal function or mild dysfunction of left ventricle. *Cardiol. J.* **2020**, *27*, 246–253. [CrossRef] [PubMed]
76. Janion-Sadowska, A.; Turek, Ł.; Dudek, A.; Andrychowski, J.; Sadowski, M. Atrial fibrillation and flutter—The state of the art. Part 2. *Med. Stud./Stud. Med.* **2021**, *37*, 239–249. [CrossRef]
77. Janion-Sadowska, A.; Turek, Ł.; Dudek, A.; Andrychowski, J.; Sadowski, M. Atrial fibrillation and atrial flutter—The state of the art. Part 1. *Med. Stud./Stud. Med.* **2021**, *37*, 151–161. [CrossRef]
78. Kiliszek, M.; Uziębło-Życzkowska, B.; Krzyżanowski, K.; Jurek, A.; Wierzbowski, R.; Smalc-Stasiak, M.; Krzesiński, P. Value of Left Atrial Strain in Predicting Recurrence after Atrial Fibrillation Ablation. *J. Clin. Med.* **2023**, *12*, 4034. [CrossRef] [PubMed]
79. Krizanovic-Grgic, I.; Anwer, S.; Steffel, J.; Hofer, D.; Saguner, A.M.; Spengler, C.M.; Breitenstein, A.; Tanner, F.C. 3D Atrial Strain for Predicting Recurrence of Atrial Fibrillation after Pulmonary Vein Isolation. *J. Clin. Med.* **2023**, *12*, 3696. [CrossRef]

Disclaimer/Publisher's Note: The statements, opinions and data contained in all publications are solely those of the individual author(s) and contributor(s) and not of MDPI and/or the editor(s). MDPI and/or the editor(s) disclaim responsibility for any injury to people or property resulting from any ideas, methods, instructions or products referred to in the content.

MDPI AG
Grosspeteranlage 5
4052 Basel
Switzerland
Tel.: +41 61 683 77 34

Journal of Clinical Medicine Editorial Office
E-mail: jcm@mdpi.com
www.mdpi.com/journal/jcm

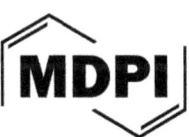

Disclaimer/Publisher's Note: The statements, opinions and data contained in all publications are solely those of the individual author(s) and contributor(s) and not of MDPI and/or the editor(s). MDPI and/or the editor(s) disclaim responsibility for any injury to people or property resulting from any ideas, methods, instructions or products referred to in the content.

www.ingramcontent.com/pod-product-compliance
Lightning Source LLC
LaVergne TN
LVHW070150100526
838202LV00015B/1927